The Science of Mental Health

Volume 5

Addiction

Series Content

Volume 1
BIPOLAR DISORDER

Volume 2
AUTISM

Volume 3
SCHIZOPHRENIA

Volume 4
ATTENTION-DEFICIT HYPERACTIVITY DISORDERS

Volume 5
ADDICTION

Volume 6
DEPRESSION

Volume 7
PERSONALITY AND PERSONALITY DISORDER

Volume 8
COMPULSIVE DISORDER AND TOURETTE'S SYNDROME

Volume 9
STRESS AND THE BRAIN

Volume 10
FEAR AND ANXIETY

The Science of Mental Health

Volume 5

Addiction

Edited with introductions by

Steven Hyman
National Institute of Mental Health

ROUTLEDGE
New York/London

Published in 2001 by

Routledge
29 West 35th Street
New York, NY 10001

Published in Great Britain by
Routledge
11 New Fetter Lane
London EC4P 4EE

Routledge is an Imprint of Taylor & Francis Books, Inc.

Printed in the United States of America on acid-free paper.

10 9 8 7 6 5 4 3 2 1

Library of Congress Cataloging-in-Publication Data

The science of mental health / edited with introductions by Steven Hyman.
p. cm.
Includes bibliographical references.
ISBN 0-8153-3743-4 (set)
1. Mental health. I. Hyman, Steven E.
RA790 .S435 2002
616.89--dc21

2001048491

ISBN 0-8153-3743-4 (set)
ISBN 0-8153-3744-2 (v.1)
ISBN 0-8153-3745-0 (v.2)
ISBN 0-8153-3746-9 (v.3)
ISBN 0-8153-3747-7 (v.4)
ISBN 0-8153-3748-5 (v.5)
ISBN 0-8153-3749-3 (v.6)
ISBN 0-8153-3750-7 (v.7)
ISBN 0-8153-3751-5 (v.8)
ISBN 0-8153-3752-3 (v.9)
ISBN 0-8153-3753-1 (v.10)

Contents

vii Introduction

Epidemiology

1 Prevalence and Correlates of Drug Use and Dependence in the United States: Results from the National Comorbidity Survey
L. A. Warner, R. C. Kessler, M. Hughes, J. C. Anthony, and C. B. Nelson

Genetics

13 Replication of the Stockholm Adoption Study of Alcoholism: Confirmatory Cross-Fostering Analysis
S. Sigvardsson, M. Bohman, and C. R. Cloninger

21 Familial Transmission of Substance Use Disorders
K. R. Merikangas, M. Stolar, D. E. Stevens, J. Goulet, M. A. Preisig, B. Fenton, H. Zhang, S. S. O'Malley, and B. J. Rounsaville

Natural History

29 Drug Dependence, a Chronic Medical Illness: Implications for Treatment, Insurance, and Outcomes Evaluation
A. T. McLellan, D. C. Lewis, C. P. O'Brien, and H. D. Kleber

37 A Long-Term Follow-up of Male Alcohol Abuse
G. E. Vaillant

Evolution

45 An Evolutionary Perspective on Substance Abuse
Randolph M. Nesse

Neurobiology of Disease

55 Conditioning Factors in Drug Abuse: Can They Explain Compulsion?
C. P. O'Brien, A. R. Childress, R. Ehrman, and S. J. Robbins

63 The Neural Basis of Drug Craving: An Incentive-Sensitization Theory of Addiction
T. E. Robinson and K. C. Berridge

109 A Cognitive Model of Drug Urges and Drug-Use Behavior: Role of Automatic and Nonautomatic Processes
S. T. Tiffany

132 Decreased Striatal Dopaminergic Responsiveness in Detoxified Cocaine-Dependent Subjects
N. D. Volkow, G. J. Wang, J. S. Fowler, J. Logan, S. J. Gatley, R. Hitzemann, A. D. Chen, S. L. Dewey, and N. Pappas

137 What Is the Role of Dopamine in Reward: Hedonic Impact, Reward Learning, or Incentive Salience?
K. C. Berridge and T. E. Robinson

199 Acute Effects of Cocaine on Human Brain Activity and Emotion
H. C. Breiter, R. L. Gollub, R. M. Weisskoff, D. N. Kennedy, N. Makris, J. D. Berke, J. M. Goodman, H. L. Kantor, D. R. Gastfriend, J. P. Riorden, R. T. Mathew, B. R. Rosen, and S. E. Hyman

221 Illicit Psychoactive Substance Use, Heavy Use, Abuse, and Dependence in a US Population-Based Sample of Male Twins
K. S. Kendler, L. M. Karkowski, M. C. Neale, and C. A. Prescott

231 Predictive Reward Signal of Dopamine Neurons
W. Schultz

259 Prediction of Reinforcing Responses to Psychostimulants in Humans by Brain Dopamine D2 Receptor Levels
N. D. Volkow, G. J. Wang, J. S. Fowler, J. Logan, S. J. Gatley, A. Gifford, R. Hitzemann, Y. S. Ding, and N. Pappas

264 Addictive Drugs as Reinforcers: Multiple Partial Actions on Memory Systems
N. M. White

293 Acknowledgments

Introduction

Abuse of and addiction to alcohol, tobacco, and illegal drugs are highly prevalent (Warner et al., 1995) and represent one of the most serious public health problems facing many of the world's countries, including the United States. Drug abuse and addiction result in medical illnesses, serious problems for individuals and families, and lost productivity. Because drug abuse and addiction often have their roots in teen years, they seriously compromise development and, ultimately, work potential. In addition, alcohol and illegal drugs are powerful contributors to serious social ills, including accidents, crime, family violence, suicide, homicide, and transmission of infectious diseases, including HIV.

One confusion in the thinking about drug addiction is that there is a scientific or biomedical distinction between illegal drugs such as heroin and cocaine and legal drugs such as alcohol and tobacco. There is not. The division into legal and illegal categories has a historical and social basis rather than a medical one. Indeed, the morbidity and mortality stemming from tobacco and alcohol far surpass those from illegal drugs, reflecting the far greater access of the population to these legal drugs. Although not intoxicating, nicotine is highly addictive; through their multiple health risks, tobacco products have a greater impact on morbidity and mortality worldwide than any other drug.

This volume contains papers addressing various aspects of drug abuse and addiction, but the major focus is on addiction itself. There is now broad agreement that the central, defining characteristic of addiction is compulsive, out-of-control drug use, despite negative consequences. This means that the life of an addicted person is focused on obtaining, using, and recovering from the effects of drugs, despite serious drug-related problems such as medical illness, disrupted relationships, and failures in life roles.

In addition to producing compulsive use, addictive drugs may produce other well-known pharmacologic effects: tolerance, dependence, and withdrawal symptoms. Tolerance is defined as a decrease in drug effect despite a constant dose, or a need for increased dosage in order to maintain a stable effect. Tolerance often develops to the desired pleasurable effects of cocaine, heroin, and other drugs, leading to increased drug use. Dependence, narrowly defined, refers to an adapted state of body that occurs in response to excessive drug stimulation. Such compensatory adaptation or "homeostasis" can occur at the level of cells, brain circuits, or organ systems. Depending on the particular drug, tolerance and dependence may affect different organ systems in the body. Dependence itself may produce no symptoms while drug use continues, but when this adapted state is unmasked by decreasing or stopping a drug, withdrawal symptoms may occur.

When a drug is psychoactive, these symptoms may be cognitive and emotional. When a drug affects the neural control of bodily functions (as do alcohol and opiates) or affects bodily organs directly (as opiates affect the bowel), physical withdrawal symptoms may occur. It is important to recognize that many drugs used therapeutically in medical practice may produce tolerance, dependence, and withdrawal symptoms involving different organ systems. These include some drugs for hypertension and drugs that treat asthma. While dependence and withdrawal may make it difficult to terminate use of a medication, this difficulty should not be confused with addiction, characterized as it is by intense compulsion. Unfortunately, because the term "addiction" was thought by some to have become pejorative, the American Psychiatric Association's *Diagnostic and Statistical Manual,* 4th edition, uses the term "dependence" in place of "addiction."[1] This choice has led to substantial confusion.

A major problem for the addicted person is the persistence of relapse risk. Even long after drug discontinuation, and long after any withdrawal symptoms have abated, relapse to drug use remains a substantial risk once a person has developed an addiction. Relapse is most often initiated by cues in the environment or bodily feelings that serve as reminders of drug use (O'Brien et al., 1998).

The question is often raised as to whether behaviors such as compulsive gambling, sex, or shopping might justifiably be called addictions. There is early evidence that behaviors related to gambling may activate circuits in the brain similar to those activated by addictive drugs. One paper is included that demonstrates such findings for neural circuitry utilized by expectancy and experience of monetary gains (Breiter, 2001). Overall, however, data are still in their earliest stages on the neural underpinnings of compulsive behaviors unrelated to drug use. At the clinical levels, important similarities in the clinical course and outcomes of drug addiction and compulsive gambling are emerging, but even clinical description of other compulsive behaviors remains fragmentary. Overall, there has been far more research on addiction to drugs of abuse than on any other compulsive behaviors that are candidates for being thought of as addictions. Thus the focus of this volume is on drug addiction.

As in other volumes in this series, papers have been included that discuss the epidemiology (Warner et al., 1995), genetics, natural history (longitudinal course) of illness, evolutionary hypotheses (Nesse, 1994), relevant neurobiology, and treatment. Powerful personal descriptions of addiction can be found in other sources.[2]

Addiction is now generally understood as a chronic medical illness (McLellan et al., 2000). There have been debates about the appropriateness of a medical model for addiction, particularly because of concern that such a model might diminish the sense of personal responsibility that addicted individuals must embrace in order to get well. In fact the medical model does not negate personal responsibility for engaging in treatment any more than it does for heart disease or diabetes. A medical model for addiction is based on the existence of identifiable risk factors, a well-characterized natural history (Vaillant, 1996), an increasingly well understood pathophysiology, and evidence-based treatments.

It has long been recognized that risk of addiction runs in families. Studies using a variety of strategies have been performed to understand the basis of familial risk. These include studies of individuals adopted away from their biological families early in life (Sigvardsson et al., 1996), studies comparing monozygotic (identical) and dizygotic (fraternal) twins (Kendler et al., 2000), and studies of transmission within families (Merikangas et al., 1998). The conclusion is that family resemblance results from the action of genes rather than from shared environment. The most extensive studies have been on alcoholism, where adoption studies performed in multiple countries have found that individuals resemble their biological, not their adoptive, parents. While these findings confirm an important role for genes, they do not negate a role for the environment. Relevant environmental factors that might occur outside the shared family environment are a matter of current research but may include the influence of peer groups and opportunities to use drugs.

The genes in which particular variants (alleles) might produce risk of addiction remain to be discovered. It will be interesting to determine whether these genetic variants are involved in the modulation of general risk-taking behavior, behavior more specific to drug taking, or in risk of being "captured" by drugs upon experimentation. What is already clear, based on family studies and initial attempts to discover risk genes by linkage methods, is that, like other significant behavioral phenotypes, risk of drug addiction is genetically complex. This means that multiple genes and nongenetic factors interact to produce addiction. While genes play a substantial role in risk, simple deterministic notions do not fit the data.

Individuals initially use drugs to alter their emotional and cognitive state for diverse reasons, including curiosity, pleasure, peer culture, or self-medication of distress. Initial experimentation often occurs during the teenage years, with onset of addiction in vulnerable individuals following after several years of drug use. After a period of experimentation, the pattern of drug use often changes. A subset of users begin to lose control, and compulsive use sets in. Addiction then behaves as a chronic disorder, with remissions and relapses initiated by drug-related cues or stress (O'Brien et al., 1998).

The major classes of addictive drugs were originally derived from natural plant products. Opiates (including semisynthetic opiates such as heroin) initially came from the opium poppy, cocaine from coca leaf, nicotine from tobacco, alcohol from the fermentation of grain, and marijuana from the cannabis plant. By ingesting natural products, humanity has collectively exposed itself and, more to the point, the human brain to a very large number of chemicals. What is it about chemicals derived from the opium poppy or coca leaf, for example, that can literally capture human behavior, whereas hundreds of thousands of other plant-derived chemicals exert no such effect? The answer appears to be that within all addictive substances, the active chemicals mimic particular chemicals in the brain, specifically certain neurotransmitters. The opiates mimic the peptide neurotransmitters collectively described as "endogenous opiates," or endorphins; cocaine looks enough like dopamine to bind to and block the protein that normally clears dopamine from synapses (leading to a massive accumulation of dopamine); alcohol activates receptors for the major inhibitory neurotransmitter in the brain; GABA blocks a subset of receptors for the major excitatory transmitter, glutamate; and marijuana mimics endogenous cannabinoids that bind the CB1 cannabinoid receptors. Each of these neurotransmitters plays a role in the regulation of a critical neural pathway that normally functions to motivate the pursuit of goals with positive survival value, such as obtaining food and sexual partners. This pathway extends from the ventral tegmental area (VTA) of the midbrain to the nucleus accumbens (NAc) in the limbic system of the brain, a term given to a collection of structures that regulate emotion and motivation. The major neurotransmitter in this pathway is dopamine, but all of the other neurotransmitters acted upon by addictive drugs modulate the effect of dopamine in this pathway. This dopaminergic pathway is often called the "brain reward pathway." In fact, drugs or experiences that stimulate this pathway are likely to prove both rewarding (that is, they are interpreted by the brain as intrinsically positive) and reinforcing (that is, behaviors associated with such drugs tend to be repeated). Herein lies the trap of the addictive process. These drugs are defined as reinforcing precisely because they are used repetitively by vulnerable individuals (and also by normal animals in experimental settings). This repetitive use induces molecular changes in the brain that promote continued drug taking that becomes increasingly difficult for the individual to control.

The neurobiology of disease section provides a variety of current views of this process. While there is not full agreement on the pathogenesis of addiction, far more is known in this area than in that of most other mental disorders. Dopamine, the key neurotransmitter in the reward pathway, is likely not involved in pleasure itself (Berridge and Robinson, 1998) but is a "learning signal", shaping the behavior of an organism so that rewards can be predicted and sought. By causing excessive dopamine release in this circuit, drugs of abuse mimic the action of powerful natural reinforcers and gain the ability to control behavior. Based on such data and on behavioral observation that drug-associated cues have a powerful effect in stimulating drug use (O'Brien et al., 1998), it has been hypothesized that drug addiction represents a usurpation of normal learning mechanisms in which dopamine plays a critical role. The critical circuits that are remodeled during the addictive process are not yet entirely clear. Robinson and Berridge (2000) argue that the key change is an alteration in the incentive salience of drugs and drug-related cues in which an intense "wanting" (rather than "liking") maintains drug use. Others (Tiffany, 1990) adduce evidence that other circuits are also critical, such as those involved in the consolidation of behavioral repertoires involved in drug foraging and drug taking. Once these behaviors are deeply ingrained, cues may activate them in a way that can become highly automatized.

Recently noninvasive neuroimaging using functional magnetic resonance imaging (MRI) and positron emission tomography (PET) has begun to extend the neurobiology of addiction to the human brain. Papers included here examine direct effects of cocaine on the brain (Breiter et al., 1997) as well as the effects of drug-related cues. Neuroimaging studies have also begun to examine neural risk factors for drug use, such as the density of key dopamine receptors (Volkow et al., 1999) and the long-term impact of drugs on dopamine systems.

Treatment of drug addiction is in early stages of development. For some drugs pharmacologic treatments have shown some efficacy, but for all drugs psychological and social interventions remain critically important. The first effective medical treatment for addiction was the use of the long-acting opiate methadone, administered under controlled circumstances, to block heroin use. For other drugs replacement strategies are not available, but alternative pharmacologic strategies have been developed based on our increasing understanding of neurotransmitter interactions in the brain reward pathway. One such advance is the use of opiate antagonists (blockers) to decrease the likelihood of relapse in detoxified alcoholics. Similar strategies are being explored for a wide range of addictive drugs. Finally, the understanding of the role of associative learning in addiction has led to the development of specific cognitive and behavioral treatments for addiction. One such approach is represented here by a paper from O'Brien et al. (1990). Addiction research is an area in which basic understanding of brain and behavior is having an increasing impact on clinical practice.

References

1. American Psychiatric Association. *Diagnostic and Statistical Manual of Mental Disorders,* 4th ed. Washington, D.C.: American Psychiatric Press, 1994.
2. W. Burroughs. *Junky.* 1953.

ORIGINAL ARTICLE

Prevalence and Correlates of Drug Use and Dependence in the United States

Results From the National Comorbidity Survey

Lynn A. Warner, MPP; Ronald C. Kessler, PhD; Michael Hughes, PhD; James C. Anthony, PhD; Christopher B. Nelson, MPH

Objectives: To analyze nationally representative data on the lifetime and 12-month prevalences of use of and dependence on illegal drugs (marijuana/hashish, cocaine/crack, heroin, hallucinogens), nonmedical prescription psychotropic drugs (sedatives, tranquilizers, stimulants, analgesics), and inhalants; and to examine data on the sociodemographic correlates of use and dependence.

Methods: The data come from the National Comorbidity Survey, a structured diagnostic interview administered to persons aged 15 to 54 years that generates reliable diagnoses according to the definitions and criteria of *DSM-III-R*.

Results: Of the respondents, 51.0% used one of the above drugs at some time in their lives, and 15.4% did so in the past 12 months. These estimates are similar to those obtained in the 1991 National Household Survey of Drug Abuse, where lifetime prevalence was 45.2% and 12-month prevalence was 16.7% among respondents in the age range 15 to 54 years. Of National Comorbidity Survey respondents, 7.5% (14.7% of lifetime users) were dependent at some time in their lives and 1.8% were dependent in the past 12 months. The prevalence estimate for lifetime dependence was reduced to 5.3% when calculated the percentage of respondents in the age range of 28 to 54 years who reported an onset of dependence as of 10 years earlier (ie, when they were 18 to 44 years old) was computed. This is similar to the Epidemiologic Catchment Area Study estimate of 5.1% among respondents in the age range 18 to 44 years, a comparison that matches the two studies on year of assessment, age of risk, and cohort. Males were significantly more likely to report both lifetime and 12-month use and dependence. Use and dependence were found to be more common in cohorts born after World War II than those born before the end of the war. The demographic predictors of lifetime use differed from the predictors of lifetime dependence among users, and these, in turn, differed from the predictors of recent dependence among people with a lifetime history of dependence.

Conclusions: Drug use and dependence are highly prevalent in the general population. The fact that there are differences in the correlates of first use, dependence among users, and persistence of dependence means that future research aimed at pinpointing modifiable risk factors must be based on disaggregated analyses of separate stages of progression.

(Arch Gen Psychiatry. 1995;52:219-229)

From the Institute for Social Research (Ms Warner, Dr Kessler, and Mr Nelson) and the Department of Sociology (Dr Kessler), The University of Michigan, Ann Arbor; Department of Sociology, Virginia Polytechnic Institute and State University, Blacksburg (Dr Hughes); and Department of Mental Hygiene, The Johns Hopkins University, Baltimore, Md (Dr Anthony).

SEVERAL ONGOING national data collection systems are currently in place to gauge drug use levels and trends.[1] These include the Drug Abuse Warning Network,[2] which tracks the prevalence of drug mentions in emergency department admissions and medical examiners' death records; the National Household Survey on Drug Abuse,[3] which tracks the prevalence of drug use in the total national household population aged 12 years and over; and the High School Senior Survey,[4] which tracks the prevalence of drug use among junior high, high school, college, and young adult populations and, beginning in 1993, school dropouts. While all of these systems include some information about problems caused by drug use, they have been criticized because none produces accurate estimates of the prevalence of drug abuse or drug dependence.[5,6] Without such information, it is difficult to assess the full magnitude of the nation's drug problem.

Although a number of surveys have reported estimates of drug abuse or dependence in particular communities and regions,[7,8] the landmark Epidemiologic Catchment Area (ECA) Study is the only large-scale general population survey to have produced national esti-

See Materials and Methods on next page

MATERIALS AND METHODS

SAMPLE

The NCS is based on a stratified, multistage area probability sample of persons aged 15 to 54 years in the noninstitutionalized civilian population in the 48 coterminous states as well as a representative supplemental sample of students living in campus group housing. Fieldwork was carried out by the staff of the Survey Research Center at the University of Michigan, Ann Arbor, between September 14, 1990, and February 6, 1992. Interviewers were carefully trained and closely monitored throughout the data collection period. The response rate was 82.4%, with a total of 8098 participants. A more detailed discussion of the NCS sampling design is presented elsewhere.[11]

Because of previous evidence that survey nonrespondents have more psychiatric disorders than respondents,[12,13] a supplemental nonresponse survey was conducted in tandem with the main NCS survey. A financial incentive was offered to a random sample of initial nonrespondents to complete a short form of the diagnostic interview. The 353 completed short forms disclosed higher rates of both lifetime and current psychiatric disorders among initial nonrespondents than among initial respondents. These results were used to construct a nonresponse adjustment weight for the main survey data to compensate for this systematic nonresponse. A second weight was used to adjust for variation in probabilities of selection both within and between households. A third weight, finally, was used to poststratify the data to approximate the national population distribution of the cross-classification of age, sex, race/ethnicity, marital status, education, living arrangement, region, and urbanicity as defined by the 1989 US National Health Interview Survey.[14] Comparisons between the NCS and National Health Interview Survey results are presented in **Table 1**.

DIAGNOSTIC ASSESSMENT

The NCS questions on illicit drug use and nonmedical use of prescription drugs were based on those asked in the National Household Survey on Drug Abuse (NHSDA).[3] The question series began by defining nonmedical use as use (1) without a physician's prescription, (2) in greater amounts than prescribed, or (3) more frequently than prescribed. Respondents were then asked about their lifetime and recent nonmedical use of each of four categories of prescription drugs (sedatives, tranquilizers, stimulants, and analgesics). This was followed by questions concerning the use of four categories of illicit drugs (marijuana/hashish, cocaine/crack, hallucinogens, and heroin) and inhalants. The procedures of the NHSDA were followed in providing a detailed verbal definition and illustrative list of qualifying drugs in each category before inquiring about use.

The NCS deviated from the procedures of the NHSDA in three major respects. First, questions were interviewer-administered rather than self-administered. This change in procedures was dictated by the requirement that the interviewer know about the respondent's drug use to administer subsequent questions about dependence. Second, we did not use the colored pill card employed in the NHSDA in asking about use of prescription psychotropic drugs. Third, we included a screening question that does not exist in the NHSDA concerning dependence in the absence of nonmedical use of prescription drugs, namely, whether persons who used prescription drugs under the supervision of a physician ever believed that they could not stop or that they were dependent even though they were following the physician's directions concerning amount and frequency of use.

Lifetime use of a drug, for purposes of this article, was defined as having tried at least one of the above drugs at least one time, excluding medical use that did not lead to feelings of dependence. As in the ECA Study, further questions that assess dependence were asked only of lifetime users. Our NCS definition of use, however, was more inclusive than the ECA definition in two ways. First, the ECA did not include people who were using a prescription drug under the supervision of a physician even if the patient felt dependent. Second, the ECA assessed dependence only among those who had used a drug more than five times in their lives, while the NCS considered a respondent a user even if he or she had used only one time.

Dependence was defined according to the definitions and criteria of *DSM-III-R*.[15] The NCS questions used to generate this diagnosis are based on the Composite International Diagnostic Interview,[16] a state-of-the-art structured diagnostic instrument designed for use by trained

mates of the prevalence of these disorders.[9] Unfortunately, representativeness of these estimates can be called into question because the five community samples that made up the ECA were not nationally representative.[10] Furthermore, the ECA estimates are now more than a decade old.

This article presents updated estimates of the prevalence of drug use and dependence in the US household population on the basis of the National Comorbidity Survey (NCS). The NCS was designed to take the next step beyond the ECA by administering a structured psychiatric diagnostic interview to a nationally representative sample of the noninstitutionalized population and using these data to calculate the prevalence of and risk factors for psychiatric disorders in the United States.

RESULTS

THE PREVALENCE OF LIFETIME AND 12-MONTH USE

The NCS estimates of lifetime and 12-month prevalence of drug use are presented in **Table 2** separately by age and sex of respondents. Overall, somewhat more than half of respondents (51.0%) reported using an illegal drug or nonmedically using a prescription drug at least once in their lives, and 15.4% reported having done so in the past 12 months. Males were significantly more likely than females to have used a controlled substance both in their lifetimes (55.8% vs 46.4%, $t=4.7$, $P<.001$) and in the past 12 months interviewers who are not clinicians.[17] World Health Organization field trials of the Composite International Diagnostic Interview have documented high interrater reliability,[18,19] test-retest reliability,[20,21] and validity of the diagnosis of psychoactive substance dependence.[22-28]

A lifetime diagnosis of dependence, generated by the Composite International Diagnostic Interview diagnostic computer program,[29] requires the respondent to have at least three of nine *DSM-III-R* criterion A symptoms at some time in his or her life (eg, developing tolerance; experiencing withdrawal; unsuccessfully attempting to control use; continuing use despite the recognition that it is related to social, psychological, or physical problems) and to fulfill the requirements of criterion B by endorsing two or more Composite International Diagnostic Interview questions concerning duration of symptoms over a period of at least 1 month or repeatedly over a longer period. Consistent with *DSM-III-R*, no requirement is imposed for the criterion A symptoms to cluster in time for a diagnosis of lifetime dependence. Our definition of 12-month prevalence, in comparison, required a clustering of three or more criterion A symptoms in the 12 months before the interview in the subsample of respondents who qualified for lifetime diagnosis.

ANALYSIS PROCEDURES

Data analyses included the estimation of lifetime and 12-month prevalences, the estimation of cohort-specific cumulative age-at-onset prevalence curves, and the estimation of demographic correlates of use and dependence. Prevalence analyses were stratified by sex on the basis of well-documented evidence of a sex difference in drug use and disorder rates.[3,9,30-35]

Because of the complex sample design and weighting, SEs of the estimates could not be based on conventional methods. In the case of the lifetime and 12-month prevalences, SEs were obtained by means of the Taylor series linearization method.[36] The PSRATIO program in the OSIRIS IV software package[37] was used to make these calculations. We calculated *t* tests for sex differences in proportions of use and dependence on the basis of these SEs.

Cumulative age-at-onset curves were generated by means of the survival analysis methods operationalized in the SURVIVAL program in the SPSS-X software package.[38] Prevalences were estimated within 10-year cohorts for 5-year age intervals (eg, cumulative lifetime prevalences by the ages of 4, 9, 14, 19, and 24 years among respondents in the age range 15 to 24 years at the time of the interview). Cumulative prevalences for ages that exceeded the current ages of some cohort members (eg, cumulative prevalence by age 24 years in the cohort currently between the ages of 15 and 24 years) were based on the at-risk subsample of the cohort at the beginning of the 5-year interval (eg, the subsample of the 15- to 24-year-old cohort currently between the ages of 19 and 24 years). Individuals in this subsample were assumed to have experienced half of the year in which they were censored. Among those with a first onset in the interval, this meant assuming that they had an onset in the middle of the year of their reported age at onset, while among those with no lifetime history, it meant assuming that they were in the middle of the year of risk corresponding to their age at interview. Discrete-time (person-year) survival files[39] were analyzed to generate *z* statistics to assess significant intercohort differences in the slopes of the cumulative onset curves. The survival models were conceptualized as nested logistic regression equations,[40] in which age, cohort, and age-by-cohort interactions were treated as predictors. Design-based estimates of the SEs were obtained by the method of balanced repeated replications in 44 balanced subsamples.[41,42] The balanced repeated replication estimates take into account the clustering and weighting of the data without the linearization constraint required in the Taylor series method, yielding somewhat less biased estimates of SEs and confidence intervals in nonlinear models, such as logistic regression.[43] The LOGISTIC module in SAS-UNIX (version 6.07) was used to make these calculations, while a SAS macro was used to compute the SEs on the basis of comparison of estimates across the replicates.

Odds ratios for the demographic correlates of use and dependence were derived by exponentiating the logistic regression coefficients, and design-based estimates of the confidence intervals were generated by the same balanced repeated replication methods described above. An odds ratio of 1.0, or indistinguishable from 1.0 as bounded by the 95% confidence interval, was considered insignificant. Significance tests were made without adjustments for multiple tests.

(18.4% vs 12.4%, t=4.9, P<.001). There was also a powerful inverse relationship between age and 12-month use, from a high of 23.8% among respondents in the age range 15 to 24 years to a low of 5.5% among respondents in the age range 45 to 54 years.

The association between age and lifetime use was complicated by the fact that there was both a positive association between age and years of risk and a negative association between cohort and age-specific risk. A disaggregation of this complex pattern is presented in **Figure 1**, where respondent reports on their age of first use are presented in curves for the age-specific cumulative probabilities of lifetime use separately for each of the four 10-year birth cohorts in the NCS. Cohort 1 (born in 1966 to 1975) includes the youngest NCS respondents, while cohort 4 (born in 1936 to 1945) includes the oldest. It is useful to recognize, in studying Figure 1, that respondents in cohort 4, the only NCS respondents born before the end of World War II, would normally have completed high school by the mid-1960s, before the widespread introduction of marijuana and subsequently other illicit drugs into youth culture.[30,44-46] Cohort 3 went through adolescence in the early years of the youth drug culture, cohort 2 at its height, and cohort 1 during the years of downturn in drug use that has taken place during the last decade.

These differences in cohort experience are reflected in the cohort-specific age trends in Figure 1. The age-at-onset curve in cohort 4 shows that cumulative prevalence of drug use did not begin to rise until middle adolescence (15- to 19-year age range), at the end of which only about 7% of the cohort had any experience with drugs. Cumulative prevalence increased to approximately 13% by the end of late adolescence (20- to 24-year age range) and continued in roughly linear fashion through the present. The curves in the three more recent cohorts, in comparison, show uniform evidence of a dramatic rise in first use between early adolescence (10- to 14-year age range) and late adolescence, at which time 48% of cohort 3, 63% of cohort 2, and 57% of cohort 1 had used drugs at least once. The slopes of the onset curves become flatter after late adolescence. Consistent with the fact that respondents in cohort 2 were adolescents during the height of the youth drug culture, the onset curve is consistently higher in cohort 2 than in either cohort 1 or cohort 3 beginning in the age range 15 to 19 years.

Significance tests for intercohort differences in the slope of the onset curve between early adolescence and late adolescence (10- to 24-year age range) documented a significantly less steep slope among respondents in cohort 4 than in the three more recent cohorts (z=3.2, P=.001) as well as a significant difference between the two most recent cohorts, with the slope for cohort 2 significantly more steep than that for cohort 1 (z=2.4, P=.004). Contrasts between cohorts 1 and 3 and cohorts 2 and 3 in the survival models failed to show significant differences. An evaluation of differences in the cumulative probability of use as of the end of late adolescence (ages 20 to 24 years) showed that differences were significant between all pairs of cohorts (z tests between 2.1 and 22.4 for pairwise comparisons, with P between .009 and .001). This means that the lower cumulative probability of use in cohort 1 compared with cohort 2 at this age likely represents a genuine decrease rather than a sampling artifact. There are also significant differences in the survival models in the slopes of the onset curves in the years after late adolescence (cohort 2 vs cohort 4, z=2.1, P=.009; cohort 3 vs cohort 4, z=3.6, P<.001; cohort 2 vs cohort 3, z=1.3, P=.05), showing that first use after late adolescence was more common in cohort 4 than the more recent cohorts.

Sex-specific cohort differences in drug use are presented in **Table 3**. For both males and females the probability of use by age 24 years was lower in the youngest cohort (cohort 1) than cohort 2 (63% vs 68% for males; 51% vs 58% for females). The table also indicates that for both sexes in the three youngest cohorts, most first use occurred in the age range 15 to 19 years, with little initiation after the age of 20 years. For members of the oldest cohort, initiation was less dramatic in the 15- to 19-year age range and continued through the age of 34 years.

Table 1. Characteristics of National Comorbidity Survey (NCS) Respondents Compared With Total US Population

	US Population, % (N=65 244)*	NCS, % (N=8098) Weighted	NCS, % (N=8098) Unweighted
Sex			
M	49.1	49.5	47.5
F	50.9	50.5	52.5
Race			
White	75.0	75.3	75.1
Black	11.9	11.5	12.5
Hispanic	8.6	9.7	9.1
Other	4.5	3.5	3.3
Education, y			
0-11	22.5	22.3	18.2
12	36.8	37.4	33.1
13-15	21.2	21.7	26.3
≥16	19.5	18.6	22.4
Marital status			
Married	59.8	62.9	54.4
Separated, widowed, divorced	10.1	10.0	15.5
Never married	30.1	27.1	30.1
Region			
Northeast	20.0	20.2	19.2
Midwest	24.6	23.8	25.6
South	33.7	36.4	35.6
West	21.7	19.6	19.6
Age, y			
15-24	25.5	24.7	21.8
25-34	30.8	30.1	32.4
35-44	25.9	27.1	27.7
45-54	17.8	18.1	18.1
Urbanicity			
Metropolitan	71.2	67.8	68.9
Other urban	8.1	7.5	6.5
Nonurban	20.7	24.7	24.6

**The US population characteristics are based on results from the 1989 US National Health Interview Survey.*

THE PREVALENCE OF LIFETIME DEPENDENCE

The results in **Table 4** show that 7.5% of NCS respondents had a lifetime history of psychoactive substance dependence. Males were significantly more likely than females to have a lifetime history of dependence (9.2% vs 5.9%, t=3.8, P<.001). This is not merely because males were more likely to use drugs. They were also signifi-

Table 2. Lifetime and 12-Month (1990 to 1992) Drug Use, by Sex and Age

	%±SE					
	Males		Females		Total	
Age, y	Lifetime Use	12-mo Use	Lifetime Use	12-mo Use	Lifetime Use	12-mo Use
15-24	46.4±2.3	29.5±2.2	38.9±2.8	17.6±1.8	42.8±1.8	23.8±1.4
25-34	69.8±2.3	21.8±1.8	60.4±1.9	14.4±1.3	64.7±1.7	17.8±1.2
35-44	64.1±2.4	13.5±1.8	48.6±2.3	9.7±1.3	56.4±1.6	11.6±1.0
45-54	35.5±3.0	5.4±1.3	27.4±2.7	5.6±1.3	31.5±1.8	5.5±0.8
Total	55.8±1.3	18.4±1.0	46.4±1.5	12.4±0.7	51.0±1.0	15.4±0.6

cantly more likely than females to be dependent in the subsample of lifetime users (16.4% vs 12.6%, t=2.4, P=.004).

There was also an age-cohort effect in Table 4. In the sample as a whole, respondents in cohort 4 were significantly less likely to report a lifetime history of dependence than those in more recent cohorts (2.9% vs 7.3% to 9.5% in more recent cohorts, t tests between 3.2 and 5.5 for pairwise comparisons, all of them significant at P<.001). Among females, this lower prevalence resulted entirely from respondents in cohort 4 being much less likely than younger respondents to have ever used a drug, as shown by the fact that there was no significant association between age and lifetime dependence in the subsample of females who ever used a drug (cohort-specific prevalences between 11.7% and 14.1%, t tests between 0.1 and 0.5 for pairwise comparisons, with .15<P<.23). The situation was different for males, though, among whom prevalence of lifetime dependence was substantially lower for cohort 4 than more recent cohorts in the subsample of lifetime users (5.8% vs 16.7% to 19.7%, t=3.2 to 3.8 for pairwise comparisons, P<.001).

A disaggregated analysis of age and cohort effects is presented in **Figure 2**, where we show the cohort-specific cumulative probabilities of lifetime dependence among respondents who used drugs by specified ages. There was a consistent trend for higher prevalence of dependence among users in successively more recent cohorts. For example, whereas only 2.1%±1.2% (SE) of those respondents in cohort 4 who reported using drugs by the age of 24 years had a lifetime history of dependence by that age, the comparable percentages in more recent cohorts increased consistently to 10.0%±1.2% in cohort 3, 12.3%±1.4% in cohort 2, and 17.3%2.3% in cohort 1. Not only was this trend significant (z=6.3, P<.001) but, equally important for current policy purposes, the percentage was significantly larger in the most recent cohort (cohort 1) than the second most recent cohort (cohort 2; 17.3% vs 12.3%, z=1.9, P=.01), suggesting either a continuation of the trend among respondents currently in the age range 15 to 24 years or a systematic association between age and recall bias concerning age at first onset.

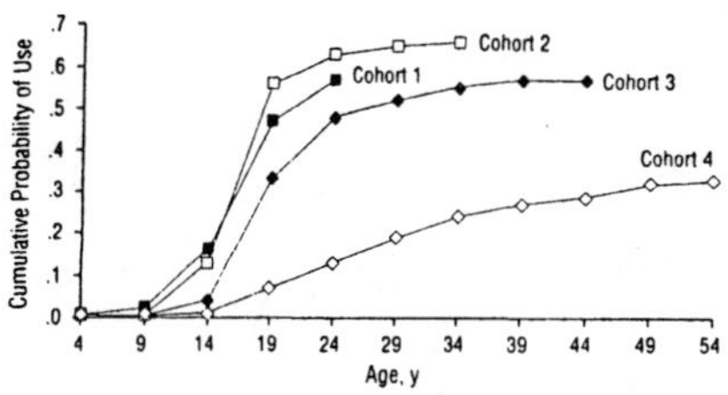

Age, y

		4	9	14	19	24	29	34	39	44	49	54
Cohort 1	CP	0	.02	.16	.47	.57						
	SE	0	0	.01	.02	.02						
Cohort 2	CP	0	0	.13	.56	.63	.65	.66				
	SE	0	0	.01	.02	.02	.02	.02				
Cohort 3	CP	0	0	.04	.33	.48	.52	.55	.57	.57		
	SE	0	0	.01	.01	.02	.02	.02	.02	.02		
Cohort 4	CP	0	0	.01	.07	.13	.19	.24	.27	.29	.32	.33
	SE	0	0	0	.01	.01	.01	.02	.02	.02	.02	.02

Figure 1. *Cumulative probability (CP) of drug use, by cohort.*

A disaggregation of these cohort differences by sex is presented in **Table 5**. Three intriguing patterns can be seen in this table. First, there was a consistent trend for the probability of lifetime dependence to be higher among female than male users at all ages in the oldest cohort. Second, there was an equally consistent trend for the probability of lifetime dependence to be higher among males than females in more recent cohorts. Third, there was a consistent sex difference in the age range at first onset of dependence. Among males, the vast majority of dependence occurred by the age of 24 years. Among females, in comparison, dependence had a later age at onset, with more than a doubling of the number of females who became dependent between the ages of 25 and 34 years compared with those with a history of dependence as of age 24 years. It is important to note that this sex difference in the age distribution of onset appears consistently across all cohorts.

THE PREVALENCE OF 12-MONTH DEPENDENCE

The results in **Table 6** show that 1.8% of NCS respondents were drug dependent during the 12 months before the interview. This represents 3.5% of lifetime users and 23.8% of persons with a lifetime history of dependence. It is worth repeating that our definition of 12 month dependence requires the respondent to meet full *DSM-III-R* A criteria within the past 12 months. If we relax this requirement and include persons with a lifetime history of dependence and at least one dependence

Table 3. Cumulative Probability of Drug Use, by Sex and Cohort

		Cumulative Probability±SE by Age Category, y								
Sex	Cohort	10-14	15-19	20-24	25-29	30-34	35-39	40-44	45-49	50-54
M	1	.19±.02	.51±.02	.63±.02	...	...	...	...	...	...
	2	.16±.02	.62±.02	.68±.02	.70±.02	.71±.02	...	...	...	...
	3	.05±.01	.43±.02	.58±.02	.62±.03	.64±.02	.64±.02	.64±.02	...	...
	4	.01±.01	.09±.02	.15±.02	.22±.02	.27±.03	.31±.03	.34±.03	.36±.03	.36±.03
F	1	.13±.02	.43±.03	.51±.03	...	...	...	...	...	...
	2	.10±.01	.51±.02	.58±.02	.61±.02	.62±.02	...	...	...	...
	3	.02±.01	.24±.02	.37±.02	.42±.02	.47±.02	.49±.02	.50±.02	...	...
	4	.01±.01	.05±.01	.10±.01	.16±.02	.20±.02	.23±.02	.25±.02	.28±.03	.29±.03

Table 4. Lifetime Drug Dependence in the Total Sample and Among Lifetime Users, by Sex and Age

	%±SE					
	Males		Females		Total	
Age, y	Total Sample	Lifetime Users	Total Sample	Lifetime Users	Total Sample	Lifetime Users
15-24	9.1±1.5	19.7±2.8	5.5±1.1	14.1±2.7	7.3±1.1	17.3±2.3
25-34	12.4±1.3	17.8±1.5	7.1±1.0	11.7±1.5	9.5±0.9	14.7±1.2
35-44	10.8±1.6	16.7±2.4	6.1±0.8	12.5±1.3	8.5±0.9	14.9±1.5
45-54	2.1±0.9	5.8±2.4	3.8±1.2	13.8±3.8	2.9±0.8	9.2±2.5
Total	9.2±0.7	16.4±1.2	5.9±0.5	12.6±1.0	7.5±0.4	14.7±0.7

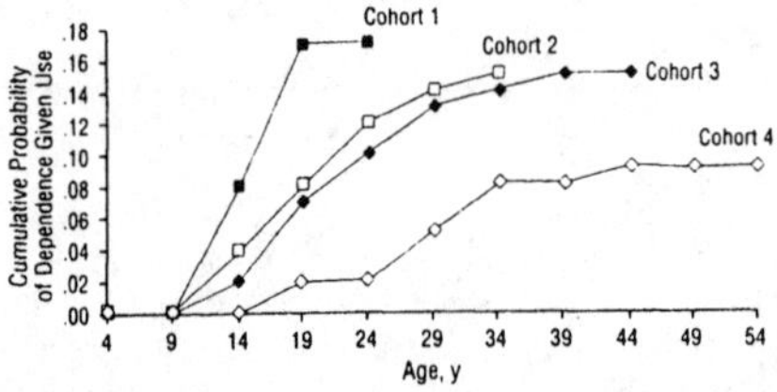

		Age, y										
		4	9	14	19	24	29	34	39	44	49	54
Cohort 1	CP	.00	.00	.08	.17	.17						
	SE	0	0	.02	.02	.02						
Cohort 2	CP	.00	.00	.04	.08	.12	.14	.15				
	SE	0	0	.01	.01	.01	.01	.01				
Cohort 3	CP	.00	.00	.02	.07	.10	.13	.14	.15	.15		
	SE	0	0	.01	.01	.01	.01	.02	.02	.02		
Cohort 4	CP	.00	.00	.00	.02	.02	.05	.08	.08	.09	.09	.09
	SE	0	0	0	.01	.02	.02	.02	.02	.02	.03	.03

Figure 2. *Cumulative probability (CP) of drug dependence, given use, by cohort.*

symptom in the past 12 months, the prevalence increases to 2.8%±0.2%, equivalent to 5.4%±0.5% of lifetime users and 37.9%±3.2% of persons with a lifetime history of dependence.

As in earlier tables, the overall proportion of respondents with 12-month dependence shown in Table 6 is significantly greater among males than females (2.3% vs 1.3%, t=2.2, P=.007). This is because males are both more likely than females to use drugs at some time in their lives and more likely to become dependent once they use them. In comparison, there was no significant sex difference in 12-month dependence in the subsample of persons with a lifetime history of dependence (24.9% vs 22.2%, t=0.5, P=.15).

Table 6 shows that 12-month dependence was significantly more prevalent among respondents in the 15- to 24-year age range (3.3%) than among those who were 25 to 34 years old (1.6%, t=2.2, P=.007), 35 to 44 years old (1.3%, t=2.6, P=.002), or 45 to 54 years old (0.7%, t=3.2, P<.001). A less obvious result captured in the last two columns of the table is that this association largely results from young people being more likely to be recent users. That is, there was no meaningful association between age and 12-month dependence in the subsample of 12-month users (eg, 13.0% among 15- to 24-year-old males vs 11.9% among 45- to 54-year-old males, t=0.1, P=.23).

DEMOGRAPHIC CORRELATES OF USE AND DEPENDENCE

The prevalence estimates reported above document the existence of significant age and sex differences in both drug use and dependence. A broader set of demographic correlates is considered in this section of the article. While a number of different contrasts are of potential interest, we focus on three stages of progression: (1) the predictors of first use (lifetime use in the total sample); (2) the predictors of first onset of dependence among users (lifetime dependence in the subsample of lifetime users); and (3) the predictors of persistence of dependence (12-month dependence in the subsample of persons with a lifetime history of dependence). The analysis is based on a series of three sets of univariate logistic regression equations in which a single demographic variable is treated as a predictor and the dichotomous measures of use or dependence are treated as outcomes.

Results are reported in **Table 7**. Whites were significantly more likely than nonwhites to use drugs at some time in their lives. Among lifetime users, there was no significant association between race and dependence. Among respondents with a lifetime history of dependence, blacks were significantly more likely than whites to have 12-month dependence. Respondents in the "other" (largely Asian) racial category, finally, had the lowest odds ratios (ORs) in all the contrasts.

There was a generally positive association between education and lifetime use of drugs. This pattern reversed, though, in predicting progression to dependence, where the ORs for respondents with 0 to 11 (OR, 2.30) or 12 (OR, 1.69) years of education were significantly greater than 1.0. The ORs of recent dependence among respondents with a lifetime history of dependence were also elevated in the subsamples with 0 to 11 and 12 years of education, although these coefficients were not statistically significant.

There was no association between family income and lifetime use in the NCS. Among users, however, there was a negative relationship between income and lifetime dependence. This was particularly pronounced among respondents in the lowest income category.

Lifetime probability of drug use was significantly higher in the Northeast and West than the Midwest or South. Given use, respondents in regions other than the Midwest had a higher odds of lifetime dependence, but

Table 5. Cumulative Probability of Drug Dependence Given Use, by Cohort and Sex

		Cumulative Probability±SE by Age Category, y								
Sex	Cohort	10-14	15-19	20-24	25-29	30-34	35-39	40-44	45-49	50-54
M	1	.06±.02	.19±.03	.20±.03	...	...	...	...	...	...
	2	.03±.01	.11±.01	.16±.02	.18±.02	.19±.02	...	...	...	...
	3	.00±.0	.09±.02	.12±.02	.15±.02	.16±.02	.17±.02	.17±.02	...	...
	4	.00±.0	.01±.01	.01±.01	.02±.01	.05±.03	.05±.02	.06±.03	.06±.03	.06±.02
F	1	.11±.04	.14±.03	.14±.03	...	...	...	...	...	...
	2	.05±.01	.06±.02	.09±.02	.11±.02	.12±.02	...	...	...	...
	3	.03±.01	.03±.01	.06±.02	.10±.01	.12±.01	.13±.01	.13±.01	...	...
	4	.00±.0	.04±.02	.04±.02	.10±.05	.10±.04	.10±.04	.13±.04	.14±.04	.14±.04

Table 6. Twelve-Month (1990 to 1992) Drug Dependence in the Total Sample, Among Lifetime Users, Among Respondents With Lifetime Dependence, and Among 12-Month Users, by Sex and Age

		%±SE			
Sex	Age, y	Total Sample	Lifetime Users	Lifetime Dependent	12-mo Users
M	15-24	4.5±1.1	9.6±2.2	48.8±8.7	13.0±3.0
	25-34	2.2±0.5	3.2±0.7	17.8±4.1	9.9±2.2
	35-44	1.4±0.4	2.0±0.7	13.3±3.7	9.7±3.0
	45-54	0.6±0.5	1.8±1.4	30.6±21.1	11.9±8.8*
	Total	2.3±0.4	4.0±0.6	24.9±3.9	11.3±1.9
F	15-24	2.1±0.5	5.4±1.4	38.1±7.7	10.6±2.5
	25-34	1.2±0.3	1.9±0.6	16.6±4.5	8.1±2.1
	35-44	1.1±0.4	2.2±0.8	17.8±6.4	11.1±4.3
	45-54	0.8±0.7	2.9±2.5	21.3±15.8	0.4±0.4*
	Total	1.3±0.2	2.8±0.5	22.2±3.8	9.0±1.4
Total	15-24	3.3±0.7	7.8±1.5	45.0±6.1	12.2±2.3
	25-34	1.6±0.3	2.5±0.5	17.3±3.1	9.1±1.6
	35-44	1.3±0.3	2.1±0.5	14.9±3.3	10.3±2.6
	45-54	0.7±0.4	2.3±1.4	24.7±11.7	6.1±4.4
	Total	1.8±0.2	3.5±0.5	23.8±3.1	10.3±1.4

* *Low precision.*

residents of the West comprised the only group for whom this difference was significant. There were no significant regional differences in the persistence of dependence.

Urbanicity was examined at the county level by distinguishing major metropolitan counties (metropolitan), urbanized counties that are not in major metropolitan areas (urban), and rural counties. There was a significant positive association between urbanicity and lifetime drug use. Given use, however, urbanicity was not significantly related to either lifetime dependence or persistence of dependence. Readers who are interested in the effect of a particular demographic correlate when the others are controlled for may request multivariate analysis results from us.

COMMENT

PREVALENCE ESTIMATES

The NCS drug use prevalence estimates are generally similar to those obtained in the 1991 NHSDA.[1] The NHSDA lifetime prevalence estimate among respondents in the age range of 15 to 54 years is 45.2% compared with the NCS estimate of 51.0%, whereas the NHSDA 12-month prevalence estimate is 16.7% compared to the NCS estimate of 15.4%.

Methodologic studies carried out by NHSDA staff show that willingness to admit drug use is reduced in the NHSDA when questions are administered by interviewers, as they are in the NCS, rather than self-administered.[47] On the basis of this evidence, the 1991 NHSDA drug use questions were self-administered. It is somewhat surprising, in light of this methodologic research, that the NCS estimate (based on interviewer-administered questions rather than self-administered questionnaires) is higher than the NHSDA estimate for lifetime use and only slightly lower than the NHSDA estimate for 12-month use. We have no way of investigating the reasons for this with our data, but we suspect that it has something to do with the fact that the NCS was a health survey rather than a drug survey. Because of our focus on health, the NCS asked about drug use in the context of other health-relevant behaviors, such as exercise and diet, and it is possible that this difference in context led to a reduction in respondent hesitation to admit drug use.

It is difficult to make direct comparisons to assess the consistency of the NCS estimates of the prevalence

Table 7. Demographic Correlates of Lifetime Drug Use in the Total Sample, Lifetime Dependence Among Users, and 12-Month Dependence Among Those With Lifetime Dependence*

	Lifetime Use (Total Sample)		Lifetime Dependence (User Subsample)		12-mo Dependence (Lifetime Dependent Subsample)	
	OR	95% CI	OR	95% CI	OR	95% CI
Race						
White	1.00	...	1.00	...	1.00	...
Black	0.62†	0.51-0.74	0.69	0.46-1.03	3.05†	1.05-8.84
Hispanic	0.70†	0.50-0.98	1.05	0.65-1.69	2.38	0.77-7.33
Other	0.37†	0.25-0.56	0.97	0.39-2.42	0.22	0.04-1.05
Education, y						
0-11	0.53†	0.45-0.63	2.30†	1.60-3.29	2.25	0.74-6.85
12	0.81†	0.70-0.93	1.69†	1.21-2.37	2.11	0.80-5.62
13-15	1.07	0.91-1.26	1.30	0.88-1.91	1.27	0.46-3.52
≥16	1.00	...	1.00	...	1.00	...
Income, ×$1000						
0-19	1.00	0.80-1.26	2.24†	1.43-3.52	1.81	0.57-5.80
20-34	0.96	0.78-1.19	1.51	0.90-2.54	1.00	0.33-3.03
35-69	0.91	0.74-1.12	1.29	0.76-2.21	0.84	0.27-2.69
≥70	1.00	...	1.00	...	1.00	...
Region						
Northeast	1.47†	1.17-1.84	1.22	0.86-1.71	1.16	0.40-3.35
Midwest	1.00	...	1.00	...	1.00	...
South	0.93	0.78-1.12	1.24	0.89-1.73	1.57	0.68-3.62
West	1.76†	1.34-2.32	1.64†	1.23-2.19	1.39	0.59-3.25
Urbanicity						
Metropolitan	1.85†	1.46-2.35	1.40	0.98-2.00	1.17	0.47-2.90
Other urban	1.54†	1.13-2.11	1.38	0.92-2.08	1.28	0.56-2.91
Nonurban	1.00	...	1.00	...	1.00	...

**OR indicates odds ratio; CI, confidence interval.*
†An odds ratio with a confidence interval that does not include 1.0 is statistically significant.

of drug dependence with those of previous surveys because the latter have usually been based on either health maintenance organization or treatment samples[8,48] and have often used measures of dependence that are not comparable with the *DSM-III-R* criteria used in the NCS.[49] It is possible, however, to compare the NCS estimate of dependence with that of the ECA Study. Before the NCS, the ECA Study provided the most up-to-date estimate of the national prevalence of drug dependence. The NCS estimate of 7.5% lifetime dependence is somewhat higher than the 5.1% estimate obtained in the ECA Study for lifetime prevalence of *DSM-III* drug dependence among respondents in the age range of 18 to 44 years.[9] However, when we focus on NCS respondents who are currently in the age range of 28 to 54 years and compute the percentage who reported an onset of dependence as of 10 years earlier (ie, when they were 18 to 44 years old)—a comparison that matches NCS data with ECA Study data on year of assessment, age of risk, and cohort—the NCS prevalence estimate for lifetime dependence is reduced to 5.3%±0.6%, very similar to the ECA Study estimate of 5.1%.

SEX, AGE, AND COHORT EFFECTS

The NCS finding that males are more likely than females to use and to be dependent on drugs is consistent with previous research.[3,9,30-32] The finding that male drug users are more likely than female users to become dependent is inconsistent with the ECA Study finding that lifetime drug use disorders are equally prevalent among male and female extramedical drug users.[9] Additionally, our finding of no sex difference in 12-month dependence among respondents with a lifetime history of dependence is at odds with the ECA Study finding that men are significantly more likely than women to experience current problems associated with lifetime abuse or dependence.[9]

Our finding of an inverse relationship between age and use has been repeatedly found in previous research,[3,46] as has our finding that use and dependence are both much more common in cohorts born after World War II.[9,30,44-46,50] The decrease in the cumulative probability of use by age 24 years in cohort 1 compared with cohort 2 is consistent with recent trends from the data that show decreases in use over the last several years for 12th graders.[51]

The interaction found in the NCS between sex and cohort in predicting lifetime dependence was also found in weaker form in the ECA Study, where women in the 45- to 64-year age range were slightly more likely than men to qualify for lifetime dependence (0.4% vs 0.2%, $t=.07$, $P=.24$), while men had higher lifetime dependence than women in other age groups.[9] Males in the NCS had a higher lifetime prevalence of dependence than females among respondents in the cohorts born after the end of World War II but a lower prevalence than females in the cohort born in the decade before the end of

World War II, despite the fact that older males are more likely than older females to have a history of drug use. This result may be related to a finding in previous studies that females predominate among people who are dependent on psychotherapeutic medicines, while males predominate among people who are dependent on other drugs.[52-54] The former would be expected to be responsible for a larger proportion of drug dependence among persons in cohort 4, as they are the only NCS cohort to go through adolescence before the introduction of marijuana and other drugs into youth culture. Consistent with this possibility, disaggregated cohort-specific analyses of NCS dependence data by type of drug reported elsewhere shows that men are more likely than women to use psychotherapeutic drugs but female users are more likely than male users to become dependent.[55] More complex analyses are needed to determine whether this accounts for the sex-by-cohort interaction in dependence among users found here. Another plausible interpretation is that the interaction between sex and cohort comes about because of greater selection bias among males than females with a history of dependence, possibly because of a stronger association between dependence and early mortality among males than females.

We are unaware of any previous research documenting that the conditional probability of dependence among users has increased among respondents who are currently in the age range 15 to 24 years (cohort 1) compared with earlier cohorts (Figure 2), despite the fact that the probability of lifetime use is lower in cohort 1 than cohort 2 (Figure 1). A methodologic interpretation of this increased probability of dependence among users is possible, emphasizing some combination of differential recall bias, differential willingness to admit use, and differential sample selection bias in cohort 1 compared with earlier cohorts. A substantive interpretation is also possible, emphasizing the possibility that the people who are selected into use of drugs during a time when use is becoming less prevalent are likely to be more vulnerable (eg, more likely to have a history of psychopathology) and, as a result, more likely to become dependent.[56,57] It would be possible to evaluate this interpretation in more detailed analyses by studying cohort differences in retrospective reports concerning history of other disorders before the onset of drug use.

The findings regarding a significantly higher prevalence of 12-month dependence among the youngest respondents but no cohort difference in 12-month dependence among 12-month users is somewhat surprising in light of evidence that use is more likely to be experimental during the teenage years[51] and the likelihood that younger users are less likely to be using drugs associated with a high risk of dependence.[58] However, it has been argued that early age at onset contributes to an increased likelihood of dependence.[46] We also found a sex difference in the relationship between cohort and prevalence of lifetime dependence. The lower prevalence among females born before vs after the end of World War II results entirely from their lower probability of ever using a drug, whereas the lower prevalence of lifetime dependence among males born before vs after World War II results from a combination of lower probability of ever using a drug and lower probability of dependence among users. This might reflect a sex difference in drug of choice or in the changing centrality of drug use to other aspects of male and female life-styles across cohorts.

A sex difference in drug of choice could also help explain our finding that the curves for age at onset of dependence differ for males and females, with the lifetime prevalence of dependence among females doubling in the age range of 25 to 34 years, while virtually all dependence among males occurred by the age of 24 years. This difference is consistent with evidence that prescription drugs are responsible for a larger part of female than male dependence.[44] It also suggests the possibility that there may be a longer time between first use and onset of dependence among females than males.

OTHER DEMOGRAPHIC CORRELATES OF USE AND DEPENDENCE

Our results concerning other demographic correlates are broadly consistent with previous research in finding that drug use is positively associated with being white rather than nonwhite,[4,59] well educated rather than poorly educated,[30,60] urban rather than rural,[30,32] and a resident of the Northeast or West rather than the South or Midwest.[30,32]

We also documented that the predictive power of demographic variables often differs from one stage of disorder to the next. For example, whites are significantly more likely than blacks ever to use one of the drugs considered here, indistinguishable from blacks in their probability of lifetime dependence after first use, and significantly less likely than blacks to have persistent dependence. These results are consistent with Kandel's finding[61] that blacks are less likely than whites to experiment with most drugs but more likely than whites to persist in their use. Results such as these underscore the complexity of the issues surrounding substance use disorders and support the argument made nearly two decades ago by Robins[62] that an adequate understanding of risk factors for substance use disorders requires a decomposition of risk factors into stages.

LIMITATIONS

The NCS prevalence estimates probably underestimate the true prevalence of drug use and dependence in the total population because the sampling frame (the household population) excludes the homeless and residents of institutional settings and group housing and because reporting errors among respondents are likely to be in the direction of underreporting rather than overreporting these experiences.

Many results hinge on respondent recall of ages when use first occurred or they first became dependent. Recall bias in reporting these dates could lead to errors in the age-at-onset analyses. If these errors differ by current age, they could distort intercohort comparisons. This, in turn, could lead to the impression that there are substantive cohort differences when, in fact, these differences result from differential recall bias.[63] As a result, caution is needed in interpreting results concerning cohort differences.

Finally, the results concerning demographic correlates should be taken as descriptive rather than as evidence concerning risk factors because these results are all based on univariate prediction equations. It is likely that some of the significant associations would disappear in more complex multivariate analyses. Anthony,[64] for example, showed no significant association between being black and drug dependence when a control was introduced for neighborhood. Even when results hold up after the introduction of controls, the causal order of associations is not always clear. For example, the significant association between low educational attainment and lifetime dependence in the subsample of lifetime users could result from an effect of educational failure on subsequent onset of dependence, an effect of dependence on subsequent school dropout, an effect of other variables on both education and dependence, or some combination of these effects. Future analyses of the NCS data will rely on survival models in which age at onset of use and disorder are treated as outcome variables, and predictors that may be reciprocally related to the outcomes are treated as time-varying covariates to clarify this temporal uncertainty in the predictors of the progression from first use to dependence.

Accepted for publication November 15, 1994.

The NCS is a collaborative epidemiologic investigation of the prevalence, causes, and consequences of psychiatric morbidity and comorbidity in the United States supported by the US Alcohol, Drug Abuse, and Mental Health Administration (grant 5 R01 MH46376) with supplemental support from the W. T. Grant Foundation (grant 90135190), Ronald C. Kessler, principal investigator. Preparation for this report was also supported by Research Scientist Development Award 1 K01 MH00507 (Dr Kessler).

The Addiction Research Foundation, Toronto, Ontario (Robin Room, PhD), Duke University Medical Center, Durham, NC (Dan Blazer, MD, and Marvin Swartz, MD), The Johns Hopkins University, Baltimore, Md (James Anthony, PhD, William Eaton, PhD, and Philip Leaf, PhD), Max Planck Institute of Psychiatry, Munich, Germany (Hans-Ulrich Wittchen, PhD), the Medical College of Virginia, Richmond (Kenneth Kendler, MD), The University of Michigan, Ann Arbor (Lloyd Johnston, PhD, and Ronald Kessler, PhD), the National Institute of Mental Health, Bethesda, Md, (Darrell Kirch, MD, and Darrel Regier, MD), New York (NY) University (Patrick Shrout, PhD), State University of New York, Stony Brook (Evelyn Bromet, PhD), The University of Toronto (Ontario) (R. Jay Turner, PhD), and Washington University School of Medicine, St Louis, Mo (Linda Cottler, PhD). A complete list of NCS publications can be obtained from the NCS Study Coordinator, Room 1006, Institute for Social Research, The University of Michigan, Box 1248, Ann Arbor, MI 48106-1248.

We appreciate the helpful comments of Lloyd Johnston, PhD, and Denise Kandel, PhD.

Reprints not available.

REFERENCES

1. Kozel NJ. Epidemiology of drug abuse in the United States: a summary of methods and findings. *Bull Pan Am Health Organ.* 1990;24:53-62.
2. US Dept of Health and Human Services. *Annual Emergency Room Data, 1990.* Rockville, Md: National Institute on Drug Abuse; 1991b.
3. US Dept of Health and Human Services. *National Household Survey on Drug Abuse, Population Estimates 1991.* Rockville, Md: National Institute on Drug Abuse; 1991a.
4. Johnston LD, O'Malley PM, Bachman JG. *Smoking, Drinking, and Illicit Drug Use Among American Secondary School Students, College Students, and Young Adults, 1975-1991: Volume 1, Secondary School Students.* Rockville, Md: US Dept of Health and Human Services; 1992.
5. Harrison LD. Trends in illicit drug use in the United States: conflicting results from national surveys. *Int J Addict.* 1992;27:817-847.
6. Kozel NJ, Adams EH. Epidemiology of drug abuse: an overview. *Science.* 1986; 234:970-974.
7. Kandel DB, Davies M. Decline in the use of illicit drugs by high school students in New York State: a comparison with national data. *Am J Public Health.* 1991;81:1064-1067.
8. Kilbey MM, Breslau N, Andreski P. Cocaine use and dependence in young adults: associated psychiatric disorders and personality traits. *Drug Alcohol Depend.* 1992;29:283-290.
9. Anthony JC, Helzer JE. Syndromes of drug abuse and dependence. In: Robins LN, Regier DA, eds. *Psychiatric Disorders in America: The Epidemiologic Catchment Area Study.* New York, NY: Free Press; 1991:116-154.
10. Robins LN, Regier DA, eds. *Psychiatric Disorders in America: The Epidemiologic Catchment Area Study.* New York: Free Press; 1991.
11. Kessler RC, McGonagle KA, Zhao S, Nelson CB, Hughes M, Eshleman S, Wittchen H-U, Kendler KS. Lifetime and 12-month prevalence of *DSM-III-R* psychiatric disorders in the United States: Results from the National Comorbidity Survey. *Arch Gen Psychiatry.* 1994;51:8-19.
12. Allgulander C. Psychoactive drug use in a general population sample, Sweden: correlates with perceived health, psychiatric diagnoses, and mortality in an automated record-linkage study. *Am J Public Health.* 1989;79:1006-1010.
13. Eaton WW, Anthony JC, Tepper S, Dryman, A. Psychopathology and attrition in the Epidemiologic Catchment Area Study. *Am J Epidemiol.* 1992;135:1051-1059.
14. US Dept of Health and Human Services. *National Health Interview Survey, 1989.* Hyattsville, Md: National Center for Health Statistics; 1992. Computer file.
15. American Psychiatric Association. *Diagnostic and Statistical Manual of Mental Disorders, Revised Third Edition.* Washington, DC: American Psychiatric Association; 1987.
16. World Health Organization. *Composite International Diagnostic Interview (CIDI, Version 1.0).* Geneva, Switzerland: World Health Organization; 1990.
17. Robins LN, Wing J, Wittchen H-U, Helzer JE. The Composite International Diagnostic Interview: an epidemiologic instrument suitable for use in conjunction with different diagnostic systems and in different cultures. *Arch Gen Psychiatry.* 1988;45:1069-1077.
18. Wittchen H-U, Robins LN, Cottler LB, Sartorius N, Burke JD, Regier DA, participants in the Multicenter WHO/ADAMHA Field Trials. Cross-cultural feasibility, reliability and sources of variance in the Composite International Diagnostic Interview (CIDI). *Br J Psychiatry.* 1991;159:645-653.
19. Cottler LB, Robins LN, Grant BF, Blaine J, Towle LH, Wittchen H-U, Sartorius N, participants in the WHO/ADAMHA Field Trials. The CIDI-core substance abuse and dependence questions: cross-cultural and nosological issues. *Br J Psychiatry.* 1991;159:653-658.
20. Semler G, von Cranach M, Wittchen H-U, eds. *Comparison Between the Composite International Diagnostic Interview and the Present State Examination: Report to the WHO/ADAMHA Task Force on Instrument Development.* Geneva, Switzerland; World Health Organization; February 1987.
21. Wacker HR, Battegay R, Mullejans R, Schlosser C. Using the CIDI-C in the general population. In: Stefanis CN, Rabavilas AD, Soldatos CR, eds. *Psychiatry: A World Perspective.* Amsterdam, the Netherlands: Elsevier Science Publishers BV; 1990:138-143.
22. Semler G, ed. *Reliabilitat und Validitat des Composite International Diagnostic Interview: Inaugural-Dissertation zur Erlangung des akademischen Grades eines Doktors der Philosophie.* Mannheim, Germany: Universitat Mannheim; 1989.
23. Spengler P, Wittchen H-U. Procedural validity of standardized symptom questions for the assessment of psychotic symptoms: a comparison of the CIDI with two clinical methods. *Compr Psychiatry.* 1989;29:309-322.
24. Janca A, Robins LN, Cottler LB, Early TS. Clinical observation of CIDI assessments: an analysis of the CIDI field trials—wave II at the St. Louis site. *Br J Psychiatry.* 1992;160:815-818.

25. Leitmeyer P, ed. *Zur Symptomerfassung mit dem standarisierten Interview CIDI-C in der Allgemeinpraxis: Inaugural dissertation zur Erlangung des medizinischen Doktorgrades fur Klinische Medizin.* Mannheim, Germany: Universitat Mannheim; 1990.
26. Farmer AE, Katz R, McGuffin P, Bebbington P. A comparison between the Present State Examination and the Composite International Diagnostic Interview. *Arch Gen Psychiatry.* 1987;44:1064-1068.
27. Farmer AE, Jenkins PL, Katz R, Ryder L. Comparison of CATEGO-derived *ICD-8* and *DSM-III* classifications using the Composite International Diagnostic Interview in severely ill subjects. *Br J Psychiatry.* 1991;158:177-182.
28. Wittchen H-U, Burke JD, Semler G, Pfister H. Recall and dating of psychiatric symptoms: test-retest reliability of time-related symptom questions in a standardized psychiatric interview. *Arch Gen Psychiatry.* 1989;46:437-443.
29. World Health Organization. *Composite International Diagnostic Interview.* Geneva, Switzerland: World Health Organization; 1991. Computer program.
30. Abelson HI, Miller JD. A decade of trends in cocaine use in the household population. In: Kozel NJ, Adams EH, eds. *Cocaine Use in America. Epidemiologic and Clinical Perspectives.* Washington, DC: National Institute on Drug Abuse; 1985:35-49. Research monograph 61.
31. Kandel DB, Yamaguchi K. Developmental patterns of the use of legal, illegal, and medically prescribed psychotropic drugs from adolescence to young adulthood. In: Jones CL, Battjes RJ, eds. *Etiology of Drug Abuse: Implications for Prevention.* Washington, DC: National Institute on Drug Abuse; 1985:193-235. Research monograph 56.
32. O'Malley PM, Johnston LD, Bachman JG. Quantitative and qualitative changes in cocaine use among American high school seniors, college students, and young adults. In: Schober S, Schade C, eds. *The Epidemiology of Cocaine Use and Abuse.* Washington, DC: National Institute on Drug Abuse; 1991:19-43. Research monograph 110.
33. Boyd CJ, Blow F, Orgain LS. Gender differences among African-American substance users. *J Psychoactive Drugs.* 1993;25:301-305.
34. Lex BW. Some gender differences in alcohol and polysubstance users. *Health Psychol.* 1991;10:121-132.
35. Thomas SM, Fick AC, Henderson J, Doherty K. Tobacco, alcohol, and marijuana use among black adolescents: a comparison across gender, grade, and school environment. *J La State Med Soc.* 1990;142:37-42.
36. Woodruff RS, Causey BD. Computerized method for approximating the variance of a complicated estimate. *J Am Stat Assoc.* 1976;71:315-321.
37. University of Michigan. *OSIRIS VII.* Ann Arbor, Mich: Institute for Social Research, University of Michigan; 1981.
38. Norusis MJ, ed. *SPSS/PC+ Advanced Statistics 4.0 for the IBM PC/XT/AT and PS/2.* Chicago, Ill: SPSS Inc; 1990.
39. Kalbfleisch JD. *The Statistical Analysis of Failure Time Data.* New York, NY: John Wiley & Sons Inc; 1980.
40. Willett JB, Singer JD. Investigating onset, cessation, relapse and recovery: why you should, and how you can, use discrete-time survival analysis to examine event occurrence. *J Consult Clin Psychol.* 1993;61:952-965.
41. Kish L, Frankel MR. Balanced repeated replications for standard errors. *J Am Stat Assoc.* 1970;65:1071-1094.
42. Koch GG, Lemeshow S. An application of multivariate analysis to complex sample survey data. *J Am Stat Assoc.* 1972;67:780-782.
43. Kalton G. Practical methods for estimating survey sampling errors. *Bull Int Stat Inst.* 1977;47:495-514.
44. Clayton RR, Voss HL, Robbins C, Skinner WF. Gender differences in drug use: an epidemiological perspective. In: Ray BA, Braude MC, eds. *Women and Drugs: A New Era for Research.* Washington, DC: National Institute on Drug Abuse; 1986:80-99. Research monograph 65.
45. Johnston LD. The etiology and prevention of substance use: what can we learn from recent historical changes? In: Jones CL, Battjes RJ, eds. *Etiology of Drug Abuse: Implications for Prevention.* Washington, DC: National Institute on Drug Abuse; 1985:155-177. Research monograph 56.
46. Robins LN, Przybeck TR. Age of onset of drug use as a factor in drug and other disorders. In: Jones CL, Battjes RJ, eds. *Etiology of Drug Abuse: Implications for Prevention.* Washington, DC: National Institute on Drug Abuse; 1985:178-192. Research monograph 56.
47. Turner CF, Lessler JT, Gfroerer JC. Future directions for research and practice. In: Turner CF, Lessler JT, Gfroerer JC, eds. *Survey Measurement of Drug Use: Methodological Studies.* Washington, DC: National Institute on Drug Abuse; 1992:299-306.
48. Rapaport MH, Tipp JE, Schuckit MA. A comparison of *ICD-10* and *DSM-III-R* criteria for substance abuse and dependence. *Am J Drug Alcohol Abuse.* 1993;19:143-151.
49. Anglin MD, Hser Y-I, McGlothlin WH. Sex differences in addict careers, 2: becoming addicted. *Am J Drug Alcohol Abuse.* 1987;13:59-71.
50. Burke KC, Burke JD, Rae DS, Regier DA. Comparing age at onset of major depression and other psychiatric disorders by birth cohorts in five U.S. community populations. *Arch Gen Psychiatry.* 1991;48:789-795.
51. Johnston LD, O'Malley PM, Bachman JG. *Smoking, Drinking, and Illicit Drug Use Among American Secondary School Students, College Students, and Young Adults, 1975-1991.* Rockville, Md: US Dept of Health and Human Services; 1992.
52. Almog YJ, Anglin MD, Fisher DG. Alcohol and heroin use patterns of narcotics addicts: gender and ethnic differences. *Am J Drug Alcohol Abuse.* 1993;19:219-238.
53. Bell DS. Dependence on psychotropic drugs and analgesics in men and women. In: Kalant OJ, ed. *Alcohol and Drug Problems in Women.* New York, NY: Plenum Press; 1980;5:423-463.
54. Cooperstock R, Parnell P. Research on psychotropic drug use: a review of findings and methods. *Soc Sci Med.* 1982;16:1179-1196.
55. Anthony JC, Warner LA, Kessler RC. Comparative epidemiology of dependence on tobacco, alcohol, controlled substances, and inhalants: basic findings from the National Comorbidity Survey. *Exp Clin Psychopharmacol.* 1994;2:244-268.
56. Weiss RD, Mirin SM, Griffin ML, Michael JL. Psychopathology in cocaine abusers: changing trends. *J Nerv Ment Dis.* 1988;176:719-725.
57. Kessler RC. The epidemiology of psychiatric comorbidity. In: Tsaung M, Tohan M, Zahner G, eds. *Textbook of Psychiatric Epidemiology.* New York, NY: John Wiley & Sons Inc; 1995:179-197.
58. Kandel DB, Faust R. Sequences and stages in patterns of adolescent drug use. *Arch Gen Psychiatry.* 1975;32:923-932.
59. US Dept of Health and Human Services. *National Household Survey on Drug Abuse, Population Estimates 1992.* Rockville, Md: National Institute on Drug Abuse; 1993.
60. Adams EH, Gfroerer JC, Rouse BA. Epidemiology of substance abuse including alcohol and cigarette smoking. *Ann N Y Acad Sci.* 1989;562:14-20.
61. Kandel DB. The social demography of drug use. In: Bayer R, Oppenheimer GM, eds. *Confronting Drug Policy: Illicit Drugs in a Free Society.* New York, NY: Cambridge University Press; 1993:24-77.
62. Robins LN. Estimating addiction rates and locating target populations: how decomposition into stages helps. In: Rittenhouse JD, ed. *The Epidemiology of Heroin and Other Narcotics.* Washington, DC: National Institute on Drug Abuse; 1977:78-559. Research monograph series 16. Dept of Health, Education, and Welfare publication 1 (ADM).
63. Simon GE, VonKorff M. Reevaluation of secular trends in depression rates. *Am J Epidemiol.* 1992;135:1411-1422.
64. Anthony JC. The epidemiology of drug addiction. In: Miller NS, ed. *Comprehensive Handbook of Drug and Alcohol Addiction.* New York, NY: Marcel Dekker Inc; 1991:55-86.

ORIGINAL ARTICLE

Replication of the Stockholm Adoption Study of Alcoholism

Confirmatory Cross-Fostering Analysis

Sören Sigvardsson, PhD; Michael Bohman, MD; C. Robert Cloninger, MD

Background: Two forms of alcoholism with distinct clinical features and mode of inheritance were first distinguished in the Stockholm Adoption Study. This involved a large sample of children born in Stockholm, Sweden, who were adopted at an early age and reared by nonrelatives. Type 1 alcoholism had adult onset and rapid progression of dependence without criminality, whereas type 2 had teenage onset of recurrent social and legal problems from alcohol abuse.

Methods: A replication study was carried out with 577 men and 660 women born in Gothenburg, Sweden, and adopted at an early age by nonrelatives. The genetic and environmental backgrounds of the adoptees were classified by the exact procedures calibrated by discriminant analysis in the original study.

Results: Both type 2 and severe type 1 alcoholism were confirmed as independently heritable forms of alcoholism in male adoptees. The lifetime risk of severe alcoholism was increased 4-fold in adopted men with both genetic and environmental risk factors characteristic of type 1 alcoholism compared with the others (11.4% vs 3.0%). Neither genetic nor environmental risk factors for type 1 alcoholism by themselves were sufficient to cause alcoholism. In contrast, the risk of type 2 alcoholism was increased 6-fold in adopted sons with a type 2 genetic background compared with others, regardless of their postnatal environment (10.7% vs 2.0%). The sons with a type 2 genetic background in the replication sample had no excess of type 1 alcoholism, and vice versa. There was no increased risk of mild abuse in adopted men regardless of their genetic or environmental background.

Conclusion: Type 1 and type 2 alcoholism are clinically distinct forms of alcoholism with causes that are independent but not mutually exclusive.

Arch Gen Psychiatry. 1996;53:681-687

TWO FORMS of alcoholism with distinct clinical features and modes of inheritance were first distinguished in the Stockholm Adoption Study.[1,2] This subdivision was identified in a large population of consecutive births by means of multivariate methods of classification. The inheritance of alcoholism was studied in 913 Swedish women and 862 Swedish men adopted by nonrelatives at an early age. Lifetime records of alcohol abuse and related behaviors were available for the adoptees and all their biological and adoptive parents. Information about the biological parents and the postnatal environments of the adoptees disclosed clinical and etiological heterogeneity among the alcoholics. Type 1 alcoholism was clinically characterized by adult onset (age of 20 years or older) and rapid progression from mild abuse to severe alcohol dependence with little or no criminality. Type 2 alcoholism was associated with teenage onset of recurrent social and legal problems from alcohol abuse. These 2 forms of alcoholism were initially distinguished in terms of their pattern of inheritance.[1-3] The risk of type 1 alcoholism was increased only when there was a combination of a characteristic genetic background and a characteristic environmental background. Consequently, the average effect of genetic factors on type 1 alcoholism was weak, accounting for 38% of the variability of liability in mild cases and 25% in severe cases. In contrast, the liability to type 2 alcoholism was 90% heritable in men but was seldom expressed in women. The type of alcoholism in the biological parents increased the risk of the same type

From the Department of Social Medicine, University of Umeå, Umeå, Sweden (Drs Sigvardsson and Bohman), and the Departments of Psychiatry and Genetics, Washington University School of Medicine, St Louis, Mo (Dr Cloninger).

See Subjects and Methods on next page

SUBJECTS AND METHODS

SAMPLE AND DESCRIPTIVE DATA

The same sampling and assessment methods used in the original Stockholm Adoption Study[1,2] were applied in this replication study except that the children selected were born elsewhere in Sweden. The replication population includes all children born to single women in Gothenburg, Sweden, from 1930 through 1949 who were adopted at an early age by nonrelatives. No subjects in this study were part of the original Stockholm study. Subjects were excluded because of placement after 3 years of age, placement with relatives, or uncertain paternity, as in the previous work. This yielded a replication sample of 577 adopted men and 660 adopted women. The adoptees ranged in age from 28 to 47 years at the time of last information, which was 1977, as in the original study.

Data about the adoptees and their biological and adoptive background were obtained from multiple sources, as detailed in previous work.[1-3] Briefly, these included (1) data about the ages, occupations, and places of residence of both biological and adoptive parents from a register of child welfare officer appointments; (2) registrations of alcohol abuse, supervision, and treatment of alcoholics as kept by the Temperance Board; (3) registrations for criminal convictions in the criminal register; and (4) registrations about diagnoses and hospitalization as kept by local agencies of the National Health Insurance, as in the Stockholm Adoption Study. Temperance Board registrations for illegal manufacture or sale of alcohol were not considered evidence of alcohol abuse in either the original or the replication study. This multisource method has been estimated to have a sensitivity of 70% and high specificity for alcoholism diagnosed by all sources, including personal psychiatric interviews.[9]

CLASSIFICATION OF THE ADOPTEE'S ALCOHOL ABUSE

Adoptees were classified according to their lifetime record of alcohol abuse in exactly the same manner as defined in the Stockholm Adoption Study based on the clinical studies by Kaij.[7] Adoptees with 4 or more Temperance Board registrations, compulsory treatment, or psychiatric hospitalization with a diagnosis of alcoholism were classified as severe type 1 alcoholics. Adoptees with only a single Temperance Board registration and no treatment were classified as mild type 1 alcoholics. Adoptees with 2 or 3 Temperance Board registrations without treatment for alcoholism were classified as type 2 alcoholics.

CLASSIFICATION OF THE GENETIC AND ENVIRONMENTAL BACKGROUNDS

The genetic background of each adoptee in the replication sample was classified by means of information about the biological parents only and according to the discriminant function derived in original Stockholm population (the calibration sample). The genetic background was classified as type 1 (mild or severe), type 2 (moderate), or neither based on information about the biological parents' alcohol abuse, criminality, and occupational status, as specified in the original report.[1] Briefly, type 1 genetic background was characterized by adult onset of recurrent alcohol abuse with little or no criminality in biological mothers and fathers, whereas type 2 genetic background was characterized by teenage onset of both recurrent criminality and recurrent alcohol abuse in the biological father.

The postnatal environmental background was classified as mild type 1, severe type 1, and type 2 based on information about the adoptive parents and the adoptee's preplacement experiences, as specified in the original report.[1] Briefly, the rearing environment predicted to increase the risk of severe type 1 alcoholism was characterized by the adoptive father having an unskilled occupation. The environment predicted to be associated with mild type 1 alcoholism was characterized by early adoptive placement into a middle-class home. The environment predicted to increase risk of type 2 alcoholism was characterized by little preplacement medical care and late placement in the adoptive home.

STATISTICAL ANALYSES

Discriminant analysis was used to classify both the genetic and environmental backgrounds in accord with the functions derived in previous research.[1] All individuals in the population were assigned to their most probable background group by the Fisher linear classification method. The classification functions were derived (ie, calibrated) in the Stockholm Adoption Study and applied without modification to the replication sample.[24] Version 4.0 of the SPSS program for personal computers was used for discriminant analysis.[24]

Odds ratios (ORs) and their 95% confidence intervals (CIs) were computed by means of PROC FREQ in the SAS computer program, version 6.07.[25] The logit estimate of the 95% CI was computed. The tests of predicted hypotheses were considered confirmed as significant only if their probability of occurring by chance was less than 5%. We report significance levels based on 2-tailed tests, which is conservative in a replication study, but no other observed differences would have been judged significant by 1-tailed tests. Hence, ORs are significantly greater than unity when the lowest point of the 95% CI is greater than 1.0.

of alcoholism and no other forms of psychopathology in their adopted-away children, with 1 exception; type 2 alcoholic fathers increased the risk of somatization disorder, but not alcoholism or other psychopathology, in the daughters.[1-4]

The hypothesis of 2 alcoholic subtypes stimulated widespread interest and was extensively cited for its strengths. One important strength of the study was that the sample was large and based on an entire population of consecutive birth cohorts. In contrast, earlier adoption studies of alcoholism[5,6] involved comparisons of fewer than 100 cases and highly selected controls, and had produced contradictory results that could be attributed to selection artifacts.[3] A second important strength was that the adoptees and all their parents were assessed for their entire lifetime for alcohol abuse by means of systematic records. Third, the classification of alcohol abuse in the adoptees used multiple sources of data that were highly accurate in classifying alcohol abuse. This multisource method was validated by detailed clinical studies, including personal psychiatric interviews.[7-9] Fourth, the genetic and environmental backgrounds were classified by multivariate methods that are statistically efficient and similar to the polythetic criteria approach adopted in modern diagnostic systems beginning with *DSM-III*.[10]

Despite these strengths, the evidence for the hypothesis was criticized in 2 major ways.[11] First, the diagnosis of alcoholism was based on multivariate analysis of registry data, rather than conventional diagnostic criteria for alcoholism based on direct interviews.[12,13] Nevertheless, later clinical studies that used interviews confirmed the validity of the distinction by means of standard diagnostic criteria[14-17] and showed its utility for prediction of individual differences in clinical course,[18] response to treatment,[19] personality,[15,20,21] and neurobiological markers.[21,22]

The second major criticism was that it was implausible, or at least surprising, that qualitatively different types of alcoholics could be distinguished by separating a group of adoptees who were intermediate in severity of alcohol abuse (ie, the type 2 alcoholics with a moderate number of problems) from others who were more extreme in severity (mild type 1 or severe type 1).[11,13] After clinical observations about the relations between registration for problems and clinical diagnosis, the adoptees' alcohol abuse had been divided into subgroups with mild, moderate, and severe problems.[7] An unexpected empirical finding of the Stockholm Adoption Study was that the genetic background of the mild abusers was the same as that of the severe abusers, whereas the moderate abusers had a different genetic background.[1] To explain this unexpected finding, we hypothesized that individuals with a type 1 genetic background, which was characteristic of both mild and severe abusers, were predisposed to progress rapidly from mild to severe alcohol dependence if they continued drinking frequently to relieve anxiety.[21,23] In contrast, we hypothesized, individuals with a type 2 genetic background, which was characteristic of moderate abusers, were predisposed to seek euphoriant stimulation from alcohol, leading to recurrent social problems and only gradual development of severe dependence. Skeptics questioned this hypothesis, but independent clinical studies showed that type 1 alcoholism often progressed rapidly to dependence accompanied by medical complications, such as liver disease. Such progression is characteristic of female alcoholics and male relatives of female alcoholics.[15] The differences between subtypes in course of illness and response to treatment were confirmed in Sweden and the United States.[16-19] Despite this corroborating evidence, the differences in genetic and environmental backgrounds of these groups were questioned as possible artifacts of complex multivariate classification procedures, which always require independent replication before they should be accepted.[11,13]

In this study, we tested the replicability of the original findings and interpretations of the Stockholm Adoption Study by carrying out a strict replication trial. Subjects were selected and classified according to exactly the same procedures as in the original experiment. The findings and conclusions of the original and the replication experiments are presented side by side to facilitate comparison.

Table 1. Inheritance of Susceptibility to Alcohol Abuse in Stockholm and Replication Adoption Studies

Alcohol Abuse in Biological Parents		Alcohol Abuse in Adoptees, No. (%)	
Father	Mother	Stockholm	Replication
		Adopted Men	
No	No	571 (14.7)	409 (12.0)
Yes	No	259 (22.4)*	78 (23.1)*
No	Yes	23 (26.0)*	22 (31.8)*
Yes	Yes	9 (33.3)*	8 (12.5)*
		Adopted Women	
No	No	577 (2.8)	546 (1.1)
Yes	No	285 (3.5)	106 (0.9)
No	Yes	29 (10.3)†	7 (0.0)
Yes	Yes	22 (9.1)†	1 (0.0)

**Sons with alcoholic biological parents were more likely than others to abuse alcohol in the Stockholm study (odds ratio, 1.7; 95% confidence interval, 1.2-2.5) and in the replication study (odds ratio, 2.2; 95% confidence interval, 1.3-3.6).*

†Daughters with alcoholic biological mothers were more likely than others to abuse alcohol in the Stockholm study (9.8% vs 2.8%; P<.01).

RESULTS

The relationship between any lifetime alcohol abuse in the biological parents and their adopted-away sons is shown in **Table 1** for the original Stockholm study and for the replication sample. According to the Stockholm study, the 291 sons with alcoholic biological parents were more likely than the 571 others to abuse alcohol (23.0% vs 14.7%; OR, 1.7; 95% CI, 1.2-2.5). This prediction was confirmed in the replication sample. The 108 adopted-away sons with at least 1 alcoholic parent had a higher risk of alcohol abuse (24.1%) than the 469 other sons (12.8%), giving an OR in men of 2.2 (95% CI, 1.3-3.6).

The inheritance of lifetime alcohol abuse was also examined in the 660 adopted-away daughters (Table 1). In the Stockholm study, alcohol abuse in only the biological father did not increase the risk of alcohol abuse in the 285 adopted-away daughters compared with the risk in daughters of parents with no abuse (3.5% vs 2.8%). This prediction was confirmed in the replication sample: the 106 adopted-away daughters of alcoholic fathers had no increased risk of alcohol abuse compared with the daughters of 2 nonabusing parents (0.9% vs 1.1%). Furthermore, in the Stockholm study, the daughters of alcoholic mothers were more likely than other daughters to abuse alcohol (9.8% vs 2.8%; $P<.01$). There were too few such daughters (n=8) to test this prediction in the replication sample.

In the Stockholm study, the 99 sons with a type 2 genetic background were more likely to have type 2 abuse than the 763 others (17.2% vs 2.5%; OR, 8.1; 95% CI, 4.1-16.2) but not type 1 abuse (12.1% vs 13.5%; OR, 0.9; 95% CI, 0.5-1.7). Both of these predictions were con-

Table 2. Confirmatory Cross-Fostering Analysis: Risk of Type 2 Alcohol Abuse in 577 Men From Replication Study Classified According to Stockholm Study Discriminant Functions

Type 2 Genetic Background	Type 2 Environmental Background	Stockholm Men			Replication Men		
		No.	% Type 1	% Type 2	No.	% Type 1	% Type 2
No	No	567	14.4	1.9	333	11.4	2.4
No	Yes	196	10.7	4.1	160	10.6	1.3
Yes	No	71	9.9	16.9*	59	16.9	6.8*
Yes	Yes	28	17.9	17.9*	25	8.0	20.0*

Sons with type 2 genetic background were more likely to be type 2 abusers than others in the Stockholm calibration sample (odds ratio, 8.1; 95% confidence interval, 4.1-16.2) and in the replication sample (odds ratio, 5.8; 95% confidence interval, 2.3-14.7).

Table 3. Confirmatory Cross-Fostering Analysis: Severe Type 1 Alcohol Abuse in 577 Men From Replication Study Classified According to Stockholm Study Discriminant Functions

Type 1 Genetic Background	Severe Environmental Background	Stockholm Men		Replication Men	
		No.	% Severe	No.	% Severe
No	No	376	4.3	363	3.0
No	Yes	72	4.2	44	2.3
Yes	No	328	6.7	135	3.0
Yes	Yes	86	11.6*	35	11.4*

Risk was significantly increased compared with all others in the Stockholm study (odds ratio, 2.4; 95% confidence interval, 1.1-4.9) and in the replication study (odds ratio, 4.2; 95% confidence interval, 1.3-13.5).

Table 4. Confirmatory Cross-Fostering Analysis: Mild Type 1 Alcohol Abuse in 577 Men From Replication Study Classified According to Stockholm Study Discriminant Functions

Type 1 Genetic Background	Mild Environmental Background	Stockholm Men		Replication Men	
		No.	% Mild	No.	% Mild
No	No	341	6.7	295	7.8
No	Yes	107	5.6	112	9.8
Yes	No	323	6.5	121	7.4
Yes	Yes	91	15.4*	49	8.2†

Risk was significantly increased compared with all others in the Stockholm study (15.4% vs 6.5%; P<.01), but not in the replication study (8.2% vs 8.1%).

†Risk was not increased compared with all others in the replication study (8.2% vs 8.1%).

firmed in the replication sample (**Table 2**). The 84 adopted sons with a type 2 genetic background were more often type 2 abusers than were the 493 others (10.7% vs 2.0%; OR, 5.8; 95% CI, 2.3-14.7). Likewise, the sons with a type 2 genetic background in the replication sample had no excess of type 1 alcoholism (14.3% vs 11.2%; OR, 1.3; 95% CI, 0.7-2.6).

In the Stockholm study, the adopted-away sons were at increased risk for severe type 1 alcoholism only if they had *both* a type 1 genetic background and a severe environmental background (**Table 3**). In the Stockholm study, the risk was significantly increased in those with both genetic and environmental risk compared with all others (11.6% vs 5.3%; OR, 2.4; 95% CI, 1.1-4.9). This prediction was confirmed in the replication study. The risk of severe type 1 alcoholism was increased in the 35 adopted-away men with both genetic and environmental risk factors compared with all others (11.4% vs 3.0%; OR, 4.2; 95% CI, 1.3-13.5).

Likewise, in the Stockholm study, the adopted sons were at increased risk for mild type 1 alcoholism only if they had both a type 1 genetic background and a mild environmental background (**Table 4**). The risk of mild abuse was significantly increased in those with both genetic and environmental risk compared with all others in the Stockholm study (15.4% vs 6.5%; *P*<.01). However, this prediction was *not* confirmed in the replication study. There was no increased risk of mild abuse in the 49 adopted-away men predicted to have both the type 1 genetic background and mild environmental risk based on the Stockholm classification functions (8.2% vs 8.1%).

To understand this discrepancy, the risk of mild type 1, severe type 1, and type 2 alcoholism was examined in detail in those predicted to have a type 1 genetic background according to the Stockholm classification functions. **Table 5** shows that there was the predicted increase in severe type 1 alcoholism and the predicted lack of differences in the risk of type 2 alcoholism. Nevertheless, there was no increase in mild abuse regardless of genetic or environmental background in the replication sample with the use of the original Stockholm classification functions.

This discrepancy might be explained by possible unreliable detection of mild type 1 abuse, which was defined by a single Temperance Board registration. Alternatively, men with type 1 genetic backgrounds in the replication sample may have been influenced by other genetic or environmental factors, leading to severe abuse. To test these possibilities, an exploratory cross-fostering analysis was carried out to identify the genetic and environmental factors that might predict mild type 1 alcoholism in the replication sample. In other words, the weights of the possible explanatory variables were optimized in the replication sample, rather than using the weights estimated in the original study in Stockholm. The classification based on only the replication sample is summarized in **Table 6**. This showed that the measured variables about the

Table 5. Confirmatory Cross-Fostering Analysis: Mild and Severe Type 1 Alcohol Abuse in 577 Men From Replication Study Classified According to Stockholm Study Discriminant Functions

Type 1 Genetic Background	Mild or Severe Environmental Background	Male Adoptees Observed			
		No.	% Mild	% Severe	% Type 2
No	No	251	6.8	2.8	3.6
No	Mild	112	9.8	3.6	4.5
No	Severe	44	13.6	2.3	2.3
Yes	No	86	9.3	1.2	2.3
Yes	Mild	49	8.2	6.1	2.0
Yes	Severe	35	2.9	11.4*	2.9

*The 35 men with both genetic and environmental backgrounds were more often severe type 1 abusers than others were.

Table 6. Exploratory Cross-Fostering Analysis: Mild Type 1 Alcohol Abuse in 577 Men From Replication Study

Type 1 Genetic Background	Mild Environmental Background	Male Adoptees Observed	
		a/N*	% Mild Abuse
No	No	41/509	8.1
No	Yes	2/22	9.1
Yes	No	4/45	8.8
Yes	Yes	0/1	0.0

*a denotes number of abusers; N, total number at risk.

biological and adoptive parents were not predictive of mild abuse in the adopted children, even when they were optimized in the replication sample itself. Essentially, those with a type 1 genetic background in the replication sample were mainly at risk for severe, but not mild, alcoholism.

Besides the type 1 genetic background, the only variable associated with severe abuse in the Stockholm Adoption Study was low occupational status in the adoptive father. In the Stockholm sample, the occupational status of the biological fathers of the type 1 alcoholics did not differ from that of the biological fathers of nonalcoholics. However, among the 46 men with a type 1 genetic background in the replication study, 36 also had at least 1 father (biological and/or adoptive) who was an unskilled laborer (**Table 7**). This difference is noteworthy because the occupational status of adult adoptees was equally correlated with that of their biological father and of their adoptive father ($r=0.12$, $P<.01$), both in the Stockholm study and in the replication study. The confounding of predisposition to both type 1 alcoholism and low occupational status in the replication sample may account for the adopted men with a type 1 genetic background in the replication sample having an increased risk for severe, but not mild, alcoholism.

COMMENT

This is the first time that the distinction between genetic subtypes of any psychiatric disorder has been validated by a strict confirmatory test of an explicit multivariate classification procedure. Specifically, this replication study confirms that type 1 and type 2 alcoholism are clinically distinct forms of alcoholism that are inherited as a consequence of independent processes. In our replication study of adoptees, the original conclusions of the Stockholm Adoption Study[1] about type 2 alcoholism and severe type 1 alcoholism were confirmed. Both type 2 alcoholism and severe type 1 alcoholism [illegible] adoptees. Severe alcoholism was shown to result from the combination of a type 1 genetic background and factors predisposing to unskilled occupational status. Neither low social status nor a type 1 genetic background alone was sufficient to cause alcoholism. Other conclusions of the Stockholm Adoption Study about the inheritance of alcoholism in women and mild alcoholism in men could not be tested because of inadequate numbers of subjects with relevant predisposing factors.

There was no excess of type 2 alcoholism in adopted children with type 1 backgrounds, or vice versa, in either the original Stockholm study or this replication study. However, this independence does not mean that type 1 and type 2 alcoholism are discrete and separate diseases. Although there was no *increase* in the risk of type 1 alcoholism in those with backgrounds characteristic of type 2, neither was there a *decrease* in its risk. In fact, given the substantial risk of type 1 alcoholism in the general population, both alcoholic subtypes are expected to occur often in the same families, as shown in Tables 2 and 5.

In this replication study, mild alcohol abuse was not predictably increased in the adopted men regardless of their genetic or environmental backgrounds. The simplest explanation would be that mild alcohol abuse, which is defined by single registrations by the Temperance Board, is not reliably measured or consistently heritable. This is supported by exploratory cross-fostering analysis in the replication sample (Table 6) showing that mild abuse was not significantly predicted by measured information about the biological or adoptive parents, even when variable weights were optimized in the replication sample itself. However, mild abuse was significantly heritable in the adoptees born in Stockholm, who also had a higher prevalence of type 1 alcoholism in their biological parents than adoptees born in Gothenburg. Alternatively, the adopted men with type 1 genetic backgrounds in Gothenburg may have also inherited other characteristics that predisposed them to an increased severity of alcoholism. For example, there are suggestions (see Table 7) in the Gothenburg replication sample that men with a type 1 genetic background were more likely to be lacking in heritable capacity and/or socially mediated opportunities for [illegible] Stockholm sample.

In any case, recurrent type 1 or recurrent type 2 alcohol abuse in biological parents was predictive of

Table 7. Interaction of Type 1 Genetic Background With Unskilled Occupational Status of Biological and Adoptive Parents and Risk of Severe Type 1 Abuse in Replication Study

Type 1 Genetic Background	Unskilled Genetic Background	Unskilled Environmental Background	Male Adoptees Observed a/N*		% Severe
No	No	No	5/199		2.5
No	Yes	No	3/197	8/332	2.4
No	No	Yes	1/53		
No	Yes	Yes	4/82		
Yes	No	No	0/10		0.0
Yes	Yes	No	4/19	7/36	19.4†
Yes	No	Yes	1/3		
Yes	Yes	Yes	2/14		

**a denotes number of abusers; N, total number at risk.*

†The 36 sons with type 1 alcoholic background who also had biological and/or adoptive parents who were unskilled workers were more likely to be severe alcoholics than others were (odds ratio, 9.8; 95% confidence interval, 3.6-26.4).

recurrent alcohol abuse of the same type in their adopted-away sons in both the Stockholm and Gothenburg samples. The replication findings strongly demonstrate that type 1 and type 2 alcoholism are influenced by independent, but not mutually exclusive, processes. If type 1 and type 2 alcoholism are not separate diseases, what is meant by our conclusion that they are clinically distinct forms of alcoholism caused by independent neuroadaptive processes? Elsewhere we have shown that the initiation, maintenance, and cessation of drinking and smoking have different causal antecedents. The initiation of drinking at an early age is associated with the heritable temperament traits of high novelty seeking, low harm avoidance, and low reward dependence.[21,26,27] This configuration of temperaments is characteristic of the antisocial temperament type,[28] which is associated with increased risk of type 2 alcoholism,[26] early conduct disorder,[29,30] and adolescent multiple-substance abuse.[31] Such individuals begin and continue drinking alcohol for its euphoriant effects.[18] In contrast, high harm avoidance inhibits the initiation of drinking but increases the risk of becoming dependent after heavy drinking has become frequent.[27] Such individuals with high harm avoidance usually drink alcohol for relief of anxiety, as is characteristic of type 1 alcoholics.

These temperament dimensions have been shown to be independently inherited.[32-34] Accordingly, it was expected and confirmed that all possible combinations of temperament dimensions occur,[28,35,36] providing extensive heterogeneity in the emotional predisposition for drinking and other activities.[27] Harm avoidance and novelty seeking appear to have predominant roles in predisposing to type 1 and type 2 alcoholism, respectively, but interact with other aspects of temperament, character, and the environment in the development of alcoholism and related psychopathology.[37,38] The psychobiology of personality in relation to alcoholic subtypes has been reviewed elsewhere.[39,40]

Some limitations of this study should be considered. Gothenburg is second to Stockholm in population size and was the most comparable available site for a replication study. Nevertheless, less registered alcohol abuse in the biological parents was identified in Gothenburg than in Stockholm, as shown in Table 1. In particular, type 1 alcoholism was much less frequent in parents in Gothenburg (29%) than in those in Stockholm (48%) (Table 4). Also, the adopted women from Gothenburg were more often reared in areas with less alcohol abuse regardless of genetic background than were the women from Stockholm (Table 1). Fortunately, cross-fostering analysis stratifies both the genetic and environmental risk factors so that such differences are taken into account. Cross-fostering analysis minimizes the impact of such distributional differences or selective placement on the observed pattern of inheritance. The replicability of our findings in men encourages future use of multivariate cross-fostering analysis. However, there were too few alcoholic mothers and adopted women in the Gothenburg sample to allow tests of the replicability of findings from the Stockholm Adoption Study about maternal inheritance of alcoholism in women,[4] but the heritability of alcoholism in women has been confirmed in female twins in the United States.[41,42]

In summary, the distinction between type 1 and type 2 alcoholism in Swedish adoptees is replicable. Similar evidence of genetic heterogeneity has also been demonstrated in male and female twins in the United States.[42] Our adoption data indicate that the subtypes are clinical manifestations of independent but not mutually exclusive etiological processes. The relief of anxiety and activation of euphoria are complementary neuroadaptive mechanisms that can each promote the development of alcoholism. The differences in age at onset, symptoms, course, and mode of inheritance of type 1 and type 2 forms of alcoholism can be well explained in terms of the interactions of individual experiences with the heritable dimensions of personality.

Accepted for publication February 13, 1996.

This study was supported in part by the Swedish Medical Research Council and by grants AA-7982 and AA-8028 from the National Institute on Alcoholism and Alcohol Abuse and grants MH-31302 and MH-46276 from the National Institute of Mental Health, National Institutes of Health, Bethesda, Md.

We thank Tordh Ohlsson for assistance in data management and Thomas R. Przybeck, PhD, for assistance in statistical analysis.

Reprints: C. Robert Cloninger, MD, 4940 Children's Pl, St Louis, MO 63110.

REFERENCES

1. Cloninger CR, Bohman M, Sigvardsson S. Inheritance of alcohol abuse: cross-fostering analysis of adopted men. *Arch Gen Psychiatry.* 1981;38:861-868.
2. Bohman M, Sigvardsson S, Cloninger CR. Maternal inheritance of alcohol abuse: cross-fostering analysis of adopted women. *Arch Gen Psychiatry.* 1981;38:965-969.
3. Cloninger CR, Bohman M, Sigvardsson S, von Knorring A-L. Psychopathology in adopted-out children of alcoholics: the Stockholm Adoption Study. *Recent*

Dev Alcohol. 1985;3:37-51.
4. Bohman M, Cloninger CR, von Knorring A-L, Sigvardsson S. An adoption study of somatoform disorders, III: cross-fostering analysis and genetic relationship to alcoholism and criminality. *Arch Gen Psychiatry.* 1984;41:872-878.
5. Roe A, Burks B. Adult adjustment of foster children of alcoholic and psychotic parentage and the influence of the foster home. In: *Memoirs of the Section on Alcohol Studies.* New Haven, Conn: Yale University; 1945.
6. Goodwin DW, Schulsinger F, Moeller N, Hermansen L, Winokur, G, Guze SB. Drinking problems in adopted and non-adopted sons of alcoholics. *Arch Gen Psychiatry.* 1974;31:164-169.
7. Kaij L. *Alcoholism in Twins: Studies on the Etiology and Sequels of Abuse of Alcohol.* Stockholm, Sweden: Almqvist & Wiksell; 1960.
8. Kaij L. Biases in a Swedish social register of alcoholics. *Soc Psychiatry.* 1970; 5:216-218.
9. Ojesjo L. Prevalence of known and hidden alcoholism in the revisited Lundby population. *Soc Psychiatry.* 1980;15:81-90.
10. Committee on Nomenclature and Statistics, American Psychiatric Association. *Diagnostic and Statistical Manual of Mental Disorders, Third Edition.* Washington, DC: American Psychiatric Association; 1980.
11. Searles JS. The role of genetics in the pathogenesis of alcoholism. *J Abnorm Psychol.* 1988;97:153-167.
12. Murray RM, Clifford CA, Gurling HMD. Twin and adoption studies: how good is the evidence for a genetic role? *Recent Dev Alcohol.* 1983;1:25-48.
13. Littrell J. The Swedish studies of the adopted children of alcoholics. *J Stud Alcohol.* 1988;49:491-515.
14. Gilligan SB, Reich T, Cloninger CR. Etiologic heterogeneity in alcoholism. *Genet Epidemiol.* 1987;4:395-414.
15. Gilligan SB, Reich T, Cloninger CR. Alcohol-related symptoms in heterogeneous families of hospitalized alcoholics. *Alcohol Clin Exp Res.* 1988;12: 671-678.
16. Cloninger CR, Sigvardsson S, von Knorring A-L, Bohman M. The Swedish studies of the adopted children of alcoholics: reply to Littrell. *J Stud Alcohol.* 1988; 49:516-521.
17. Babor TF, Hofmann M, DelBoca FK, Hesselbrock V, Meyer RE, Dolinsky ZS, Rounsaville B. Types of alcoholics, I: evidence for an empirically derived typology based on indicators of vulnerability and severity. *Arch Gen Psychiatry.* 1992;49:599-608.
18. Nordstrom G, Berglund M. Different patterns of successful long-term adjustment in genetically defined subtypes of alcoholics. *Alcohol Alcohol.* 1987; suppl 1:401-405.
19. Litt MD, Babor TF, DelBoca FK, Kadden RM, Cooney NL. Types of alcoholics, II: application of an empirically derived typology to treatment matching. *Arch Gen Psychiatry.* 1992;49:609-614.
20. Von Knorring L, von Knorring A-L, Smigan L, Lindberg U, Edholm M. Personality traits in subtypes of alcoholics. *J Stud Alcohol.* 1987;48:523-527.
21. Cloninger CR. Neurogenetic adaptive mechanisms in alcoholism. *Science.* 1987; 236:410-416.
22. Von Knorring A-L, Bohman M, von Knorring L. Oreland L. Platelet MAO activity as a biological marker in subgroups of alcoholism. *Acta Psychiatr Scand.* 1987;72:51-58.
23. Sigvardsson S. *Alcohol Abuse and Criminality: A Cross-fostering Study of Gene-Environment Interaction.* Umeå, Sweden: Umeå University; 1982. Dissertation.
24. SPSS Inc. *Statistical Package for the Social Sciences for Personal Computers (SPSS/PC): Version 4.0.* Chicago, Ill: SPSS Inc; 1989.
25. SAS Institute Inc. *SAS Technical Report P-229, SAS/STAT Software: Changes and Enhancements, Release 6.07.* Cary, NC: SAS Institute Inc; 1992.
26. Cloninger CR, Sigvardsson S, Bohman M (1988). Childhood personality predicts alcohol abuse in young adults. *Alcohol Clin Exp Res.* 1988;12:494-505.
27. Cloninger CR, Sigvardsson S, Przybeck TR, Svrakic DM. Personality antecedents of alcoholism in a national area probability sample. *Eur Arch Psychiatry Clin Neurosci.* 1995;245:239-244.
28. Cloninger CR. A systematic method for clinical description and classification of personality variants. *Arch Gen Psychiatry.* 1987;44:573-588.
29. Sigvardsson S, Bohman M, Cloninger CR. Structure and stability of childhood personality: prediction of later social adjustment. *J Child Psychol Psychiatry.* 1987;38:929-946.
30. Tremblay RE, Pihl RO, Vitaro F, Dobkin PL. Predicting early onset of male antisocial behavior from preschool behavior. *Arch Gen Psychiatry.* 1994;54:732-739.
31. Wills TA, Vaccaro D, McNamara G. Novelty seeking, risk taking, and related constructs as predictors of adolescent substance use: an application of Cloninger's theory. *J Subst Abuse.* 1994;6:1-20.
32. Heath AC, Cloninger CR, Martin NG. Testing a model for the genetic structure of personality: a comparison of the personality systems of Cloninger and Eysenck. *J Pers Soc Psychol.* 1994;66:762-775.
33. Svrakic NM, Svrakic DM, Cloninger CR. A general quantitative theory of personality: fundamentals of a self-organizing psychobiological complex. *Dev Psychopathol.* 1996;8:247-272.
34. Stallings MC, Hewitt JK, Cloninger CR, Heath AC, Eaves LJ. Genetic and environmental structure of the Tridimensional Personality Questionnaire: three or four primary temperament dimensions? *J Pers Soc Psychol.* In press.
35. Cloninger CR, Przybeck TR, Svrakic DM. The Tridimensional Personality Questionnaire: U.S. normative data. *Psychol Rep.* 1991;69:1047-1057.
36. Svrakic DM, Whitehead C, Przybeck TR, Cloninger CR. Differential diagnosis of personality disorders by the seven-factor model of temperament and character. *Arch Gen Psychiatry.* 1993;50:991-999.
37. Cloninger CR. A unified biosocial theory of personality and its role in the development of anxiety states. *Psychiatr Dev.* 1986;3:167-226.
38. Cloninger CR, Svrakic DM, Przybeck TR. A psychobiological model of temperament and character. *Arch Gen Psychiatry.* 1993;50:975-989.
39. Cloninger CR. The psychobiology of social cooperation. *Nat Med.* 1995;1:623-625.
40. Cloninger CR, Adolfsson R, Svrakic NM. Mapping genes for human personality. *Nat Genet.* 1996;12:3-4.
41. Pickens RW, Svikis DS, McGue M, Lykken DT, Heston LL, Clayton PJ. Heterogeneity in the inheritance of alcoholism: a study of male and female twins. *Arch Gen Psychiatry.* 1991;48:19-28.
42. Kendler KS, Neale M, Heath AC, Kessler RC, Eaves LJ. A twin-family study of alcoholism in women. *Am J Psychiatry.* 1994;151:707-715.

ORIGINAL ARTICLE

Familial Transmission of Substance Use Disorders

Kathleen R. Merikangas, PhD; Marilyn Stolar, MA; Denise E. Stevens, PhD; Joseph Goulet, MS; Martin A. Preisig, MD; Brenda Fenton, PhD; Heping Zhang, PhD; Stephanie S. O'Malley, PhD; Bruce J. Rounsaville, MD

Background: There is increasing evidence that substance use disorders are familial and that genetic factors explain a substantial degree of their familial aggregation. To perform a controlled family study of probands with several different predominant drugs of abuse, including opioids, cocaine, cannabis, and/or alcohol.

Methods: The subjects for the present study included 231 probands with dependence on opioids, cocaine, cannabis, and/or alcohol and 61 control probands, and their 1267 adult first-degree relatives. Diagnostic estimates were based on semistructured diagnostic interviews and/or structured family history interviews regarding each proband, spouse, and adult first-degree relative. The interview data were reviewed blindly and independently by clinicians with extensive experience in the evaluation and treatment of substance use disorders.

Results: There was an 8-fold increased risk of drug disorders among the relatives of probands with drug disorders across a wide range of specific substances, including opioids, cocaine, cannabis, and alcohol, which is largely independent from the familial aggregation of both alcoholism and antisocial personality disorder. There was also evidence of specificity of familial aggregation of the predominant drug of abuse.

Conclusions: Elevation in risk of this magnitude places a family history of drug disorder as one of the most potent risk factors for the development of drug disorders. These results suggest that there may be risk factors that are specific to particular classes of drugs as well as risk factors that underlie substance disorders in general.

Arch Gen Psychiatry. 1998;55:973-979

THE FAMILIAL aggregation of alcoholism has been well established.[1,2] Although the results of numerous studies suggest that drug abuse is familial, there is a lack of adequate evidence from studies that use contemporary family study methods, including comparable control probands and direct interviews of relatives, in investigating the familial patterns of drug abuse.[3-14]

See also pages 964, 967, and 982

Although most twin studies of substance abuse have focused on alcoholism, an increasing number have investigated twin concordance for drug use and abuse.[9-11,15-19] In fact, several studies have found greater levels of heritability for drug abuse than for alcoholism.[18] Studies of twin registries have demonstrated the importance of genetic factors in both the quantity and frequency of use and degree of abuse of specific drugs, including nicotine, caffeine, tranquilizers, and sedatives.[9-11,18] Results of a recent large-scale twin study of male Vietnam-era veterans suggest that substance abuse is highly heritable, and that the contribution of genetic factors is more significant for frequent use or abuse than for nonproblematic use.[17] Of particular interest was the finding that the subjective effects of marijuana, including suspiciousness and agitation, are also under genetic control.[19] Likewise, the classic adoption studies of Cadoret et al[20-23] provide further evidence of the importance of the role of genetic factors in the development of drug disorders, with a far greater impact on the transition from drug use to abuse than on drug use itself.

The present study was designed to investigate the familial aggregation of drug and alcohol disorders across a broad range of drugs, including opioids, cocaine, mari-

From the Departments of Epidemiology and Public Health (Drs Merikangas, Stevens, and Zhang, Ms Stolar, and Mr Goulet) and Psychiatry (Drs Merikangas, O'Malley, and Rounsaville), Yale University School of Medicine, New Haven, Conn; Department of Psychiatry, University of Lausanne, Lausanne, Switzerland (Dr Preisig); and Department of Psychiatry, University of Geneva, Geneva, Switzerland (Dr Fenton).

This article is also available on our Web site: www.ama-assn.org/psych.

SUBJECTS AND METHODS

SAMPLE CHARACTERISTICS

Probands

The sample of 299 probands was composed of a total of 149 probands with drug dependence (87 probands with opioid, 27 probands with cocaine, and 35 probands with cannabis dependence) and 89 probands with alcohol dependence, recruited from outpatient specialty clinics for substance disorders, and 61 control probands with no evidence of a lifetime history of any diagnosis in *DSM-III-R*.[24] The controls were recruited through a random-digit dialing procedure in the greater New Haven, Conn, area. Study criteria were presented in detail by Merikangas et al.[25]

Relatives

There were a total of 1267 first-degree relatives, primarily composed of parents and siblings (42% parents, 51% siblings, and 7% offspring). Overall, 57% of the relatives of probands who met study criteria were interviewed directly, either in person or by telephone (approximately 25% of the total number of relatives). Twenty percent of the first-degree relatives who refused direct interviews were assessed via informant reports. The interview rates did not significantly differ by proband diagnostic group and are in accordance with previous family studies of substance abuse.[3,4,13]

OVERVIEW OF PROCEDURES

The procedures of the current study included the following: (1) interviewers with experience in substance abuse or clinical psychiatry interviewed relatives blindly with respect to the disorder of the index family member; (2) direct semistructured diagnostic interviews were applied, with expanded information on the correlates and course of patterns of drug use, particularly with respect to polysubstance use and abuse; (3) semistructured informant interviews were used, with expanded sections on substance abuse to obtain family history information; and (4) standardized diagnostic criteria based on information from both clinical material and informant reports were used in conjunction with the direct interview to assess diagnostic criteria for substance disorders and other psychiatric disorders (ie, best-estimate diagnoses).

Diagnostic Interview

The diagnostic interview for adults was the semistructured Schedule for Affective Disorders and Schizophrenia, current and lifetime versions,[26] modified to obtain *DSM-III*[27] and *DSM-III-R*[24] criteria. With respect to substance abuse, the interview was modified to obtain more detailed information on the patterns of use of each drug class and their interrelationship, and on the course of alcohol and drug use and abuse.

Kappas derived from joint ratings of individual interviews were generally quite high for substance abuse (0.72-0.94) and somewhat lower for anxiety or affective disorders (0.54-0.78) across the first 3 series of training sessions. Comparison of diagnoses obtained through direct face-to-face interview and those from telephone interviews in both the present study and previous studies[28-31] showed high levels of agreement across all diagnostic categories.

Family History Information

Family history information was obtained by means of a modified version of the Family History–Research Diagnostic Criteria developed by Andreasen et al[32] for data collected by the family history method designed to obtain both *DSM-III* and *DSM-III-R* diagnoses in adults and children. The family history interview was modified to obtain more extensive information on patterns and sequelae of drug and alcohol use as well as extent of knowledge by the informant about the index subject.

Diagnostic Procedures

The probands were assigned to the 5 lifetime diagnostic substance disorder groups based on the predominant type of substance disorder through a blind and independent review by clinicians with extensive experience in the evaluation and treatment of substance abuse (K.R.M., S.S.O., B.J.R.). The predominant substance of abuse of probands and relatives was determined through a review of the following information on the life chart of substance use based on the diagnostic interview, treatment records where relevant, and family history information: age at onset, order of onset, quantity, frequency, chronicity, substance of choice, number of symptoms, and severity.

Statistical Analysis

To assess the demographic homogeneity of the proband groups and their relatives, χ^2 tests for contingency tables with discrete demographic variables and 1-way analyses of variance for continuous measures were applied.

To account for familial clustering, mixed-effects multinomial logistic regression models were run with a program called MIXNO.[33] MIXNO provides maximum marginal likelihood estimates of parameters for mixed-effects logistic regression of correlated nominal response data. In the present analyses, mixed-effects multinomial logistic regression models were used to investigate the association between (1) a 3-level substance disorder diagnosis variable (drug dependence ± alcohol dependence; alcohol dependence only; neither) in probands and relatives and (2) a 4-level predominant drug disorder variable (opioid, cocaine, cannabis, none) in probands (independent variable) and relatives (dependent variable), while adjusting for model covariates and correlated within family observations across all outcomes.

juana, and alcohol. Specifically, we examined the following patterns of familial associations: (1) the association between substance disorders in probands and relatives (ie, familial aggregation); (2) the association between drug disorders in probands and alcoholism in relatives and vice versa (ie, independence); and (3) the association between the predominant drug disorder in probands and relatives (ie, specificity).

Table 1. Demographic Distribution of Probands and Relatives

	Predominant Drug Disorder in Probands					Test for Homogeneity of Percentages or Means, *P*
	Opioid (n = 87)	Cocaine (n = 27)	Cannabis (n = 35)	Alcohol (n = 89)	Controls (n = 61)	
Probands (n = 299)						
Sex, % male	37	41	60	71	43	χ^2_4 = 24.966, <.001
Mean ± SD age, y	35.3 ± 5.3*	34.1 ± 5.1*	35.9 ± 4.2*	40.4 ± 6.7	40.8 ± 5.9	$F_{4,294}$ = 16.20, <.001
Socioeconomic status, Hollingshead Score >III, %	82	77	01	53	25	χ^2_4 = 40.211, <.001
Marital status, married or remarried, %	39	44	63	60	97	χ^2_4 = 53.071, <.001
Relatives (n = 1267)						
No.	332	94	178	408	255	
Sex, % male	49	50	50	51	49	χ^2_4 = 0.225, .99
Mean ± SD age, y	49.2 ± 17.3	50.1 ± 17.4	45.8 ± 15.8*	49.0 ± 17.3	50.1 ± 18.7	$F_{4,1262}$ = 1.81, .13

*Dunnett *t* test, df = 1; adjusted *P*<.05 for significant difference from controls.

RESULTS

DEMOGRAPHIC AND CLINICAL CHARACTERISTICS OF PROBANDS AND RELATIVES

Demographic characteristics of probands and relatives are presented in **Table 1**. Although the sex and age composition of the drug-abusing probands differed from that of the controls, there were no statistically significant differences in the age and sex distribution of the relatives.

There were no significant differences in the mean number of relatives of probands when compared with controls (ie, 4.5 relatives per proband). Of the 1267 first-degree biological relatives, 42% were parents, 51% were siblings, and 7% were offspring older than 18 years.

FAMILIAL AGGREGATION OF ALCOHOLISM AND DRUG DISORDERS

The familial aggregation of alcoholism and drug disorders is presented in **Table 2** and **Table 3**. Table 2 presents the proportions of substance use disorders across broad categories of drugs, including "hard" drugs (ie, opioids, cocaine, stimulants, hallucinogens, or inhalants), "soft" drugs (ie, cannabis, sedatives, benzodiazepines, or barbiturates), alcohol, and nicotine among relatives by the predominant drug disorder of probands. Rates of hard drug disorders increased according to the deviance of the predominant drug among probands. Rates of abuse or dependence on hard drugs were greatest among the relatives of probands with opioid disorders (14.5%), moderately elevated among relatives with cocaine or cannabis disorders (9.6% or 8.4%, respectively), and lowest among relatives of probands with alcoholism (4.4%) when compared with relatives of controls (1.2%). In contrast, rates of alcoholism were increased only among the relatives of probands with cannabis or alcohol dependence compared with those of either the opioid or cocaine groups or the controls. Finally, rates of nicotine dependence were elevated among the relatives of all of the substance use disorder proband groups compared with those of controls. Approximately two thirds of the relatives reported a history of dependence on nicotine.

Table 3 presents the proportions of relatives with drug and/or alcohol disorders according to the presence or absence of drug and alcohol disorders in probands. The main effects of the familial aggregation of all alcoholism and drug disorders were highly significant: the relatives of probands with drug disorders had a 4.5-fold greater rate of drug disorders themselves than relatives of controls. Likewise, relatives of probands with alcohol disorders had a 2.0-fold greater rate of alcohol disorders than relatives of controls.

Statistically significant pairwise differences of proportions and their respective SEs, *z* scores, and *P* values are shown in the footnotes to Table 3. The proportions of relatives with both drug and alcohol disorders did not differ between those of probands with pure drug disorders (8.1%) and relatives of probands with comorbid drug disorders and alcohol disorders (9.1%) The lack of differences between rates of drug disorders among relatives of probands with comorbid drug disorders and alcoholism compared with relatives of probands with drug disorders only suggests that alcoholism and drug disorders are independent and that comorbidity is not an indicator of severity of substance disorders in probands.

Likewise, no significant evidence of coaggregation of pure forms of alcoholism and drug disorders emerged. Rates of pure drug disorders were increased among relatives of probands with pure drug disorders when compared with those of probands with alcohol only (*P* = .003); conversely, rates of pure alcoholism in the relatives were significantly elevated among relatives of probands with alcoholism only vs those with drug-only diagnoses (*P*<.001). Because similar patterns of familial aggregation of substance disorders emerged among relatives of probands in the drug and alcoholism group vs those in the drug-only group (see Table 3), these groups were collapsed in subsequent analyses.

Table 4 examines the association between drug and alcohol disorders in probands and relatives cross-classified according to the presence or absence of drug and alcohol disorders after controlling for demographic and clinical covariates. A mixed-effects generalized logit model, which allows for both adjustment for correlated observations (within families) and the simultaneous investigation of the 3 levels of the outcome variable (drug

Table 2. Proportions of Relatives With Drug Disorders by Predominant Substance in Probands

Proband Drug Disorder	No. of Relatives	Drug Disorders in Relatives, %*				
		"Hard" Drugs†	"Soft" Drugs‡	All Drugs	Alcohol	Nicotine
Opioid	332	14.5	11.5	20.5	14.5	68.1
Cocaine	94	9.6	8.5	14.9	18.1	78.3
Cannabis	178	8.4	18.5	21.3	36.0	60.0
Alcohol	408	4.4	7.1	8.3	35.5	61.2
Controls	255	1.2	3.5	3.5	14.9	44.1
Total	**1267**	7.3	9.2	12.9	24.6	60.7

Categories are not mutually exclusive.
†*Opioids, cocaine, hallucinogens, inhalants.*
‡*Cannabis, sedatives, barbiturates.*

Table 3. Alcoholism and Drug Abuse in Probands and Relatives

Probands	No. of Relatives	Relatives With Drug and Alcohol Disorders, %*			
		Drug and Alcohol†	Drug Only‡	Alcohol Only§	Neither
Drug and alcohol	431	**9.1**	9.1	15.0	66.8
Drug only	173	8.1	**8.7**	6.3	76.9
Alcohol only	408	7.8	2.0	**27.7**	62.5
Control	255	3.1	0.8	11.8	**84.3**

**For the proportion of relatives with the indicated disorders, statistically significant contrasts among proband groups, α = .05;* P *values are not adjusted for multiple comparisons. Boldface cells indicate specificity of concordance between probands and relatives.*
†*Drug and alcohol vs controls, percentage difference (% diff) = 6.0, SE = 1.8, z = 3.36,* P<.001; *alcohol vs controls, % diff = 4.7, SE = 1.7, z = 2.73,* P=.006.
‡*Drug and alcohol vs alcohol only, % diff = 7.1, SE = 1.5, z = 4.60,* P<.001; *drug and alcohol vs controls, % diff = 8.3, SE = 1.5, z = 5.56,* P<.001; *drug only vs alcohol only, % diff = 6.7, SE = 2.2, z = 2.99,* P=.003; *and drug only vs controls, % diff = 7.9, SE = 2.2, z = 3.47,* P<.001.
§*Drug and alcohol vs drug only, % diff = 8.7, SE = 2.5, z = 3.44,* P<.001; *drug and alcohol vs alcohol only, % diff = −12.7, SE = 2.8, z = −4.50,* P<.001; *drug only vs alcohol only, % diff = −21.4, SE = 2.9, z = −7.38,* P<.001; *drug only vs controls, % diff = −5.5, SE = 2.7, z = −1.97,* P=.049; *and alcohol only vs controls, % diff = 15.9, SE = 3.0, z = 5.32,* P<.001.

disorder with or without alcoholism; alcoholism alone; neither) was used. Applying the analyses presented in Table 4 to the subset of directly interviewed relatives yielded similar results. The intraclass correlations for familial clustering derived by the MIXNO program for nominal logistic regression analysis were 0.17 for alcoholism only vs none, and 0.04 for drug with or without alcoholism vs none.

After potential confounders were considered, these results were consistent with those in Table 3; alcoholism and drug disorders aggregated independently in families, since there was no effect modification of the association between drug disorders in probands and relatives by the presence of alcoholism in the proband, nor was the association between alcoholism in probands and relatives modified by the presence of drug disorders in the proband. The strongest association between proband and relatives' drug and/or alcohol disorders emerged for drug disorders with or without alcoholism in relatives of probands with drug disorders (adjusted odds ratio, 7.9). Likewise, there was a significant association between alcoholism only in probands and relatives (adjusted odds ratio, 4.2). Cross comparisons indicated that drug disorders in probands were associated with a significantly *lower* magnitude of alcoholism in relatives than that among relatives of probands with alcoholism only. Finally, there was also a significantly elevated odds ratio of drug disorders (with or without alcoholism) among the relatives of probands with alcoholism compared with those of control probands. Although this would appear to suggest a lack of specificity of the familial aggregation of drug and alcohol disorders, the elevation in this group of relatives was found to be most strongly attributable to comorbid alcohol and drug disorders rather than to drug disorders alone.

FAMILIAL PATTERNS OF SPECIFIC DRUGS

The association between rates of the predominant drug disorder in probands and relatives is shown in **Table 5**. The statistically significant differences in the proportions between the predominant drug disorder in probands and the same predominant drug disorder in relatives are presented in the footnotes to Table 5, along with test statistics and *P* values.

The results in Table 5 show that there was a strong association between the predominant drug disorder in probands and relatives. The rates shown on the diagonal exceed the off-diagonal rates of all of the drug disorders and alcoholism. Inspection of the *P* values of the *z* scores comparing rates of the predominant drug in probands and relatives vs other proband drug groups showed significant levels of specificity for opioids, cannabis, and alcohol, with a weaker trend toward specificity of cocaine. Similar trends emerged when this analysis was applied to the subset of directly interviewed relatives.

Table 6 presents the results of the mixed-effects generalized logit model of the associations between the predominant drug disorders in probands and relatives after controlling for the effects of relevant covariates. The results in Table 6 confirm the findings of a direct associa-

Table 4. Adjusted Odds Ratios of Drugs and Alcohol Disorders in Relatives by Proband Diagnostic Group

	Relatives: Adjusted Odds Ratio (95% Confidence Interval)	
	Drug ± Alcohol	Alcohol Only
Proband group		
Drug ± alcohol vs alcohol only	1.3 (0.9-2.2)	0.3 (0.2-0.6)*
Drug ± alcohol vs controls	7.0 (3.6-17.1)*	1.4 (0.8-2.5)
Alcohol only vs controls	6.0 (2.6-13.1)*	4.2 (2.3-5.7)*
Covariates		
Sex of proband, female vs male	2.0 (1.3-3.2)†	1.4 (0.9-2.1)
Antisocial in proband	0.8 (0.5-1.3)	1.4 (0.8-2.2)
Antisocial in relative	7.6 (4.1-14.0)*	2.4 (0.6-3.4)
Sex of relative, female vs male	0.4 (0.2-0.6)*	0.3 (0.2-0.5)*
Age of relative, <50 y vs >50 y	8.2 (4.8-14.5)*	0.8 (0.5-1.1)
Interview status	3.5 (2.2-5.7)*	1.9 (1.3-3.0)†

*P<.001.
†P<.01.

tion between the predominant drug disorders in probands and relatives reported in Table 5. For each of the specific drugs investigated, the adjusted odds ratio was greatest for the same drug disorder in the relatives (ie, 10.2 for opioids, 4.4 for cocaine, and 5.8 for cannabis) compared with the cross-drug associations. However, the overlapping and wide confidence intervals in the specific vs cross-drug comparisons also suggest that specificity should be considered as a trend rather than a conclusive finding.

COMMENT

The results of the present study show a remarkable degree of familial aggregation of substance abuse. There was an 8-fold increased risk of drug disorders among relatives of probands with drug disorders across a wide range of specific substances, including opioids, cocaine, cannabis, and sedatives, compared with that of relatives of controls. Elevation in risk of this magnitude demonstrates that a family history of drug abuse is one of the most potent risk factors for the development of drug abuse.

The increased risk of both drug disorders and alcoholism in male relatives across all proband groups is in accordance with the sex ratio for these disorders reported in large-scale epidemiological studies.[34,35] The results of the present study confirm those of previous family studies of alcoholism,[36,37] concluding that genetic factors appear to operate similarly in men and women. With respect to drug disorders, however, the small number of female probands in most previous studies has diminished the power to detect sex differences.[37] For example, Pickens et al[16] concluded that the lack of significance of heritability of drug abuse in female twins was attributable to the low number of female pairs, since the magnitude of increase in concordance rates between monozygotic and dizygotic twins was similar in male and female twin pairs. The adoption studies of Cadoret et al[22,23] also demonstrated equivalent genetic pathways underlying substance abuse in males and females. The familial aggregation of drug disorders was greater among relatives of women than men in the present study, suggesting greater familial loading among women. The greater tendency for assortative mating among female than male substance abusers is one possible explanation for this finding.[38]

The familial aggregation of drug disorders was largely independent of that of both alcoholism and antisocial personality disorder, thereby confirming the results of previous family[6,8,13,39] and twin studies that suggest independence of genetic factors predisposing to alcohol and drug disorders.[15-18] In the present study there was no evidence of cross-transmission of drug disorders and alcoholism, nor did the presence of alcoholism modify the association between drug disorders in probands and relatives and vice versa.

The specificity of familial aggregation of the predominant drug disorder, particularly cannabis and alcohol, and to some extent the opioids, was unexpected. Several previous studies have shown a specific association between parental and offspring marijuana and nicotine use.[7,40,41] Even more surprising in these earlier studies was the conclusion that parental and offspring resemblance was not attributable to direct exposure to parental substance use. These findings suggest that there may be some genes or environmental factors that predispose to the use of specific drugs rather than contributing to a deviant pattern of behavior or substance abuse in general.

In addition to some evidence for specificity of familial aggregation of the predominant drug disorder, the results also suggest that alcoholism and the specific drug disorders investigated herein appear to represent a continuum of severity. There was a direct increase in rates of serious drug disorders among relatives with increasing levels of "deviance" of substance disorders in probands ranging from alcoholism (4% drug disorders in relatives) to cannabis (8% in relatives) to cocaine (10% in relatives) to opioid abuse or dependence (15% in relatives) as compared with 1% among control relatives. Therefore, familial factors may be associated with increasing levels of progression along this continuum of severity of substance abuse rather than to the preference for a particular salient substance of abuse.

Familial clustering of drug abuse could be attributable to either common genetic or environmental factors that influence the development of drug disorders. Genetic factors could influence vulnerability to the development of drug abuse through individual differences in the effects of the drugs themselves, including metabolism, sensitivity, tolerance, side effects, and cognitive or psychological effects, or in alteration of affective, emotional, or cognitive states, such as reduction of stress, depression, or anxiety.[42,43]

Families may convey an increased risk of substance disorders through both specific (eg, increasing environmental exposure to drugs or facilitating drug availability[44-46]) and nonspecific (eg, impaired parenting behavior, exposure to marital discord, acute or chronic stress, negative life events, disrupted family structure, social deprivation, and physical, sexual, and emotional abuse) mechanisms.[47-56] However, most of these family factors are not specific to drug disorders, since they also have been shown to characterize families of individuals with alcoholism as well as other psychiatric disorders.

There are several unique aspects of the design and methods of the present study that enhance its contribu-

Table 5. Specific Drug Disorders in Probands and Relatives

Proband Drug Disorder	No. of Relatives	Predominant Drug Disorder in Relatives, %* Opioid†	Cocaine‡	Cannabis§	Alcohol‖	All Drugs
Opioid	332	**10.2**	4.2	6.0	19.9	14.4
Cocaine	94	2.1	**7.5**	5.3	22.3	9.6
Cannabis	178	6.2	2.3	**12.9**	20.2	8.4
Alcohol	408	1.7	2.7	3.9	**28.4**	4.4
Controls	255	0.4	0.8	2.4	11.0	1.2

For the proportion of relatives with the indicated specific drug disorder, statistically significant contrasts among proband groups, $\alpha = .05$; P values are not adjusted for multiple comparisons. Boldface cells indicate specificity of concordance between probands and relatives.

†*Opioid vs cocaine, percentage difference (% diff) = 8.1, SE = 2.2, z = 3.63, P<.001; opioid vs alcohol, % diff = 8.5, SE = 1.8, z = 4.78, P<.001; and opioid vs controls, % diff = 9.8, SE = 1.7, z = 5.76, P<.001.*

‡*Cocaine vs controls, % diff = 6.7, SE = 2.8, z = 3.93, P<.001.*

§*Cannabis vs opioid, % diff = 6.9, SE = 2.8, z = 2.44, P = .02; cannabis vs cocaine, % diff = 7.6, SE = 3.4, z = 2.22, P = .03; cannabis vs alcohol, % diff = 9.0, SE = 2.7, z = 3.34, P<.001; and cannabis vs controls, % diff = 10.5, SE = 2.7, z = 3.93, P<.001.*

‖*Alcohol vs opioid, % diff = 8.5, SE = 3.1, z = 2.73, P = .006; alcohol vs cannabis, % diff = 8.2, SE = 3.7, z = 2.19, P = .03; and alcohol vs controls, % diff = 17.4, SE = 3.0, z = 5.88, P<.001.*

Table 6. Adjusted Odds Ratios for Associations Between Predominant Drug Disorder in Probands and Relatives

	Predominant Drug Disorders in Relatives, Adjusted Odds Ratio (95% Confidence Interval)* Opioids (n = 55)	Cocaine (n = 38)	Cannabis (n = 70)
Predominant drug disorders in probands			
Opioids (n = 87)	**10.2 (3.2-32.6)**†	2.8 (1.1-7.2)‡	2.4 (1.1-5.9)‡
Cocaine (n = 27)	2.2 (0.3-15.8)	**4.4 (1.5-13.2)**§	1.8 (0.5-6.3)
Cannabis (n = 35)	8.2 (1.7-39.1)§	1.9 (0.4-8.5)	**5.8 (2.6-12.9)**†
Effects of confounders			
Antisocial personality in proband	0.4 (0.2-1.2)	0.5 (0.2-1.7)	1.0 (0.5-2.1)
Antisocial personality in relative	79.9 (26.9-237.4)†	7.0 (1.4-35.4)‡	7.4 (2.3-23.4)†
Sex of proband, female vs male	1.1 (0.4-3.0)	2.8 (1.1-7.0)‡	1.4 (0.7-2.6)
Sex of relative, female vs male	0.7 (0.3-1.7)	0.4 (0.1-0.9)‡	0.5 (0.3-0.9)‡
Age of relative, <50 y	8.1 (3.1-21.1)†	49.7 (2.9-86.1)§	12.1 (4.5-32.7)†
Interview status of relative	0.4 (0.1-1.7)	0.9 (0.3-3.1)	2.5 (1.3-4.7)§

Boldface cells indicate specificity of concordance between probands and relatives.
†P<.001.
‡P<.05.
§P<.01.

tion to current knowledge regarding familial factors and drug disorders. Design features include (1) a control group in which similar diagnostic and assessment methods were used; (2) probands with a range of drugs of abuse that strengthens the generalizability of the results; (3) a sufficient number of female probands to allow investigation of familial patterns of substance abuse among women; and (4) application of a statistical method that examines multinomial classification of probands and relatives simultaneously while controlling for the effects of clustered observations in families.

Limitations include (1) the lack of direct interview data on some of the relatives, necessitating the derivation of best-estimate diagnoses from family history information; (2) the imprecision of retrospective data in characterization of patterns of drug use and abuse (particularly among polysubstance abusers); (3) the lack of power to test adequately patterns of cross-transmission of specific drugs with such low base rates; and (4) possible selection biases with respect to clinical sampling of probands and recruitment of families with offspring, which may limit generalizability of the results.

Because the family has been shown to play a critical role in the etiology of drug use and abuse, it is important to obtain a deeper understanding of the complex mechanisms through which the family exerts its influence. Additional controlled family and twin studies are critical to identify patterns of expression of substance disorders and comorbid psychiatric disorders, to test the classic modes of genetic transmission of substance abuse, to determine the role of sex-specific patterns of transmission of substance abuse, and to elucidate the role of genetic and environmental factors and their interaction in its development.

Specificity of familial aggregation of some classes of drugs as well as independence from alcoholism suggests that research and treatment should focus on specific drugs of abuse and patterns of concurrent use to determine whether different genetic, biological, and environmental risk factors underlie their development.

In terms of prevention, these findings support a shift in drug prevention programs from the universal level to programs that target the families of substance abusers.

Accepted for publication May 26, 1998.

This work was supported primarily by grant DA05348 and in part by grants AA07080, AA09978, DA09055, and MH36197 and by Research Scientist Development Awards K02 DA00293 (Dr Merikangas) and K05 DA00059 (Dr Rounsaville) from the Alcohol, Drug Abuse and Mental Health Administration of the US Public Health Service; and by MH14235 training awards (Drs Stevens and Fenton, Mr Goulet, and Ms Stolar). The Swiss National Science Foundation (grant 8238-033242) provided support to Dr Preisig.

We thank Donald Hedeker, PhD, Division of Epidemiology and Biostatistics, School of Public Health, University of Illinois at Chicago, for making available to us his Fortran program MIXNO.

Reprints: Kathleen R. Merikangas, PhD, Genetic Epidemiology Research Unit, Yale University School of Medicine, 40 Temple St, New Haven, CT 06510 (e-mail: kathleen.merikangas@yale.edu).

REFERENCES

1. Merikangas KR. The genetic epidemiology of alcoholism. *Psychol Med.* 1990;20:11-22.
2. McGue M. Genes, environment, and the etiology of alcoholism. In: Zucker R, Boyd G, Howard J, eds. *The Development of Alcohol Problems: Exploring the Biopsychosocial Matrix. NIAAA Research Monograph No. 26.* Rockville, Md: US Dept of Health and Human Services, Public Health Service, National Institutes of Health, National Institute on Alcohol Abuse and Alcoholism; 1994:1-39.
3. Croughan JL. The contributions of family studies to understanding drug abuse. In: Robins L, ed. *Studying Drug Abuse.* New Brunswick, NJ: Rutgers University Press; 1985:240-264.
4. Rounsaville BJ, Kosten TR, Weissman MM, Prusoff BA, Pauls D, Foley S, Merikangas KR. Psychiatric disorders in the relatives of probands with opiate addiction. *Arch Gen Psychiatry.* 1991;48:33-42.
5. Gordon HW. Human neuroscience at National Institute on Drug Abuse: implications for genetics research. *Am J Med Genet.* 1994;54:300-303.
6. Hill SH, Cloninger CR, Ayre FR. Independent familial transmission of alcoholism and opiate abuse. *Alcohol Clin Exp Res.* 1977;1:335-342.
7. Gfroerer J. Correlation between drug use by teenagers and drug use by older family members. *Am J Drug Alcohol Abuse.* 1987;13:95-108.
8. Meller W, Rinehart R, Cadoret R, Troughton E. Specific familial transmission in substance abuse. *Int J Addict.* 1988;23:1029-1039.
9. Claridge G, Ross E. Sedative drug tolerance in twins. In: Claridge G, Canter S, Hume W, eds. *Personality Differences and Biological Variations: A Study of Twins.* Oxford, England: Pergamon Press; 1978:115-131.
10. Pedersen N. Twin similarity for usage of common drugs. In: Gredda L, Paris P, Nance W, eds. *Twin Research 3: Epidemiological and Clinical Studies.* New York, NY: Alan R Liss Inc; 1981:53-59.
11. Gurling H, Grant S, Dangl J. The genetic and cultural transmission of alcohol use, alcoholism, cigarette smoking and coffee drinking: a review and an example using a log linear cultural transmission model. *Br J Addict.* 1985;80:269-279.
12. Mirin S, Weiss R, Michael J. Psychopathology in substance abusers: diagnosis and treatment. *Am J Drug Alcohol Abuse.* 1988;14:139-157.
13. Mirin SM, Weiss RD, Griffin ML, Michael JL. Psychopathology in drug abusers and their families. *Compr Psychiatry.* 1991;32:36-51.
14. Merikangas KR, Rounsaville BJ, Prusoff BA. Familial factors in vulnerability to substance abuse. In: Glantz MD, Pickens RW, eds. *Vulnerability to Drug Abuse.* Washington, DC: American Psychological Association; 1992:75-98.
15. Grove W, Eckert E, Heston L, Bouchard T, Segal N, Lykken D. Heritability of substance abuse and antisocial behavior. *Biol Psychiatry.* 1990;27:1293-1304.
16. Pickens R, Svikis D, McGue M, Lykken D, Heston L, Clayton P. Heterogeneity in the inheritance of alcoholism. *Arch Gen Psychiatry.* 1991;48:19-28.
17. Tsuang MT, Lyons MJ, Eisen SA, Goldberg J, True W, Nang L, Meyer JM, Eaves L. Genetic influences on abuse of illicit drugs. *Am J Med Genet.* 1996;5:473-477.
18. Jang KL, Livesley WJ, Vernon PA. Alcohol and drug problems: a multivariate behavioural genetic analysis of co-morbidity. *Addiction.* 1995;90:1213-1221.
19. Lyons MJ, Toomey R, Meyer JM, Green AI, Eisen A, Goldberg J, True WR, Tsuang MT. How do genes influence marijuana use? the role of subjective effects. *Addiction.* 1997;92:409-417.
20. Cadoret R, Troughton E, O'Gorman T, Heywood E. An adoption study of genetic and environmental factors in drug abuse. *Arch Gen Psychiatry.* 1986;43:1131-1136.
21. Cadoret RJ. Genetic and environmental factors in initiation of drug use and the transition to abuse. In: Glantz M, Pickens R, eds. *Vulnerability to Drug Abuse.* Washington, DC: American Psychological Association; 1992:99-113.
22. Cadoret RJ, Yates WR, Troughton E, Woodworth G, Stewart MA. Adoption study demonstrating two genetic pathways to drug abuse. *Arch Gen Psychiatry.* 1995;52:42-52.
23. Cadoret RJ, Yates WR, Troughton E, Woodworth G, Stewart MA. An adoption study of drug abuse/dependency in females. *Compr Psychiatry.* 1996;37:88-94.
24. American Psychiatric Association. *Diagnostic and Statistical Manual of Mental Disorders, Third Edition, Revised.* Washington, DC: American Psychiatric Association; 1987.
25. Merikangas KS, Stevens D, Fenton B, O'Malley S, Woods S, Stolar M, Risch M. Comorbidity of alcoholism and anxiety disorders. *Psychol Med.* In press.
26. Endicott J, Spitzer R. A diagnostic interview: the Schedule for Affective Disorders and Schizophrenia–Lifetime version. *Arch Gen Psychiatry.* 1978;35:837-844.
27. American Psychiatric Association. *Diagnostic and Statistical Manual of Mental Disorders, Third Edition.* Washington, DC: American Psychiatric Association; 1980.
28. Colombotos J. Personal vs. telephone interviews. *Public Health Rep.* 1969;84:773-782.
29. Weeks M, Kulka R, Lessler J, Whitmore R. Personal versus telephone surveys for collecting household data at the local level. *Am J Public Health.* 1983;73:1389-1394.
30. Aneshensel C, Frerichs R, Clark V, Yokopanic P. Telephone vs. in-person surveys of community health surveys. *Am J Public Health.* 1982;72:1017-1021.
31. Rhode P, Lewinsohn P, Seeley R. Comparability of telephone and face-to-face interviews in assessing axis I and II disorders. *Am J Psychiatry.* 1997;154:1593-1598.
32. Andreasen NC, Endicott J, Spitzer RL, Winokur G. The family history method using diagnostic criteria. *Arch Gen Psychiatry.* 1977;34:1229-1235.
33. Hedeker D. *MIXNO: A Computer Program for Mixed-Effects Nominal Logistic Regression.* Chicago: University of Illinois at Chicago, School of Public Health and Prevention Research Center; 1998. Technical Report.
34. Regier D, Farmer M, Rae D, Locke BZ, Keith SJ, Judd LL, Goodwin FK. Comorbidity of mental disorders with alcohol and other drug abuse: results from the Epidemiologic Catchment Area (ECA) Study. *JAMA.* 1990;264:2511-2518.
35. Warner L, Kessler R, Hughes M, Anthony J, Nelson C. Prevalence and correlates of drug use and dependence in the United States. *Arch Gen Psychiatry.* 1995;52:219-229.
36. Cloninger CR, Christiansen KO, Reich T, Gottesman II. Implications of sex differences in the prevalence of antisocial personality, alcoholism, and criminality for familial transmission. *Arch Gen Psychiatry.* 1978;35:941-951.
37. Hill SY, Smith TR. Evidence for genetic mediation of alcoholism in women. *J Subst Abuse.* 1991;3:159-174.
38. Merikangas K, Brunetto W. Assortative mating and psychiatric disorders. In: Papadimitriou G, Mendlewicz J, eds. *Bailliere's Clinical Psychiatry: International Practice and Research.* London, England: Bailliere Tindall; 1996:175-185.
39. Annis H. Patterns of intra-familial drug use. *Br J Addict.* 1974;69:361-369.
40. Bauman KE, Foshee VA, Linzer MA, Koch GG. Effect of parental smoking classification on the association between parental and adolescent smoking. *Addict Behav.* 1990;15:413-422.
41. Duncan TE, Duncan SC, Hops H, Stoolmiller M. An analysis of the relationship between parent and adolescent marijuana use via generalized estimating equation methodology. *Multivariate Behav Res.* 1995;30:317-339.
42. Khantzian EJ. The self-medication hypothesis of addictive disorders: focus on health and cocaine dependence. *Am J Psychiatry.* 1985;142:1259-1264.
43. Weiss R, Griffin M, Mirin S. Drug abuse as self-medication for depression: an empirical study. *Am J Drug Alcohol Abuse.* 1992;18:121-129.
44. Barnes G, Welte J. Patterns and predictors of alcohol use among 1-12th grade students in New York State. *J Stud Alcohol.* 1986;47:53-62.
45. Brook JS, Whiteman M, Gordon AS, Cohen P. Some model mechanisms for explaining the impact of maternal and adolescent characteristics on adolescent stage of drug use. *Dev Psychol.* 1986;22:460-467.
46. Bailey SL, Hubbard RL. Developmental variation in the context of marijuana initiation among adolescents. *J Health Soc Behav.* 1990;31:58-70.
47. Robins LN. The natural history of drug abuse. *Acta Psychiatr Scand Suppl.* 1980;284:7-20.
48. Farrington DP. Longitudinal research strategies: advantages, problems and prospects. *J Am Acad Child Adolesc Psychiatry.* 1991;30:369-374.
49. Brown SA. Life events of adolescents in relation to personal and parental substance abuse. *Am J Psychiatry.* 1989;146:484-489.
50. Holden MG, Brown SA, Mott MA. Social support network of adolescents: relation to family alcohol abuse. *Am J Drug Alcohol Abuse.* 1988;14:487-498.
51. Roosa MW, Beals J, Sandler IN, Pillow DR. The role of risk and protective factors in predicting symptomatology in adolescent self-identified children of alcoholic parents. *Am J Community Psychol.* 1990;18:725-741.
52. McCarthy WJ, Anglin MD. Narcotics addicts. *J Drug Issues.* 1990;20:99-123.
53. Brook JS, Brook DW, Gordon AS, Whiteman M, Cohen P. The psychosocial etiology of adolescent drug use. *Genet Soc Gen Psychol Monogr.* 1990;116:111-267.
54. Kandel DB, Andrews K. Processes of adolescent socialization by parents and peers. *Int J Addict.* 1987;22:319-342.
55. Kumpfer KL, Hopkins R. Recent advances in addictive disorders: prevention: current research and trends. *Psychiatr Clin North Am.* 1993;16:11-20.
56. Simcha-Fagan O, Schwartz J. Neighborhood and delinquency: an assessment of contextual effects. *Criminology.* 1986;24:667-703.

Drug Dependence, a Chronic Medical Illness
Implications for Treatment, Insurance, and Outcomes Evaluation

A. Thomas McLellan, PhD
David C. Lewis, MD
Charles P. O'Brien, MD, PhD
Herbert D. Kleber, MD

The effects of drug dependence on social systems has helped shape the generally held view that drug dependence is primarily a social problem, not a health problem. In turn, medical approaches to prevention and treatment are lacking. We examined evidence that drug (including alcohol) dependence is a chronic medical illness. A literature review compared the diagnoses, heritability, etiology (genetic and environmental factors), pathophysiology, and response to treatments (adherence and relapse) of drug dependence vs type 2 diabetes mellitus, hypertension, and asthma. Genetic heritability, personal choice, and environmental factors are comparably involved in the etiology and course of all of these disorders. Drug dependence produces significant and lasting changes in brain chemistry and function. Effective medications are available for treating nicotine, alcohol, and opiate dependence but not stimulant or marijuana dependence. Medication adherence and relapse rates are similar across these illnesses. Drug dependence generally has been treated as if it were an acute illness. Review results suggest that long-term care strategies of medication management and continued monitoring produce lasting benefits. Drug dependence should be insured, treated, and evaluated like other chronic illnesses.

JAMA. 2000;284:1689-1695 www.jama.com

Many expensive and disturbing social problems can be traced directly to drug dependence. Recent studies[1-4] estimated that drug dependence costs the United States approximately $67 billion annually in crime, lost work productivity, foster care, and other social problems.[2-4] These expensive effects of drugs on all social systems have been important in shaping the public view that drug dependence is primarily a social problem that requires interdiction and law enforcement rather than a health problem that requires prevention and treatment.

This view is apparently shared by many physicians. Few medical schools or residency programs have an adequate required course in addiction. Most physicians fail to screen for alcohol or drug dependence during routine examinations.[5] Many health professionals view such screening efforts as a waste of time. A survey[6] of general practice physicians and nurses indicated that most believed no available medical or health care interventions would be "appropriate or effective in treating addiction." In fact, 40% to 60% of patients treated for alcohol or other drug dependence return to active substance use within a year following treatment discharge.[7-9] One implication is that these disappointing results confirm the suspicion that drug dependence is not a medical illness and thus is not significantly affected by health care interventions. Another possibility is that current treatment strategies and outcome expectations view drug dependence as a curable, acute condition. If drug dependence is more like a chronic illness, the appropriate standards for treatment and outcome expectations would be found among other chronic illnesses.

To explore this possibility, we undertook a literature review comparing drug dependence with 3 chronic illnesses: type 2 diabetes mellitus, hypertension, and asthma. These examples were selected because they have been well studied and are widely believed to have effective treatments, although they are not yet curable. Our review searched all English-language medical and health journals in MEDLINE from 1980 to the present using the following key words: *heritability, pathophysiology, diagnosis, course, treatment, compliance, ad*

Author Affiliations: The Treatment Research Institute, Philadelphia, Pa (Dr McLellan); The Penn/VA Center for Studies of Addiction at the Veterans Affairs Medical Center and the University of Pennsylvania, Philadelphia (Drs McLellan and O'Brien); The Brown University Center for Alcohol and Addiction Studies, Providence, RI (Dr Lewis); and The National Center on Addiction and Substance Abuse at Columbia University, New York, NY (Dr Kleber).
Corresponding Author and Reprints: A. Thomas McLellan, PhD, The Treatment Research Institute, 150 S Independence Mall W, Suite 600, Philadelphia, PA 19106-3475 (e-mail: tmclellan@tresearch.org).

herence, relapse, and *reoccurrence.* Importantly, our definition of *drug* and our review criteria included all over-the-counter (alcohol and nicotine), prescription (benzodiazepines, amphetamines, opiates), and illegal (heroin, marijuana, cocaine) drugs.

The review is presented in 2 parts. The first part considers some characteristic aspects of chronic illness, such as diagnosis, heritability, etiology, and pathophysiology. The second part reviews recent advances in the medical treatment of drug dependence and considers treatment response, particularly medication adherence and relapse or recurrence. Although we are aware that arguments by analogy are limited, we believe this comparative analysis of drug dependence with other chronic illnesses offers some instructive and provocative implications.

DIAGNOSIS, HERITABILITY, ETIOLOGY, AND PATHOPHYSIOLOGY

Diagnosis

Most adults have used alcohol and/or other drugs, sometimes heavily to the point of abuse but rarely to the point where that use could reasonably be called an illness. There is no laboratory test for dependence, but the diagnostic differentiation of use, abuse, and dependence has been operationally refined and repeatedly shown to be reliable and valid.[10,11]

Dependence or what is commonly called *addiction* is operationally defined in the *Diagnostic and Statistical Manual of Mental Disorders, Fourth Edition*[10] as a pathologic condition manifested by 3 or more of 7 criteria. Two of these criteria, tolerance and withdrawal, indicate neurologic adaptation or so-called physiologic dependence. However, as has been pointed out,[12] physiologic adaptation (tolerance or withdrawal) by itself is neither necessary nor sufficient for a diagnosis of substance dependence. Indeed, those receiving a dependence diagnosis are required to show a "compulsive desire for and use of the drug(s) despite serious adverse consequences" such as "use instead of or while performing important responsibilities."[10,11]

There are several short (<5 minutes of patient or practitioner time) questionnaires that can screen for alcohol and other drug dependence disorders with high rates of sensitivity and specificity.[13] Following a positive screening result, standardized diagnostic checklists can be applied during the medical evaluation. Diagnoses that result from these standardized and easily applied criteria have been reliable and valid across a range of clinical and nonclinical populations.[11]

Genetic Heritability

One of the best methods for estimating the level of genetic contribution is to compare the rates of a disorder in monozygotic and dizygotic twins. Heritability estimates from twin studies[14,15] of hypertension range from 0.25 to 0.50, depending on the sample and the diagnostic criteria used. Twin studies of diabetes offer heritability estimates of approximately 0.80 for type 2[16] and 0.30 to 0.55 for type 1 diabetes mellitus.[17] Finally, twin studies[18,19] of adult-onset asthma have produced a somewhat broader range of heritability estimates, ranging from 0.36 to 0.70.

Several twin studies[20-23] have been published in the substance dependence field, all showing significantly higher rates of dependence among twins than among nontwin siblings and higher rates among monozygotic than dizygotic twins. Published heritability estimates include 0.34 for males dependent on heroin, 0.55 for males dependent on alcohol, 0.52 for females dependent on marijuana, and 0.61 for cigarette-dependent twins of both sexes.[20-23] More studies of heritability are needed across drug types and sexes, but the evidence suggests significant genetic contribution to the risk of addiction comparable to that seen in other chronic illnesses.

Role of Personal Responsibility

Since the use of any drug is a voluntary action, behavioral control or willpower is important in the onset of dependence. Thus, at some level an addicted individual is at fault for initiating the behaviors that lead to a dependence disorder. Doesn't this voluntary initiation of the disease process set drug dependence apart, etiologically, from other medical illnesses?

There are many illnesses in which voluntary choice affects initiation and maintenance, especially when these voluntary behaviors interact with genetic and cultural factors. For example, among males, salt sensitivity is a genetically transmitted risk factor for the eventual development of one form of hypertension.[24,25] However, not all of those who inherit salt sensitivity develop hypertension. This is because the use of salt is determined by familial salt use patterns and individual choice. Similarly, risk factors such as obesity, stress level, and inactivity are products of familial, cultural, and personal choice factors.[24,25] Thus, even among those with demonstrated genetic risk, a significant part of the total risk for developing hypertension can be traced to individual behaviors.

There are also involuntary components embedded within seemingly volitional choices. For example, although the choice to try a drug may be voluntary, the effects of the drug can be influenced profoundly by genetic factors. Those whose initial, involuntary physiologic responses to alcohol or other drugs are extremely pleasurable will be more likely to repeat the drug taking than those whose reaction is neutral or negative. Work by Schuckit[26] and Schuckit and Smith[27] has shown that sons of alcohol-dependent fathers inherit more tolerance to alcohol's effects and are less likely to experience hangovers than sons of non–alcohol-dependent fathers. In contrast, the inherited presence of an aldehyde dehydrogenase genotype (associated with alcohol metabolism) causes an involuntary skin "flushing" response to alcohol.[28-30] Individuals who are homozygous for this allele (approximately 35% of the Chinese population, and 20% of Jewish males in Israel) have an especially unpleasant initial reaction to voluntary alcohol use to the point where there are virtually no alcoholics found with this genotype.[28-30]

Pathophysiology

The acute effects of alcohol and other drugs have been well characterized. However, even a complete understanding of these acute effects cannot explain how repeated doses of alcohol and other drugs produce paradoxically increasing tolerance to the effects of those drugs concurrent with decreasing volitional ability to forgo the drug. As suggested by Koob and Bloom,[31] the challenge is to find an internally consistent sequence by which molecular events modify cellular events and in turn produce profound and lasting changes in cognition, motivation, and behavior. Research on the neurochemical, neuroendocrine, and cellular changes associated with drug dependence has led to remarkable findings during the past decade, as summarized in the recent literature.[32-35] Herein, we summarize just 3 areas of investigation.

Addictive drugs have well-specified effects on the brain circuitry involved in the control of motivated and learned behaviors.[31-36] Anatomically, the brain circuitry involved in most of the actions of addictive drugs is the ventral tegmental area connecting the limbic cortex through the midbrain to the nucleus accumbens.[35,36] Neurochemically, alcohol, opiates, cocaine, and nicotine have significant effects on the dopamine system, although through different mechanisms. Cocaine increases synaptic dopamine by blocking reuptake into presynaptic neurons; amphetamine produces increased presynaptic release of dopamine, whereas opiates and alcohol disinhibit dopamine neurons, producing increased firing rates. Opiates and alcohol also have direct effects on the endogenous opioid and possibly the γ-aminobutyric acid systems.[31-36]

Significantly, the ventral tegmental area and the dopamine system have been associated with feelings of euphoria.[31,36] Animals that receive mild electrical stimulation of the dopamine system contingent on a lever press will rapidly learn to press that lever thousands of times, ignoring normal needs for water, food, or rest.[36] Cocaine, opiates, and several other addictive drugs produce supranormal stimulation of this reward circuitry.[31-36]

Given the fundamental neuroanatomy and neuropharmacology of this system, it is understandable that addictive drugs could produce immediate and profound desire for their readministration. Less clear is why simply preventing the administration of these drugs for some period would not correct the situation, return the system to normal, and lead to a "sadder but wiser" individual who would be less instead of more likely to reuse those drugs.

It is known that use of these drugs at some dose, frequency, and chronicity will reliably produce enduring and possibly permanent pathophysiologic changes in the reward circuitry, in the normal levels of many neurochemicals, and in the stress response system.[31,35,37-41] Volkow et al[37,42] found impairments in the dopamine system of abstinent former cocaine users 3 months after their last use. Other studies[39,40] have documented sustained changes in the stress response system following abstinence from opiate or cocaine dependence. Researchers do not know how much drug use is required to create these changes or whether these effects ever return to normal. Somatic signs of withdrawal last several days, motivational and cognitive impairments may last several months,[33] but the learned aspects of tolerance to the drug may never return to normal.[35,36,41]

A second explanation for the enduring pathology seen among drug-dependent persons and their tendency to relapse lies in the integration of the reward circuitry with the motivational, emotional, and memory centers that are colocated within the limbic system. These interconnected regions allow the organism not only to experience the pleasure of rewards but also to learn the signals for them and to respond in an anticipatory manner.[36,41,43] Repeated pairing of a person (drug-using friend), place (corner bar), thing (paycheck), or even an emotional state (anger, depression) with drug use can lead to rapid and entrenched learning or conditioning. Thus, previously drug-dependent individuals who have been abstinent for long periods may encounter a person, place, or thing that previously was associated with their drug use, producing significant, conditioned physiologic reactions, such as withdrawal-like symptoms and profound subjective desire or craving for the drug.[43,44] These responses can combine to fuel the "loss of control" that is considered a hallmark of drug dependence.[10]

These conditioned physiologic responses have been shown in laboratory studies[41,45,46] of currently abstinent former opiate, cocaine, and alcohol-dependent individuals. Childress et al,[43] using positron emission tomography, examined limbic and control brain regions of detoxified, male, cocaine-dependent subjects and cocaine-naive controls during videos of cocaine-related scenes. During the video, these currently abstinent former cocaine-dependent subjects experienced increased craving and showed a pattern of limbic increases and basal ganglia decreases in regional cerebral blood flow that mimicked the effects of the drug itself. This pattern did not occur in cocaine-naive controls or among the formerly cocaine-dependent patients in response to a neutral video.[43] Thus, even artificial video scenes of cocaine-related stimuli, presented in the sterile context of a positron emission tomography laboratory, produced excitation of brain reward regions and triggered drug craving.

TREATMENT RESPONSE

A central question in the comparison of drug dependence with other illnesses is whether dependence will decrease without treatment and whether it will respond to medications and other interventions. There is a large research literature on drug dependence treatment outcomes.[7-9,34,35,47-49] The treatment of addiction has been described in a manual[50] and 2 detailed volumes.[51,52] Space permits only a few examples from that literature, addressing questions of particular import to physicians.

Untreated Persons

Examinations of untreated, dependent persons offer some indication of the natural course of addiction. For example, Metzger et al[53] measured drug use, needle-sharing practices, and human immunodeficiency virus (HIV) infection rates of 2 large samples of opiate-dependent persons in Philadelphia, Pa. The in-treatment (IT) group included 152 patients randomly selected at admission to a methadone maintenance program. Out-of-treatment (OT) subjects were also heroin-dependent individuals matched to the IT group by age, race, sex, neighborhood, and other relevant background factors, although none of the 103 OT subjects had received treatment. Both groups were interviewed and tested for HIV status every 6 months for 7 years. At the initial assessment, 13% of the IT sample and 21% of the OT sample were HIV positive. By 7 years, 51% of the OT group but only 21% of the IT group tested HIV positive.[53] Of course, even this substantial between-group difference does not prove that treatment participation was the causal agent. It is likely that the OT subjects lacked the motivation for change found among the treated patients. Thus, lack of desire for personal change, rather than the effects of the treatment itself, could have produced the differences seen.

One way to separate the effects of drug dependence treatment from the effects of motivation is to compare treated and untreated substance-dependent individuals who were explicitly not interested in treatment. Booth and colleagues[54] studied 4000 intravenous drug users seeking HIV testing as part of a multisite acquired immunodeficiency syndrome initiative in 15 cities. Subjects were randomly assigned to either standard HIV testing alone or to standard testing plus 3 sessions of motivational counseling from a health educator. At 6-month follow-up, those who received additional counseling showed half the rate of drug injection (20% vs 45%), 4 times the likelihood of abstinence (confirmed by urinalysis), and significantly lower arrest rates (14% vs 24%) than those randomly assigned to receive just HIV testing.[54] Studies of other illnesses show that screening and brief advice from physicians can affect the motivation for change among patients and the longer-term course of their health. The data of Booth et al suggest this is true even for seriously addicted individuals.

Svikis et al[55] studied drug abuse treatment in pregnant, cocaine-dependent women who did not originally apply for treatment. All women had simply applied for prenatal care and were found to be positive for cocaine use on a routine drug screen. They were compared with 46 pregnant, demographically matched women who tested positive for cocaine use and received standard prenatal care during the year before the opening of the experimental treatment program. Drug dependence treatment consisted of 1 week of residential care followed by twice-weekly addiction counseling in the context of the scheduled prenatal visits.

At delivery, 37% of the treated patients tested positive for cocaine use compared with 63% of the untreated women. Infants of the treated women averaged higher birth weights (2934 vs 2539 g) and longer gestational periods (39 vs 34 weeks) than those of the comparison group. Following delivery, 10% of infants in the treated group required care in the neonatal intensive care unit (mean, 7 days). In comparison, 26% of infants in the untreated group required intensive care (mean, 39 days). Average costs of care were $14500 for the treated group and $46700 for the comparison group. These data indicate that drug-dependent women can be screened and motivated during prenatal care and that drug dependence treatment can be combined with traditional prenatal care in an extremely cost-effective manner.

Medications

In addition to medications for nicotine dependence, such as nicotine gum and patch and bupropion hydrochloride, medications for alcohol and opiate addiction have been developed under Food and Drug Administration guidelines, have been researched in randomized clinical trials, and have reached the market. Herein, we discuss a few recent developments, but a complete review has been published by the Institute of Medicine.[35]

Opioid Dependence. Opioid agonists, partial agonists, and antagonists are the 3 primary types of medications available for the treatment of opioid dependence, all acting directly on opioid receptors, particularly μ-receptors.[35] Agonist medications, such as methadone hydrochloride, are prescribed in the short-term as part of an opioid detoxification protocol or in the long-term as a maintenance regimen. Double-blind, placebo-controlled trials[56,57] have shown methadone to be effective in both inpatient and outpatient detoxification, although the long-term effects of detoxification alone, without continuing treatment, have been uniformly poor. As a maintenance medication, methadone's oral route of administration, slow onset of action, and long half-life have been effective in reducing opiate use, crime, and the spread of infectious diseases, as was recently validated by a National Institutes of Health Consensus Conference.[58]

The partial agonist buprenorphine hydrochloride is administered sublingually and is active for approximately 24 to 36 hours.[59] Large double-blind, placebo-controlled trials of buprenorphine have shown reductions in opiate use comparable with methadone but with fewer withdrawal symptoms on discontinuation.[60] Importantly, the combination of buprenorphine plus naloxone hydrochloride, designed to reduce injection use, will soon be released for prescription in primary care settings.[61]

Opioid antagonists such as naltrexone block the actions of heroin through competitive binding for 48 to 72 hours, producing neither euphoria nor dysphoria in abstinent patients.[62,63] Naltrexone is used as a maintenance medication, designed as an "insurance policy" in situations where the patient is likely to be confronted with relapse risks. Naltrexone in combination with social or criminal justice sanctions is routinely used in the monitored treatment of physicians, nurses, and other professionals.[63] In a recent controlled trial, Cornish and colleagues[64] showed that naltrexone added to standard federal probation produced 70% less opiate use and 50% less reincarceration than standard probation alone.

Alcohol Dependence. Naltrexone has been found effective at 50 mg/d for reducing drinking among alcohol-dependent patients.[65,66] It works by blocking at least some of the "high" produced by alcohol's effects on μ-opiate receptors. More recently, European researchers have found encouraging results using the γ-aminobutyric acid agonist acamprosate to block craving and relapse to alcohol abuse.[67] Alcohol-dependent patients prescribed acamprosate showed 30% higher abstinence rates at 6-month follow-up than those randomized to placebo. Furthermore, those who returned to drinking while receiving acamprosate reported less heavy drinking (≥5 drinks per day) than those receiving placebo.[67]

Stimulant Dependence. Although there are not yet effective medications for the treatment of cocaine or amphetamine dependence,[35] there are proven behavioral treatments.[68-71] There also are promising animal studies of a potential vaccine that binds to and inactivates metabolites of cocaine,[72] but clinical trials will not be scheduled for several years.

Comparing Treatments for Drug Dependence With Treatments for Other Chronic Diseases

There is no reliable cure for drug dependence. Dependent patients who comply with the recommended regimen of education, counseling, and medication have favorable outcomes during and usually for at least 6 to 12 months following treatment.[47-50] Favorable outcomes typically continue in patients who remain in methadone maintenance or in abstinence maintenance through participation in Alcoholics Anonymous (AA) or other self-help programs.[48,50-52] However, because of insurance restrictions, many patients receive only detoxification or acute stabilization with no continuing care.[3,6,9] Others drop out of rehabilitation-oriented treatment and/or they ignore physician advice to continue taking medications and participating in AA. Thus, 1-year, postdischarge follow-up studies[47-52,73] have typically shown that only about 40% to 60% of discharged patients are continuously abstinent, although an additional 15% to 30% have not resumed dependent use during this period. Problems of low socioeconomic status, comorbid psychiatric conditions, and lack of family and social supports are among the most important predictors of poor adherence during addiction treatment and of relapse following treatment.[47-52,74]

Hypertension, diabetes, and asthma are also chronic disorders, requiring continuing care throughout a patient's life. Treatments for these illnesses are effective but heavily dependent on adherence to the medical regimen for that effectiveness. Unfortunately, studies have shown that less than 60% of adult patients with type 1 diabetes mellitus fully adhere to with their medication schedule,[75] and less than 40% of patients with hypertension or asthma adhere fully to their medication regimens.[76,77] The problem is even worse for the behavioral and diet changes that are so important for the maintenance of gains in these chronic illnesses. Again, studies indicate that less than 30% of patients with adult-onset asthma, hypertension, or diabetes adhere to prescribed diet and/or behavioral changes that are designed to increase functional status and to reduce risk factors for recurrence of the disorders.[75-78] Across all 3 of these chronic medical illnesses, adherence and ultimately outcome are poorest among patients with low socioeconomic status, lack of family and social supports, or significant psychiatric comorbidity.[75-79]

Perhaps because of the similarity in treatment adherence, there are also similar relapse rates across these disorders. Outcome studies indicate that 30% to 50% of adult patients with type 1 diabetes and approximately 50% to 70% of adult patients with hypertension or asthma experience recurrence of symptoms each year to the point where they require additional medical care to reestablish symptom remission.[75-80]

COMMENT

Few persons who try drugs or regularly use drugs become dependent. However, once initiated, there is a predictable pathogenesis to dependence marked by significant and persistent changes in brain chemistry and function. It is not yet possible to explain the physiologic and psychological processes that transform controlled, voluntary use of alcohol and other drugs into uncontrolled, involuntary dependence. Twin studies indicate a definite role for genetic heritability. Nonetheless, personal choice and environmental factors are clearly involved in the expression of dependence. In terms of vulnerability, onset, and course, drug dependence is similar to other chronic illnesses, such as type 2 diabetes, hypertension, and asthma.

Our review of treatment response found more than 100 randomized controlled trials of addiction treatments, most showing significant reductions in drug use, improved personal health, and reduced social pathology but not cure.[7-9,34,35,47-52,81,82] Recent treatment advances include potent, well-tolerated medications for nicotine, alcohol, and opioid dependence[35,58,61,65-67] but not marijuana or stimulant dependence. There is little evidence of effectiveness from detoxification or short-term stabilization alone without maintenance or monitoring such as in methadone maintenance or AA.[47-52,57] However, as in treatments for other chronic disorders, we found major problems of medication adherence, early drop-out, and relapse among drug-dependent patients. In fact, problems of poverty, lack of family support, and psychiatric comorbidity were major and approximately equal predictors of noncompliance and relapse across all chronic illnesses examined.[74-83]

Thus, our review suggests that drug dependence shares many features with other chronic illnesses. We are aware that arguments by analogy are limited, and even marked similarities to other illnesses are not proof that drug dependence is a chronic illness. Nonetheless, these similarities in heritability, course, and particularly response to treatment raise the question of why medical treatments are not seen as appropriate or effective when applied to alcohol and drug dependence. One possibility is the way drug dependence treatments have traditionally been delivered and evaluated.

Many drug dependence treatments are delivered in a manner that is more appropriate for acute care disorders. Many patients receive detoxification only.[3,35,48,49] Others are admitted to specialty treatment programs, where the goal has been to rehabilitate and discharge them as one might rehabilitate a surgical patient following a joint replacement.[47] Outcome evaluations are typically conducted 6 to 12 months following treatment discharge. The usual outcome evaluated is whether the patient has been continuously abstinent after leaving treatment.

Imagine this same strategy applied to the treatment of hypertension. Hypertensive patients would be admitted to a 28-day hypertension rehabilitation program, where they would receive group and individual counseling regarding behavioral control of diet, exercise, and lifestyle. Very few would be prescribed medications, since the prevailing insurance restrictions would discourage maintenance medications. Patients completing the program would be discharged to community resources, typically without continued medical monitoring. An evaluation of these patients 6 to 12 months following discharge would count as successes only those who had remained continuously normotensive for the entire postdischarge period.

In this regard, it is interesting that relapse among patients with diabetes, hypertension, and asthma following cessation of treatment has been considered evidence of the effectiveness of those treatments and the need to retain patients in medical monitoring. In contrast, relapse to drug or alcohol use following discharge from addiction treatment has been considered evidence of treatment failure. The best outcomes from treatments of drug dependence have been seen among patients in long-term methadone maintenance programs[49,50,58,83] and among the many who have continued participating in AA support groups.[84,85]

IMPLICATIONS

For primary care physicians, this review suggests that addiction screening, diagnosis, brief interventions, medication management, and referral criteria should be taught as part of medical school and residency curricula and routinely incorporated into clinical practice.[86,87] For those in health policy, our review offers support for recent insurance parity initiatives.[88] Like other chronic illnesses, the effects of drug dependence treatment are optimized when patients remain in continuing care and monitoring without limits or restrictions on the number of days or visits covered. Although it is unknown whether care delivered in a specialty program or coordinated through primary care will provide the maximal benefits for patients and society, it is essential that practitioners adapt the care and medical monitoring strategies currently used in the treatment of other chronic illnesses to the treatment of drug dependence.

Funding/Support: This review was supported by grants from the Department of Veterans Affairs, the National Institute on Drug Abuse, the Center for Substance Abuse Treatment, The Robert Wood Johnson Foundation, and the Office of National Drug Control Policy.

Acknowledgment: The manuscript was reviewed (but not supported financially) by the Physician Leadership for National Drug Policy before submission, and Dr Lewis is a member of that organization.

REFERENCES

1. Rice DP, Kelman S, Miller LS. Estimates of the economic costs of alcohol, and drug abuse and mental illness, 1985 and 1988. *Public Health Rep*. 1991;106:280-292.
2. *Behind Bars: Substance Abuse and America's Prison Population*. New York, NY: National Center for Addiction and Substance Abuse at Columbia University; 1998.
3. *Alcohol and Health: Tenth Special Report to the U.S. Congress*. Washington, DC: US Dept of Health and Human Services; 1997.
4. French MT, Rachal JV, Harwood HJ, Hubbard RL. Does drug abuse treatment affect employment and earnings of clients? *Benefits Q*. 1998;6:58-67.
5. Fleming MF, Barry KL. The effectiveness of alcoholism screening in an ambulatory care setting. *J Stud Alcohol*. 1991;52:33-36.
6. Weisner CM, Schmidt L. Alcohol and drug problems among diverse health and social service populations. *Am J Public Health*. 1993;83:824-829.
7. Finney JW, Moos RH. The long-term course of treated alcoholism, II: predictors and correlates of 10-year functioning and mortality. *J Stud Alcohol*. 1992;53:142-153.
8. Hubbard RL, Craddock G, Flynn PM, Anderson J, Etheridge R. Overview of 1-year follow-up outcomes in the Drug Abuse Treatment Outcome Study (DATOS). *Psychol Addict Behav*. 1997;11:261-278.
9. McLellan AT, McKay J. The treatment of addiction: what can research offer practice? In: Lamb S, Greenlick M, McCarty D, eds. *Bridging the Gap: Forging New Partnerships in Community-Based Drug Abuse Treatment*. Washington, DC: National Academy Press; 1998.
10. *Diagnostic and Statistical Manual of Mental Disorders, Fourth Edition*. Washington, DC: American Psychiatric Association; 1994:175-272.
11. Schuckit MA, Hesselbrock V, Tipp J. A comparison of DSM-III, DSM-IV and ICD-10 substance use disorders diagnoses in 1992 men and women subjects in the COGA study. *Addiction*. 1994;89:1629-1638.
12. Glass RM. Caffeine dependence: what are the implications? *JAMA*. 1994;272:1065-1066.
13. Babor TF, Kranzler HR, Lauerman RJ. Early detection of harmful alcohol consumption. *Addict Behav*. 1989;14:139-157.
14. Williams RR, Hunt SC, Hasstedt SJ, et al. Are there interactions and relations between genetic and environmental factors predisposing to high blood pressure? *Hypertension*. 1991;18(suppl):129-137.
15. Fagard R, Brguljan J, Staessen J, et al. Heritability of conventional and ambulatory blood pressures: a study in twins. *Hypertension*. 1995;26:919-924.
16. Kaprio J, Tuomilehto J, Koskenvuo M, et al. Concordance for type 1 (insulin-dependent) and type 2 (non-insulin-dependent) diabetes mellitus in a population-based cohort of twins in Finland. *Diabetologia*. 1992;35:1060-1067.
17. Kyvik KO, Green A, Beck-Nielsen H. Concordance rates of insulin dependent diabetes mellitus. *BMJ*. 1995;311:913-917.
18. Duffy DL, Martin NG, Battistutta D, et al. Genetics of asthma and hay fever in Australian twins. *Am Rev Respir Dis*. 1990;142:1351-1358.
19. Nieminen MM, Kaprio J, Koskenvuo M. A population-based study of bronchial asthma in adult twin pairs. *Chest*. 1991;100:70-75.
20. Tsuang MT, Lyons MJ, Eisen S, et al. Genetic influences on DSM-III-R drug abuse and dependence: a study of 3,372 twin pairs. *Am J Med Genet*. 1996;67:473-477.
21. Kendler KS, Prescott C. Cannabis use, abuse and dependence in a population-based sample of female twins. *Am J Psychiatry*. 1998;155:1016-1022.
22. VandenBree M, Johnson E, Neale M, Pickens R. Genetic and environmental influences on drug use and abuse/dependence in male and female twins. *Drug Alcohol Depend*. 1998;52:231-241.
23. True WR, Xian H. Common genetic vulnerability for nicotine and alcohol dependence in men. *Arch Gen Psychiatry*. 1999;56:655-661.

24. Mitchell BD, Kammerer CM, Blangero J, et al. Genetic and environmental contributions to cardiovascular risk factors in Mexican Americans. *Circulation*. 1996;94:2159-2170.
25. Svetkey LP, McKeown SP, Wilson AF. Heritability of salt sensitivity in black Americans. *Hypertension*. 1996;28:854-858.
26. Schuckit MA. Low level of response to alcohol as a predictor of future alcoholism. *Am J Psychiatry*. 1994; 151:184-189.
27. Schuckit MA, Smith TL. An 8-year follow-up of 450 sons of alcoholics and controls. *Arch Gen Psychiatry*. 1996;53:202-210.
28. Thomasson HR, Edenberg HJ, Crabb DW, et al. Alcohol and aldehyde dehydrogenase genotypes and alcoholism in Chinese men. *Am J Hum Genet*. 1991; 48:667-681.
29. Newmark YD, Friedlander Y, Thomasson HR. Association of the ADH2*2 allele with reduced alcohol consumption in Jewish men in Israel: a pilot study. *J Stud Alcohol*. 1998;59:133-139.
30. Chao YC, Kiou SR, Chung YY, et al. Polymorphism of alcohol and aldehyde dehydrogenase genes and alcoholic cirrhosis in Chinese patients. *Hepatology*. 1994;19:360-366.
31. Koob GF, Bloom FE. Cellular and molecular mechanisms of drug dependence. *Science*. 1998;242:715-723.
32. Special issue. *Science*. 1997;278:1-211.
33. Series on addiction. *Lancet*. 1996;347:31-36, 97-100, 162-166, 237-240, 301-305, 373-376.
34. National Academy of Sciences, Institute of Medicine. *Dispelling the Myths About Addiction*. Washington, DC: National Academy Press; 1995.
35. Institute of Medicine, Fulco CE, Liverman CT, Earley LE, eds. *Development of Medications for the Treatment of Opiate and Cocaine Addictions: Issues for the Government and Private Sector*. Washington, DC: National Academy Press; 1995.
36. Wise RA, Bozarth MA. Brain substrates for reinforcement and drug-self-administration. *Prog Neuropsychopharmacol*. 1981;5:467-474.
37. Volkow ND, Fowler JS, Wolf AP, et al. Changes in brain glucose metabolism in cocaine dependence and withdrawal. *Am J Psychiatry*. 1991;148:621-626.
38. London ED, Cascella NG, Wong DF, et al. Cocaine-induced reduction of glucose utilization in human brain: a study of positron emission tomography and [flourine 18]-fluorodeoxyglucose. *Arch Gen Psychiatry*. 1990;47:567-574.
39. Kreek MJ, Koob GF. Drug dependence: stress and dysregulation of brain reward pathways. *Drug Alcohol Depend*. 1998;51:23-48.
40. Self DW, Nestler EJ. Drug dependence: stress and dysregulation of brain reward pathways. *Drug Alcohol Depend*. 1998;51:49-60.
41. Weiss F. Neurochemical adaptation in brain reward systems during drug addiction. In: *Institute of Medicine Symposium on Neuroscience Research: Advancing Our Understanding of Drug Addiction*. Washington, DC: National Academy of Sciences; 1996.
42. Volkow ND, Hitzemann R, Wang DJ, et al. Long-term frontal brain metabolic changes in cocaine abusers. *Synapse*. 1992;11:184-190.
43. Childress AR, McElgin W, Mozley PD, et al. Limbic activation during cue-induced cocaine craving. *Am J Psychiatry*. 1999;156:1, 11-18.
44. Holman BL, Mendelson J, Garada B, et al. Regional cerebral blood flow improves with treatment in chronic cocaine polydrug users. *J Nucl Med*. 1993; 34:723-727.
45. Pearlson GD, Jeffery PJ, Harris GJ, et al. Correlation of acute cocaine-induced changes in local cerebral blood flow with subjective effects. *Am J Psychiatry*. 1993;150:495-497.
46. O'Brien CP. Experimental analysis of conditioning factors in human narcotic addiction. *Pharmacol Rev*. 1975;27:533-543.
47. McLellan AT, Metzger DS, Alterman AI, et al. Is addiction treatment "worth it"? public health expectations, policy-based comparisons. In: Fox JS, ed. *Proceedings of Josiah Macy Conference on Medical Education*. New York, NY: Josiah Macy Foundation; 1995: 165-212.
48. Moos RH, Finney JW, Cronkite RC. *Alcoholism Treatment: Context, Process and Outcome*. New York, NY: Oxford University Press; 1990.
49. Gerstein D, Harwood H, eds. *Treating Drug Problems: A Study of the Evolution, Effectiveness, and Financing of Public and Private Drug Treatment Systems*. Washington, DC: National Academy Press; 1990.
50. National Institute on Drug Abuse. *Principles of Drug Addiction Treatment: A Research Based Guide*. Bethesda, Md: National Institutes of Health; 1999. NIH publication 99-4180.
51. American Society of Addiction Medicine. *Principles of Addiction Medicine*. 2nd ed. New York, NY: Harcourt Brace Press; 1998.
52. Lowinson J, Ruiz P, Millman RB, eds. *Substance Abuse, A Comprehensive Textbook*. 2nd ed. Baltimore, Md: Williams & Wilkins; 1992:56-69.
53. Metzger DS, Woody GE, McLellan AT, et al. HIV seroconversion among intravenous drug users in and out of treatment. *AIDS*. 1993;6:1049-1056.
54. Booth RE, Crowley TJ, Zhang Y. Substance abuse treatment entry, retention and effectiveness. *Drug Alcohol Depend*. 1996;42:11-20.
55. Svikis DS, Golden AS, Huggins GR, et al. Cost effectiveness of treatment for drug abusing pregnant women. *Drug Alcohol Depend*. 1997;45:105-113.
56. Gossop M, Johns A, Green L. Opiate withdrawal: inpatient versus outpatient programmes and preferred versus random assignment to treatment. *BMJ*. 1986;293:103-104.
57. Mattick RP, Hall W. Are detoxification programmes effective? *Lancet*. 1996;347:97-100.
58. National Consensus Development Panel on Effective Medical Treatment of Opiate Addiction. Effective medical treatment of opiate addiction. *JAMA*. 1998;280:1936-1943.
59. Bickel WK, Amass L. Buprenorphine treatment of opioid dependence: a review. *Exp Clin Psychopharmacol*. 1995;3:477-489.
60. O'Connor PG, Oliveto AH, Shi JM, et al. A randomized trial of buprenorphine maintenance for heroin dependence in a primary care clinic for substance users versus a methadone clinic. *Am J Med*. 1998;105: 100-105.
61. O'Connor PG, Fiellin DA. Pharmacologic treatment of heroin-dependent patients. *Ann Intern Med*. 2000;133:234-241.
62. O'Brien CP, Greenstein RA, Mintz J, Woody GE. Clinical experience with naltrexone. *Am J Drug Alcohol Abuse*. 1975;2:365-377.
63. Ling W, Wesson DR. Naltrexone treatment for addicted health care professionals. *J Clin Psychiatry*. 1984; 45:46-48.
64. Cornish J, Metzger D, Woody G, et al. Naltrexone pharmacotherapy for opioid dependent federal probationers. *J Subst Abuse Treat*. 1998;13:477-489.
65. Volpicelli JR, Alterman AI, Hayashida M, O'Brien CP. Naltrexone in the treatment of alcohol dependence. *Arch Gen Psychiatry*. 1992;49:876-880.
66. O'Malley SS, Jaffe AJ, Chang G, et al. Naltrexone and coping skills therapy for alcohol dependence. *Arch Gen Psychiatry*. 1992;49:881-887.
67. Sass H, Soyka M, Mann K, Zieglgasberger W. Relapse prevention by acamprosate. *Arch Gen Psychiatry*. 1996;53:673-680.
68. Carroll KM, Rounsaville BJ, Gordon LT, et al. Psychotherapy and pharmacotherapy for ambulatory cocaine abusers. *Arch Gen Psychiatry*. 1994;51:177-187.
69. Carroll KM, Power MD, Bryant K, et al. One-year follow-up status of treatment-seeking cocaine abusers: psychopathology and dependence severity as predictors of outcome. *J Nerv Ment Dis*. 1993;181: 71-79.
70. Alterman AI, McLellan AT, O'Brien CP, et al. Effectiveness and costs of inpatient versus day hospital cocaine rehabilitation. *J Nerv Ment Dis*. 1994;182: 157-163.
71. Higgins ST, Delaney DD, Budney AJ, et al. A behavioral approach to achieving initial cocaine abstinence. *Am J Psychiatry*. 1991;148:1218-1224.
72. Fox BS. Development of a therapeutic vaccine for the treatment of cocaine addiction. *Drug Alcohol Depend*. 1997;48:153-158.
73. O'Brien CP, McLellan AT. Myths about the treatment of addiction. *Lancet*. 1996;347:237-240.
74. McLellan AT, Alterman AI, Metzger DS, et al. Similarity of outcome predictors across opiate, cocaine and alcohol treatments. *J Clin Consult Psychol*. 1994;6: 1141-1158
75. Graber AL, Davidson P, Brown A, McRae J, Woolridge K. Dropout and relapse during diabetes care. *Diabetes Care*. 1992;15:1477-1483.
76. Clark LT. Improving compliance and increasing control of hypertension: needs of special hypertensive populations. *Am Heart J*. 1991;121:664-669.
77. Dekker FW, Dieleman FE, Kaptein AA, Mulder JD. Compliance with pulmonary medication in general practice. *Eur Respir J*. 1993;6:886-890.
78. Kurtz SM. Adherence to diabetic regimens: empirical status and clinical applications. *Diabetes Educ*. 1990;16:50-59.
79. Sinnock P. Hospitalization of diabetes. In: *Diabetes Data: National Diabetes Data Group*. Bethesda, Md: National Institutes of Health Press; 1985.
80. Schaub AF, Steiner A, Vetter W. Compliance to treatment. *J Clin Exp Hypertens*. 1993;15:1121-1130.
81. Institute of Medicine. *Managing Managed Care: Quality Improvement in Behavioral Health*. Washington, DC: National Academy Press; 1996.
82. Ball JC, Ross A. *The Effectiveness of Methadone Maintenance Treatment*. New York, NY: Springer-Verlag; 1991.
83. Ouimette PC, Moos RH, Finney JW. Influence of outpatient treatment and 12-step group involvement on one-year substance abuse treatment outcomes. *J Stud Alcohol*. 1998;59:513-522.
84. Vaillant GE. *The Natural History of Alcoholism Revisited*. Cambridge, Mass: Harvard University Press; 1995.
85. Vaillant GE. A long-term follow-up of male alcohol abuse. *Arch Gen Psychiatry*. 1996;53:243-249.
86. Lewis DC. The role of the generalist in the care of the substance abusing patient. *Med Clin North Am*. 1997;81:831-843.
87. Fleming MF. Who teaches residents about the prevention and treatment of substance abuse disorders? a national survey. *J Fam Pract*. 1999;48:725-729.
88. US Office of Personnel Management, Office of Insurance Programs, FEHB Program Carrier Letter, No. 1999-027. June 7, 1999.

ORIGINAL ARTICLE

A Long-term Follow-up of Male Alcohol Abuse

George E. Vaillant, MD

Background: This study attempted to determine the course of male alcohol abuse from the age of 40 years to 60 or 70 years, to estimate the duration of abstinence required for stable remission and to study the hypothesis of progression of symptoms in chronic alcohol abuse.

Methods: The subjects were 268 former Harvard University (Cambridge, Mass) undergraduates (college sample) and 456 nondelinquent inner-city adolescents (core city sample) who had been repeatedly studied in multidisciplinary fashion since 1940. Since 47 years of age, these men have been followed up biennially by questionnaire and every 5 years by physical examination. At some point during their lives, 55 (21%) of the college and 150 (33%) of the core city men met *DSM-III* criteria for alcohol abuse. The college cohort has been followed until the age of 70 years, the core city cohort until age 60 years. The dependent variables were mortality and alcohol abuse status every 5 years.

Results: By 60 years of age, 18% of the college alcohol abusers had died, 11% were abstinent, 11% were controlled drinkers, and 59% were known to be still abusing alcohol. By 60 years of age, 28% of the core city alcohol abusers had died, 30% were abstinent, 11% were controlled drinkers, and only 28% were known to be still abusing alcohol.

Conclusions: In three respects the two socially divergent samples resembled each other. After abstinence had been maintained for 5 years, relapse was rare. In contrast, return to controlled drinking without eventual relapse was unlikely. Alcohol abuse could continue for decades without remission or progression of symptoms. The samples differed in that the core city men began to abuse alcohol when younger and, although they were more likely than the college men to become alcohol dependent, the core city men were twice as likely to achieve stable abstinence.

(Arch Gen Psychiatry. 1996;53:243-249)

Approximately 100 000[1] deaths in the United States each year can be attributed directly or indirectly to alcohol; thus, alcohol abuse vies with strokes and accidents as the third most important cause of death in this country. Nevertheless, we know far more about the natural course of most cancers than we do of alcohol abuse. A major reason for our ignorance is the scarcity of long-term prospective follow-up studies.

Indeed, there are three unanswered questions regarding the clinical course of alcoholism that can be answered only by prolonged follow-up. First, why does the prevalence of alcohol abuse decline sharply with age?[2] Is the explanation for this decline stable abstinence, or return to asymptomatic drinking, or high mortality, or poor case finding among the elderly? Second, if alcohol abuse persists over the life course, does it really progress inexorably, as investigators such as Jellinek[3] believed? Or, over time, do some individuals without remission remain chronic alcohol abusers without progressing to dependence? Third, how long must abstinence or return to controlled drinking persist before an individual's recovery can be considered secure? In cancer, remission must often last for 5 years before relapse is considered unlikely. In alcohol treatment studies, however, investigators often speak of recovery after the alcohol abuser has been symptom-free for 6 months or 1 year.

To the extent that the natural course of alcoholism can be addressed from a 50-year study confined to white

See Subjects and Methods on next page

From Harvard Medical School and Brigham and Women's Hospital, Boston, Mass.

SUBJECTS AND METHODS

A prospective cohort study of two socially contrasting samples of men has been conducted since 1940.

STUDY PARTICIPANTS

The core city sample (mean±SD date of birth, 1929±2) included 456 men first studied from early adolescence until age 31 years as a nondelinquent control group for Glueck and Glueck's well-known studies of juvenile delinquents.[5,6] Ninety percent of these men came from working-class or welfare families; 61% of their parents were foreign-born. They resided in high-crime inner-city Boston, Mass, neighborhoods. Their mean IQ was 95±12; 48% graduated from high school and 7% from college. Their 1976 mean income was approximately $15 000. The sample included no African Americans.

At the time of original study, the men, their parents, and their teachers were interviewed individually. More than 90% of the surviving participants were reinterviewed at 25 and 31 years of age.[6] At these interviews alcohol abuse or its absence was specifically recorded. When the men reached age 47 years, a 2-hour semistructured interview with a detailed 23-item section on lifetime problem drinking was used to reinterview 87% of the surviving men.[4]

The college sample (mean±SD date of birth, 1921±2) included 268 Harvard University sophomores selected for a study of "normal" development from 1938 to 1942. Selection criteria required the absence of known physical or mental illness and a freshman grade average above C.[7] Although half of the sample worked during college to help pay tuition and/or were on scholarships, most of their parents were upper or middle class and were born in this country. Their estimated mean IQ was 130; 76% attended graduate school; and their 1976 mean income was approximately $50 000. Up to 47 years of age, the college sample was studied in roughly the same fashion as the core city sample; after age 47 years the college sample was studied in an identical manner to the core city sample.[4,8]

DATA COLLECTION

From age 47 years until the present, both groups were followed up by biennial questionnaires and by obtaining reports of physical examinations every 5 years. Besides gathering information regarding health, work, and relationships, the biennial questionnaires inquired about alcohol use. In addition to describing quantity and frequency of alcohol use, the men were asked five questions: whether (1) they, (2) their friends, (3) their families, or (4) their physicians had been concerned about their drinking, and (5) whether and for how long they had stopped drinking.

MEASUREMENT OF ALCOHOL ABUSE

Presence or Absence of Alcohol Abuse by Age 47 Years

For both samples, 2-hour interviews at age 48±3 years were performed by clinicians, most with two or more years of experience in alcohol clinics. Interviews at age 31 years and recent psychiatric, medical, and arrest records also were reviewed. These records confirmed the participants' self-reports and documented alcohol-related problems. On the basis of all of the available data, clinicians rated the men on two scales of alcohol abuse. (The core city men were also rated on an 11-point scale, developed by Cahalan,[9] to assess alcohol-related social deviance.)

The first scale from the American Psychiatric Association's *DSM-III*[10] reflected a three-category medical model for diagnosing alcoholism, where 1 represents no alcohol abuse; 2, alcohol abuse; and 3, alcohol dependence (tolerance or withdrawal symptoms from alcohol *in addition* to alcohol abuse). Diagnosis was made by consensus of two clinicians; the extensive evidence for convergent validity of diagnosis is discussed elsewhere.[4,8]

The second scale used was the Problem Drinking Scale, an equally weighted 16-point scale (similar to the Michigan Alcoholism Screening Test)[11] devised to combine the emphasis of the *DSM-III* on physiologic dependence and the emphasis of the Cahalan scale on social deviance. The scale assigned points for social, legal, medical, and employment problems caused by alcohol abuse and points for blackouts, going on the wagon, seeking treatment, and admitting to problems with control and withdrawal symptoms. Measurement of alcohol in a breath sample and laboratory drug screens were not performed.

Presence or Absence of Alcohol Abuse After Age 47 Years

Since age 47 years, if any man who was not previously classified as an alcohol abuser reported two or more of the four alcohol-related problems (eg, wife or physician complains, participant feeling guilty, etc) on the biennial questionnaire for two consecutive questionnaires (see the "Data Collection" section), he was reclassified as an alcohol abuser. Because the follow-up depended largely on questionnaires, after age 47 years no further attempt was made to distinguish alcohol abuse from dependence. Progression

men, this report will attempt to provide answers to the three questions posed above. The report prospectively builds on a 1976 follow-up study[4] of two contrasting community samples: 456 underprivileged inner-city adolescents and 268 Harvard University (Cambridge, Mass) sophomores. In the current study, all the alcohol abusers identified in those samples were followed up until 60 years of age (the core city men) and 70 years of age (the college men).

RESULTS

AGE AT ONSET OF ALCOHOL ABUSE

By age 70 years, 52 (21%) of the 249 college men who remained in the study at age 47 years had met *DSM-III* criteria for alcohol abuse (as had three of the 13 who dropped out of the study). At some point, 21 (38%) of the 55 men also met *DSM-III* criteria for dependence. By of symptoms, however, could be determined from the serial physical exams and assessments of social functioning.

Age at Onset of Alcohol Abuse

The age at which each participant first met criteria for alcohol abuse was estimated from the repeated interviews and questionnaires. Age at development of dependence was not determined.

SMOKING

Pack-years of cigarette smoking were estimated by review of all information at age 47 years and at age 60 years. Age at stable smoking cessation was estimated.

OUTCOME DEFINITIONS

Quinquennial alcohol use status was determined by estimating the use or abuse status of each alcohol abuser every 5 years. This status estimate was based on the questionnaires administered every 2 years and physical examinations obtained every 5 years.

Alcohol use or abuse status was categorized as follows: (1) *abstinent:* less than one drink (0.5 oz of alcohol) per month for more than a year; (2) *social drinker:* not yet an abuser, or follow-up suggests that original diagnosis of *DSM-III* alcohol abuse could be challenged because of brief duration (<5 years) *and* minimal symptoms (Problem Drinking Scale score <5) *and* subsequent problem-free drinking for 10 years or more; (3) *return to controlled drinking:* a former alcohol abuser consuming more than one drink per month for at least 2 years but with no reported problems; (4) *continued alcohol abuse:* clear history of sustained alcohol abuse and one or more acknowledged problems caused by drinking in the past 2 years; relapse to *alcohol abuse* from a status of *stable abstinence* or of *stable return to controlled drinking* required reporting at least *two* or more problems caused by alcohol use; and (5) *dead:* death certificates were obtained for all alcohol abusers (and nonabusers) categorized as deceased.

Complete physical examinations were sought for all subjects every 5 years. Data from physical examinations and death certificates were used to determine presence or absence of *cancer* and *heart disease.*

Final outcome status was determined as follows. At the most recent follow-up or at the time of death or long-term institutionalization, each alcohol abuser was assigned to one of four categories: (1) *stable abstinence* in the community (3 years or more); (2) *stable return to controlled drinking* (3 years or more); (3) *reclassified social drinker* (original diagnosis of previous alcohol abuse open to question because of brevity, minimal symptoms (Problem Drinking Scale score <5), and 10 to 40 years of return to social drinking; and (4) *chronic alcohol abuse,* which was alcohol abuse, usually chronic, during the last 3 years of follow-up or during the 3 years before death or institutionalization. (Although this broad definition theoretically could include men who had abused alcohol for only 1 year, 83 of the 86 men assigned to this outcome category had abused alcohol for 6 to 40 years. The three exceptions died after 1, 3, and 5 years of alcohol abuse, respectively.)

ATTRITION

Before age 47 years, 19 (7%) of the 268 men from the college sample could not be classified for presence or absence of alcohol abuse because of nonparticipation or death in World War II. Before age 47 years, 23 (5%) of the 456 core city men could not be classified because of early death, nonparticipation, or difficulty in location.

Since age 47 years, the alcohol-abusing subjects in both samples were less likely than nonabusers to return questionnaires, but not significantly so. In an average mailing, 61% of non–alcohol abusers and 53% of abusers returned questionnaires. Questionnaire nonresponders were interviewed by telephone or in person. Subjects with whom contact was lost and nonresponding subjects were traced through credit agencies and departments of motor vehicles. During any given 5-year period, no more than 2% to 3% of participants were unavailable, and only 1% of the sample appeared permanently unavailable. Alcohol-abusing participants were somewhat more likely to withdraw from the study. As of 1992, 21 of the known 150 alcohol-abusing core city men and two of the known 52 alcohol-abusing college men had dropped out. The mortality of nonresponders and dropouts was monitored through the National Death Index.

STATISTICAL ANALYSIS

The significance of differences between groups was determined by the χ^2 test for categoric predictors or Student's t test for continuous predictors. All tests were two tailed, with a P value of .05 considered significant. The log-rank test was used to contrast age at onset of alcohol abuse between the two groups. Logistic regression was employed to determine whether alcohol abuse was a risk factor for mortality even after controlling for multiple hypothesized risk factors (obesity, blood cholesterol level, blood pressure, and smoking). Results are presented as odds ratios and are accompanied by 95% confidence intervals.

age 60 years, 150 (35%) of the 433 core city men who remained in the study at age 47 years whose alcohol abuse status was known had met *DSM-III* criteria for alcohol abuse. At some point, 77 (51%) of the core city alcohol abusers also met criteria for alcohol dependence. The average age at onset of alcohol abuse was a decade later for the 51 college men who developed alcohol abuse by age 60 years (mean, 40.2±9.9 years) than it was for the 149 core city men (mean, 29.2±9.5 years). **Figure 1** illustrates graphically the differing age at onset between the two groups. The difference was highly significant (log-rank statistic=38.5, df=1, P<.01).

OUTCOME STATUS OF ALCOHOL ABUSERS

Table 1 summarizes the outcome status for the two cohorts at age 60 years. As noted, 21 of the 150 core city alcohol abusers dropped out of the study after age 47 years.

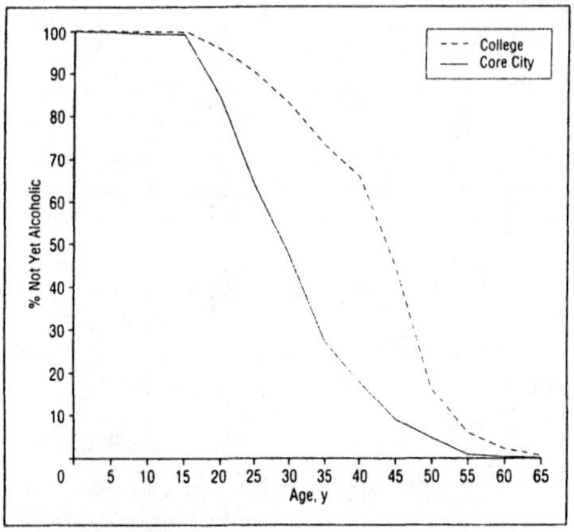

Figure 1. *Approximate age at which each of the 150 core city and the 52 college alcohol abusers with complete data sets first met the* DSM-III *criteria for alcohol abuse. Age at onset before age 45 years was based in part on retrospective data.*

Roughly half of the men in both samples achieved stable remission, but stable abstinence was significantly more common in the core city cohort. Of the 129 core city men whose alcoholic careers were known, only 31% (n=19) of the 62 core city men who met criteria for alcohol abuse achieved stable abstinence, in contrast to 43% (n=29) of the 67 core city men classified as dependent. However, this difference did not reach statistical significance (χ^2=2.2, *df*=1, *P*=.14). Of the 18 core city men who returned to controlled drinking, nine (50%) had met criteria for alcohol dependence. An equal proportion, 28 (51%), of the 55 men who continued to abuse alcohol until age 60 years or death were alcohol dependent.

Table 1 also shows that by age 60 years, 38 (25%) of the 150 core city alcohol abusers had died. In contrast, only 37 (14%) of the 264 core city non–alcohol abusers had died (χ^2=8.3, *df*=1, *P*<.01). For the same period (20 to 60 years of age), the comparable mortality for white men living in the United States was also 14%.[12] Of the 78 core city men who met criteria for alcohol dependence, 25 (32%) died; this was significantly more than the 13 (18%) of the 72 alcohol abusers who died by age 60 years (χ^2=3.9, *df*=1, *P*<.05).

At age 60 years, the comparable mortality for the 194 nonalcoholic college men was only 5%—much lower than the national rate and only a third of the 15% mortality noted for alcohol-abusing college men. By age 70 years, 13 (62%) of the 21 alcohol-dependent college men were dead, contrasted to 17% of the 228 non–alcohol-dependent college men (χ^2=23.4, *df*=1, *P*<.01). For comparison, 40% of 20-year-old white men living in the United States would be dead by age 70 years.[12]

In both samples, the risk of heart disease and cancer was roughly two times the risk for alcohol abusers as for non–alcohol abusers. Heavy smoking greatly increased the mortality of alcohol abusers in both groups. Thirty (31%) of the 97 core city alcohol abusers with sustained one-pack-per-day smoking habits died before age

Table 1. Final Outcome Status for the Two Cohorts of Alcohol Abusers at Last Contact or Time of Death ...

	No. (%)	
	College (n=52)*	**Core City (n=129)†**
Stable abstinence (≥3 y)	10 (19)	48 (37)‡
Return to controlled drinking (≥3 y)	5 (10)	18 (14)
Reclassified as social drinker	6 (11.5)	8 (6)
Chronic alcohol abuse	31 (59.5)	55 (43)
Total	**52 (100)**	**129 (100)**
Dead by age 60 y	8 (15)	38 (25)
Dead by age 70 y	22 (40)§	...

**N=52 because data sets for three alcohol abusers are incomplete.*

†N=129 because data sets for 21 core city alcohol abusers are incomplete.

‡χ^2=5.5, df=2, P=.02.

§The death rate for 55 college alcohol abusers was significantly greater than the 16% of 194 college nonalcoholics who had died by age 70 years (χ^2=15.6, df=1, P<.01).

60 years; 24 (22%) of the 111 similarly heavy-smoking but non–alcohol-abusing core city participants died before age 60 years. Only 16 (11%) of the 146 non–heavy-smoking, non–alcohol-abusing core city men were dead. Among the 52 college alcohol abusers, 15 of the 22 deaths by age 70 years occurred among the 23 alcohol abusers with the heaviest (≥50 pack-year) smoking habits. When the effect of smoking was controlled by logistic regression, the odds ratio for mortality among the alcohol abusers remained clinically and statistically significant in the college sample (odds ratio, 3.32 [95% confidence interval, 1.40 to 7.91]) and in the core city sample (odds ratio, 2.71 [95% confidence interval, 1.30 to 5.63]).

Alcohol abuse appeared associated with failure to stop smoking. For example, by age 65 years, 54 (84%) of the 64 heavy-smoking but nonalcoholic college men had stopped smoking. In contrast, only 15 (37%) of the 41 heavy-smoking *and* alcohol-abusing college men had stopped smoking. This difference between the two groups in smoking cessation was significant (χ^2=25.6, *df*=1, *P*<.01).

PROGRESSION OF SYMPTOMS

Figure 2 depicts the life course of alcohol abuse among the core city alcohol abusers who have continued to participate in the study. The number of subjects is 121 and not 129 because the eight core city alcohol abusers who were reclassified as social drinkers in Table 1 were excluded. At age 60 years, data were missing for nine of these 121 core city alcohol abusers. Only 30 (27%) of the remaining 112 men were still classified as alcohol abusers at age 60 years. This reduction in prevalence of alcohol abuse resulted more from high mortality (n=31 [28%]) and stable abstinence (n=34 [30%]) than from return to controlled drinking (n=12 [11%]).

Figure 3 demonstrates that the life course of alcohol abuse for the college men was similar to that for the core city men, except that the core city men began abusing alcohol at a younger age and appeared more likely to achieve stable abstinence. At age 60 years, excluding

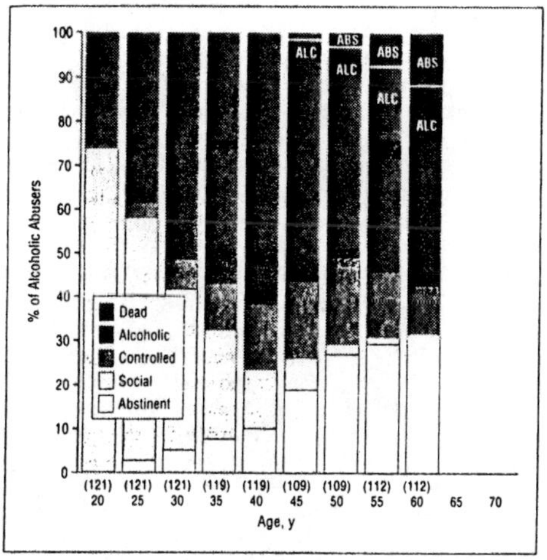

Figure 2. *Quinquennial alcohol use status of the 121 core city men who remained active in the study and met the criteria for* DSM-III *alcohol abuse. (The eight men who were reclassified as social drinkers because of brief duration of alcohol abuse and minimal symptoms have been excluded.) ALC indicates the proportion of deaths that occurred among alcohol abusers; ABS, the proportion among stably abstinent men.*

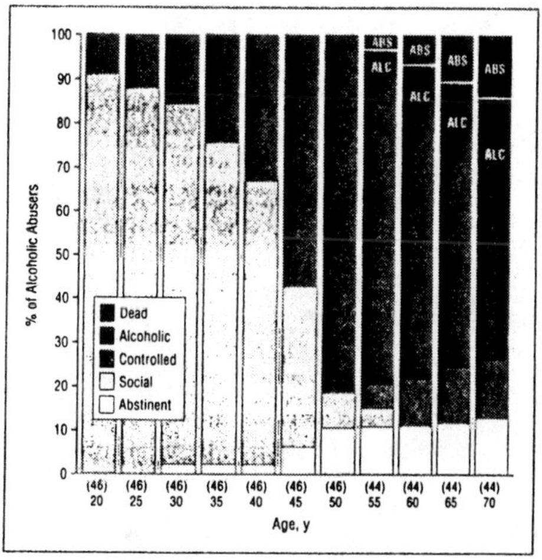

Figure 3. *Quinquennial alcohol use status of the 46 college men who met* DSM-III *criteria for alcohol abuse. (The six alcohol abusers reclassified as social drinkers and the three alcohol abusers with incomplete data sets have been excluded.) ALC indicates the proportion of deaths that occurred among alcohol abusers; ABS, the proportion among stably abstinent men.*

six men reclassified as social drinkers and two men with missing data, eight (18%) of the remaining 44 college men were dead, five (11%) were classified as abstinent, and five (11%) were classified as controlled drinkers. At age 60 years, 26 (59%), and at age 70 years, only 14 (32%), of the college men were still abusing alcohol. Just as the mean age of alcohol abuse onset was a decade later for the college sample, their mean age of peak prevalence and then their steady decline in alcohol abuse appeared to occur a decade later.

Many members of the surviving college sample spent the last 20 years (ages 50 to 70 years) alternating between periods of controlled drinking and periods of alcohol abuse. They reported continued alcohol-related problems with their health, self-esteem, and families. Yet, despite decades of observation, their sustained patterns of alcohol abuse seldom progressed to job loss, dependence, or the need for detoxification.

It is possible that alcohol dependence contributes to the likelihood of stable abstinence. None of the 34 college men who met criteria only for alcohol abuse achieved five or more years of abstinence, in contrast to 10 (48%) of the 21 college men classified dependent (χ^2=11.0, df=1, P<.01). As noted previously, the alcohol-dependent core city men were also more likely to become abstinent, but the difference was not statistically significant. About 40% of men with stable abstinence in each cohort attended Alcoholics Anonymous for a year or more.

DURATION OF ABSTINENCE REQUIRED FOR STABLE REMISSION

The association between length of abstinence and probability of relapse was examined for the 10 college and 46 core city alcohol abusers who reported at least 2 years of abstinence and who subsequently survived for at least 8 years. Eventual relapse to alcohol abuse occurred in 23 (41%) of the 56 men who reported 2 years of abstinence. Nine relapses occurred in year 3, five relapses in year 4, six relapses during years 5 through 7, and three relapses during years 8 through 13. After 6 years of abstinence, subsequent relapse to abuse of alcohol seemed unlikely. The mean length of recorded abstinence among the 33 men not reporting relapse was 18 years (range, 9 to 33 years).

Table 2 shows that if 5 to 6 years of abstinence was adequate to predict stable future abstinence, return to controlled drinking was a much less stable state. In 1977, at the end of the age 20 to 47 years follow-up period, 21 of the core city men had been classified as having achieved stable abstinence of 3 years or more, and 22 men had been classified as returned to controlled drinking for 3 years or more.[4] Of the 21 core city men with 3 or more years of abstinence in 1977, 18 (86%) were still abstinent in 1992 or at death. The mean length of known abstinence for these 18 men was 20 years (range, 3 to 37 years). Of the 22 men with 3 or more years of controlled drinking, only eight men (including three who were reclassified as social drinkers) were *still* known to be drinking in a controlled fashion in 1992 or at death. Three others became stably abstinent and four withdrew from the study. For the seven controlled drinkers who relapsed to sustained alcohol abuse, the mean duration of alleged controlled drinking before relapse was 12 years (range, 5 to 28 years).

COMMENT

Longitudinal studies appear necessary to understand alcohol abuse. First, some studies have suggested that in-

Table 2. Long-term Course of Core City Men Identified in 1977 as Practicing Stable Abstinence or Return to Controlled Drinking

	1977 Status	
1992 Status	≥3 y of Abstinence (<1974-1977) (n=21)	≥3 y of Controlled Drinking (<1974-1977) (n=22)
Abstinent	18	3
Controlled drinking	1	8*
Relapse	1†	7
Dropped out or contact lost	1†	4‡

*Three of these eight men abused alcohol only briefly, with minimal symptoms, and were reclassified as social drinkers.

†Before relapse or loss of contact, both these men were abstinent for 13 years.

‡The mean length of controlled drinking before loss of contact was 8 years.

dividual alcohol abuse is unstable and fluctuates greatly over time.[4] Such a picture is derived from cross-sectional "snapshots" obtained over too short a time frame. In the present study of men's lives examined in 5-year blocks rather than in 1-month blocks, alcohol abuse appeared relatively stable. Men identified as alcohol abusers, when contrasted to social drinkers, appeared to continue to experience far more alcohol-related problems, not the least of which was a twofold increase in mortality. In part, the increased mortality may be mediated by the failure of alcohol abusers to stop smoking.[13]

Nevertheless, as the alcohol abusers aged, the prevalence of alcohol abuse steadily declined. At age 60 years, only 28% of the surviving core city abusers whose status was known were still symptomatic. At age 70 years, only 32% of the surviving college abusers were still symptomatic. The reasons for this decline were both stable abstinence *and* high mortality.

By studying only the severely alcohol-dependent clients of detoxification centers, clinicians often believe that Jellinek[3] was right in asserting that alcoholism is a "progressive disease." However, the long-term evidence from a community sample such as the present one suggests that, rather than progressing, chronic alcohol abuse often appears merely to fluctuate in severity. Analogous to the reported eating habits of the chronically obese, the reported daily alcohol consumption of many of the college alcohol abusers fell within normal limits. However, analogous to the obese, alcohol abusers in concert with their friends, relatives, and physicians continue to perceive their alcohol use as problematic.

Since systematic follow-ups of abstinent alcohol abusers are seldom undertaken, the long-term stability of abstinence has been unclear. However, data from the few existing follow-up studies support the finding from this study that 2 years of abstinence is inadequate to provide a basis for long-term prognosis. Reanalysis of data from a previously reported 8-year follow-up[14] noted that, when followed up from 4 to 14 years (mean, 8 years), 45% of 33 alcohol-dependent men and women relapsed after 2 years of abstinence. However, after 5 years of follow-up, only 9% relapsed, and none relapsed after 6 years. In another follow-up of 29 alcohol abusers already abstinent for 2 years, six (21%) relapsed within the next 2 years.[15]

Finally, short-term epidemiologic studies such as the RAND report have suggested that return to controlled drinking is relatively common.[16] However, long-term follow-up studies of controlled drinking[17-19] have confirmed the findings in Table 2 that return to a stable pattern of trouble-free drinking among chronic alcohol abusers is unlikely.

Since these contrasting cohorts of white men born between 1917 and 1932 are small and hardly representative of the general population, the above conclusions may not be broadly applicable. However, controlling for birth cohort and sex, the lifetime rate of alcohol abuse in the two cohorts is roughly the same as that observed for United States population samples.[2,4] In addition, most findings from the study were similar for the two socioeconomically very different samples.

The findings are limited by the absence of information from significant others. The fact that the follow-up data in this article were obtained by self-report does not control for heavy drinkers who manifested but failed to acknowledge alcohol-related problems. Such men would have been incorrectly classified as having returned to controlled drinking. Three factors mitigate this limitation. First, some men undoubtedly were alcohol abusers who denied problems, but their total number cannot be large. Of the 181 alcohol abusers in the study who were assigned final outcome status in Table 1, only 23 (13%) were actually classified as having returned to controlled drinking. Second, the self-reports of sustained abstinence (mean duration, 19 years) and of active alcohol abuse can be considered relatively reliable. Third, the study depended on "CAGE"-type questions[20] to identify alcohol-related problems on the biennial questionnaire. (CAGE is an acronym for questions about cutting down on drinking, annoyance at others' concern about drinking, feeling guilty about drinking, and using alcohol as an eye-opener in the morning.) Although the present data and data from other studies suggest that alcohol abusers underreport daily alcohol consumption by about 50%,[21] studies that have used the CAGE-type questions yield relatively reliable data that are superior to biochemical tests and roughly comparable with data obtained from significant others.[22,23]

Because of their highly selective nature, the samples enjoyed two serendipitous advantages that may actually help to elucidate the course of alcoholism for the general population. First, both samples were selected as normal nondelinquent adolescents in subcultures and during historical epochs in which alcohol was the principal drug of abuse. Thus, the confounding problems of dual diagnosis (eg, sociopathy, polydrug abuse, and schizophrenia) that obscure the natural course of alcohol abuse were minimized. Second, since the men shared the same contemporary culture and historical epoch, they experienced similar federal controls, alcohol cost structure, and drinking mores. Recovery from alcohol abuse could be viewed as a function of the natural course of the disorder rather than the result of changes in social mores.

The significant differences in age at onset of alcohol abuse between the college and core city samples were probably a result of the fact that familial disorganization, late adolescent delinquency, and dropping out of school—far more common among the core city sample—all lead to increased risk for early onset of drug abuse of all kinds and to rapid progression of alcohol abuse to dependence.[24]

This report has not discussed predictors of recovery nor reviewed other long-term studies of the natural course of alcohol abuse. However, these topics are reviewed at length in a recently published book.[25] As in the long-term follow-up by Edwards et al,[26] variables as promising as alcoholic heredity, family disorganization, number and severity of alcohol problems, and alcohol clinic treatment fail to predict long-term outcome. In part, this failure of prediction is because alcohol abusers with the best prognosis come from two divergent groups. On the one hand, socially disadvantaged men, in part as a function of the early onset of severe alcohol dependence, often become stably abstinent. However, because of poor health habits (especially smoking and diet), they are also more likely to die. On the other hand, alcohol abusers with excellent social supports, high education, good health habits, and late onset of minimal alcohol abuse are more likely to survive and resume problem-free drinking, but such men also appeared more likely to maintain a pattern of lifelong intermittent alcohol abuse. Thus, as Figure 3 illustrates, the college sample despite their educational and social advantages were less likely to abstain from their alcohol abuse than were the disadvantaged core city sample.

Accepted for publication July 10, 1995.

This work was supported by research grants KO5-MH00364 and MH42248 from the National Institute of Mental Health, Bethesda, Md.

I am indebted to John Orav, PhD, for helpful advice. As is evident in my coauthored articles, the bibliography, and the acknowledgments in my cited books, at least a score of individuals, living and dead, could be included as coauthors in this 50-year study.

Reprint requests to Division of Psychiatry, Brigham and Women's Hospital, 75 Francis St, Boston, MA 02115 (Dr Vaillant).

REFERENCES

1. McGinnis JM, Foege WH. Actual causes of death in the United States. *JAMA.* 1993;270:2207-2212.
2. Robins LN, Regier DA. *Psychiatric Disorders in America.* New York, NY: Free Press; 1991.
3. Jellinek EM. *The Disease Concept of Alcoholism.* New Haven, Conn: Hillhouse Press; 1960.
4. Vaillant GE. *The Natural History of Alcoholism: Paths to Recovery.* Cambridge, Mass: Harvard University Press; 1983.
5. Glueck S, Glueck E. *Unraveling Juvenile Delinquency.* New York, NY: Commonwealth Fund; 1950.
6. Glueck S, Glueck E. *Delinquents and Nondelinquents in Perspective.* Cambridge, Mass: Harvard University Press; 1968.
7. Heath CW. *What People Are.* Cambridge, Mass: Harvard University Press; 1945.
8. Vaillant GE, Schnurr PP, Baron JA, Gerber PD. A prospective study of the effects of cigarette smoking and alcohol abuse on mortality. *J Gen Intern Med.* 1991;6:299-304.
9. Cahalan D. *Problem Drinkers: A National Survey.* San Francisco, Calif: Jossey Bass Inc; 1970.
10. American Psychiatric Association, Committee on Nomenclature and Statistics. *Diagnostic and Statistical Manual of Mental Disorders, Third Edition.* Washington, DC: American Psychiatric Association Press; 1980.
11. Selzer ML. The Michigan alcoholism screening test: the quest for a new diagnostic instrument. *Am J Psychiatry.* 1971;127:1653-1658.
12. *Vital Statistics of the United States, Volume II—Mortality.* Washington, DC: US Dept of Health Statistics; 1988.
13. DiFranza J, Guerrera M. Alcoholism and smoking. *J Stud Alcohol.* 1990;51:130-135.
14. Vaillant GE, Clark W, Cyrus C, et al. Prospective study of alcoholism treatment: eight-year follow-up. *Am J Med.* 1983;75:455-463.
15. Loosen PT, Dew BW, Prange AJ. Long-term predictors of outcome in abstinent alcoholic men. *Am J Psychiatry.* 1990;147:1662-1666.
16. Armor DJ, Polich JM, Stanbul HB. *Alcoholism and Treatment.* New York, NY: John Wiley & Sons Inc; 1978.
17. Pendery ML, Maltzman IM, West LJ. Controlled drinking by alcoholics? New findings and a reevaluation of a major affirmative study. *Science.* 1982;217:169-175.
18. Edwards G. A later follow-up of a classic case series: D. L. Davies' 1962 report and its significance for the present. *J Stud Alcohol.* 1985;46:181-190.
19. Miller WR, Leckman AL, Delaney HD, Tinkcom M. Long-term follow-up of behavioral self-control training. *J Stud Alcohol.* 1992;53:249-261.
20. Ewing JA. Detecting alcoholism: the CAGE questionnaire. *JAMA.* 1984;252:1905-1907.
21. Smith PF, Remington PL, Williamson DF, Anda RF. A comparison of alcohol sales data with survey data on self-reported alcohol use in 21 states. *Am J Public Health.* 1990;80:309-312.
22. Moore RD, Bone LR, Geller G, Mamon JA, Stokes EJ, Levine DM. Prevalence, detection, and treatment of alcoholism in hospitalized patients. *JAMA.* 1989;261:403-407.
23. Cyr MG, Wortman SA. The effectiveness of routine screening questions in the detection of alcoholism. *JAMA.* 1988;259:51-54.
24. Vaillant GE. Evidence that the type 1/type 2 dichotomy in alcoholism must be re-examined. *Addiction.* 1994;89:1049-1057.
25. Vaillant GE. *The Natural History of Alcoholism Revisited.* Cambridge, Mass: Harvard University Press; 1995.
26. Edwards G, Brown D, Oppenheimer E, Sheehan M, Taylor C, Duckitt A. Long-term outcome for patients with drinking problems: the search for predictors. *Br J Addict.* 1988;83:917-927.

An Evolutionary Perspective on Substance Abuse

Randolph M. Nesse
Department of Psychiatry, University of Michigan, Ann Arbor, Michigan

This article describes how recent advances in understanding the evolutionary functions of emotions can help to reconcile diverse approaches to substance abuse. Emotions can be understood as specialized states that prepare individuals to cope with opportunities and threats. Drugs that artificially induce pleasure or block normal suffering disrupt these evolved mechanisms, and thus should tend to interfere with adaptive behavior, even if the drugs are medically safe. Nonetheless, we routinely use drugs quite safely to block defenses like pain, cough, and anxiety. This apparent contradiction is explained by the relatively small costs of defenses compared to the potentially huge costs of not expressing a defensive response when it is needed. An evolutionary perspective has implications for substance abuse research, treatment, and social policy. This perspective suggests that the search for etiology needs to address the human tendency to abuse drugs separately from individual differences in these tendencies, that clinical treatments that take account of the broad range of patients' emotional life are well justified, and that social policies need to address substance use and abuse not as diseases to be cured but as human tendencies that need to be managed. To prepare for future drugs that will likely alter emotions safely, we urgently need a better understanding of the adaptive function of the emotions.

KEY WORDS: Substance abuse; Evolution; Adaptation; Drugs; Psychiatry

INTRODUCTION

Over 18,000 articles have been published about substance abuse in the past 25 years. Despite this huge outpouring of facts and theory, fundamental questions remain unresolved (Shaffer 1986; Brower et al. 1989). Disagreements continue concerning whether substance abuse is a disease, a behavior, a psychological problem, a social problem, or a moral issue. Arguments rage over such issues as whether substance abuse is caused mainly by genetic factors, life experi-

Received December 16, 1993; revised September 17, 1994.

Address reprint requests and correspondence to: Randolph M. Nesse, M.D., Department of Psychiatry, University of Michigan, Med-Inn Building, Room C440, Ann Arbor, MI 48109-0840, U.S.A., randolph.nesse@med.umich.edu

Ethology and Sociobiology 15: 339–348 (1994)

655 Avenue of the Americas, New York, NY 10010

ences, social situations, or some combination. Divergent answers to these questions arise not so much from disagreement about facts but from different ways of thinking about substance abuse.

This article develops an evolutionary framework for thinking about substance abuse that can encompass otherwise divergent approaches. While natural selection has not directly shaped a trait that motivates substance abuse, it has shaped the behavior regulation mechanisms on which psychotropic drugs act, most specifically, the emotions. Understanding the origins and functions of emotional pleasures and pains leads to insights about why people use psychoactive substances. These insights have implications for treatment, research and public policy.

THE EVOLUTION OF EMOTIONS

The utility of the emotions as communications, motivations, and influences on future behavior has long been recognized, but a modern evolutionary approach specifies more precisely how the capacities for particular emotions increased the reproductive success of individuals in past generations. By emotion, I mean a pattern of coordinated changes in physiology, cognition, behavioral tendencies, and subjective experience that prepare an individual to cope especially well with a particular kind of situation. The capacities for emotions and their regulating mechanisms have been shaped by natural selection, which maximizes reproductive success, not survival (Daly and Wilson 1983), and maximizes individual fitness, not that of groups or species (Williams 1966; Dawkins 1976). It is widely recognized that emotional capacities evolved for life in hunter-gatherer bands and may be maladaptive in a modern setting (Konner 1983).

An evolutionary approach increasingly is providing a foundation for research on the emotions (Plutchik and Kellerman 1980; McNaughton 1989; Nesse 1990). Previously, many authors tried to specify the adaptive function for each emotion, just as one would for the turtle's shell or the bluebird's song. For instance, fear was said to motivate avoidance of danger, and romantic love to increase the success of courtship. Such explanations are limited, however, because one emotion may serve many functions (e.g., fear causes physiological arousal, communicates danger to others, inhibits socially unacceptable behavior, and motivates escape and avoidance), and several emotions may unite to serve one function (e.g., fear, envy, and anger combine to prevent the loss of a mate). Emotions are different from other traits in that they correspond not to specific functions but to specific situations. They have been shaped by the adaptive challenges of certain situations that have repeatedly influenced fitness during the course of evolution.

An important characteristic of the emotions is that they are all, to some degree, pleasurable or painful. There are no hedonically neutral emotions because the force of natural selection acts only when fitness is increased or decreased. In general, opportunities and satisfactions induce pleasure, and threats and losses induce pain. People abuse drugs mainly to seek pleasure and to avoid pain. Understanding the adaptive significance of painful and pleasurable aspects of the emotions is an essential first step for understanding why people abuse drugs and how drug use interferes with adaptation.

PAIN, PLEASURE, AND DRUGS

The aversiveness of painful emotions motivates escape from danger and avoidance of threats. Physical pain motivates withdrawal from situations that are damaging bodily tissues, and the arousal associated with pain mobilizes the ability to escape and prevents reoccurrence. Congenital lack of capacity for pain is a serious handicap that results in severe orthopedic problems in early adulthood (Osuntokun et al. 1968). Diarrhea expels toxins from the gastrointestinal tract. Patients with shigellosis who receive antidiarrheal drugs have slower recoveries and more complications (DuPont and Hornick 1973). Cough clears foreign material from the respiratory tract. A depressed cough reflex increases susceptibility to pneumonia. Each of these capacities is aversive, but useful. Blocking such defensive responses generally decreases fitness (Williams and Nesse 1991).

The aversive emotions seem to serve similar functions. Fear, guilt, anger, grief, and low mood protect against threats to relationships, resources, and social status, in addition to threats to bodily integrity (Thornhill and Thornhill 1989). Social dangers reduce reproductive success by their influence on mating opportunities and position in the group. Impairment of the capacities for mental pain is often maladaptive. For instance, a person without the capacity for fear would not likely survive long among the predators on the savannah (Marks 1987). Phobic avoidance of the rock that last month hid a tiger might seem senseless, but would nonetheless be wise if there is even a small chance that the tiger is there again. We usually experience some anxiety because most of the time we face some threat or another. Calm contentment is not the normal state of the organism.

Experiences that tend to increase Darwinian fitness tend to arouse pleasure, and pleasure tends to generate future actions that repeat such experiences (Nesse 1990). Good food, sex, friendship, having children, being admired, having insight—these experiences bring pleasure, and people who successfully pursue them have a reproductive advantage. Psychoactive drugs short-circuit these evolved mechanisms. Cocaine and opium by-pass perception and cognition to directly stimulate the brain mechanisms that regulate pleasure. The mind signals that this experience is strongly increasing fitness, hence the tendency to repeat such experiences. Compared to such pleasure, most ordinary life satisfactions are feeble. Furthermore, continued drug use both desensitizes brain pleasure mechanisms and disrupts normal behavior regulation mechanisms; so ordinary life becomes doubly less rewarding. Compared to what everyday life can offer, satisfactions provided by drugs become greater and greater, in the well-known feedback spiral of chronic substance abuse (Alexander and Hadaway 1982, p. 376).

WHY NOT USE DRUGS?

"If drugs make people feel better, why not use them?" It is a fair question, and one that substance abusers often ask. They receive many answers. Drugs can cause disease or death or brain damage. Drugs are addicting and become the center of the user's existence. Drugs have withdrawal effects. Such answers emphasize addiction and medical dangers. Are these the only reasons not to use drugs? As new agents without these dangers become available, will there be any medical reasons to avoid their use?

An evolutionary view emphasizes a different danger. In a manner of speaking, drugs are like magnets near the compass of the mind. Any drug that disrupts the emotional guidance system shaped by natural selection an be expected to impair the person's ability to behave adaptively. No matter how medically safe and nonaddicting, all psychotropic drugs should, for this reason alone, be considered potentially harmful.

OVERPROTECTIVE MOTHER NATURE

How, then, can we explain the seeming safety of many drugs? Many drugs we take for everyday ailments—cough, fever, pain, nausea, and diarrhea—seem to cause little harm. And caffeine, alcohol, and nicotine in moderate amounts seem not to interfere with our ability to act adaptively. In fact, they can increase our ability to perform certain tasks (Hanna and Hornick 1977; Pomerleau and Pomerleau 1987; Thayer 1989). If these drugs block normal evolved systems, why don't they cause harm?

Consider the selective forces that shaped the regulation of defensive responses. Every control system makes some errors of excessive response and some errors of deficient response. Defenses are usually inexpensive, while failure to express a defense when it is needed can be catastrophic. Natural selection therefore tends to shape control mechanisms that err on the side of over-responsiveness for inexpensive actions that may prevent great harm. This is why cough suppressants, aspirin, and antianxiety agents can so often be used safely.

A slightly different argument applies to pleasure. While it is important that positive emotions usually accompany behaviors that increase fitness, occasional impairment of pleasure is not catastrophic. If, however, intense pleasure accompanies behaviors that don't increase fitness, much time and effort may be wasted. Modern life provides so many such pleasures—playing video games is an example—that we tend not to recognize that the pleasure they provide is artificial and usually unrelated to fitness.

Selection seems to have created a mind that cannot be satisfied. We no sooner accomplish one goal than satisfaction fades and we are driven towards another. It is possible to get enough food and water, for a time, at least, but no amount of social status seems to be enough. To the extent that status increases fitness, genes that code for acting in ways that increase status will tend to spread; genes that result in lack of such striving will be gradually eliminated. The systems that motivate us were shaped to benefit our genes, not our selves. Our minds were shaped to maximize fitness, not happiness.

ETIOLOGY OF SUBSTANCE ABUSE

An evolutionary framework suggests that two separate questions need to be asked about the etiology of substance abuse: (1) Why do all humans have the capacity for substance abuse? (2) Why do people differ in their susceptibility to substance abuse?

An answer to the first question is straightforward: We all have a capacity for substance abuse because our motivational systems can be directly influenced by chemicals (Frye 1980). The seeking of certain chemicals is one manifestation of the generally adaptive tendency to repeat behaviors that bring pleasure. In this sense, trying to explain why humans use drugs is like trying to explain why people eat. The difference, of course, is that food intake is useful and selection has shaped specialized brain mechanisms that regulate food intake, while no mechanisms have evolved specifically to regulate psychotropic drug intake. An evolutionary view supports Siegel's suggestion that substance abuse is best approached as a normal human tendency, but it flatly contradicts his suggestion that drug seeking is a "fourth drive" (Siegel 1989).

In the debate about whether substance abuse should be considered a medical disease, an evolutionary view supports a medical model in that substance abuse is not just socially unacceptable, but is biologically maladaptive. Also, patterns of substance abuse can be viewed as syndromes with typical courses that result from exposure to novel agents. However, as we shall see, an evolutionary approach also suggests that the search for a specific medical etiology for substance abuse may well prove fruitless.

INDIVIDUAL SUSCEPTIBILITY TO SUBSTANCE ABUSE

Differences in individual susceptibility to substance abuse result in part from genetic differences. Twin studies (Goodwin 1986), family history studies (Cloninger 1981), and adoption studies (Schuckit 1985) show an increased risk of substance abuse for male offspring of alcoholics. Being raised by an alcoholic parent seems not to increase the risk, but the genetic offspring of alcoholics have alcoholism rates four times as high as those in the general population, even when they are reared in a nonalcoholic family (Goodwin). In a prospective study, the quality of the childhood environment, I.Q., and the parental social class were extremely weak predictors of adult alcohol abuse, while a family history of alcoholism and the absence of Mediterranean ancestry were strong predictors (Vaillant 1983). One study is currently following 470 men from their college years through midlife to determine the factors that predict substance abuse (Schuckit 1987). Those with a strong family history of alcoholism have relatively reduced reactions to alcohol intake in the laboratory, but data on their relative rates of alcoholism are not yet available.

Although criticism of the methods and conclusions of the studies cited above makes their significance uncertain (Murray et al. 1983; Searles 1988), genetic factors certainly do influence individual susceptibility to substance abuse. This does not mean however, that substance abuse is a "genetic disease." Many inherited characteristics could increase susceptibility to substance abuse, including differences in emotional reactions to different substances, ability to control impulses, abilities to get satisfactions in socially acceptable ways, tendencies to low mood or anxiety, and susceptibility to social influences. Personality traits are moderately heritable (Plomin et al. 1980), and it would be surprising if they did not contribute to the heritability of substance abuse. In the natural environment, which does not offer access to a variety of concentrated drugs and routes of administration, most people with traits that increased the tendency to substance abuse would not have any substance abuse disorder. Even if specific genes are found to predispose some people to substance abuse (Mullen 1989), these will not be "genes for substance abuse" but genes that have been selected because they offer some kind of benefit, perhaps a benefit entirely distinct from behavioral regulation.

In certain populations, selection may have shaped protection against alcoholism. Low rates of alcoholism in Orientals have been attributed to a change in a single gene nucleotide. This change makes an inactive form of alcohol dehydrogenase so that drinking results in the rapid accumulation of toxic acetaldehyde, which causes nausea and vomiting like that caused by Antabuse (Smith 1986; Mullen 1989). It is difficult to say if this characteristic is an adaptation shaped by natural selection in Orientals, or merely a quirk that is adaptive. More clear is the selective force of alcohol preference today. Alcohol-caused motor vehicle accidents are a major cause of death in the early reproductive years, so natural selection should gradually decrease the human preference for alcohol. The time course of changes from natural selection is so slow, however, that cars will likely be extinct before such selection eliminates our taste for alcohol.

CLINICAL IMPLICATIONS

The greatest clinical benefit of an evolutionary view of substance abuse may be its explanation of why drug use is often inadvisable, even when it is not addicting or medically dangerous. Some patients will be helped by knowing that psychotropic drugs interfere with the evolved mechanisms that regulate behavior.

An evolutionary perspective also supports the principle that cessation of drug use is, as many clinicians have long recognized, the first step in treatment. Whatever methods accomplish abstinence—behavioral, psychotherapeutic, and social—are indicated. Also indicated are more general strategies that increase the person's ability to get normal satisfactions from social life. Bad feelings, and lack of good feelings, are significant factors in the return to drug use. Helping people to feel better, whether by psychotherapy, marital counselling, employment change, or the use of medications, is essential, not adjunctive treatment. An evolutionary view also supports matching different treatments to the needs of individual patients (Brower 1989). Finally, it encourages both clinician and client to view some suffering as normal and even useful.

There are also implications for the use of psychotropic drugs in general. Some people say new drugs will bring an age of human happiness, while others oppose almost all psychotropic drug use. Although an evolutionary perspective tends to support the conservative side of this argument, it also can specify some situations in which drug use is clearly warranted.

First, there are situations, already discussed, in which defensive systems overreact. Dampening the responses of these systems can sometimes relieve suffering with little risk. The use of benzodiazepines to control anxiety would be a perfect example, except for the major problems of dependence and withdrawal.

Psychotropic drugs are also appropriately used to block outmoded responses. Our minds were shaped for an environment vastly different from that in which we live. The constraints on aggression in a bureaucracy, the vicissitudes of modern marriages, the possibility of working long into the night—our emotions do not guide us reliably in these circumstances.

Drugs are also used to adjust arousal. Stimulants increase alertness for study or long-distance driving, and sedatives adjust sleep to changes in time zones (Thayer 1989). Such uses are exceptions to the principle that drugs are used for their subjective effects. In this case, they mainly adjust the timing of arousal to match the challenges of our unnatural world.

Drugs can also correct brain abnormalities. It remains difficult to tell, however, when psychotropic drugs are correcting neurophysiological abnormalities, and when they are simply blocking normal aversive emotions. It is tempting, but erroneous, to conclude that finding neurophysiologic correlates of a mental condition implies that the condition is caused by a brain abnormality. Many neurophysiologic correlates of mental states have nothing to do with the etiology of the state, they are merely aspects of the operation of normal brain mechanisms. Evidence of a "biological disorder" is not needed, however, to justify the drug treatment of mental distress. Psychiatry is, in this respect, like the rest of medicine. A general practitioner routinely diagnoses and treats conditions like fever and pain that do not represent any defect in the body, but only the arousal of normal defenses against infection or trauma. Drugs that dampen the body's defensive responses can often safely relieve discomfort, whether the response is cough, pain, anxiety, or sadness.

IMPLICATIONS FOR SOCIAL POLICY

An evolutionary perspective suggests that it will be impossible to "solve the drug problem." Substance abuse is not a rare phenomenon of a few people in a few societies, but of many otherwise-normal people in most societies. Although a social phenomenon, it consists, ultimately, of the actions of individuals. A difficult responsibility of any government is to set and enforce rules about drug use. In modern Western society, this effort is particularly difficult because of our wealth, freedom, leisure, travel, and the constant discovery of new drugs and routes of administration.

Frustration about the failure to control drug use and recognition of the socially corrosive effect of a large illicit economy had led to calls for legalization of some abused substances (Nadelmann 1989). The tacit argument seems to be that society is paying too high a price for protecting deviant individuals from actions that harm mainly themselves. An evolutionary view suggests, however, that all of us, not just deviants, are susceptible to substance abuse and that legalization might result in substance abuse by many more people.

This view does not necessarily imply that legalizing certain drugs is unwise. The debate about how the law should view drug use should be based on controlled studies and pragmatic experience, not on the erroneous notions that substance abusers are fundamentally different from other people, that substance abuse is a genetic disease, or that substance abuse is created only by social environment. If drug abuse is seen as an intrinsic human tendency, instead of a disease with a specific explanation and a specific cure, then the control of substance abuse can be expected to require substantial and continuing public expenditures for a variety of interventions. Even modest control of drug use will need every available cost-effective strategy—education, establishment of social norms, treatment, police enforcement, legal sanctions, political influence on suppliers, and others still to be developed.

THE FUTURE

Although it seems that our society is awash with drugs, the drug age may just be beginning. Private entrepreneurs and pharmaceutical companies are steadily inventing new agents. Recently introduced antidepressants seem to induce confidence and a mild euphoria even in those without a depressive disorder. We will likely soon have drugs that relieve anxiety safely without the withdrawal and side effects that limit the use of present agents. Soon, we may have drugs that stop grief, increase self-esteem, arouse the feeling of love, and make people feel that their lives are more meaningful. Some argue that the invention of such drugs is the solution to our current dilemmas about substance abuse (Siegel 1989).

How will we make decisions about how to use these agents? Should we treat people with drugs whenever a safe agent is available that will make them feel better? Or, to put it more realistically, should society try to prohibit people from using such agents? Prepared or not, we soon will confront these questions. We will be better able to answer them if we have a deeper understanding of the evolutionary functions of the emotions.

This manuscript benefited substantially from comments from members of the Evolutionary Psychiatry Seminar at the University of Michigan, and from James Abelson, Cynthia Pomerleau, Nathan Wolf, and especially Fred Glaser and Helena Cronin. Its preparation was supported by the University of Michigan Evolution and Human Behavior Program.

REFERENCES

Alexander, B.K., and Hadaway, P.F. Opiate addiction: the case for an adaptive orientation *Psychological Bulletin* 92: 367–381, 1982.

Brower, K.J., Blow, F.C., et al. Treatment implications of chemical dependency models: an integrative approach. *Journal of Substance Abuse Treatment* 6: 147–157, 1989.

Cloninger, C.R. Inheritance of alcohol abuse. *Archives of General Psychiatry* 38: 861–868, 1981.

Daly, M., and Wilson, M. *Sex, Evolution, and Behavior,* Boston: Willard Grant Press, 1983.

Dawkins, R. *The Selfish Gene,* Oxford: Oxford University Press, 1976.

DuPont, H.L., and Hornick, R.B. Adverse effect of Lomotil therapy in shigellosis. *Journal of the American Medical Association* 226: 1525–1528, 1973.

Frye, R.V. The sociobiological paradigm: a new approach to drug using behavior. *Journal of Psychedelic Drugs* 12: 21–25, 1980.

Goodwin, D.W. Genetic factors in the development of alcoholism. *PCNA* 9: 427, 1986.

Hanna, J.M., and Hornick, C.A. Use of cocoa leaf in southern Peru: adaptation or addiction? *Bulletin on Narcotics* 29: 63–73, 1977.

Konner, M. *The Tangled Wing: Biological Constraints on the Human Spirit,* New York: Harper Colophon Books, 1983.

Marks, I.M. *Fears, Phobias, and Rituals,* New York: Oxford University Press, 1987.

McNaughton, N. *Biology and Emotion,* Cambridge, England: Cambridge University Press, 1989.

Mullen, M. Alcoholism and the "new genetics." *British Journal of Addiction* 84: 1433–1440, 1989.

Murray, R.M., Clifford, C.A., et al. Twin and adoption studies: how good is the evidence for a genetic role? *Recent Developments in Alcoholism,* New York: Academic Press, 1983.

Nadelmann, E.A. Drug prohibition in the United States: costs, consequences, and alternatives. *Science* 245: 939–946, 1989.

Nesse, R.M. Evolutionary explanations of emotions. *Human Nature* 1: 261–289, 1990.

Osuntokun, B.O., Odeku, E.L., et al. Congenital pain asymoblia and auditory imperception. *Journal of Neurology, Neurosurgery, and Psychiatry* 31: 291–296, 1968.

Plomin, R., DeFries, J.C., et al. *Behavioral Genetics: A Primer,* San Francisco: W.H. Freeman, 1980.

Plutchik, R., and Kellerman, H. *Theories of Emotion,* Orlando: Academic Pres, Inc., 1980.

Pomerleau, O.F., and Pomerleau, C.S. A biobehavioral view of substance abuse and addiction. *Journal of Drug Issues* 17: 111–131, 1987.

Schuckit, M.A. Genetics and the risk for alcoholism. *Journal of the American Medical Association* 254: 2614–2617, 1985.

Schuckit, M.A. Biological vulnerability to alcoholism. *Journal of Consulting and Clinical Psychology* 55: 301, 1987.

Searles, J.S. The role of genetics in the pathogenesis of alcoholism. *Journal of Abnormal Psychology* 97: 153–167, 1988.

Shaffer, H.J. Conceptual crises and the addictions: a philosophy of science perspective. *Journal of Substance Abuse Treatment* 3: 285–296, 1986.

Siegel, R.K. *Intoxication: Life in Pursuit of Artificial Paradise,* New York: E.P. Dutton, 1989.

Smith, M. Genetics of human alcohol and aldehyde dehydrogenases. *Advances in Human Genetics* 15: 249–290, 1986.

Thayer, R.E. *The Biopsychology of Mood and Arousal,* New York: Oxford University Press, 1989.

Thornhill, R., and Thornhill, N.W,. The evolution of psychological pain. In *Sociobiology and the Social Sciences.* Lubbock, TX: Texas Tech University Press, 1989.

Vaillant, G.E. *The Natural History of Alcoholism,* Cambridge, MA: Harvard University Press, 1983.

Williams, G.C. *Adaptation and Natural Selection: A Critique of Some Current Evolutionary Thought,* Princeton, NJ: Princeton University Press, 1966.

Williams, G.W., and Nesse, R.M. The dawn of Darwinian medicine. *Quarterly Review of Biology* 66: 1–22, 1991.

Journal of Psychopharmacology 12(1) (1998) 15–22

SAGE Publications, London, Thousand Oaks, CA and New Delhi
0269-8811 [199803] 12:1; 15–22; 003051

Conditioning factors in drug abuse: can they explain compulsion?

Charles P. O'Brien, Anna Rose Childress, Ronald Ehrman and Steven J. Robbins
Veterans Affairs Medical Center, University of Pennsylvania 3900 Chestnut Street, Philadelphia PA 19104-6178, USA

There is a good deal of clinical evidence suggesting that compulsion to resume drug taking is an important part of the addiction syndrome. The symptoms comprising motivation to resume drug use, namely craving and compulsion, have been studied experimentally in human subjects. While much work remains to be done, there is evidence showing that these symptoms are influenced by learning. The research has been guided by animal studies demonstrating that drug effects can be conditioned. Much attention has been directed toward demonstrating the existence of drug conditioning in human addicts and exploring the neurological structures that may underlie such learned responses. We do not yet know the relative importance of learning in the overall phenomenon of relapse, and treatments based on conditioning principles are still under investigation.

Key words: addiction; conditioning; craving; dependence

Introduction

Compulsion is an integral part of the phenomenon of addiction. It is defined in the *American Heritage Dictionary* as 'an irresistible impulse to act regardless of the rationality of the motivation'. Compulsion to use drugs in a person diagnosed with a substance-use disorder does not depend on the presence of the drug; it can occur long after drug taking has stopped and long after any evidence of physical dependence or withdrawal syndrome has disappeared.

Consider this quote from a perplexed patient in treatment for the fourth time who was confirmed 5 weeks free of cocaine and was shown a videotape of simulated cocaine use: 'Doc, I don't understand what's going on. I really meant it when I told my therapy group yesterday that I never wanted to touch cocaine again. Now after seeing that video, I want cocaine more than anything and I feel the urge to go out and get it. What's the real me?'

Compulsion implies a loss of control, an inability to resist an urge. There is a memory trace that is unconscious which can be activated unexpectedly. The patient, not understanding what is going on inside their own brain, usually makes up an explanation: 'I'm just not a nice person if I don't smoke. I need nicotine in my body. It's best for those around me if I start smoking again'.

From a clinical standpoint, the most striking cases of compulsion are seen in patients who persist in drug-taking behavior even while undergoing treatment for the life-threatening consequences of that behavior. For example, consider the heavy smoker with severe emphysema, impaired oxygen diffusion and symptoms of air hunger who persists in smoking despite this most uncomfortable situation. Even more tragic are the individuals who may actually try to smoke through the tracheotomy tube after a laryngectomy for cancer. It is difficult to conceive of an animal experiment that truly addresses these striking aspects of compulsion to relapse well-known to clinicians. The best analog would be a study in which drug-free, formerly dependent animals were tested on the amount of shock they were willing to endure in order to self-administer a drug choice. However, most studies of drug self-administration in animals do not incorporate such a punishment contingency.

It is important to make the distinction between compulsive behavior occurring in a state of withdrawal and compulsion that occurs long after the withdrawal syndrome has disappeared. The long-lasting compulsion appears to be triggered by environmental stimuli and may be one of the most important problems faced by a clinician trying to treat drug dependence. It is not so difficult to get individuals to stop using a drug; the problem is to keep them from re-starting. Responses elicited by drug-related events may be one of the important factors producing high rates of relapse following treatment.

Cycles of remissions and relapses

Cessation of an addicting drug typically results in a withdrawal syndrome that is either mild as in the case of stimulants or dramatic as in the case of opiates or alcohol. The severity depends on the dose of drug typically administered and on the duration of the dependence. Medical detoxification consists of gradually reducing the dose of the addicting drug or providing a substitute from the same drug category. For the alcoholic, this can be a critical step because sedative withdrawal can be dangerous. However, the long-term success of treatment depends on the quality of the program for rehabilitation and prevention of relapse. Such programs have traditionally involved group or individual counseling or psychotherapy. After leaving the hospital or rehabilitation center, the treated, drug-free former addict may report occasional unexpected episodes of a sudden compulsion or urge to consume the drug. In these instances the relapse may appear paradoxical. However, anecdotes such as those cited at the beginning of this paper suggest that learning produced by repetitive drug use may play a role in relapse. While it is possible that some of these patients are making up stories to evade responsibility for the relapse, many of them appear sincere and there is a consistency to their reports.

From the perspective of the clinician, cessation of drug use (detoxification) is just the beginning of treatment. Even a 28-day rehabilitation program has little impact unless there is some program to deal with the proneness to relapse when the former addict leaves the hospital or residential treatment program and returns to their usual environment. As is the case with chronic medical illnesses such as arthritis or asthma, addictive behavior has a proclivity to return repeatedly, even after apparently successful short-term treatment (O'Brien and McLellan, 1996). Of course there are many reasons why relapse after a period of abstinence may occur. Both psychosocial and biological factors probably contribute to the phenomenon of relapse. A critical part of treatment is analyzing those factors that increase the likelihood of relapse and devising strategies to deal with them.

In follow-up studies, we have examined the factors associated with relapse in our patients over the years. For drug-dependence disorders in general, multiple factors have been found to be important in influencing long-term outcome. The presence of a psychiatric disorder in addition to addiction significantly worsens prognosis (McLellan *et al.*, 1983) and clinical observations suggest that social and economic conditions and drug availability in the community play a role. Withdrawal symptoms that persist for months (Martin and Jasinski, 1969) may also increase the risk of relapse. As discussed later, learned responses may also be a contributing factor.

Drug-related conditioning

The clinical data clearly indicate that something has changed in the brains of individuals who have engaged in repeated use of drugs of abuse. This residual 'habit or compulsion' does not depend on the presence of the drug in the body, because, as stated earlier, it persists long after drug use has stopped. The behavior comprising this compulsion can be precipitated by environmental stimuli in both animals and humans. Abraham Wikler first noticed the similarity of this phenomenon to a classically conditioned response and conducted studies in rats showing that opiate withdrawal signs could be conditioned (Wikler and Pescor, 1967). At the Penn/VA Center, we began conditioning experiments in human subjects in the early 1970s and we have focused on the four most important drugs of abuse. In order of clinical importance, these are nicotine, alcohol, heroin and cocaine. We have examined three central questions regarding drug conditioning:

(1) Do stimuli associated with persistent drug use acquire conditioned properties?
(2) Do such drug-related stimuli motivate drug taking?
(3) Can the risk of relapse be reduced by reducing the potential impact of drug stimuli?

We have also begun to investigate the neurochemical substrates of responding to drug-related stimuli. All drugs of abuse have in common the production of subjective responses that human users describe as pleasant or even euphoric. Furthermore, these drugs all serve as reinforcers in animal self-administration studies. Drugs of abuse also all appear to produce increases in extracellular dopamine (DA) in brain reward pathways (particularly the nucleus accumbens); this shared neurochemical effect has received much attention as a possible brain substrate of drug reward effects (see Wise, 1996 for a recent review). This DA increase is accomplished via different mechanisms for each drug category and it is still unclear whether it plays a causal role in drug reward. Nevertheless, this interest in DA function in the limbic system has served as a starting point for recent attempts to uncover the mechanisms underlying craving and compulsive drug taking, including the possible role of learned drug cues.

How does drug-related learning occur?

Drugs are used excessively producing a rapid onset of pleasant feelings in the user. In addition to reliable and prompt changes in affect (feelings), these drugs cause changes in numerous organ systems which may or may not be perceptible to the drug user. Some of these effects (e.g. tachycardia, cortisol increases) may simply contribute to an overall feeling of excitement. Many investigators have proposed that environmental cues which are associated with drug effects may begin to produce automatic changes in various organ systems *in advance* of the drug being received (e.g. Wikler, 1965; Siegel, 1979; Stewart *et al.*, 1984). Over time, these cues may also provoke a desire for the drug, even a craving or compulsion to use the drug. In principle, *any* stimuli associated with drug use (e.g. drug paraphernalia, people and places associated with use, particular odors, mood states, etc.) may develop learned properties.

Although different theories of drug-related learning describe the process in different ways, they all postulate the same primary path to continued drug use. According to conditioning models, environmental cues associated with past drug use become classically conditioned stimuli which evoke conditioned physiological changes. Experienced users also report drug-related effects such as high, withdrawal, or craving in response to drug cues. These stimulus-induced symptoms then motivate voluntary drug-seeking (operant) behaviors. If the drug seeker succeeds in obtaining the drug, the chain of behaviors is reinforced by the pleasurable drug state caused by the pharmacological effects of the drug on the brain and various other organ systems.

The ability of drug-related events to evoke both physiological responses and self-reported craving and withdrawal is well-established (see O'Brien *et al.*, 1986; Baker *et al.*, 1987; Sherman *et al.*, 1988; Drummond *et al.*, 1990; Robbins and Ehrman, 1992 for reviews). However, it has proved much more difficult to definitively establish either that such responses result from a past history of conditioning or that they motivate continued drug use. Studies which present drug users with naturalistic cues under laboratory conditions have been unable to conclusively demonstrate that the observed responses have a conditioned origin. Such studies suffer both from our inability to measure cue reactivity prior to the subject's drug-use history and our inability to directly observe the acquisition of presumed conditioned responses. Laboratory studies of drug conditioning solve these problems by allowing the learning process to be observed directly. However, such studies have typically lacked many of the control procedures used to rule out non-associative effects such as sensitization and pseudoconditioning. Furthermore, the demonstration that conditioning can occur under the ideal learning conditions of a laboratory does not prove that such learning typically occurs under the far less consistent conditions of drug use in the natural environment (see Sherman *et al.*, 1988; Robbins and Ehrman, 1992 for more discussion). The role of cue reactivity in motivating drug taking also requires further study. A few studies have documented increases in smoking behavior (Rickard-Figueroa and Zeichner, 1985; Droungas *et al.*, 1995) and in alcohol consumption (Ludwig *et al.*, 1974; Kaplan *et al.*, 1983) following exposure to drug cues. However, more work is needed, particularly to demonstrate the role of cues in motivating use of illicit drugs such as heroin and cocaine.

Theories of drug conditioning

Two general models of drug conditioning have received the most attention over the years. One model proposes that drug-related events evoke conditioned responses which are the opposite of the direct effects of the drug. Such responses produce tolerance to the effects of the drug and may be perceived as withdrawal symptoms when drug use is abruptly terminated (e.g. Siegel, 1979). A second model proposes that drug cues will produce conditioned drug-like responses (e.g. euphoria) which provide incentive motivation for further drug taking (e.g. Stewart *et al.*, 1984). Although the two classes of model differ as to the predicted form of conditioned drug responses, they are similar in two important respects. First, both postulate that environmental events associated with drug use will acquire conditioned properties. Second, both assume that these properties provide some of the motivation to continue drug taking and to relapse following a period of abstinence. The first model holds that drug seeking is motivated by the desire to escape aversive conditioned withdrawal-like states, while the second views drug use as driven by the pleasurable anticipation of drug effects produced by drug-like conditioned responses.

Opiate conditioning

The first drugs of abuse subjected to studies of conditioning in human addicts were the opiate group. One of the reasons commonly given by opiate users for continuing opiate use is the avoidance of withdrawal symptoms. Since in most opioid addicts, some withdrawal symptoms will occur several times per day, there may be thousands of pairings of environmental stimuli and withdrawal symptoms during the life of a patient before they seek treatment. In the laboratory, we have shown that after as few as *seven* pairings between mild naloxone-induced withdrawal symptoms and a neutral stimulus such as a peppermint odor, humans begin to show signs of withdrawal when exposed to the odor alone (O'Brien *et al.*, 1975, 1977). Some of the responses were relatively unique to opiate withdrawal such as lacrimation, rhinorrhea and nausea while others were consistent with autonomic nervous system arousal. While these results are consistent with a conditioning interpretation, control groups/stimuli were not included to rule out non-associative learning. For example, it is possible that responses to the odor resulted from general sensitization which, after training, would have produced withdrawal on exposure to any salient stimulus.

Opiate-opposite responses have also been seen in response to videotapes of drug use shown to addicts in a laboratory situation. Subjects typically respond to such naturalistic cues with decreases in skin temperature and skin resistance, and self-reports of withdrawal and craving (Ternes *et al.*, 1980; Childress *et al.*, 1986a,b). Non-addict controls showed no significant responses (Ternes *et al.*, 1980). Such data are consistent with a conditioning model. Although the data from laboratory studies of opiate cues do not conclusively demonstrate the existence of drug conditioning, they do provide a likely mechanism to explain the anecdotes concerning onset of withdrawal symptoms when a drug-free patient returns to an environment in which withdrawal symptoms had occurred in the past.

Drug-opposite responses to environmental cues may also underlie the development of tolerance. For example, opiate injections produce *elevations* in skin temperature in human subjects, but stimuli that have repeatedly preceded opiate injections reliably produce *reductions* in skin temperature when presented to experienced opiate users. There are many other examples of 'drug-opposite' responses that can be demonstrated by polygraphic measurement of physiological changes, by ratings of effects that subjects perceive (subjective effects) or by observer ratings of subject behavior. If these responses occur just before the drug is taken, then they will serve to reduce the effects of the drug. This attenuation of drug effects produced by conditioned responses can be thought of as a form of 'tolerance' and it may form a partial explanation for the diminished drug effects commonly seen with repeated administration of the same dose of a drug in a constant environment (i.e. environment-specific tolerance, see Siegel, 1979). Conditioned tolerance to the analgesic properties of opiates has been demonstrated experimentally in rats (Siegel, 1975; Siegel *et al.*, 1978; Siegel and MacRae, 1984). Cue-induced tolerance to heart rate and skin temperature changes caused by opiates has been demonstrated in human opiate addicts (Ehrman *et al.*, 1992b).

Alcohol conditioning

Probably the largest body of data on drug cue reactivity has centered around the use of alcohol. Many studies have examined responding to naturalistic alcohol cues, while many others have attempted to produce conditioned responses to novel stimuli paired with alcohol consumption in the laboratory (see Niaura *et al.*, 1988; Sherman *et al.*, 1988; Drummond *et al.*, 1990 for reviews and critical comments). As with the opiate studies, there is good evidence that naturalistic alcohol cues can produce physiological and self-report responses in the laboratory and that novel stimuli will elicit responding following pairings with alcohol consumption. However, some difficulties for a conditioning interpretation of such responses remain. Naturalistic cue studies have produced inconsistent results; not all studies have documented cue responding and those that have do not always report the same patterns of responding (see the above review papers for more discussion). Furthermore, studies that do show robust responding do not conclusively demonstrate that such effects result from a past history of conditioning. Studies which pair novel stimuli with alcohol ingestion in the laboratory have similarly failed to provide the control conditions necessary to conclusively attribute observed responding to conditioning (see Sherman *et al.*, 1988; Robbins & Ehrman, 1992 for more discussion of design issues).

Animal studies show that the augmentation of DA in the nucleus accumbens produced by alcohol is readily conditioned. Animals placed in a chamber where they have previously been able to self-administer alcohol show an augmentation of DA prior to alcohol availability (Weiss *et al.*, 1993). Other studies have shown that the augmentation of DA in animals directly produced by alcohol must be mediated by endorphinergic pathways because it is blocked by naloxone (Holman *et al.*, 1987). Therefore, the conditioned release of DA in rats may also be blocked by opiate receptor antagonists, but the critical experiment has not yet been done.

These animal results suggest a potential explanation of some of the effects of the opiate receptor antagonist naltrexone in the therapy of alcoholics. In double-blind studies naltrexone has been shown to significantly reduce the rate of relapse in abstinent alcoholics enrolled in a rehabilitation program (Volpicelli *et al.*, 1990, 1992; O'Malley *et al.*, 1992). Craving to drink alcohol is reported to be diminished and the effects of alcohol are likewise diminished if the individual does 'slip' and take a drink. Our hypothesis is that some of the reports of craving to resume drinking reported by alcoholics are actually conditioned phenomena. Just as in rats, stimuli previously associated with drinking in human alcoholics may provoke an augmentation of DA in specific limbic regions. We postulate that in alcoholic humans this form of conditioned responding is blocked or diminished by naltrexone. If the individual does drink, a further augmentation of DA by the alcohol itself is also blocked by the presence of naltrexone. Thus, the patient reports reduced reward from alcohol. This account is purely hypothetical at present; studies need to be done both to document a role of DA transmission in cue-elicited craving for alcohol and to demonstrate that such craving can be blocked by naltrexone.

Cocaine conditioning

The responses produced by cocaine users in response to laboratory cocaine cues are quite similar to those reported in studies of opiate users. More specifically, subjects at our treatment center show decreases in skin temperature and resistance and increases in heart rate when exposed to cocaine-related cues (e.g. Childress *et al.*, 1988; O'Brien *et al.*, 1990; Ehrman *et al.*, 1992a, 1996; Robbins *et al.*, 1992, 1996). In earlier studies of opiates, such physiological responses were interpreted as representing drug-opposite withdrawal responses. A parallel interpretation in the present case would view these responses as drug-like appetitive responses (they are similar to the stimulant properties of cocaine). Alternatively, these responses could be construed as non-specific arousal in both cases. It is not yet possible to separate these interpretations. Subjectively, subjects report increases in high, withdrawal and craving in response to cocaine cues, and many subjects report increases in two or three measures simultaneously. Furthermore, the magnitudes of physiological responses to the cues are not correlated with reported levels of high, withdrawal, or craving (Robbins *et al.*, 1996). Therefore, while cocaine cues produce robust physiological and subjective state changes, it is difficult to characterize these changes as reflecting a particular motivational central state such as drug high or withdrawal.

Some evidence exists suggesting that responses to cocaine cues have a conditioned origin. Drug-free former cocaine addicts report craving for cocaine and exhibit increases in heart rate and decreases in skin temperature and skin resistance when exposed to videotapes of cocaine use and cocaine paraphernalia. Cocaine users do not show similar responses to opiate or non-drug cues, and non-addicts do not differentially respond to the three stimulus types. These data suggest that responses to the cocaine stimuli may have a conditioned origin rather than representing unconditioned responses to naturally arousing events (Ehrman *et al.*, 1992a).

Animal studies show clear conditioning of cocaine-induced hyperactivity, a drug-like response. If the stimulant is given in a consistent environment, the environment alone acquires the ability to produce behavioral activation (Post *et al.*, 1981, 1987). Some intriguing evidence for conditioned neurochemical effects following cocaine administration comes from direct brain studies using the microdialysis technique in the region of the nucleus accumbens in rats (Kalivas and Duffy, 1990). Increased DA was recorded in this region after each dose of i.p. cocaine. The DA responses increased with successive cocaine doses (sensitization). After repeated exposure to cocaine injections, the animals were given a saline (placebo) injection under similar conditions on a different day. The response in the nucleus accumbens was a small but significant augmentation of DA, presumably conditioned by the prior experiences with cocaine.

This work raises the possibility that former cocaine-using patients experience a similar augmentation of limbic DA when they are exposed to cocaine-related stimuli. The peripheral measures of arousal would be consistent with this interpretation. It has long been known that cocaine self-administration in animals can be reinstated following small doses of the same or a similar drug, a phenomenon known as priming (Stewart, 1984). Priming doses of cocaine have also been shown to produce increases in craving in humans in a laboratory setting (Jaffe *et al.*, 1989). Therefore, increases in limbic DA might underlie priming effects as well. The possibility of such a shared mechanism leads to the suggestion that a conditioned increase in central DA could provide a priming effect which cocaine users might experience as craving prior to reinitiation of cocaine use.

While we cannot directly measure changes in brain chemistry in our human subjects (Childress *et al.*, 1993a,b), the O^{15}-labeled water positron emission tomography (PET) technique enables us to measure changes in regional cerebral blood flow as a rapid reaction measure of localized brain activity (Childress *et al.*, 1994, 1995). We postulated that limbic areas would show an increase in activity in response to cocaine-related stimuli in former cocaine users compared to normal controls. We showed subjects videotapes of cocaine buying and using while measuring blood flow. Former cocaine users reported cue-elicited increases in craving even though they were confined in a PET scanner. As postulated, these subjects also showed significant increases in blood flow to amygdala, anterior cingulate and temporal poles during the same 10-min period. There was no activation observed in the dorsolateral prefrontal cortex nor in the hippocampal areas (Childress *et al.*, 1996). Neutral stimuli did not produce this effect nor was stimulus-specific limbic activation observed in non-addict controls.

The marked amygdalar activation provoked by cocaine-related stimuli in our laboratory is consistent with recent data showing that the basolateral amygdala is probably involved in the development of instrumental responses for cocaine reinforcement (Whitelaw *et al.*, 1996). However, our findings are inconsistent with a recent report by Grant *et al.* (1996) who examined metabolic activity in 18 brain regions of interest in cocaine users and non-addict controls during exposure to cocaine and non-drug cues. They failed to find significant responding in amygdala or anterior cingulate of cocaine users, but did find increased activity in a number of other areas including the dorsolateral prefrontal cortex, a region which did not show differential activation in our study. Although stimulus-specific responding was not observed in the amygdala for the cocaine users, activation in this area was significantly correlated with subject-reported levels of craving. Full understanding of these different patterns of results awaits further research, but it is possible that differences in the nature of the drug stimuli or measures of brain activity employed might have played a role.

One difficulty with existing studies of cue-elicited brain activation lies in the complex nature of the drug cues employed. It is extremely difficult to produce neutral, control cues which are precisely matched to the drug cues in terms of sensory activation, emotional content, and so on. In other words, brain activation evoked by drug cues could reflect anxiety or other emotional states produced by the videotape rather than the effects of specific conditioned drug states such as craving. Future studies are needed to further refine the nature of control stimuli to better isolate the drug-related content of drug cues as the factor responsible for brain activation effects.

Nicotine conditioning

Our work with the most important addictive drug, nicotine, has been facilitated by the ease of obtaining drug-dependent subjects. Of all the addicting drugs, nicotine has the highest proportion of users who lose control and become dependent. It is also, arguably, the most difficult addiction to treat. However, because nicotine is a legal drug, it can be studied without the constraints placed on studies of illegal substances. Therefore, we can directly study the effects of smoking-related cues on smoking behavior. Using techniques similar to those developed for the studies of opiate, cocaine and alcohol, we and others have demonstrated that smoking-related stimuli provoke self-reports of craving and withdrawal compared to neutral events (Rickard-Figueroa and Zeichner, 1985; Abrams *et al.*, 1988; Niaura *et al.*, 1989; Tiffany and Drobes, 1990; Droungas *et al.*, 1995; Drobes and Tiffany, 1997). Moreover, we have been able to demonstrate that smoking behavior is provoked by exposure to smoking-related stimuli. After sessions in which the subjects viewed either smoking or control videotapes, they were unobtrusively observed in a situation in which they knew that smoking was permissible and their latency to smoke was measured. Prior exposure to smoking-related cues significantly reduced their latency to smoke. Thus, we not only have reports of increased craving for cigarettes, but also a quantifiable behavior, latency to smoke, that was significantly affected by smoking-related stimuli, but not by neutral stimuli (see also Rickard-Figueroa and Zeichner, 1985). Such results represent some of the best evidence to date that drug-related cues motivate increases in levels of drug taking.

Clinical relevance

One way of answering the question concerning whether a conditioning mechanism underlies the compulsions observed in addicts is by assessing the clinical effects of procedures aimed at extinguishing or reducing the responses to drug-related cues. In several different populations we have randomly assigned patients to a behavioral treatment aimed at reducing cue reactivity or to a control group receiving equal attention but without focused attempts at extinguishing conditioned responses. We first studied the conditioned responses associated with chronic opioid use, speculating that some of these responses could lead to resumption of drug use after the patient has achieved abstinence. The responses that we targeted in our extinction treatment program included cue-induced subjective responses such as craving, feelings of high, and feelings of drug withdrawal. We also studied the effects of the extinction program on autonomic responses such as changes in heart rate, skin resistance and skin temperature. The procedure for modifying these responses was based on a process of systematic, gradual exposure to drug-associated cues without the possibility of pharmacological reinforcement. The general approach in this series of studies has been to first select cues that reliably elicit subjective and physiological responses in the target population, and then to attempt to reduce these responses through repeated, non-reinforced exposure (extinction).

We first studied detoxified and long-term drug-free opiate patients, some of whom were therapeutic community graduates. Subjects were asked to perform repeated unreinforced self-injections under laboratory conditions. This procedure was generally ineffective; subjects reported increasing withdrawal and craving in response to the injections and many found the injections so unpleasant that they dropped out of the study (O'Brien *et al.*, 1974, 1980). In later work, we exposed drug-free, opiate-addicted subjects to repeated presentations of a videotape of opiate use. This procedure was better tolerated and produced significant reductions in both reported withdrawal and craving (Childress *et al.*, 1986a). Subjects enrolled in methadone treatment similarly showed increases in self-reported withdrawal and craving in response to opiate cues and subsequent reductions in craving responses during extinction (Childress *et al.*, 1984, 1986b). Both extinction and control groups showed significant improvement in drug use and other symptoms but there was no evidence for a specific effect of extinction treatment on outcome. However, it is possible that the failure to find a treatment effect could have been the result of inadequate extinction training (Childress, 1986b).

Similar difficulties have plagued more recent attempts at cue-exposure treatments for opiate addicts. For example, Powell *et al.* (1993) reported that opiate addicts repeatedly exposed to drug cues (extinction training) showed a greater reduction in cue-elicited craving than did control subjects. However, the lack of outcome data on drug use prevented an assessment of the significance of this extinction effect for treatment. A later study showed equal reductions in reactivity for extinction and control groups and demonstrated no differences in clinical outcome (Dawe *et al.*, 1993). Thus, the efficacy of cue-reduction strategies for reducing opiate use remains to be adequately tested. When significant reduction in reactivity has been achieved, no outcome measures have been available. Conversely, when outcome has been measured, there has been little evidence that the extinction treatment differentially reduced responding.

Cue-exposure treatments have been applied to other substance abuse populations as well. One recent study assigned alcoholics to either cue-exposure treatment or a relaxation control group (Drummond and Glautier, 1994). Subjects in the cue-exposure group showed longer latencies to relapse to drinking than controls. Unfortunately, the two groups showed equivalent reduction in cue reactivity during the trial, calling into question the mechanism of the observed treatment effects. Similar results were obtained in a study in our laboratory on extinction treatment for cocaine abusers. Preliminary analyses suggested that a group receiving repeated cue exposure had fewer cocaine positive urines than a randomly assigned control group receiving equal attention (O'Brien *et al.*, 1990). As in the alcohol study, however, control subjects showed as great a reduction in cue reactivity as did subjects receiving systematic exposure to cues over an 8-week period. The artificial nature of repeated viewing of laboratory videotapes makes the results difficult to compare to reactivity in the natural environment. Because the two groups showed no differences in cue reactivity at the end of the exposure period, the mechanism underlying any observed differences in treatment outcome is again unclear.

In an attempt to improve the efficacy of the extinction-based treatment, we recently developed a menu of active strategies that the patient could learn in order to cope with conditioned craving whenever and wherever it might be evoked. The protocol called for the patient to recall a craving episode in the clinic on each of several appointments. The patient then practiced reducing the resulting craving and arousal with one of several behavioral interventions. The menu of options that was most effective for each individual was worked out in the clinic and included systematic relaxation, behavioral alternatives, visual imagery and cognitive interventions. Patients randomly assigned to a control group received only the standard treatment provided to both groups. Preliminary data from the 8-week outpatient trial showed more clean urines for the experimental group, but this effect was small and both groups tended to relapse over time (Childress *et al.*, 1993a). Because the technique has face validity, it has been copied as a treatment manual by the National Institute on Drug Abuse (Childress with NIDA contractors, 1993).

We have also investigated the use of medications to reduce responses to drug-related cues. Ultimately, a combination of behavior therapy and medication may be the most effective treatment. The first medication we tested in the cue-reactivity paradigm was amantadine, a DA agonist which actually increased the physiological response to cocaine-related cues (Robbins *et al.*, 1992). In contrast, a DA receptor (D_2) antagonist (haloperidol) did reduce cocaine cue-elicited craving (Berger *et al.*, 1996), but for a variety of reasons, this medication would not be useful in the treatment of cocaine addiction. Most recently, we found that ritanserin, a 5-HT_2 receptor antagonist, failed to block cocaine cue reactivity in a randomized, double-blind, placebo-controlled trial (Ehrman *et al.*, 1996).

Conclusion

The question posed by the title of this article still cannot be answered with certainty despite a good deal of research using animal models and human subjects. There is no question that environmental events associated with drug use do produce robust physiological and subjective state changes in abstinent drug users. However, whether these responses reflect a specific history of conditioning and/or explain the compulsive nature of addiction still remains open to question. Future research will be needed to more conclusively determine if we can clearly reduce or eliminate compulsion to relapse by focusing on blocking responses to drug-related events.

Acknowledgments

This work was supported by NIH/NIDA grants RO 1 DA 000586 and P50 DA 5186 and by the Department of Veterans Affairs.

Address for correspondence

C. P. O'Brien
Veterans Affairs Medical Center
University of Pennsylvania
3900 Chestnut Street
Philadelphia, PA 19104-6178
USA
Email: obrien@research.trc.upenn.edu

References

Abrams D B, Monti P M, Carey K B, Pinto R P, Jacobus S I (1988) Reactivity to smoking cues and relapse: two studies of discriminant validity. Behav Res Ther *26*: 225–233

Baker T B, Morse E, Sherman J (1987) The motivation to use drugs. A psychobiological analysis of urges. In Rivers C (ed.) The Nebraska symposium on motivation: alcohol use and abuse. University of Nebraska Press, Lincoln, NE, pp. 257–323

Berger S P, Hall S, Mickalian J D, Reid M S, Crawford C A, Delucchi K, Carr K, Hall S (1996) Haloperidol antagonism of cue-elicited cocaine craving. Lancet *347*: 504–508

Childress A R with NIDA contractors (1993) Cue extinction: in-service training curriculum. NIH Pub. No. 93-3692. US Government Printing Office, Washington, DC

Childress A R, McLellan A T, O'Brien C P (1984) Measurement and extinction of conditioned withdrawal-like responses in opiate dependent patients. NIDA Research Monograph 49. US Government Printing Office, Washington, DC, pp. 212–219

Childress A R, McLellan A T, O'Brien C P (1986a) Abstinent opiate abusers exhibit conditioned craving, conditioned withdrawal and reduction in both through extinction. Br J Addict *81*: 644–660

Childress A R, McLellan A T, O'Brien C P (1986b) Conditioned responses in a methadone population: a comparison of laboratory, clinic and natural setting. J Substance Abuse Treat *3*: 173–179

Childress A R, McLellan A T, Ehrman R, O'Brien C P (1987) Extinction of conditioned responses in abstinent cocaine or opioid users. NIDA Research Monograph 76. US Government Printing Office, Washington, DC, pp. 189–195

Childress A R, Ehrman R N, McLellan A T, O'Brien C P (1988) Conditioned craving and arousal in cocaine addiction: a preliminary report. NIDA Research Monograph 81. US Government Printing Office, Washington, DC, pp. 74–80

Childress A R, Hole A V, Ehrman R N, Robbins S J, McLellan A T, O'Brien C P (1993a) Cue reactivity and cue reactivity interventions in drug dependence. NIDA Research Monograph 137. US Government Printing Office, Washington, DC, pp. 73–95

Childress A R, Kung H, Mallison R T, Alavi A, Mozley D, Fitzgerald J, Kushner S, O'Brien C P (1993b) Brain correlates of induced cocaine craving. Paper presented at 23rd Annual Meeting of the Society for Neuroscience, Washington, DC, 762.8

Childress A R, Mozley D, Fitzgerald J, Reivich M, Jaggi J, O'Brien C P (1994) Regional brain blood flow during cue-induced cocaine craving. Paper presented at 24th Annual Meeting of the Society for Neuroscience, Miami Beach, FL, 666.2

Childress A, Mozley D, Fitzgerald J, Reivich M, Jaggi J, O'Brien C P (1995) Limbic activation during cue-induced cocaine craving. Paper presented at 25th Annual Meeting of the Society for Neuroscience, San Diego, CA, 767.1

Childress A E, McElgin W, Mozley D, Reivich M, O'Brien C P (1996) Brain correlates of cue induced cocaine and opiate craving. Paper presented at 26th Annual Meeting of the Society for Neuroscience, Washington, DC, 365.5

Dawe S, Powell J, Richards D, Gossop M, Marks I, Strang J, Gray J A (1993) Does post-withdrawal cue exposure improve outcome in opiate addiction? a controlled trial. Addiction *88*: 1233–1245

Drobes D J, Tiffany S T (1997) Induction of smoking urge through imaginal and *in vivo* procedures: physiological and self-report manifestations. J Abnorm Psychol *106*: 15–25

Droungas A, Ehrman R, Childress A R, O'Brien C P (1995) Effect of smoking cues and cigarette availability on craving and smoking behavior. Addict Behav *20*: 657–673

Drummond D C, Glautier S (1994) A controlled trial of cue exposure treatment in alcohol dependence. J Cons Clin Psychol *62*: 809–817

Drummond D C, Cooper T, Glautier S P (1990) Conditioned learning in alcohol dependence: implications for cue exposure treatment. Br J Addict *85*: 725–743

Ehrman R N, Robbins S J, Childress A R, O'Brien C P (1992a) Conditioned responses to cocaine-related stimuli in cocaine abuse patients. Psychopharmacology *107*: 523–529

Ehrman R, Ternes J, O'Brien C P, McLellan A T (1992b) Conditioned tolerance in human opiate addicts. Psychopharmacology *108*: 218–224

Ehrman R N, Robbins S J, Cornish J W, Childress A R, O'Brien C P (1996) Failure of ritanserin to block cocaine cue reactivity. Drug Alcohol Depend *42*: 167–174

Grant S, London E D, Newlin D B, Villemagne V L, Liu X, Contoreggi C, Phillips R L, Kimes A S, Margolin A (1996) Activation of memory circuits during cue-elicited cocaine craving. Proc Natl Acad Sci USA *93*: 12040–12045

Holman R B, Snape B M, Widdowson P S (1987) Naloxone elicits dose-dependent changes in alcohol-induced increases in endogenous dopamine release from rat striatum. Alcohol *1*: 737–741

Jaffe J H, Cascella N G, Kumo K M, Sherer M A (1989) Cocaine-induced cocaine craving. Psychopharmacology *97*: 59–64

Kalivas P W, Duffy P (1990) Effect of acute and daily cocaine treatment on extracellular dopamine in the nucleus accumbens. Synapse *5*: 48–58

Kaplan R F, Meyer R E, Stoebel C F (1983) Alcohol dependence and responsivity to an ethanol stimulus as predictors of alcohol consumption. Br J Addict *78*: 259–267

Ludwig A M, Wikler A, Stark L H (1974) The first drink: psychobiological aspects of craving. Archs Gen Psychiat *30*: 539–547

Martin W, Jasinski D (1969) Physiological parameters of morphine dependence in man—tolerance, early abstinence and protracted abstinence. J Psychiat Res *7*: 9–17

McLellan A T, Luborsky L, Woody G E, O'Brien C P (1983) Predicting response to alcohol and drug abuse treatment: role of psychiatric severity. Archs Gen Psychiat *40*: 620–625

Niaura R S, Rosenhow D J, Binkoff J A, Monti P M, Pedraza M, Abrams D B (1988) Relevance of cue reactivity to understanding alcohol and smoking relapse. J Abnorm Psychol *97*: 133–152

Niaura R S, Abrams D B, Demuth B, Pinto R P, Monti P M (1989) Responses to smoking-related stimuli and early relapse to smoking. Addict Behav *14*: 419–428

O'Brien C P, McLellan A T (1996) Myths about the treatment of addiction. Lancet *347*: 237–240

O'Brien C P, Chaddock B, Woody G, Greenstein R (1974) Systematic extinction of narcotic drug use using narcotic antagonists. Psychosom Med *36*: 458

O'Brien C P, O'Brien T J, Mintz J (1975) Conditioning of narcotic abstinence symptoms in human subjects. Drug Alcohol Depend *1*: 115–123

O'Brien C P, Testa T, O'Brien T J, Brady J P, Wells B (1977) Conditioned narcotic withdrawal in humans. Science *195*: 1000–1001

O'Brien C P, Greenstein R, Ternes J, McLellan A T, Grabowski J (1980) Unreinforced self-injections: effects on rituals and outcome in heroin addicts. NIDA Research Monograph 27. US Government Printing Office, Washington, DC, pp. 275–281

O'Brien C P, Ehrman R, Ternes J (1986) Classical conditioning in human opioid dependence. In Goldberg S R, Stolerman I P (eds), Behavioral analysis of drug dependence. Academic Press, Orlando, FL, pp. 329–356

O'Brien C P, Childress A R, McLellan A T, Ehrman R (1990) Integrating systematic cue exposure with standard treatment in recovering drug dependent patients. Addict Behav *15*: 355–365

O'Malley S S, Jaffe A J, Chang G, Schottenfeld R S, Meyer R E, Rounsaville B (1992) Naltrexone and coping skills therapy for alcohol dependence. Archs Gen Psychiat *49*: 881–887

Post R M, Lockfeld A, Squillace K M, Contel N R (1981) Drug–environment interaction: context dependency of cocaine-induced behavioral sensitization. Life Sci *28*: 755–760

Post R M, Weiss S R B, Pert A, Uhde T W (1987) Chronic cocaine administration: sensitization and kindling effects. In Fisher S, Raskin A, Uhlenhuth E (eds), Cocaine: clinical and biobehavioral aspects. Oxford University Press, New York

Powell J, Gray J, Bradley B (1993) Subjective craving for opiates: Evaluation of a cue exposure protocol for use with detoxified opiate addicts. Br J Clin Psychol *32*: 39–53

Rickard-Figueroa K, Zeichner A (1985) Assessment of smoking urge and its concomitants under an environmental smoking cue manipulation. Addict Behav *10*: 249–256

Robbins S J, Ehrman R N (1992) Designing studies of drug conditioning in humans. Psychopharmacology *106*: 143–153

Robbins S J, Ehrman R N, Childress A R, O'Brien C P (1992) Using cue reactivity to screen medications for cocaine abuse: a test of amantadine hydrochloride. Addict Behav *17*: 491–499

Robbins S J, Ehrman R N, Childress A R, O'Brien C P (1996) Relationships among physiological and self-report responses produced by cocaine-related cues. Addict Behav *22*: 1–11

Sherman J E, Jorenby M S, Baker T B (1988) Classical conditioning with alcohol: acquired preferences and aversions, tolerance and urges/craving. In Wilkinson D A, Chaudron D (eds), Theories of alcoholism. Addiction Research Foundation, Toronto, pp. 173–237

Siegel S (1975) Evidence from rats that morphine tolerance is a learned response. J Comp Physiol Psychol *89*: 498–506

Siegel S (1979) The role of conditioning in drug tolerance and addiction. In Keehn J D (ed.), Psychopathology in animals: research and treatment implication. Academic Press, New York, pp. 143–168

Siegel S, MacRae J (1984) Environmental specificity of tolerance. Trends Neurosci *7*: 140–142

Siegel S, Hinson R, Krank M (1978) The role of predrug signals in morphine analgesic tolerance: support for a Pavlovian conditioning model of tolerance. J Exp Psychol: Anim Behav Proc *4*: 188–196

Stewart J (1984) Reinstatement of heroin and cocaine self-administration behavior in the rat by intracerebral application of morphine in the ventral tegmental area. Pharmac Biochem Behav *20*: 917–923

Stewart J, deWit H, Eikelboom R (1984) The role of unconditioned and conditioned drug effects in the self-administration of opiates and stimulants. Psychol Rev *91*: 251–268

Ternes J W, O'Brien C P, Grabowski J, Wellerstein H, Jordan-Hayes J (1980) Conditioned drug responses to naturalistic stimuli: problems of drug dependence. NIDA Research Monograph 27. US Government Printing Office, Washington DC, pp. 282–288

Tiffany S T, Drobes D J (1990) Imagery and smoking urges: the manipulation of affective content. Addict Behav *15*: 531–539

Volpicelli J, Alterman A, Hayashida M, Muentz L, O'Brien C (1990) Naltrexone and the treatment of alcohol dependence. In: Reid L (ed.), Opioids, bulimia and alcoholism. Springer, New York, pp. 195–214

Volpicelli J R, Alterman A I, Hayashida M, O'Brien C P (1992) Naltrexone in the treatment of alcohol dependence. Archs Gen Psychiat *49*: 876–880

Weiss F, Lorang M T, Bloom F E, Koob G F (1993) Oral alcohol self-administration stimulates dopamine release in the rat nucleus accumbens: genetic and motivational determinants. J Pharmac Exp Ther *267*: 250–267

Whitelaw R B, Markou A, Robbins T, Everitt B J (1996) Excitotoxic lesions of the basolateral amygdala impair the acquisition of cocaine-seeking behaviour under a second-order schedule of reinforcement. Psychopharmacology *127*: 213–224

Wikler A (1965) Conditioning factors in opiate addiction and relapse. In Willner D I, Kassenbaum, G G (eds), Narcotics. McGraw-Hill, New York, pp. 85–100

Wikler A, Pescor F (1967) Classical conditioning of a morphine abstinence phenomenon, reinforcement of opioid-drinking behavior and relapse in morphine-addicted rats. Psychopharmacologia *10*: 255–284

Wise R A (1996) Neurobiology of addiction. Curr Opin Neurobiol *6*: 243–251

Brain Research Reviews, 18 (1993) 247–291

BRESR 90157

Full-length reviews

The neural basis of drug craving: an incentive-sensitization theory of addiction

Terry E. Robinson and Kent C. Berridge

Department of Psychology and Neuroscience Program, The University of Michigan, Neuroscience Laboratory Building, Ann Arbor, MI 48104-1687 (USA)

(Accepted 20 April 1993)

Key words: Drug addiction; Brain; Dopamine; Incentive motivation; Sensitization; Neuroadaptation; Nucleus accumbens; Striatum

This paper presents a biopsychological theory of drug addiction, the 'Incentive-Sensitization Theory'. The theory addresses three fundamental questions. The first is: why do addicts crave drugs? That is, what is the psychological and neurobiological basis of drug craving? The second is: why does drug craving persist even after long periods of abstinence? The third is whether 'wanting' drugs (drug craving) is attributable to 'liking' drugs (to the subjective pleasurable effects of drugs)? The theory posits the following. (1) Addictive drugs share the ability to enhance mesotelencephalic dopamine neurotransmission. (2) One psychological function of this neural system is to attribute 'incentive salience' to the perception and mental representation of events associated with activation of the system. Incentive salience is a psychological process that transforms the perception of stimuli, imbuing them with salience, making them attractive, 'wanted', incentive stimuli. (3) In some individuals the repeated use of addictive drugs produces incremental neuroadaptations in this neural system, rendering it increasingly and perhaps permanently, hypersensitive ('sensitized') to drugs and drug-associated stimuli. The sensitization of dopamine systems is gated by associative learning, which causes excessive incentive salience to be attributed to the act of drug taking and to stimuli associated with drug taking. It is specifically the sensitization of incentive salience, therefore, that transforms ordinary 'wanting' into excessive drug craving. (4) It is further proposed that sensitization of the neural systems responsible for incentive salience (for 'wanting') can occur independently of changes in neural systems that mediate the subjective pleasurable effects of drugs (drug 'liking') and of neural systems that mediate withdrawal. Thus, sensitization of incentive salience can produce addictive behavior (compulsive drug seeking and drug taking) even if the expectation of drug pleasure or the aversive properties of withdrawal are diminished and even in the face of strong disincentives, including the loss of reputation, job, home and family. We review evidence for this view of addiction and discuss its implications for understanding the psychology and neurobiology of addiction.

CONTENTS

Summary 247
1. Introduction 248
2. The Incentive-Sensitization Theory of Addiction: an overview 249
3. Theories of addiction 250
3.1. Negative reinforcement views of addiction (escape from distress) 250
3.1.1. Problems with negative reinforcement views 251
3.2. A positive reinforcement view of addiction (pleasure-seeking) 252
3.2.1. Problems with a positive reinforcement/euphoria view of addiction 252
3.3. Requirements of an Incentive-Sensitization Theory of Addiction 255
4. Evidence for the Incentive-Sensitization Theory of Addiction 256
4.1. Criterion 1: there should be a common neural system affected by many different addictive drugs 256
4.2. Criterion 2: the repeated administration of different addictive drugs should render a common neural system hypersensitive in a gradual and incremental fashion. 256
4.2.1. Sensitization to the psychomotor-activating effects of addictive drugs. 256
4.2.2. Sensitization to the incentive motivational effects of drugs. 257
4.2.3. The neural basis of behavioral sensitization. 258

Correspondence: T.E. Robinson, Neuroscience Building, The University of Michigan, 1103 East Huron Street, Ann Arbor, MI 48104-1687, USA. Fax: (1) (313) 936-2690; e-mail: GB92@um.cc.umich.edu.

4.3. Criterion 3: sensitization-related neuroadaptations should be very long-lasting. 258
4.4. Criterion 4: the expression of sensitization-related neuroadaptations should be amenable to conditioned stimulus control. 259
4.5. Criterion 5: the role of mesotelencephalic dopamine systems in incentive motivation. 260
4.6. Criterion 6: the effects of dopamine are on incentive salience, not pleasure. 260
4.6.1. Incentive salience. 261
4.6.2. Introspection into 'wanting' and 'liking'. 262
4.6.3. Evidence that mesotelencephalic dopamine mediates incentive salience, not pleasure. 262

5. Elaboration of the Incentive-Sensitization Theory and its implications. 265
5.1. The independence of drug craving from drug pleasure and withdrawal. 266
5.2. The development of addictive behavior. 267
5.3. Relapse: drug-induced drug craving. 267
5.4. Relapse: interactions between different drugs and the effects of drug-related stimuli. 268
5.5. Relapse: the role of stress. 269
5.6. Individual differences in the propensity to addiction. 269
5.7. Implications of the Incentive-Sensitization Theory for therapy. 270
5.7.1. Extinction training. 270
5.7.2. Pharmacotherapeutic approaches. 271
5.8. Relationship between incentive sensitization and other views of addiction. 271

6. Notes 272
6.1. Role of control and intermittency of drug administration in sensitization. 272
6.1.1. Control. 272
6.1.2. Intermittency. 273
6.2. Specific motivational effects of dopamine blockade. 273
6.3. The neural substrate of drug 'liking' (pleasure). 274
6.4. Dopamine, sensitization and incentive salience. 274
6.5. Tolerance to drug pleasure. 275
6.6. The compulsive nature of addictive behavior. 276
6.7. Benzodiazepines and sedative-hypnotics. 276
6.8. The role of dopamine in mediating the effects of conditioned incentives. 276
6.9. Stress, aversive stimuli and stimulant-induced psychoses. 277
6.10. Dopamine antagonists and therapy. 278

7. Glossary 279
Acknowledgements 282
References 282

A firm conviction of the material reality of Hell never prevented medieval Christians from doing what their ambition, lust or covetousness suggested. Lung cancer, traffic accidents and the millions of miserable and misery-creating alcoholics are facts even more certain than was, in Dante's day, the fact of the Inferno. But all such facts are remote and unsubstantial when compared with the near, felt fact of a craving, here and now, for release or sedation, for a drink or a smoke.

(Aldous Huxley, The Doors of Perception, 1951)

1. INTRODUCTION

There are three major features of addictive behavior that need to be explained by any adequate theory of drug addiction *. The first is drug craving†, by which we simply mean intensely 'wanting'† drugs[184]. Although drug addiction† is defined as a pattern of 'compulsive drug-taking behavior', drug taking does not in itself constitute addictive behavior. Only when the repeated self-administration of drugs leads to a pattern of compulsive drug-seeking and drug-taking behavior, which occurs at the expense of most other activities, is a person said to be addicted[79,148]. To understand addiction, therefore, we need to understand the process by which drug-taking behavior evolves into compulsive drug-taking behavior. Presumably this transformation in behavior occurs because addicts develop an obsessive craving for drugs, a craving that is so irresistible that it almost inevitably leads to drug seeking and drug taking. It is difficult, of course, to provide an adequate definition of subjective terms, such as 'wanting' and craving[184,363], but clinical experience suggests that drug craving is fundamental to addiction; it cannot be ignored. Any satisfactory account of addiction must explain: why do addicts want or crave drugs so much?

Drug addiction is also "a chronic relapsing disorder" (ref. 148, p. 522). The second major feature of addic-

* Many of the terms in this article are used in different ways by different authors and they are not always clearly defined. To avoid ambiguity we have provided a glossary with definitions of many of the most problematic terms. Thus, a reference to the glossary, which will be indicated by the symbol, †, refers the reader to the definition of a term. The reader may not always agree with a given definition, but we hope at least this makes it clear what we mean.

tion that must be explained, therefore, is: why drug craving often persists or can be reinstated, long after the discontinuation of drug use. An understanding of the propensity to relapse will be critical not only for understanding the process of addiction, but in developing effective therapies.

A third feature of drug addiction that requires explanation is that, as drugs come to be 'wanted' more-and-more, they often come to be 'liked' less-and-less. That is, as craving for drugs increases the pleasure derived from drugs often decreases. Why is this? What is the relationship between 'wanting' drugs and 'liking' drugs and does this relationship change during addiction?

The purpose of this article is to present a biopsychological theory of addiction, an Incentive-Sensitization Theory, that addresses these issues *. The paper is organized into four parts. In Part I the theory is summarized to give a brief overview of its major features. In Part II the theory is put into a broader context by critically discussing other theories of addiction, specifically negative reinforcement (e.g., withdrawal avoidance) and positive reinforcement (e.g., pleasure-seeking) theories. In doing so it is argued that theories based on the concepts of negative or positive reinforcement† do not adequately explain the key features of addiction discussed above. In Part III research findings that support the concept of an Incentive-Sensitization Theory are reviewed. Finally, in Part IV the theory is elaborated and its implications discussed in greater detail.

2. THE INCENTIVE-SENSITIZATION THEORY OF ADDICTION: AN OVERVIEW

The Incentive-Sensitization Theory of Addiction posits that addictive behavior is due largely to progressive and persistent neuroadaptations caused by repeated drug use. It is, if you will, a 'neuroadaptationist model'. It is proposed that these drug-induced changes in the nervous system are manifest both neurochemically and behaviorally by the phenomenon of 'sensitization', which refers to a progressive increase in a drug effect with repeated treatment[272,291]. These sensitization-related neuroadaptations have not been considered in previous theories of addiction. In fact, until recently, the phenomenon of sensitization usually was not mentioned in books and articles on addiction and if sensitization was mentioned, it was referred to only in passing, as part of a more extensive discussion of tolerance. Nevertheless, it is proposed here that *the defining characteristics of addiction (craving and relapse) are due directly to drug-induced changes in those functions normally subserved by a neural system that undergoes sensitization-related neuroadaptations.*

The neural system that is rendered hypersensitive ('sensitized') to activating stimuli is hypothesized to mediate a specific psychological function involved in the process of incentive motivation: namely the *attribution of incentive salience†* to the perception and mental representation of stimuli and actions. This makes stimuli and their representations highly salient, attractive and 'wanted'. It is the activation of this neural system that results in the experience of 'wanting', and transforms ordinary stimuli into incentive stimuli.

Sensitization of this neural system by drugs results in a pathological enhancement in the incentive salience that the nervous system attributes to the act of drug taking. The co-activation of associative learning directs the focus of this neurobehavioral system to specific targets that are associated with drugs and leads to an increasing pathological focus of incentive salience on drug-related stimuli. Thus, with repeated drug use the act of drug taking and drug-associated stimuli, gradually become more and more attractive. Drug-associated stimuli become more and more able to control behavior, because the neural system that mediates 'wanting' becomes progressively sensitized. 'Wanting' evolves into obsessive craving and this is manifest behaviorally as compulsive drug seeking and drug taking. Therefore, by this view, drug craving and addictive behavior are due specifically to sensitization of incentive salience.

But 'wanting' is not 'liking'. The neural system responsible for 'wanting' incentives is proposed to be separable from those responsible for 'liking' incentives (i.e., for mediating pleasure) and repeated drug use only sensitizes the neural system responsible for 'wanting'. Because of this, addictive behavior is fundamentally a problem of sensitization-induced excessive 'wanting' alone. This is in contrast to 'pleasure-seeking' theories of addiction, which explicitly assume that the incentive motivational properties of drugs are due directly to their subjective pleasurable effects; i.e., their ability to produce positive affective states. In colloquial language, it is usually assumed that addicts 'want' drugs because they 'like' drugs and the more they 'like'

* This paper is not a comprehensive review of the primary research literature on addiction and addictive drugs. We cite review articles to support specific points in many instances. Readers should consult these review articles for more extensive lists of citations to the primary literature.

them the more they should 'want' them. In this traditional view 'wanting' and 'liking' drugs are necessarily connected. The Incentive-Sensitization Theory is unique, however, because we propose the progressive increase in drug 'wanting' that characterizes addiction is not accompanied by an increase in the pleasure derived from drugs. Repeated drug use does not sensitize neural systems responsible for the subjective pleasurable† effects of drugs, only those responsible for incentive salience – transforming 'wanting' into craving.

In addition, the neuroadaptations underlying behavioral sensitization are long-lasting and in some cases they may be permanent. It is hypothesized that it is the persistence of sensitization-related neuroadaptations that renders addicts hypersensitive to drugs and to drug-related stimuli, even after years of abstinence. It is the permanence of sensitization that is thought to render drug-related stimuli so effective in precipitating relapse, even in detoxified, 'recovered' addicts.

Finally, it is hypothesized that the neural substrate for incentive-sensitization (that is the neural system(s) that normally attributes salience to incentive stimuli and becomes sensitized by addictive drugs) is the mesotelencephalic dopamine system. Sensitization results in an increase in the responsiveness of the dopamine system to activating stimuli, such that activating stimuli produce a greater increase in dopamine neurotransmission in sensitized than in non-sensitized individuals. The relationship between changes in dopamine neurotransmission, the subjective pleasurable effects of drugs and incentive salience, which occurs during addiction according to the Incentive-Sensitization Theory, are illustrated schematically in Fig. 1.

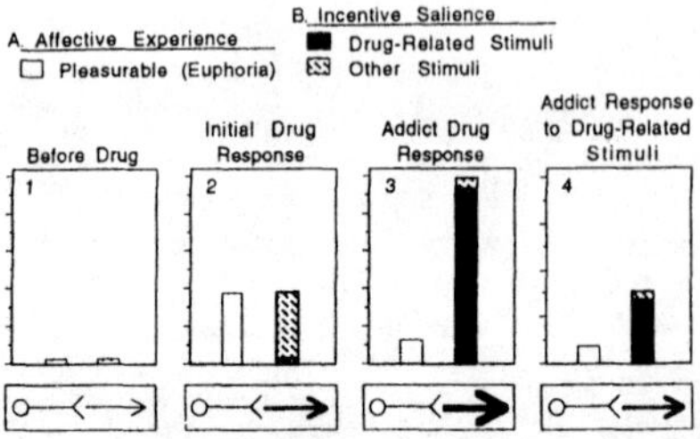

Fig. 1. A schematic illustration of changes, as addiction develops, in (A) the pleasurable affective experience produced by drugs; (B) the incentive salience attributed to drug-associated stimuli and their mental representations and to other stimuli; and (C) the activation of dopamine systems (arrows); as proposed by Incentive-Sensitization. Dopamine systems are hypothesized to provide the neural substrate for incentive salience. Panel 1 depicts the subjective experience and degree of incentive salience in a normal individual (before taking a drug). We assume the person is not depressed and therefore, the normal affective state is fairly neutral, but slightly in the positive direction (as is incentive salience). Panel 2 indicates that the initial drug experience (or first few drug experiences) results in a marked increase in subjective pleasure (the drug is 'liked') and in the attribution of salience to stimuli in the immediate environment. These are not yet 'drug-related' stimuli because they have not yet been linked associatively with the drug experience. (Note that the initial drug experience could also have aversive components, but these are not depicted here.) The initial drug experience is accompanied by an increase in dopamine neurotransmission, as indicated by an increase in the size of the arrow in the lower panel indicating 'dopamine activity'. Panel 3 shows that after many drug experiences and the development of addictive behavior, the response to the same dose of the drug shown in Panel 2 is changed. In the addict the subjective pleasurable effects of the drug are decreased due to tolerance (alternatively, they could be unchanged, as discussed in Fig. 2 and Note 5 in Ch. 6). But the incentive salience attributed to drug taking is markedly enhanced due to sensitization of the neural system responsible for the attribution of incentive salience. Due to associative conditioning there is a focus of incentive salience on what are now drug-associated stimuli. It is further hypothesized that this sensitization of incentive salience is due to sensitization of dopamine neurotransmission (large arrow in lower panel; but also see Note 4 in Ch. 6). Panel 4 shows that in the addict exposure to conditioned incentive stimuli (stimuli that have acquired incentive value through their association with drugs) may produce effects similar to the drug itself, but of lesser magnitude. It is the sensitization of incentive salience depicted in Panels 3 and 4 that is hypothesized to be responsible for excessive drug 'wanting' (craving) in the addict, leading to compulsive drug-seeking and drug-taking behavior.

The Incentive-Sensitization Theory of Addiction will be discussed in much greater detail later. Before that, however, we need to address the features of addictive behavior that are not adequately explained by other theories of addiction and thus require explanation by a new theory. The most widely accepted theories of addiction presently fall into two classes: negative reinforcement models (e.g., drugs are taken to avoid the symptoms of withdrawal) and positive reinforcement models (i.e., drugs reinforce self-administration behavior by producing pleasure). There have been many papers describing the strengths and short-comings of negative and positive reinforcement views of addiction[86,326,363,365] and it is not necessary to review this entire literature in great detail here. Instead, negative and positive reinforcement models will be only briefly summarized and their difficulty in explaining several key features of addiction (e.g., craving and relapse) will be emphasized, primarily to provide a comparison with the Incentive-Sensitization Theory. We want to stress, however, that none of these views are mutually exclusive. Pleasure-seeking, escape from distress and incentive-sensitization probably each play some role in drug-taking behavior.

3. THEORIES OF ADDICTION

3.1. Negative reinforcement views of addiction (escape from distress)

Historically, the aversive consequences of discontinuing drug use (the withdrawal syndrome) have been a central focus of research on addiction, in part because many early studies were on opiates, which produce clear tolerance and physical withdrawal symptoms. This research emphasized the action of drugs as negative reinforcers†[64,148,180,227,312,326,337,349,365]. To paraphrase Wise and Bozarth[365], negative reinforcers sustain behavior (drug seeking and drug taking in this case) not because of the state they produce, but because of the state they alleviate. According to this negative reinforcement view of addiction drug use is maintained because the aversive symptoms associated with withdrawal are alleviated by the drug. Addictive drugs that do not result in overt physical withdrawal symptoms, such as cocaine and the amphetamines, are thought to act as negative reinforcers by alleviating a 'psychological distress syndrome' produced by the discontinuation of drug use (ref. 105 for example). In addition, previously neutral environmental stimuli associated with withdrawal can themselves come to elicit withdrawal-like symptoms, by secondary conditioning[305,306,357]. Thus, drugs may not only alleviate 'primary' withdrawal symptoms, but also the conditioned withdrawal symptoms induced by exposure to drug-related stimuli. A second negative reinforcement view is that drugs are sometimes used to 'self-medicate', relieving preexistent symptoms such as pain, anxiety or depression that occur in life independent of drug use (ref. 170 for example).

The traditional focus on withdrawal and tolerance was driven by the assumption that these processes are critical for the development and maintenance of addictive behavior. It is now clear, however, that the avoidance of withdrawal is not the most important factor in the development or maintenance of addictive behavior, although certainly the avoidance of withdrawal may motivate drug-seeking and drug-taking behavior in some instances. A number of leading figures in drug addiction research have noted, for example, that "physical dependence is neither a necessary nor sufficient condition for addiction" (ref. 365, p. 470), that "for rats and monkeys physical dependence is neither a necessary nor a sufficient condition for opiates to act as reinforcers" (ref. 290, p. 186) and that "physical dependence is currently viewed not so much as a direct cause of drug dependence but as one of several factors that contribute to its development" (ref. 148, p. 527). A number of critiques of negative reinforcement theories of addiction have been published[86,149,326,363,365] and the major shortcomings of negative reinforcement theories in explaining addiction are briefly summarized below.

3.1.1. Problems with negative reinforcement views

- Both people and animals will self-administer opioids in the absence of withdrawal symptoms or physical dependence[335,372]. For example, Ternes et al.[335] found that in cynomolgus monkeys the opioid, hydromorphone, maintained self-administration at doses that produced neither tolerance nor physical dependence, the latter indicated by the absence of any effect of a naloxone challenge. Similarly, Lamb et al.[192] recently reported that former heroin addicts, who showed no withdrawal symptoms upon a naloxone challenge, nevertheless worked at high rates (lever pressed) to receive a low-dose injection of morphine.
- Maximal periods of drug self-administration often do not coincide in time with periods of maximal withdrawal distress[365]. This lack of correlation between withdrawal distress and drug-seeking behavior is also evident in comparisons made across drug classes. Jaffe (ref. 149, p. 9) notes that, although the severity of the withdrawal syndrome associated with different drugs varies dramatically, ranging from very subtle physiological signs to life-threatening consequences, "there is little correlation between the visibility or physiological seriousness of withdrawal signs and their motivational force" in maintaining addictive behavior.
- There are many drugs used medically that produce withdrawal syndromes but "are not typically self-administered for non-medical purposes", including "certain tricyclic antidepressants (imipramine, amitriptyline), anticholinergics and κ-opioid agonists" (ref. 149, p. 9).
- There are numerous reports that the "relief of withdrawal is minimally effective in treating addiction" (ref. 365, p. 470 for references).
- There is a high tendency to relapse even after an extended period of abstinence from drugs, long after overt withdrawal symptoms have subsided. This is usually explained in the context of conditioned withdrawal effects, whereby environmental stimuli associated with withdrawal come to elicit withdrawal-like symptoms[306,357]. There are, however, a number of problems with this explanation. (1) At least a third of opiate addicts deny that they experience conditioned withdrawal symptoms when they are exposured to drug-related stimuli[50]. (2) Although many opiate addicts experience conditioned withdrawal symptoms very few cite this as the reason for resuming drug use[212]. There is, in fact, a poor correlation between craving and withdrawal signs[50]. Even withdrawal-like physiological symptoms induced by drug-associated cues (e.g., temperature, skin resistance, heart rate) are not highly correlated with reports of subjective state[80]. (3) Stewart et al. (ref. 326, p. 258) have argued that "attempts to demonstrate such conditioned withdrawal symptoms increase the probability of drug taking and relapse in animals have been unsuccessful" (ref. 329 as well).

– A number of researchers have noted that self-reported craving for some drugs, such as cocaine, is often highest immediately after drug administration, when the drug is producing subjective pleasure (a 'high') and withdrawal symptoms are eliminated or are at their weakest[50,80,96,98,150,215]. If drug craving were due to a desire to relieve withdrawal symptoms (ref. 64 for example), it would be expected that craving would dramatically decrease when the drug alleviates withdrawal and is producing pleasure, not be sustained or even increase.

– Finally, animals will avidly self-administer a variety of drugs directly into brain regions that do not produce withdrawal symptoms[366]. Furthermore, the infusion of drugs into these same brain regions can 'prime' or reinstate responding in animals in which drug responding has been extinguished[326]. These studies have established that the incentive motivational effects of centrally applied drugs can be dissociated from their negative reinforcing or withdrawal-related effects.

For the reasons summarized above it is now generally accepted that the negative reinforcing effects of drugs are not necessary for the development and maintenance of addictive behavior. Escape from distress cannot explain the defining characteristics of addiction, craving and relapse. We do not wish to imply, however, that withdrawal plays no role at all in the maintenance of addictive behavior. The alleviation of withdrawal distress may indeed sometimes motivate drug-seeking and drug-taking behavior. In addition, the positive reinforcing effects of drugs may be enhanced when drugs are given during periods of withdrawal distress[86,290]. However, relief from withdrawal symptoms cannot be the sole cause or even the primary cause of drug craving and compulsive drug-taking behavior.

3.2. A positive reinforcement view of addiction (pleasure-seeking)

In part because of the shortcomings of negative reinforcement theories of addiction more recent formulations have focussed on the role of drugs as positive reinforcers†[148,326,349,363,365]. Most drugs that are self-administered by people also act as positive reinforcers for animals. Thus, a positive reinforcement view of addiction posits that drug self-administration is maintained because of the state drugs induce, not because they alleviate an unpleasant state[326,363,365].

But to state that addictive drugs are positive reinforcers does not explain addiction. As pointed out by Wise and Bozarth (ref. 365, p. 472): "To assert that all addictive drugs are reinforcers is to do little more than redefine the phenomenon of addiction."... "To identify a drug as reinforcing goes no further than to identify the drug as addicting, because it is the common observation of habitual self-administration that serves as the basis for most definitions of both drug reinforcement and drug addiction. A theory of addiction based on the concept of reinforcement would have to identify actions of drugs that are operationally independent of self-administration habits in order to offer insight as to why drugs are addictive." That is, positive reinforcement is merely a description of a behavioral effect, not an explanation of the effect[307]. The critical questions are, why are some drugs positively reinforcing (i.e., what specific actions of drugs are positively reinforcing) and why do drugs become more effective reinforcers as addiction develops? It is usually assumed that drugs act as positive reinforcers because they produce pleasure. Thus, Wise and Bozarth state[365] "the only existing positive reinforcement view of addiction that might qualify as an explanatory theory identifies positive reinforcement with drug euphoria. In this view drugs are addicting (establish compulsive habits) because they produce euphoria or positive affect" (ref. 29 and ref. 213, p. 474). Similarly, Stewart et al.[326] argued that compulsive drug use is maintained by appetitive motivational states generated by the ability of drugs to produce *positive affective states†*.

There are, however, a number of problems with the hypothesis that the subjective pleasurable (hedonic) effects of drugs are either necessary or sufficient to motivate compulsive drug-seeking and drug-taking behavior. As put by Dews[72] over 15 years ago, "it was supposed that the prediction of addiction liability was essentially equivalent to prediction of euphorigenic power. As with most self-evident ideas, the mere matter of there being essentially no evidence in favor of it and much against it, had little effect on its acceptance" (p. 75).

3.2.1. Problems with a positive reinforcement / euphoria view of addiction

– If the positive reinforcing effects of drugs are primarily due to their ability to produce pleasurable affective states (euphoria†) and if this is sufficient to produce addictive behavior, the subjective pleasurable effects of drugs must be enormous. Indeed, the subjective pleasurable effects of drugs would have to be so potent that just the memory of drug experiences would be sufficient to evoke compulsive drug-seeking and drug-taking behavior. Although addictive drugs can indeed produce extremely pleasant affective states (anonymous, personal communication) it is difficult to believe that this property of drugs alone is sufficient to account for addiction. For one, there is no clear relationship between the ability of individual drugs to produce euphoria and their addictive potential. For example, nicotine is considered highly addictive, but nicotine does not produce marked euphoria or other strong hedonic states (ref. 266 for example). Also, many addictive drugs can actually produce strong dysphoric states, especially with initial use. Second, it could be argued that in addicts the magnitude of the negative consequences of continued drug use often far outweigh the magnitude of drug pleasure or the memory of drug pleasure. In fact, to most people (including many addicts), the negative consequences of continued drug use, including loss of health, friends, family, home and job, seem enormous relative to the pleasure derived from drugs. Falk et al.[86] have pointed out (p. 58): "the apparent irrationality of these activities [drug use]. The activities seem to produce more harm than benefit for the individual. How could creatures have evolved such powerful, wasteful and even self-destructive propensities? Not only are the activities apparently irrational, but also an apparent disparity exists between the immediate consequences of the behavior and its strength. The rush of an intravenous injection is transient and with street-quality heroin, rarely dramatic. Yet, the drug somehow can support day-long hustling and determine a whole subculture".

Indeed, addicts will sometimes report that they are miserable, that their life is in ruins and that the drug is not even that great anymore – but they still want it! Addicts themselves often are bewildered by the intensity and irrationality of their own 'wanting'. It is difficult to explain this situation by just evoking short-lasting drug pleasure. If the incentive motivational effects of drugs are due only to their ability to produce transient pleasure, but the aversive consequences of continued drug use eventually come to far outweigh the pleasurable effects – and, if drug taking behavior is maintained by simple contingencies of reinforcement, self-administration behavior should extinguish. But it usually does not (although see Falk et al.[86] for a discussion of the unique effects of intermittent schedules of reinforcement).

– A positive reinforcement/euphoria view of addiction does not adequately explain drug craving or relapse elicited by environmental stimuli associated with drug taking. Both Stewart et al.[326] and Wise and Bozarth[365] have argued convincingly that drug-related stimuli can evoke 'drug-like' effects that serve to motivate further drug-seeking and drug-taking behavior. They recently termed this view a 'proponent-process theory'[329], in contrast with the 'opponent-process' view associated with negative reinforcement models[182,312]. Stewart and Wise[329] argue "it is drug-like processes rather than drug-opposite processes that whet the appetite and stimulate renewed responding. In this view it is the 'taste' of the drug or the experience of stimuli that – through Pavlovian conditioning – cause drug-like central effects that motivate drug intake in experienced subjects" (p. 80).

The question remains, however, what exactly is this 'drug-like process'? One possibility is that it resembles the positive affective state, the pleasurable state, evoked by the drug itself. That it is equivalent to what has been called a conditioned 'high'[50]. For example, Stewart et al.[326] say: "Conditioned drug effects that mimic the unconditioned drug effects, as are conditioned *positive affective states*, are elicited by the environment where these drugs are experienced." (p. 264, our italics). In this view drug-associated stimuli may evoke 'conditioned pleasure', which reminds the addict of the even greater pleasure of the drug itself, thus motivating the individual to once again obtain the drug[362].

Addicts do report conditioned 'highs', as in the example of the oft cited 'needle freak'. In laboratory studies, however, self-reports of conditioned 'highs' occur much less frequently than self-reports of either conditioned craving or conditioned withdrawal-like signs[50,229]. Self reports of conditioned craving are especially frequent. This suggests that conditioned craving is dissociable from conditioned 'highs' and therefore, in many instances, drug craving is not caused by a conditioned 'high'. How then is craving explained in the context of a positive reinforcement/euphoria view of addiction?

A second possibility is that relapse in a 'recovered' addict is triggered by cues that evoke an explicit memory or representation of past drug experiences. Unlike a 'conditioned high', which is accompanied by an affective experience similar to that produced by the drug itself, an explicit memory need not be pleasant in itself. It recalls past pleasure in a cognitive form, as a semantic proposition or as a conscious image of the act of drug taking and spurs the addict to attempt to regain the remembered experience of pleasure once again.

An 'explicit memory of past pleasure' interpretation of relapse is not implausible and may describe some instances of relapse. But an interpretation that posits explicit memories of taking drugs to be a sufficient cause for relapse finds it difficult to explain why relapse occurs only when it does. No addict who relapses after months or years of abstinence could possibly not have remembered drug experiences many times before. During the process of withdrawal every addict must often recall and dwell upon memories of the drug experience. Once withdrawal is successfully endured the circumstances of daily living would cause one to sometimes remember earlier times, when life was different and drugs were the focus. Even without any particular cue or reminder, the mere process of free association would often call to mind scenes from earlier life, including upon occasion, drug-related experiences. Why should the explicit memory of a drug experience suddenly be sufficient to trigger relapse, when a person has had innumerable previous memories of drug experiences without relapse?

An 'explicit memory of past pleasure' interpretation might reply that, because relapse is often triggered by particular situations that have been paired with drug use in the past, these situations evoke a memory that is more vivid than all the memories that have come before. Whether this is true or not is an empirical question. Certainly, vivid memories can be triggered by associative cues and there is ample evidence that associative context is a powerful modulator of conditioned behavior; although whether context modulates explicit memories in this way is less clear (ref. 259 for example). However, images or other forms of conscious remembering that occur during withdrawal, daily life or free association might also be expected to be fairly vivid at least some of the time. It is not intuitively obvious that these memories should necessarily differ in vividness or in any other subjective quality that might explain why some conscious memories provoke relapse when others do not. In other words, an 'explicit memory' hypothesis places an extraordinary explanatory burden on the crucial assumption that relapse-provoking memories are qualitatively different from the myriad other memories of drugs that do not provoke relapse. As far as we know, there is no evidence to support this assumption.

– The most compelling evidence against the idea that drug taking is necessarily motivated by the subjective pleasurable effects of drugs comes from studies showing that drug self-administration can be maintained in the *absence of subjective pleasure;* that is, subjective pleasure is not necessary to maintain drug-seeking and drug-taking behavior. A striking example of a dissociation between the incentive motivational effects of morphine and the subjective pleasurable effects of morphine was reported recently by Lamb et al.[192]. These researchers found that opiate 'postaddicts' would work (press a lever) to get an injection of a low dose of morphine, despite the fact that four of five people *could not distinguish the subjective effects of the morphine from the placebo* – but the placebo did not reinforce lever pressing (ref. 151 as well). In other words, people 'self-administered' a low dose of morphine and not the placebo, but reported that neither the drug nor the placebo produced pleasure; there was no subjective difference between them. Similar effects have been reported by Fischman and Foltin[94,95] in laboratory studies of cocaine self-administration behavior in humans. Cocaine users reliably choose a low dose of cocaine (4 mg) over placebo, although this dose produces no self-reported subjective effects or cardiovascular effects. In addition, Fischman and Foltin[95] report that within-session tolerance to many of the cardiovascular and subjective (euphoric) effects produced by higher doses of cocaine is not accompanied by changes in drug-taking behavior; that is, within a self-administration session a dissociation develops between the subjective effects of cocaine and cocaine self-administration behavior.

On the basis of their study Lamb et al.[192] concluded "*that the reinforcing effects of morphine can occur in the absence of self-reported subjective effects and thus, do not appear to be causually related to drug-liking or euphoria*" (p. 1172, our italics). Similarly, when asked to speculate what maintains the self-administration of cocaine in the absence of subjective pleasure Fischman[95] replied:

> "I think cocaine is maintaining their behavior! If you want to know what the subjects say about their self-administration of these low doses, they tell me that they were not choosing cocaine over placebo. They often insist that they were sampling equally from each of the two choice options and both were placebo. On the other hand, if you look at the data from that session, you see that they were choosing the low dose (as low as 4 mg) or the dose with no measurable effect."... "I do not believe that measuring subjective effects provides us with the information about 'what' is maintaining their cocaine-taking. The best we can say at this point is that it is the cocaine that is maintaining cocaine-taking" (p. 179).

Of course, these studies also suggest that a memory or representation of the subjective pleasurable effects of morphine or cocaine is not required to sustain drug-taking behavior either, because if that were true then there should be some subjective difference in memories during low-dose morphine or cocaine compared to the placebo and there was none. Clearly there is a difference between low-dose morphine or cocaine and the placebo, but the data suggest it is not a subjective difference; it is not explicit and does not have access to conscious awareness.

Although the effects described by Lamb et al.[192] and Fischman and Foltin[95] are particularly striking, dissociations between the subjective pleasurable effects of drugs and drug-taking behavior have been noted previously. For example, Falk et al.[86] review studies showing that "the subjective effects produced by a drug do not necessarily predict whether the drug actually will be self-administered" (p. 58). In addition, Katz and Goldberg[165] describe experiments that suggest "the reinforcing effects and the subjective reports by human volunteers are not functionally equivalent entities" (p. 24).

Similarly, studies in rats on the affective vs. reinforcing properties of opiates suggest these actions may be mediated by separable neural systems[205,355]. This was suggested, for example, by White et al.[355] on the basis of studies on the effects of morphine in a runway task, in which food was available in the goal box. They found that morphine acted as a strong positive reinforcer, leading to faster and faster running speeds. But at the same time animals learned to avoid morphine-paired food. Thus, "the aversive effects of morphine were accompanied by positive reinforcement, a paradox that is difficult to understand" (ref. 355, p. 66). White et al.[355] suggested an explanation for this paradox may be "that the reinforcing effects of morphine" do "not depend upon the affective properties of the drug, but that the drug directly activate(s) a neural mechanism of reinforcement, which facilitates learning independantly of the animal's affective state".

The studies cited above are very important because their findings directly contradict the central premise of a positive reinforcement/euphoria view of addiction. In our terms, they establish that the incentive motivational effects of drugs are not directly attributable to their subjective pleasurable effects: that is, drug 'wanting' is not equivalent to drug 'liking'.

In summary, both negative reinforcement (e.g., withdrawal avoidance) and positive reinforcement/euphoria (pleasure-seeking) views of addiction have difficulty explaining a number of important features of addictive behavior. Any plausible new theory of addiction needs to address the same issues and better explain them. Specifically, an adequate theory of addiction must explain:

(1) What accounts for drug craving elicited by drug-associated stimuli, if craving is not causally related to conditioned withdrawal signs, conditioned 'highs' or the explicit memory of past pleasure?

(2) Why is craving sometimes highest immediately after drug administration, when subjective pleasurable effects are still predominant?

(3) Why does obsessive craving for drugs persist in the face of enormous negative consequences associated with continued drug use, and relatively modest subjective pleasurable effects?

(4) How can low doses of drugs, which do not produce discernible subjective pleasure or physical dependence, maintain drug-seeking and drug-taking behavior?

(5) Why is relapse such a prevalent and persistent feature of addiction, even in 'recovered' addicts?

(6) Why can relapse be precipitated by so many different stimuli (drugs, environmental stimuli associated with drugs, mood changes)?

3.3. Requirements of an Incentive-Sensitization Theory of Addiction

Neither traditional positive reinforcement nor negative reinforcement theories of addiction provide compelling answers to the questions listed above. We will argue below that the Incentive-Sensitization Theory of Addiction does. The Incentive-Sensitization Theory was introduced as a 'neuroadaptationist' model. It posits that repeated intermittent drug use results in incremental and persistent changes in a neural system that mediates craving for drugs; to be more precise, in a neural system responsible for the attribution of incentive salience (not pleasure) to stimuli. We first need to ask, therefore, whether there is any experimental evidence that repeated exposure to addictive drugs can produce neuroadaptations that meet the relevant criteria. The criteria required of such neuroadaptations in order for the theory to be true include the following:

(1) To the extent that the excessive incentive salience elicited by drugs is mediated by a common substrate, there should be a common neural system affected by many different addictive drugs.

(2) To explain the progressive development of addictive behavior repeated drug administration should render this neural system hypersensitive in a gradual and incremental fashion.

(3) To explain the persistence of relapse these drug-induced neuroadaptations should persist for very long periods of time (if not permanently) following the discontinuation of drug use.

(4) To explain the role of drug-associated stimuli in relapse the expression of these neuroadaptations should be susceptible to conditioned stimulus or environmental control.

(5) To explain drug craving the activation of this neural system should mediate the incentive motivational effects of drugs and drug-related stimuli and the neuroadaptations produced by drugs should potentiate these motivational effects.

(6) To explain the dissociation between drug 'wanting' and drug 'liking' this neural system should not directly mediate the subjective pleasurable effects of drugs or the subjective pleasure associated with other stimuli.

Evidence that the repeated use of a number of different addictive drugs does indeed produce neuroadaptations that meet each of these criteria is presented next.

4. EVIDENCE FOR THE INCENTIVE-SENSITIZATION THEORY OF ADDICTION

4.1. Criterion 1: there should be a common neural system affected by many different addictive drugs

Addictive drugs represent a diverse group of compounds that markedly differ in their behavioral and neurochemical actions. Nevertheless, there is increasing evidence that many addictive drugs share the ability to enhance mesotelencephalic dopamine neurotransmission[73,365]. This evidence has been reviewed recently and need not be reiterated here. Suffice it to say that the following drugs have been reported to increase dopamine neurotransmission in the nucleus accumbens and dorsal striatum: amphetamine ('speed'), cathinone ('Khat'), cocaine ('coke'; 'crack'), methamphetamine ('ice'; 'crystal meth'), methylenedioxyamphetamine (MDA; 'the love drug'); methylenedioxymethamphetamine (MDMA; 'ecstasy'), methylphenidate, ethanol, fentanyl ('China white'), methadone, morphine, nicotine and phencyclidine (PCP; 'angel dust'). This common action of diverse drugs is consistent with the hypothesis that mesotelencephalic dopamine systems mediate, at least in part, the incentive motivational properties of many different drugs of abuse[362,363]. Although it cannot be said that there is a single neural system that is affected by all addictive drugs, dopamine systems and their associated structures are affected by most[179,363,365].

4.2. Criterion 2: the repeated administration of different addictive drugs should render a common neural system hypersensitive in a gradual and incremental fashion

Drug effects are known to change when drugs are given repeatedly, and some of these changes are known involve adaptations in neural elements mediating specific drug effects[148]. Much of the emphasis in the past has been on homeostatic neuroadaptations thought to underly the development of tolerance and to contribute to withdrawal symptoms. But as discussed above, tolerance and withdrawal do not account for the defining characteristics of addiction and therefore, tolerance and withdrawal-associated neuroadaptations do not meet Criterion 2 under discussion here.

4.2.1. Sensitization to the psychomotor-activating effects of addictive drugs. However, some effects of drugs are not decreased, but are actually increased by repeated intermittent drug administration. Indeed, for a given drug, some effects may decrease (show tolerance) while simultaneously other effects increase. This latter phenomenon has been referred to as behavioral sensitization, behavioral facilitation, reverse tolerance and auxoesthesia[160,162,201,257,272,291,297,354]. We will use the term 'sensitization' here.

Psychomotor stimulant drugs, such as amphetamine or cocaine, have been used in the majority of studies on drug-induced sensitization, and the effects of these drugs have been well characterized[188,250,257,269,272,291,354]. For example, the acute administration of a low-to-moderate dose of amphetamine or cocaine produces 'psychomotor activation', characterized by an increase in locomotor activity (ambulation), rearing behavior and rotational behavior[267]. Higher doses result in the emergence of focussed stereotyped behaviors, such as repetitive head movements and sniffing and a resultant decrease in locomotion and rearing[254,284]. The repeated intermittent administration of a constant, relatively low dose, produces a progressive increase in drug-induced locomotor stimulation with each successive administration. Repeated administration of a moderate dose will come to elicit the stereotyped behavior typical of a higher dose, even though it produced only ambulation the first time it was given. Furthermore, sensitization-related changes in behavior can come under strong conditioned stimulus control and this feature of sensitization is discussed in more detail below. In summary, it is the gradual and incremental increase in drug-induced 'psychomotor activation' and the emergence of increasingly stereotyped behavior, that is usually referred to as 'behavioral sensitization'. The only comparable stimulant effect that has been characterized in humans is sensitization to the psychotogenic effects of amphetamine and cocaine[250,272,280,297].

Behavioral sensitization is produced by the repeated administration of many different psychomotor stimulants, including the amphetamines[8,188,272,292], cocaine[160,250], methylphenidate[40,177,301], fencamfamine[3] and the endogenous trace amine, phenylethylamine[35]. The phenomenon is not limited, however, to classical psychomotor stimulants. Other drugs, not traditionally considered psychomotor stimulants, also produce psychomotor activation, enhance dopamine neurotransmission and produce behavioral sensitization[73,365]. These include: opioids[11,153,302], nicotine[25,52,171,186], phencyclidine[116,117,147,225], ethanol[58,61,114,208,209] and MDMA[316] (cf. Note 7 in Ch. 6).

Repeated intermittent treatment with an addictive drug not only produces sensitization to that drug, but may also produce cross-sensitization to other drugs. Although the literature is not entirely consistent, cross-sensitization has been reported between drugs in the same class (e.g., amphetamine and cocaine) and between drugs in different classes (e.g., stimulants and opioids)[159,160,268]. Furthermore, cross-sensitization is also found between drugs and stress, which led to the suggestion that drugs may induce sensitization by their action as stressors[8,9,249]. Evidence for cross-sensitization between drugs and stress comes from studies showing that animals pretreated with drugs like amphetamine, cocaine or morphine are later hyperresponsive to stress and vice versa, animals sensitized to stress are hyperresponsive to a drug challenge[8,9,160,190,196,268]. Even the repeated administration of exogenous corticosterone is reported to increase the locomotor response to a later challenge with amphetamine[70] (see also Note 9 in Ch. 6).

4.2.2. Sensitization to the incentive motivational effects of drugs. Of more direct relevance to the process of addiction are recent studies on sensitization to the incentive motivational properties of addictive drugs. There has been relatively little research on this topic, but there have been a number of recent experiments, using either self-administration procedures or the conditioned place preference paradigm, which suggest that prior exposure to amphetamine, cocaine or morphine produces sensitization to the incentive motivational effects of these drugs.

In one of the first reports of this kind Woolverton et al.[373] found that rhesus monkeys would self-administer a low dose of methamphetamine only after they had received a regimen of non-contingent injections of methamphetamine. That is, the threshold dose necessary to sustain self-administration was lowered by methamphetamine pretreatment, suggesting "an increased sensitivity to the reinforcing properties of the drug" (p. 740). There are now a number of similar reports in rats[241]. For example, Piazza and his co-workers[242,243] have reported that *d*-amphetamine pretreatment, which induces behavioral sensitization, facilitates the later acquisition of an amphetamine self-administration habit, especially in animals not predisposed to self-administer amphetamine. Similarly, pretreatment with cocaine facilitates the later acquisition of a cocaine self-administration habit[137].

Sensitization has also been observed with the conditioned place preference paradigm, in which the place where a drug is experienced becomes preferred by an animal in subsequent choice tests. For example, Lett[195] examined the influence of amphetamine, cocaine or morphine pretreatment on the later acquisition of a conditioned place preference produced by the same drug. For all three drugs, pretreated (sensitized) animals showed a significantly enhanced conditioned place preference, relative to control animals. A similar effect has been reported following pretreatment with morphine[102] or ethanol[114].

Cross-sensitization also occurs in these situations. Animals pretreated with amphetamine show an enhanced place preference for morphine, animals pretreated with morphine show an enhanced place preference for cocaine and animals pretreated with morphine show an enhanced place preference for amphetamine[195]. These latter findings suggest that the enhancement of the conditioned place preference is not due to tolerance to the drug's aversive properties, because cross-tolerance does not occur between the stimulants and morphine[195]. Similarly, cross-sensitization has been found using self-administration procedures. Noncontingent pretreatment with amphetamine, caffeine or nicotine facilitates the later acquisition of cocaine self-administration[136-138,282]. An especially intriguing example of cross-sensitization between opiates and amphetamine was reported recently by Cunningham and Kelley[62]. These researchers found that the repeated intra-accumbens application of a mu receptor agonist (morphine or DAMGO) for 4 days potentiated (sensitized) the ability of systemic amphetamine to later enhance responding for a conditioned reinforcer; i.e., a light/tone previously paired with food.

It was mentioned above that cross-sensitization to the psychomotor-activating effects of drugs can occur not only between drugs, but between drugs and stress. Therefore, the effects of prior stress on the incentive motivational effects of drugs are also of interest. Indeed, prior stress (tail pinch) facilitates the acquisition of an amphetamine self-administration habit[243]. In fact, a number of potentially stressful environmental manipulations, such as social isolation or prenatal stress, are reported to increase sensitivity to amphetamine and facilitate amphetamine or cocaine self-administration behavior[68,152,281].

In conclusion, these studies establish that not only are the 'psychomotor-activating' properties of addictive drugs sensitized by repeated drug administration, but their incentive motivational properties are sensitized as well. Animals sensitized to amphetamine, cocaine or morphine later show an enhanced preference for an environment associated with drug administration and animals sensitized to amphetamine or cocaine show enhanced vulnerability to acquire a drug self-administration habit. Obviously, sensitization to the incentive motivational properties of drugs (and drug-related stimuli) could have a profound influence on the development of addictive behavior. With more-and-more drug experience the incentive value of the act of drug-taking and of drug-related stimuli would be progressively enhanced, which would increase the probability of repeating drug-seeking and drug-taking behavior in the future (although, see Note 1 in Ch. 6 for a discussion of the role of response contingency in drug sensitization).

4.2.3. The neural basis of behavioral sensitization. The behavioral studies summarized above strongly suggest that the repeated administration of many different addictive drugs produces gradual and incremental neuroadaptations that render animals hypersensitive to these agents. The behavioral studies also provide prima facie evidence that sensitization-related neuroadaptations involve a hypersensitivity in mesotelencephalic dopamine systems. A change in dopamine neurotransmission is implicated for a number of reasons. First, the behaviors that are sensitized by addictive drugs are known to involve an activation of mesotelencephalic dopamine systems. There is considerable evidence that both the psychomotor-activating effects and the incentive motivational effects of many of these drugs requires the integrity of mesotelencephalic dopamine systems, especially dopamine projections to the ventral striatum[362]. Second, the activation of dopamine systems appears to be necessary to induce sensitization. The sensitization produced by amphetamine, cocaine or morphine is prevented by co-treatment with dopamine antagonists[121,187,344,345,352] (see ref. 160 for a review) and amphetamine sensitization is prevented by a 6-OHDA lesion[293]. Third, the application of amphetamine or morphine directly into the ventral tegmental area, where dopamine cell bodies are located, induces sensitization[160]. Fourth, a local 'challenge' injection of amphetamine into the lateral ventricle[258] or nucleus accumbens[178,233] evokes a sensitized behavioral response in animals treated previously with systemic amphetamine.

Perhaps even more importantly, behavioral sensitization is accompanied by changes in mesotelencephalic dopamine activity[160,257,269,272,354]. For example, amphetamine sensitization is accompanied by an increase in amphetamine-stimulated dopamine release from striatal tissue in vitro[48,176,178,271,358,375]. More recently, in vivo microdialysis studies have shown that although amphetamine sensitization is not accompanied by changes in the basal extracellular concentration of dopamine, it is associated with an enhanced dopamine response to a drug challenge[144,166,231,269,274,370] (cf. ref. 295). Even the local application of amphetamine into the ventral tegmental area sensitizes the dopamine release produced by a subsequent systemic challenge with amphetamine[347]. A similar enhancement in dopamine response has also been reported in association with sensitization to cocaine[5,157,167,236,238] (cf. ref. 296), ethanol[24], nicotine[25,101,123] (cf. ref. 65), morphine[154,160] (cf. ref. 155), phenylethylamine[189] and methylphenidate[177] and following cross-sensitization between different drugs[4,159,166] and between drugs and stress[156,159,160,315,320,358]. Furthermore, co-treatment with a dopamine receptor antagonist, which prevents the induction of behavioral sensitization to methamphetamine, also attenuates the dopaminergic response to a methamphetamine challenge assessed with microdialysis[121]. Although there is no convincing evidence for sensitization-related changes in dopamine receptor binding[272], there is electrophysiological evidence for an increased sensitivity of nucleus accumbens neurons to iontophoretically applied dopamine in cocaine sensitized rats[124,354]. It is possible, therefore, that sensitization produced by cocaine and amphetamine is also accompanied by changes in the transduction of dopamine receptor-mediated events[15,112,124,140,265,276].

The biophysical basis of sensitization-related changes in dopamine neurotransmission is not known. There have been a number of hypotheses proposed, including changes in autoreceptor sensitivity, changes in the intraneuronal distribution of dopamine leading to enhanced release, changes in the dopamine uptake carrier and changes in transduction mechanisms[6,160,188,226,269,354]. It is not known, however, whether the behavioral sensitization produced by different drugs involves the same or different cellular and molecular changes. Even the processes involved in the induction of sensitization differ from those involved in the expression of sensitization[160,233,269]. Furthermore, sensitization-related changes in dopamine systems have been emphasized here because only dopamine systems have been studied in any detail. But neuroadaptations in other neurotransmitter systems that interact with dopamine systems must also be considered. For example, glutamate systems have been implicated in recent studies showing that glutamate antagonists, like dopamine antagonists, prevent the induction of sensitization[161,163,164,369].

In summary, there is considerable experimental evidence in support of Criterion 2. The repeated administration of many different addictive drugs produces behavioral sensitization and behavioral sensitization is associated with hypersensitive mesotelencephalic dopamine systems.

4.3. Criterion 3: sensitization-related neuroadaptations should be very long-lasting

One of the most striking characteristics of sensitization is its persistence. A single injection of amphetamine, cocaine or morphine induces behavioral sensitization lasting for weeks to months[40,197,236,237,267,302] and animals sensitized with escalating doses of amphetamine remain behaviorally hypersensitive to an amphetamine challenge for at least 1 year[232]. In fact, Paulson et al.[232] found that rats were just as sensitized a year following the discontinuation of amphetamine pretreatment, which is over one third of their life-span, as they were at 2–4 weeks. These findings suggest that after at least some pretreatment regimens the neuroadaptations responsible for behavioral sensitization to amphetamine may be essentially permanent. Similarly, behavioral sensitization in rats is reported to persist for over 3 months following pretreatment with cocaine[304], for over 50 days following pretreatment with methylphenidate[301] and for over 8 months following pretreatment with morphine[12,17,302].

It is not known if sensitization to the incentive motivational properties of drugs persists for as long as sensitization to their psychomotor-activating effects, but this is obviously an important issue for the Incentive-Sensitization Theory. To the extent that sensitization to the psychomotor-activating effects and the incentive motivational effects of drugs have a common neural basis we would expect both effects to show comparable persistence. Neither have neurochemical studies been conducted as long as a year following drug pretreatment. But sensitization-related changes in dopamine systems have been reported to persist for months after withdrawal[269,272]. The available evidence suggests, therefore, that the neuroadaptations underlying behavioral sensitization meet the criterion of persistence.

4.4. Criterion 4: the expression of sensitization-related neuroadaptations should be amenable to conditioned stimulus control

The Incentive-Sensitization Theory of Addiction posits that drugs sensitize a neural system that mediates 'wanting'. It is also hypothesized that associative processes focus exaggerated 'wanting' (craving) specifically onto drug-related stimuli. This implies that the behavioral expression of sensitization-related neuroadaptations should be strongly influenced by associative factors.

Indeed, the environmental context in which drugs are experienced can have profound effects on the development and expression of sensitization. Stewart[323] recently reviewed the literature on the conditioned stimulus control of sensitization and the reader is referred to this paper for a more detailed and excellent discussion of such issues. In brief, Stewart[323] points out that the conditioned stimulus control of sensitization can take one of two basic forms, depending to some extent on experimental design. In one design the drug (the UCS), which produces a pharmacological effect (the UCR), is given only in association with unique environmental cues (CS). After repeated pairing of the UCS and CS, the CS alone can acquire the ability to elicit drug-like responses (CR). For example, after repeated administration of a dose of amphetamine that produces locomotor hyperactivity, just placing an animal in the environment in which it previously received amphetamine is sufficient to produce conditioned locomotor hyperactivity, in the absence of any drug. A number of researchers have reported drug-environment conditioning of this type and have suggested these conditioned effects contribute to the development of sensitization[128,283,323] (see ref. 338 for a review).

A second type of conditioned stimulus control of sensitization is the situation where, after explicit pairing of a drug and specific test environment, animals are administered a 'challenge' injection of the drug in either the drug-paired environment or in a new environment. In this case one observes the effect of the CS (the environment) on the response to the UCS (the drug). In some experiments of this type the expression of sensitization has come under complete conditioned stimulus control. For example, Post et al.[251] reported that rats given ten daily injections of 10 mg/kg of cocaine in a test environment showed a progressively greater behavioral response (locomotor activation) to the drug, but animals given daily injections of cocaine in their home cage did not show evidence of behavioral sensitization when subsequently challenged with cocaine in the test environment. Similarly, Vezina and Stewart[344] reported that repeated injections of morphine into the ventral tegmental area produced evidence of sensitization on a subsequent challenge test only when rats were tested in the environment where they received morphine. In addition, the conditioned stimulus control of sensitization may not only enhance the expression of sensitization in drug-paired environments, but may also inhibit the expression of sensitization in environments that predict the absence of the drug. For example, Vezina and Stewart[344] found that the locomotor response to an intra-ventral tegmental area challenge injection of morphine in explicitly unpaired animals was significantly depressed relative to saline-pretreated controls (also see ref. 328). Nevertheless, sensitization is not only a conditioned response, even though the expression of sensitization can come under strong conditioned stimulus control, a point that has been made by a number of authors[40,210,272,323,346].

Our discussion of the conditioned stimulus control of sensitization has focused thus far on the effects of drug-associated stimuli on the subsequent response to drugs. It is important to know, however, whether environmental stimuli associated with drugs can also influence the response to other incentive stimuli; even non-drug-related stimuli. This issue has received almost no experimental attention, despite its theoretical importance. Nevertheless, it was addressed in one study by Mitchell and Stewart[218]. In this study male rats were given morphine either in a test arena or their home cage, every other day for four injections. All rats were then placed in the test arena in the presence of a receptive female. Rats pretreated with morphine in the test arena showed more frequent female-directed behaviors than either rats pretreated with morphine in their home cage or saline-pretreated controls. The enhancement of sexual behavior produced by the drug-associated environment did not involve changes in copulatory behavior per se, but only in the appetitive behaviors leading to copulation, including more frequent "pursuit of the female, anogenital exploration and partial mounts and... shorter latencies to initiate copulation" (p. 367). That is, the female appeared to be a more salient incentive stimulus in male rats tested in the presence of morphine-associated cues. These results suggest that sensitization to drugs may change neural systems that not only modulate the incentive properties of drug-associated stimuli, but the incentive properties of 'natural incentives'†. This is important because it implies that drug-associated stimuli may potentially influence a wide range of motivated behaviors.

To summarize thus far, we have addressed the first four criteria, and reviewed evidence to establish that: (1) Many different addictive drugs activate a common neural system, the mesotelencephalic dopamine system; (2) Repeated administration of many addictive drugs causes dopamine systems to become hypersensitive and this is accompanied by a gradual and incremental increase (sensitization) in the psychomotor-activating and incentive motivational properties of drugs; (3) The neuroadaptations underlying sensitization are extremely persistent; and (4) The expression of sensitization is subject to conditioned stimulus control.

We next need to address Criteria 5 and 6. Criterion 5 requires that the neural system sensitized by repeated treatment with addictive drugs normally mediate the incentive motivational effects of drugs and drug-related stimuli. Criterion 6 requires that this neural system not mediate the subjective pleasurable effects of drugs or the pleasure associated with other stimuli.

4.5. Criterion 5: the role of mesotelencephalic dopamine systems in incentive motivation

There is a wealth of evidence implicating dopamine systems in the incentive motivational† effects of drugs, as well as of food, sex and other natural incentives[19,84,90,131,262,263,356,365,368] (cf. ref. 181). For example, signals predicting the availability of food, water or a sexual partner activate brain dopamine systems, increasing dopamine neurotransmission in the ventral striatum[51,66,126,246,376]. Addictive drugs also increase dopamine neurotransmission[73]. Indeed, in the case of drugs, a direct action on dopamine systems alone is sufficient to motivate behavior. Animals will work for microinjections of drugs directly into appropriate portions of the mesotelencephalic dopamine system[366]. Furthermore, microinjections of amphetamine or dopamine directly into the nucleus accumbens facilitates responding for conditioned incentive stimuli† (conditioned reinforcers) – stimuli that have acquired incentive properties by association with a natural incentive[†85,262,263]. In short, a common neural currency for many incentives appears to be activation of mesotelencephalic dopamine systems (see Note 4 in Ch. 6).

Consistent with this idea are studies showing that the motivational properties of natural incentives and addictive drugs are attenuated by decreasing dopamine activity[360]. Antagonist drugs that prevent the activation of dopamine receptors or the complete destruction of mesotelencephalic dopamine projections by neurochemically selective toxins, impair the instrumental performance of animals for food, for drugs and for electrical brain stimulation. A great deal of effort has been directed towards ascertaining whether the suppression of dopamine neurotransmission produces changes in behavior because of effects on the control of movement or because of effects on incentive motivation and a variety of experimental paradigms have been developed to distinguish between motor and motivational effects (see Note 2 in Ch. 6). It is now generally accepted that dopamine antagonists can have effects on behavior that are truly motivational. This is not to say they may not also have effects that are 'motor', but in many cases the effect on behavior is precisely what one would expect if dopamine antagonism reduced the motivational properties of incentives[82,360,361].

In summary, the large literature on the role of dopamine in mediating the incentive motivational effects of drugs and other stimuli satisfies Criterion 5. What of Criterion 6, which requires that dopamine not mediate the subjective pleasurable effects of drugs or the pleasure associated with natural incentives.

4.6. Criterion 6: the effects of dopamine are on incentive salience, not pleasure

The evidence that brain dopamine systems mediate the incentive motivational effects of natural incentives and addictive drugs provided the basis for Wise's[359,360,361] provocative anhedonia hypothesis: the hypothesis that mesotelencephalic dopamine systems mediate the subjective pleasure produced by food, drugs, electrical brain stimulation, etc. and that dopamine antagonists suppress the pleasure produced by these agents. The anhedonia hypothesis provided a parsimonious explanation of dopamine's motivational effects by equating it with the psychological process of subjective pleasure *.

If the motivational properties of natural incentive stimuli or drugs depended only on their ability to produce subjective pleasure, then the effects of dopamine manipulations on motivated behavior would be compelling evidence for the anhedonia hypothesis. We suggest, however, that incentive motivation depends on a number of additional psychological processes that interact with pleasure: including associative learning and the attribution of incentive salience to external events and their representations[27,28]. It is the entire complex of pleasure, learning and incentive salience† together that comprise the process of incentive motivation†.

4.6.1. Incentive salience. Of particular importance to the Incentive-Sensitization Theory of Addiction are the relative roles of 'wanting' and 'liking' in incentive motivation. The idea that there may be a psychological process (and neural substrate) responsible for 'wanting' incentives that is dissociable from the psychological process (and neural substrate) responsible for 'liking' incentives has not been considered explicitly in previous theories of incentive motivation[30,339,**]. Based on a series of studies on the relationship between taste pleasure and appetite, such a dissociation was recently proposed[27,28]. Berridge and his colleagues hypothesized that a psychological process specifically involving the attribution of salience to incentive stimuli (incentive salience) results in the experience of 'wanting'. This view of incentive motivation posits that salience attribution is a specific psychological process that is activated normally in conjunction with pleasure ('liking') and associative learning in the creation of new incentives. As new incentives are acquired particular stimuli that allow an individual to recognize an incentive (e.g., the sight of food; in nature, a flowering plant that signals the availability of food; or, in the laboratory, a tone that predicts food), become associated with the pleasure food produces by the process of classical conditioning. The stimulus features of the incentive predict the pleasure that will follow and may elicit conditioned pleasure. But conditioned stimulus features also become themselves the target of a separate and powerful motivational process – salience attribution. Salience attribution transforms the sensory features of the incentive stimulus into an especially salient percept, which 'grabs attention', becomes attractive and 'wanted' and thus guides behavior to the incentive. That is, new incentives become attractive in their own right as conditioned incentives† (also called conditioned or secondary reinforcers).

Thus, the role of salience attribution in incentive motivation is proposed to occur as the third stage of a three-stage process (see Fig. 2). First, pleasure is normally activated by an encounter with a natural incentive, such as when an hungry animal eats food. In the normal course of events, pleasure is a necessary step in the establishment of a new conditioned incentive. However, pleasure ('liking') is not by itself sufficient to motivate behavior[28]. Pleasure by itself has no object or action. Assignment of pleasure to something requires associative learning, which is the second stage in the formation of incentives.

If pleasure is assigned to an action or stimulus by associative learning, then the action or stimulus should come to predict pleasure or elicit pleasure, on its own. No doubt this often happens. But we would argue that neither the experience of pleasure nor the expectation of impending pleasure by themselves constitute 'wanting'[27,28]. 'Wanting' requires an additional process: the attribution of incentive salience to stimuli or actions. Stimuli that are attributed with incentive salience become attractive and demand attention. Like the sight of food to a starving person, they cannot be ignored. This does not necessarily make them 'liked'; the sight of food may be irresistibly attractive to the starving person, but if out of reach it may torment rather than please. But the food is still much 'wanted'. In summary, incentive motivation is proposed to involve three distinct psychological processes acting together; pleasure, associative learning and *incentive salience* and different neural systems are thought to be responsible for each[27,28,***].

Changes in any one of these three processes that

* Note, however, that in discussing his anhedonia hypothesis of dopamine blockade Wise[361] stated: "The anhedonia hypothesis is most vulnerable in its assumption that positive hedonic states such as pleasure or euphoria are attenuated by neuroleptics. This is, for the most part, speculation" (p. 184).

** Although neither Bindra nor Toates distinguished 'wanting' from 'liking', Toates[339] did distinguish the associative control of 'wanting/liking' from mere recall of past 'wanting/liking'. For example, as in the Krieckhaus effect, a stimulus that is ordinarily not 'wanted' or 'liked' may suddenly become 'wanted/liked' on the basis of its prior associations when physiological state is changed[185].

*** For a discussion of evidence that most motivated behavior is primarily controlled by incentive processes see Toates[339].

constitute incentive motivation would produce effects on instrumental or appetitive behavior indistinguishable, by most measures, from changes in another. Mesotelencephalic dopamine does not seem to be critical specifically for associative learning; i.e., for forming stimulus–stimulus associations[19,90]. For example, dopamine antagonists do not disrupt the learning of associations between a stimulus and electrical shock, as measured by a conditioned emotional response or by the defensive burying paradigm[22,23,141]. It is more likely, therefore, that the effects of dopamine on motivated behavior are due to effects on subjective pleasure or incentive salience. If mesotelencephalic dopamine systems mediate the subjective pleasurable effects of drugs, then the addictive property of drugs such as cocaine, heroin, amphetamine, etc., which sensitize dopamine systems, might be best understood in terms of the pleasure these drugs induce. But if a sensitized dopamine system enhanced the incentive salience of the act of taking drugs, rather than the subjective pleasurable effects of drugs, then the neuroadaptations underlying sensitization would cause drugs to be 'wanted' or craved, independently of the pleasure they produce.

Most animal studies on the effects of dopamine antagonists on motivated behavior (summarized in Note 2 in Ch. 6) are equally consistent with the hypothesis that dopamine mediates pleasure (the anhedonia hypothesis of Wise) and the hypothesis that dopamine mediates incentive salience[27,28]. Likewise, studies on the effects of manipulating dopamine systems on the incentive properties of conditioned reinforcers are consistent with both interpretations of dopamine function[85,262]. In these latter experiments animals must learn a new instrumental response (bar press) that is reinforced only by a stimulus (light/tone) that was previously associated with a primary incentive, such as food, water or a mate. Manipulations that increase dopamine neurotransmission in the ventral striatum potentiate the incentive properties of conditioned reinforcers and manipulations that decrease dopamine neurotransmission in the ventral striatum block these potentiating effects[44,127,168,169,264,333,334]. Barry Everitt has suggested these studies support a view that, in some way "ventral striatal dopamine makes the world brighter" (Catecholamine Symposium, Amsterdam, 1992). This view is compatible with the attribution of incentive salience hypothesis proposed here. Nevertheless, these studies could also be interpreted in support of the 'pleasure' hypothesis and therefore, they do not resolve the issue.

4.6.2. Introspection into 'wanting' and 'liking'. At first glance it seems it should be relatively easy to resolve the issue by asking people to report what effect dopamine antagonist drugs have on the subjective effects of addictive drugs. Indeed, Wise[361] challenged researchers to test this hypothesis, arguing that "it would be procedurally simple for workers using neuroleptics with human subjects to determine the effects of these drugs on the subjective effect of rewarding stimuli". Despite his challenge, the relationship between dopamine blockade and anhedonia remains equivocal and the data are inconsistent[98,298].

In light of the incentive salience hypothesis, however, assessment of the effects of dopamine blockade on subjective pleasure in humans may not be as simple as Wise thought. In fact, it may be an especially difficult task[228]. Humans may not, under normal conditions, be able to subjectively tell the difference between the two psychological processes of 'wanting' versus 'liking'. Studies of introspection and self-report have established that humans often (a) report psychological 'events' that can be shown to have not happened; (b) strongly deny the existence of psychological events that can be shown to have influenced their behavior; and (c) confuse events that are not connected[228]. Under many circumstances humans actually have very little direct access into the nature of their own psychological processes. Rather, introspection appears to interpret underlying processes in ways that seem plausible to the person[228]. Introspection does not reveal psychological processes directly. This implies that a person might mistake a change in incentive salience for a change in pleasure ('If I don't want it, then I must not like it'). It may be possible to distinguish between changes in 'wanting' and 'liking' by asking appropriate questions that tap into different aspects of a person's reaction to an incentive, but this will have to be approached with great sophistication and caution.

4.6.3. Evidence that mesotelencephalic dopamine mediates incentive salience, not pleasure. Although the studies cited above are equivocal, there are at least four lines of evidence which lead us to suggest that sensitization of dopamine neurotransmission produces enhanced incentive salience rather than enhanced pleasure. The evidence is based both on reports by human addicts of their own experience and on studies in animals on the role of dopamine in sensory pleasure and motivated behavior.

– The first line of evidence comes from animal studies that have explicitly examined the role of dopamine in mediating natural reactions to the sensory qualities of tastes. These studies have used the 'taste reactivity paradigm', which is based upon natural hedonic and aversive reactions (tongue protrusions, gapes, forelimb

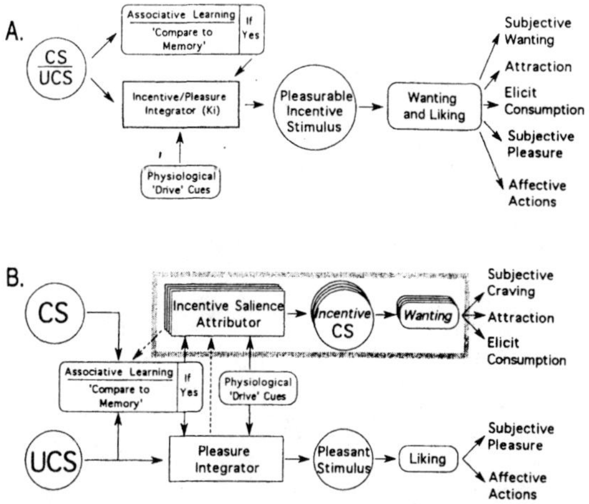

Fig. 2. A schematic illustration of a major existing model of the psychological processes that constitute incentive motivation (A, top) and our alternative model, which proposes a separate process of incentive salience and accounts for the consequences of drug-induced sensitization (B, bottom). Panel A: the 'Toates/Bindra model' of incentive motivation, on which our model is based (adapted from Toates[339]). By this model the sensory stimuli (CS and UCS) of incentive objects are both pleasant and attractive. Their ability to produce an incentive motivational state (K_i) is partly dependent on memories of previous favorable experiences with them. Physiological states (such as hunger, thirst or withdrawal) selectively potentiate the ability of particular stimuli (related to food, water or drugs) to evoke incentive processes: to become 'wanted' and 'liked' (see Toates[339] for a more complete description of this model). Panel B: in our modified model of incentive motivation the psychological process (and neural substrate) for pleasure ('liking') is separate from the psychological process (and neural substrate) responsible for incentive salience ('wanting'). We further propose that the activation of mesotelencephalic dopamine systems plays a *direct* role only in the process of 'wanting', via the attribution of incentive salience to the perception and representation of conditioned stimuli (as described by Berridge and Valenstein[27]; also see Note 4 in Ch. 6). In Panel B the portion of the model (i.e., the psychological process) that is sensitized by repeated drug administration is 'highlighted' within the shaded box. It is the hyperactivation of this specific psychological process (incentive salience), due to sensitization of its neural substrate by drugs, that results in the excessive attribution of incentive salience to drug-related stimuli. Whereas normal levels of incentive salience attribution results in normal 'wanting', we propose hyperactivation of this system results in excessive incentive salience attribution, which is experienced as craving. Craving is pathologically intense 'wanting'. The major difference between our model of incentive motivation and the traditional model is that in ours the psychological processes and neural substrates responsible for pleasure ('liking') are separate from those for incentive salience ('wanting'). Thus, in our model 'natural incentives' (UCS stimuli) produce pleasure directly, but produce incentive salience and elicit goal-directed approach behavior only indirectly (as indicated by the dashed arrow from 'pleasure integrator' to the 'incentive salience attributor'). The direction of incentive salience attribution to stimuli that preceded or accompanied incentive salience activation is determined by associative learning. Thus, activation of the incentive salience attributor by a UCS results in incentive salience being assigned to the perception of conditioned stimuli that were originally neutral (such as the sight of a syringe) and to their mental representations. This is what makes conditioned stimuli attractive and 'wanted' and able to elicit approach. Conditioned stimuli (and UCS's) are always compared against past associative memories. Without the direction provided by associative learning, incentive salience could not be focussed upon any single target. Although diffuse attribution of incentive salience would be both psychologically and behaviorally activating, without associative direction it would not be sufficient to guide behavior towards a specific goal. Familiar conditioned stimuli that have been paired with incentive salience attribution in the past are the target of incentive salience when encountered again, especially when an animal is in particular physiological states (indicated by the arrow from 'physiological drive cues'). Incentive salience assigned to conditioned stimuli must be further 'reboosted' each time they are paired again with salience activation (indicated by the dashed arrow from the incentive salience attributor to associative learning). Disruption of this reboosting, by neuroleptics for example, can produce 'extinction mimicry' or decay of incentive value. Ordinarily, incentive salience is assigned only to stimuli that have been paired with pleasure. But brain manipulations (such as drugs or electrical brain stimulation) may circumvent pleasure, by activating the neural substrate of incentive salience directly. This will result in the attribution of incentive salience to associated stimuli and actions and result in their becoming 'wanted', even in the absence of pleasure. This can be considered a kind of 'sham reward' (see glossary entry for reward). Sensitization of the neural substrate for incentive salience will lead to pathological 'wanting' (craving) for stimuli associated with its excessive activation (e.g., those involved in drug taking), even if this produces little or no pleasure. As mentioned above, the direction of incentive salience by associative learning is the primary determinant of exactly which stimuli become craved. Thus, in the addict, drug-paired stimuli, which have been experienced repeatedly in association with the excessive stimulation of dopamine systems, become the nearly exclusive targets for the attribution of incentive salience. Other contributions of associative learning are also possible in this model. For example, the pleasure elicited by a UCS can change with repeated experience, as when one develops an appreciative palate for Scotch whiskey (this is indicated in the model by the arrow from learning to the 'pleasure integrator'). Also, a CS that has been repeatedly paired with pleasure can come to itself elicit subjective pleasure, as in the example of a conditioned 'high' reported by 'needle freaks' (arrows from the CS to the 'pleasure integrator' via associative learning). But we suggest these effects are separate from the attribution of incentive salience and that they have only a relatively weak influence on motivated behavior, compared to the craving produced by the attribution of excessive incentive salience. Finally, we suggest that none of the psychological processes described in this model, except for subjective 'wanting' (craving) and subjective pleasure, are apparent to conscious awareness. The interaction among incentive salience, pleasure and associative learning is not available to introspection. Only the final products of the interaction are interpreted by cognitive mechanisms (not shown in the figure, see Nisbett and Wilson[228]) as subjective 'wanting' and 'liking'. For an addict, whose neural substrates of incentive salience have been sensitized, the subjective product is dominated by the intense experience of drug craving.

flails, etc.) that rats emit to tastes[119]. Much like the facial expressions that human infants display to sweet or bitter tastes[319], these hedonic and aversive reactions reflect the perceived pleasure or displeasure of a taste sensation. The reactions of rats to taste are altered by many of the same things that control human perceptions of taste pleasure. The sensory pleasure of sweetness to humans, for example, is enhanced by hunger and suppressed by caloric satiety[41,42]. Hedonic reactions of rats to sweet tastes are similarly enhanced by hunger and suppressed by satiety[26,43]. The taste pleasure of a palatable food for humans can be abolished and replaced with subjective aversion by associative pairing of that food with gastrointestinal illness[278]. Similarly, hedonic reactions of rats to sweetness are abolished and replaced by aversive behavioral reactions after associative pairing of that taste with illness[118]. Finally, drugs that affect opioid or GABA neurotransmitters can enhance or suppress the hedonic reactions of rats to tastes in ways that should be expected based on current theories of the role of these neurotransmitter systems in taste pleasure[75,230,340].

Application of the 'taste reactivity paradigm' to the role of mesotelencephalic dopamine systems in taste pleasure and motivated behavior leads to the conclusion that dopamine systems do not mediate taste pleasure, although they do mediate the incentive motivational properties of foods. There are three lines of evidence leading to this conclusion. (1) Dopamine antagonists do not decrease the sensory pleasure of tastes, measured by hedonic reactions, although they can decrease their incentive value. Conversely, dopamine agonists do not increase the sensory pleasure of tastes, although they can increase their incentive value[340]. (2) A bilateral neurotoxic lesion (6-OHDA), which depletes dopamine from the nucleus accumbens and caudate nucleus, does not diminish the hedonic evaluation of tastes, even though it completely abolishes the motivation to eat and renders natural incentives ineffective (ref. 28 and unpublished data). (3) Activation of the motivation to eat by electrical stimulation of the lateral hypothalamus, which is mediated in part by dopamine systems, does not potentiate the hedonic evaluation of tastes[27].

These experiments suggest, therefore, that the role of dopamine systems in behavior motivated by food is not to enhance the sensory pleasure of tastes. Or, put another way, these experiments suggest that neural systems mediating 'wanting' food can be dissociated from neural systems mediating 'liking' food and that dopamine activates 'wanting'. This is what would be expected if dopamine mediates the salience of incentive stimuli, rather than the sensory pleasure evoked by incentive stimuli (Fig. 2). These findings are precisely what would be expected on the basis of our hypothesis that dopamine systems mediate the incentive motivational effects of drugs and are dissociable from other neural systems that mediate the subjective pleasurable effects of drugs and other stimuli. This kind of dissociation would explain the findings reported by Fischman and Foltin[95] and by Lamb et al.[192] (see above). You will recall that in these studies a low dose injection of cocaine or morphine motivated drug-taking behavior in 'postaddicts', but did not produce self-reported subjective pleasure.

– The second line of evidence that dopamine mediates incentive salience rather than sensory pleasure comes from a series of electrophysiological experiments on the conditions under which dopamine neurons discharge in behaving animals[288]. When monkeys are first exposed to a novel situation dopamine neurons discharge to new, unexpected stimuli that produce orienting behavior. But these neuronal and behavioral responses soon habituate[199]. Dopamine neurons also respond when an animal encounters a natural incentive, such as when it touches food located out-of-sight or, in a learning task, when liquid in delivered to the mouth[199,287]. However, when a neutral stimulus (e.g., light) is paired with the availability of a natural incentive, dopamine neurons soon stop responding to the natural incentive and start to discharge most vigorously in response to the newly established *conditioned incentive stimulus*†[199] (also see ref. 217). Dopamine neurons do not discharge when the animal actually eats the food, which they should if dopamine mediated the sensory pleasure associated with incentives (ref. 330 as well). Similarly, Kosobud et al.[183] reported in a recent poster that in rats trained to bar press for sucrose, VTA unit activity increased prior to the presentation of sucrose. Dopamine neurons did not increase activity after sucrose presentation, when presumably the animal would experience sensory pleasure. Finally, the activity of dopamine neurons can be dissociated from non-incentive aspects of a situation and from the details of motor behavior, because their discharge is not coupled to "mnemonic or preparatory representational task components" (ref. 198, p. 337), to the execution of reaching movements to obtain and retrieve food or to a light unassociated with food[199,287,289]. Studies in cats also suggest that VTA dopamine neurons do not discharge in relation to most phasic movements[330,341].

In summary, dopamine neurons discharge under conditions consistent with an attribution of incentive salience hypothesis of dopamine function[27,28]. They change their rate of discharge to a stimulus as the incentive value of the stimulus changes; as the stimulus becomes more or less salient. Indeed, Schultz[288] concluded that their electrophysiological experiments "are consistent with the conclusion that dopamine neurons respond specifically to *salient stimuli* that have alerting, arousing and attention-grabbing properties" (p. 134, our italics) #.

– A third line of evidence that dopamine mediates incentive salience rather than sensory pleasure comes from recent studies using high speed chronamperometry to measure nucleus accumbens dopamine activity during i.v. self-administration of heroin or cocaine[115,172]. In trained animals the first few drug injections greatly elevated a dopamine-related electrochemical signal. However, detailed analysis of the time course of changes in the dopamine-related electrochemical signal, relative to subsequent injections, revealed that the dopamine-related signal increased prior to drug self-administration, peaked at the time a response was inititated and then significantly decreased immediately following drug infusion. This is consistent with the view that dopamine mediates the incentive salience attributed to a drug-associated stimulus (presumably the lever in this case), because as extracellular dopamine increased drug 'wanting' would increase, to the point that an animal would initiate another drug infusion. The results are not consistent, however, with the view that dopamine mediates subjective pleasure (in which case dopamine should rise after drug administration). Neither are they consistent with the view that drug responding is initiated by withdrawal symptoms associated with dopamine depletion, as suggested, for example, by Dackis and Gold[64]. A dopamine depletion hypothesis would predict that animals should initiate a drug infusion when the dopamine signal is at its lowest, not highest. Of course, a dopamine depletion/withdrawal hypothesis, such as that proposed by Dackis and Gold[64], also suffers from the shortcomings associated with all negative reinforcement hypotheses of addiction, which were discussed above.

– The fourth line of evidence that dopamine is more likely to produce enhanced incentive salience than enhanced drug pleasure comes from a consideration of the relative patterns of change in drug 'wanting' vs. drug 'liking' reported by human addicts during the gradual development of addictive behavior (Fig. 3). The pleasure induced by drugs does not increase if the dose of a drug is held constant over the course of repeated administrations. In fact, if pleasure changes at all it decreases with repeated administrations (although, see Note 5 in Ch. 6). If increased synaptic activity in sensitized dopamine systems were the neural substrate of pleasure, a given dose should produce more and more pleasure with repeated experience, rather than less and less (or no change).

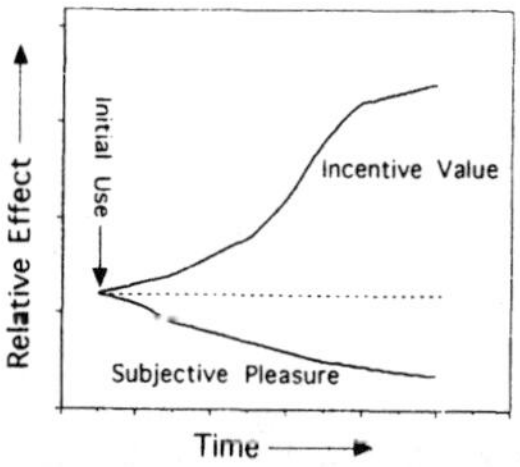

Fig. 3. A schematic illustration of the hypothetical relationship between changes in the incentive value of drugs and drug-related stimuli (drug 'wanting') vs. the subjective pleasurable effects of drugs (drug 'liking') during the development of an addiction. The development of an addiction is characterized by an increasing dissociation between the incentive properties of drugs, which gradually increase and the subjective pleasurable effects of drugs, which are shown here to slightly decrease (develop tolerance; but also see text and Note 5 in Ch. 6).

Although the pleasure produced by a drug does not increase for human addicts, the craving for the same drug does increase with repeated experience (Fig. 3). An increase in 'wanting' drugs, as evidenced by self-report and by progressively more compulsive drug-seeking and drug-taking behavior is, of course, the defining characteristic of drug addiction. An increase in drug craving without an increase in drug pleasure cannot by explained on the assumption that sensitization enhances a dopaminergic mechanism mediating the subjective pleasure of drugs (see Note 3 in Ch. 6). But this increasing dissociation between drug 'wanting' and drug 'liking' is precisely what would be expected if enhanced activity at dopamine synapses were the neural substrate responsible for incentive salience (see Note 4 in Ch. 6).

5. ELABORATION OF THE INCENTIVE-SENSITIZATION THEORY AND ITS IMPLICATIONS

In this section we will elaborate more precisely how the major features of addiction are explained by the Incentive-Sensitization Theory of Addiction and discuss implications of the theory. To summarize the

\# Schultz[288] tentatively suggested that the common psychological process underlying the discharge of dopamine neurons may be "motivational arousal", but also noted this was not completely satisfactory because "dopamine neurons respond every few seconds to the same stimuli over several tens of trials without habituation[199,275,287,289], whereas arousal should be a longer lasting state not repeatedly induced at such short intervals" (p. 135). We suggest that the conditions under which dopamine neurons discharge are better described by the hypothesis that dopamine neurons attribute incentive salience[27,28].

central elements of the theory, we posit the following. (1) Many addictive drugs have in common the ability to enhance mesotelencephalic dopamine neurotransmission and to engage related structures (but see Note 4 in Ch. 6). (2) A psychological function of this neural system is to attribute incentive salience to the perception and mental representation of stimuli and actions, especially those that have been associated with activation of the system; to cause them to become highly salient, attractive and 'wanted'. (3) Repeated and intermittent administration of addictive drugs leads to incremental neuroadaptations in this neural system, which render it increasingly and perhaps permanently hyperresponsive (sensitized). (4) Associative control of this sensitized neural system causes tremendously enhanced incentive salience to be attributed to the act of drug taking and to stimuli associated with drug taking (i.e., to the acts and stimuli most closely associated with hyperactivation of dopamine systems); and thus, in the addict, drugs come to be pathologically 'wanted' (craved). (5) Sensitization of the neural system responsible for incentive salience can motivate addictive behavior (compulsive drug seeking and drug taking) independent of other motivating factors, such as the expectation of drug pleasure or the aversive properties of withdrawal. The associative targeting of sensitized incentive salience to drug-related stimuli results in the persistence of addictive behavior even in the face of many disincentives: for example, the loss of reputation, job, home and family (see Note 6 in Ch. 6).

We have argued that addictive behavior is motivated by the excessive 'wanting' of drugs (drug craving). Therefore, the first major issue we need to address is: why do addicts crave drugs independently of drug pleasure and withdrawal? What is the neuropsychological process that results in obsessive craving for drugs, leading to compulsive drug-seeking and drug-taking behavior, even when the drug may produce little pleasure? The second fundamental question we need to address concerns why drug craving persists for so long after the discontinuation of drug use and after the cessation of withdrawal symptoms; i.e., the nature of relapse. After this we will discuss the implications of Incentive-Sensitization for individual differences in the propensity to addiction, for therapy and the relationship between Incentive-Sensitization and other views of addiction.

5.1. The independence of drug craving from drug pleasure and withdrawal

The Incentive-Sensitization Theory of Addiction provides an unique neuropsychological explanation for drug craving. Drug craving is the subjective experience that accompanies the attribution of excessive levels of incentive salience to drug-related stimuli (or their mental representations), due to sensitization of dopamine systems (see Note 4 in Ch. 6). Thus, drug craving is considered by this hypothesis to be a psychological process that is distinct from conditioned withdrawal signs and from either drug-induced pleasure or a conditioned 'high'. Other views of addiction often consider craving to be identical with or the direct result of, either conditioned withdrawal or a conditioned 'high'. For example, Childress et al.[50] state: "We have often used the terms 'conditioned withdrawal' and 'conditioned craving' almost interchangeably, with the assumption that craving might be a form of mild withdrawal" (p. 38). But Childress et al.[50] go on to say: "Our patients did not, however, always subscribe to this position; reports of craving usually showed low correlations with reports of withdrawal. To paraphrase one indignant user, 'No, doc, craving is when you want it – want it so bad you can almost taste it... but you ain't sick... sick is, well, sick' ". To this addict withdrawal sickness clearly is separable from drug craving[212]. Neither is craving equivalent to a conditioned 'high', because reports of conditioned 'highs' are uncommon and are thus dissociable from the more frequent occurrence of both conditioned withdrawal signs and conditioned craving, as discussed earlier[50,229].

The Incentive-Sensitization view of addiction is in agreement with the indignant user cited above; craving is pathological 'wanting'. It is not due to sickness. It is distinct from both the unpleasant symptoms of withdrawal and from drug pleasure. This view is supported by studies directly relating self-reported craving induced by exposure to drug-associated stimuli to ratings of withdrawal-like symptoms, drug-like effects and 'outcome expectancies'[80,253]. Although exposure to drug-related stimuli produced a significant increase in self-reported craving, as well as drug-opposite and drug-like effects "in a simple additive model the combined effects of positive outcome expectancies, cue-specific dysphoria and cue-specific drug-positive reactions were able to predict 28% of the variance in cue-specific craving."... "A much larger proportion of the variance in craving remains unexplained by these factors" (ref. 253, p. 1142–1143). We suggest the reason there is only a weak relationship between these variables and drug craving is that *they do not cause craving*. Craving is due to excessive activity in a separate and sensitized neuronal system that mediates the attribution of salience to incentives. This is a neuronal system that normally mediates the 'wanting' of things in the environment. Although this neuronal system usually functions in concert with neuronal systems that mediate pleasure ('liking'), in the addict the normal link between these systems is disrupted and pathological levels of 'wanting' become dissociated from 'liking'. We think this dissociation accounts for the unusual psychological profile of an addict: intense drug craving separated from the normal pleasures and punishments of life *.

In this light the irrationality of addictive behavior, which is discussed so eloquently by Falk et al.[86], starts to make some 'sense'. The irrationality of the behavior is due to an increasing dissociation between the incentive properties of drugs (incentive salience) and their subjective pleasurable effects. Because the process of salience attribution can be activated, independent of subjective pleasure, incentive salience can be strong even if pleasure is weak or absent. This is one reason why there is not always a strong correlation between the incentive motivational properties of drugs and their hedonic properties. It is also why people will self-administer low doses of drugs that do not produce subjective pleasure[95,192]. Furthermore, the attribution of incentive salience is not a conscious process and the introspective experience of 'wanting' or craving is only a person's interpretation of the outcome of that process. Much of the time the attribution of incentive salience may be more implicit than explicit[228]. Regardless, the addict can be only subjectively aware of the outcome of excessive incentive salience attribution, craving. The addict may have little insight into the reason for the craving and indeed, may himself be bewildered by its intensity. At a conscious level addicts may recount all of the negative consequences of continued drug use, deplore their situation, even comment that the drug does not continue to give great pleasure – and not understand why their craving persists.

5.2. The development of addictive behavior

The Incentive-Sensitization Theory can explain why the development of an addiction is typically a gradual, progressive process. The attribution of a high level of incentive salience to drug-associated stimuli and the pleasurable effects of drugs, increase the probability drug-related stimuli will attract attention and that drugs will be sought out in the future. If drug use continues, dopamine systems become progressively more sensitized. With each repetition greater and greater incentive salience is attributed to drug-related stimuli and the associative pairing of drug-related stimuli with the intense activation of dopamine systems produced by drugs leads to an increasing focus of salience attribution upon just these stimuli. Thus, 'wanting' is gradually transformed into craving, drugs become craved to the relative exclusion of all else, and drug-associated stimuli elicit this craving independent of any pleasure they produce. In short, the developing addict comes to 'want' drugs more and more because drug-related stimuli become imbued with greater and greater incentive salience, even though at the same time drugs may be 'liked' less and less.

5.3. Relapse: drug-induced drug craving

Drug craving sometimes remains high or is even increased immediately after drug administration, when the drug is producing subjective pleasure, as has been reported for alcohol, cocaine, heroin and hydromorphone[80,96,150,215,325]. This is the proverbial drink that whets the appetite and leads to relapse. Why should this be? As pointed out earlier, this is not consistent with a negative reinforcement view of craving[329], because the drug should eliminate withdrawal symptoms **. Neither is it consistent with a pleasure-seek-

* Other brain manipulations also are known to 'fracture' behavioral or psychological subsystems whose operations are so intertwined that one's subjective experience is of only one process. An example is the phenomenon of 'blindsight'[350], which refers to the ability of people rendered blind by an occipital cortex lesion to accurately localize visual stimuli presented in their blind visual field, despite having no conscious awareness of perceiving any stimulus. People have no subjective experience of separate psychological processes (and neural systems) underlying the identification vs. the localization of visual stimuli. But an occipital lesion 'fractures' these processes, revealing two distinct psychological processes where there appeared to be only one. Another example is the dissociation of declarative (explicit) and procedural (implicit) memory systems seen following damage to the medial temporal lobes[318]. We are not subjectively aware that distinct neural systems are involved in learning to solve puzzles (for example, the Tower of Hanoi puzzle) and learning facts (for example, learning a list of words). But following a bilateral medial temporal lobe lesion the ability to learn and remember facts is lost, whereas the ability to learn and remember puzzles is left intact; although the latter occurs in the absence of conscious awareness. We think that the dissociation between 'wanting' and 'liking' seen in addicts represents a 'fracture' of psychological processes akin to 'blindsight' and the implicit/explicit memory distinction. That is, repeated drug use changes the brain, as a lesion changes the brain, revealing two distinct psychological processes where there subjectively appeared to be only one. Furthermore, like the localization of visual stimuli and procedural learning, the attribution of incentive salience is 'implicit'; it often may occur in the absence of conscious awareness.

** Except according to Solomon's opponent-process theory[312], which is the only negative reinforcement theory that can successfully explain relapse induced by re-exposure to the drug. According to Solomon's theory, re-exposure to the drug elicits a moderate a-process or drug-like effect, which in turn triggers the still strong b-process or drug-opponent effect. The problems faced by the opponent-process theory, however, are: (1) it relies entirely upon withdrawal symptoms to motivate addictive behavior and is thus liable to the general criticisms that we described for negative reinforcement theories of addiction; (2) it posits the growth of an opponent-like process during addiction, for which there is no direct evidence other than the phenomena of tolerance and withdrawal themselves (and which is contradicted by evidence discussed above that the incentive properties of drugs show sensitization rather than tolerance); and (3) it posits the opponent-process to be elicited only and always by the a-process, whereas evidence exists that withdrawal and drug pleasure have separate, independent neural substrates[365].

ing view, because a dose sufficient to produce subjective pleasure should satisfy or at least reduce the craving; not exacerbate it. Drug craving at the time of drug taking is consistent, however, with an Incentive-Sensitization view. According to Incentive-Sensitization craving is the subjective experience associated with incentive salience attribution. Because many addictive drugs increase dopamine activity, which produces incentive salience, one would expect drug administration to produce drug 'wanting'.

Indeed, there is considerable evidence that re-exposure to drugs can reinstate compulsive drug-seeking and drug-taking behavior[83,325,326]. As pointed out by Stewart et al.[326]: "The idea that ingestion of a formerly abused drug induces a strong motivational state or craving for the drug and that it retains the ability to reinstate this craving over an indefinite period of abstinence from the drug is not new. One of the basic tenets of Alcoholics Anonymous (anonymous, 1939) is that people who have at one time shown uncontrolled drinking and physical dependence are permanently unable to drink moderately; one drink is said to elicit an urge to have another" (p. 257). This phenomenon is usually explained by 'priming' and Stewart et al.[326] have argued that 'priming' reinstates drug use because "the presence of the drug in the body (not its absence) activates appetitive motivational mechanisms that are involved in the reinitiation of drug seeking behavior" (p. 253). An involvement of dopamine in priming is suggested by reports that the infusion of morphine directly into the ventral tegmental area is sufficient to prime responding for i.v. heroin or cocaine, intra-accumbens amphetamine can prime responding for i.v. heroin[325,326], and haloperidol prevents priming for amphetamine[83]. It is also relevant to note that craving in long-term abstinent cocaine abusers (humans) has been associated with elevated plasma and CSF levels of the dopamine metabolite, HVA[173,206].

Stewart's view is entirely consistent with the Incentive-Sensitization Theory of Addiction presented here. We would add only two additional points. First, an Incentive-Sensitization view of addiction identifies the "appetitive motivational mechanism" mentioned by Stewart et al.[326] specifically as incentive salience and not, for example, drug pleasure. Second, we hypothesize that the ability of drugs to produce incentive salience is progressively increased (sensitized) by repeated exposure to drugs because drugs sensitize mesotelencephalic dopamine systems. Thus, in highly sensitized individuals, such as addicts, relapse is the rule rather than the exception, especially after a priming 'taste', because this acts on a hypersensitive neural system that mediates incentive salience – eliciting pathologically strong 'wanting' (craving) and thus relapse.

5.4. Relapse: interactions between different drugs and the effects of drug-related stimuli

Not only can the preferred drug of abuse reinstate addictive behavior, but often other drugs can as well; and addicts usually use more than one drug (which is significant in itself). In animals too, priming can occur across drug classes. For example, i.v. amphetamine or bromocriptine can prime the self-administration of heroin[367] and i.v. morphine can prime responding in animals trained to self-administer cocaine[326]. Furthermore, dopamine systems have been implicated in priming between drug classes. An intra-accumbens injection of amphetamine, which selectively activates the mesolimbic dopamine system, can prime responding for i.v. heroin[327] and intra-ventral tegmental area morphine can prime responding for i.v. cocaine[322].

According to the Incentive-Sensitization view of addiction, drugs can prime responding for each other because the same dopamine systems are activated by each and dopamine mediates the incentive salience attributed to many different drugs. Therefore, if dopamine systems become sensitized by past drug use it would be expected that a second, novel drug would be able to prime responding and precipitate relapse, as long as the second drug also activates hypersensitive dopamine systems. This idea was proposed previously by Stewart and Vezina[327], who argued that the ability of opiates and stimulants to prime responding for one another "may be related to the ability of opiates and stimulant drugs to cause sensitization" (p. 287), within dopamine systems. In support of this view, cross-sensitization has been reported to the psychomotor stimulant effects and to the incentive motivational effects of a number of drugs, as well as in the ability of drugs to elevate dopamine neurotransmission (see above for references).

Not only may re-exposure to drugs themselves precipitate relapse, but environmental stimuli associated with drugs are known to induce craving and precipitate relapse in humans[50,229] and prime drug responding in animals[325,326]. This evidence has been reviewed by Stewart et al.[326] and need not be reiterated here. It is consistent, however, with an Incentive-Sensitization view of addiction. In this view sensitization of a neural substrate responsible for incentive salience becomes expressed as addictive behavior largely by enhancing the incentive properties of stimuli associated with drugs. Heightened incentive salience is focussed on these stimuli and their mental representations by associative learning processes and they become the elicitors and objects of craving. Even in the absence of the drug and long after withdrawal signs have faded, drug-related stimuli remain potent conditioned incentives able to elicit the attribution of incentive salience. Indeed, in the context of an Incentive-Sensitization view of addiction this is why environmental stimuli associated with drugs are extremely effective in precipitating relapse in addicts (however, see Note 8).

This view is an alternative to both the conditioned 'high' interpretation and the 'explicit memory' interpretation of relapse discussed above in the section on positive reinforcement/euphoria theories. We suggest the effects of drug-related stimuli on relapse are independent of both drug cue elicited feelings of pleasure (a conditioned 'high') and of the explicit memories of drug taking such cues might elicit. You will recall we argued that an 'explicit memory' hypothesis of relapse places an extraordinary explanatory burden on the assumption that relapse-provoking memories are qualitatively different from the myriad other memories of drugs that do not provoke relapse. We suggest, to the contrary, that conscious remembering in response to cues may be essentially similar to explicit memories that have gone before, neither more vivid nor qualitatively different. The difference in the processes triggered by an effective drug-paired context, which results in relapse when earlier memories did not, may be in associative incentive systems that are not explicitly available to consciousness.

Incentive salience is such an associatively triggered process. It occurs in the absence of awareness and its operation requires no qualitative difference in explicitly conscious memory in order to provoke relapse. Unlike explicit memories, the attribution of incentive salience is an implicit process. It is governed by the laws of associative learning and is influenced by factors that control other forms of implicit learning. Chief among these controlling influences is the gating role of associative context[259]. Context refers to the entire configuration of situational stimuli in which the CS has been learned. Associative context can modulate the effectiveness of any CS. Why then should relapse occur at a particular moment, rather than during earlier memories or earlier encounters with drug-paired stimuli? Presumably because of variations in the completeness of the associative context. The greater the extent to which contextual factors, such as mood, environment and other situational variables, mimic the context of previous drug taking, the more likely relapse will occur.

5.5. Relapse: the role of stress

Relapse to compulsive drug use is not always precipitated by re-exposure to a drug or even by specific environmental stimuli associated with drugs, but sometimes by ill-defined environmental circumstances; including mood changes evoked by stress[49,229]. A traditional view of why stress may lead to relapse is that it prompts 'escape' from an unpleasant situation via drug taking. An alternative possibility is that sensitization of incentive salience could play a role in stress-induced relapse because addictive drugs and stress both activate dopamine systems and both sensitize dopaminc systems[8,9,160,268]. As discussed above, animals previously exposed to drugs such as amphetamine, cocaine or morphine are later hyperresponsive to stress and animals exposed to repeated intermittent stress are later hyperresponsive to the psychomotor stimulant and incentive motivational properties of drugs[243]. According to an Incentive-Sensitization view stress may induce craving and relapse because, by activating dopamine systems, stress would magnify the incentive salience attributed to environmental stimuli. Environmental stimuli that were especially potent as incentives, such as drug-associated stimuli for addicts, would be the focus of enhanced salience due to their associative history. Drug-associated events would become especially craved again as a consequence of stress (see Note 9 in Ch. 6).

It is interesting to speculate that the converse sequence of events could also occur. That is, prior exposure to repeated intermittent stress may predispose susceptible individuals to drug addiction by sensitizing those neural systems that mediate the incentive motivational effects of drugs[69,159,268]. In such individuals the incentive motivational effects of an initial drug experience may be significantly enhanced because of drug action on a previously sensitized neural substrate. This would increase the probability that these individuals would show subsequent drug-seeking and drug-taking behavior. Indeed, experimental evidence for such a phenomenon has been reported by Piazza et al.[243], who found that past experience with stress (repeated tail pinch) facilitated the subsequent acquisition of amphetamine self-administration behavior in rats.

5.6. Individual differences in the propensity to addiction

The last feature of addiction we will discuss concerns the fact that the majority of people in this country at some point experiment with drugs, but most do not become addicts. For example, over 55% of 18–34 yr olds have at one time sampled illicit drugs (e.g., marijuana, inhalents, cocaine, heroin or hallucinogens; NIDA National Household Survey on Drug Abuse, 1991). Why do the vast majority of these people not develop an addiction? Why are some individuals more susceptible to addiction than others? Social factors are important, of course, but even persons from very similar backgrounds differ greatly in their tendency to develop addictive behavior. If, as proposed here, drug-induced neuroadaptations underlying sensitization play a central role in the development of addiction: (1) there should be large individual differences in the susceptibility to sensitization and (2) individual differences in the susceptibility to sensitization should be related to the propensity to addiction.

There are indeed enormous individual differences in the susceptibility to sensitization, a point that has been emphasized by a number of researchers[190,194,268,294]. Some of this individual variation is due to genetic variation, because among animals there are marked strain differences in the susceptibility to sensitization. Strain differences in both rats and mice have been reported in the sensitization produced by repeated treatment with amphetamine[110,194,268,300], cocaine[304], ethanol[60,142,240] and morphine[302]. There are also marked strain differences in mesotelencephalic dopamine systems[14,91,145], but we know of no studies directly relating strain differences in the susceptibility to sensitization to strain differences in mesotelencephalic dopamine systems. Nevertheless, it is important that initial studies with recombinent-inbred lines of mice suggest that the genetic determinants of acute responsiveness to drugs are dissociable from those responsible for susceptibility to sensitization[304]. Many behavioral genetic studies on drug responsiveness have focussed on variation in the acute response to drugs, not susceptibility to sensitization. But the Incentive-Sensitization Theory suggests that the susceptibility to sensitization may be most relevant for the development of addictive behavior and therefore, information on genetic factors leading to high susceptibility to sensitization may be of particular importance in understanding the genetics of addiction.

A number of other factors have been reported to influence individual differences in the susceptibility to sensitization including, age[100,175,303], sex[45,46,107,250,267,273] and hemispheric differences in dopamine systems[190]. Whether the influence of these variables on the susceptibility to sensitization is causally related to the propensity to self-administer drugs or to related variation in dopamine systems is not yet known, although correlative relations have been reported[47,108,109,294].

There are, however, a number of interesting studies on behavioral traits that do predict both the susceptibility to sensitization and the propensity to self-administer amphetamine[241]. For example, responsivity to novelty is reported to predict susceptibility to sensitization[133–135,242]. Similarly, animals that eat and drink in response to electrical stimulation of the lateral hypothalamus (not all do) show an enhanced susceptibility to amphetamine sensitization[220,221]. Most importantly, these same traits are correlated with a propensity to acquire amphetamine self-administration[241] and with differences in dopamine dynamics in the nucleus accumbens[36,132]. Individual differences in reactivity to novelty, in amphetamine sensitization, and in amphetamine self-administration may involve variation in the responsiveness of the hypothalamo-pituitary-adrenal (HPA) axis. Animals that show a high response to novelty also show a prolonged elevation in plasma corticosterone in this situation, relative to low responders[190,241]. That the HPA axis may play a role in drug sensitization is suggested by experiments showing that activation of the HPA axis is necessary to induce sensitization to amphetamine or stress[54,55,69], perhaps by the action of corticosterone on glucocorticoid receptors[261] (cf. ref. 57) and by a report that repeated exposure to exogenous corticosterone sensitizes animals to a subsequent amphetamine challenge[244].

5.7. Implications of the Incentive-Sensitization Theory for Therapy

There is considerable interest in developing effective therapies for the treatment of drug addiction, but this has proven to be a very difficult problem. The Incentive-Sensitization view of addiction may provide some insight as to why effective therapies have been elusive, and potentially, may point the way to the development of more effective approaches.

5.7.1. Extinction training. A recent trend in the psychotherapeutic treatment of addiction is based on the recognition that drug-conditioned stimuli are very potent in eliciting craving and precipitating relapse[229]. There have been attempts, therefore, to 'extinguish' conditioned responses to such stimuli. Indeed, the repeated presentation of drug-related stimuli, in a laboratory setting, results in a progressive decline in drug craving elicited by drug-related stimuli[50,229]. It is interesting, however, that some of the autonomic responses to such stimuli are more resistant to extinction than the subjective effects, and non-specific changes in mood state (especially anger) can rapidly reinstate conditioned stimulus-induced drug craving[49].

In the context of the Incentive-Sensitization Theory this might occur because the neuroadaptations underlying sensitization persist, despite extinction of the conditioned stimulus control of sensitization. That is, the ability of conditioned stimuli to control the expression of sensitization may be thought of as learning-related neuroadaptations layered 'on-top' of the neuroadaptations responsible for sensitization, but which do not directly alter or reverse the neuronal changes responsible for sensitization. Also, contextual factors that control the associative attribution of incentive salience may not transfer between the clinic and the street. Thus, extinction training may extinguish responses to specific stimuli under specific circumstances, but other non-target stimuli can still access sensitized neural systems mediating incentive salience, as can environmental stress. On the positive side, the fact that the expression of sensitization can be brought under strong conditioned stimulus control[323] suggests it should be possible to develop learning strategies to control the output of sensitized neural systems. However, the persistence of the neuroadaptations underlying sensitization and their resistance to extinction[328], suggests that coping with addiction may be a very long, ongoing process. Of course, this has been recognized for many years by organizations like Alcoholics Anonymous. For example, Anonymous states: "We know that while the alcoholic keeps away from drink, as he may do for months or years, he reacts much like other men. We are equally positive that once he takes any alcohol whatever into his system, something happens, both in bodily and mental sense, which makes it virtually impossible for him to stop" (ref. 7, p. 22).

5.7.2. Pharmacotherapeutic approaches. The Incentive-Sensitization Theory of Addiction also has implications for the development of effective pharmacotherapies. The two major pharmacotherapeutic approaches at present either target the treatment of withdrawal symptoms or involve drug substitution therapy (e.g., methadone maintenance). The Incentive-Sensitization Theory predicts neither of these approaches will be very successful in eliminating addictive behavior, because neither target the fundamental neuroadaptations underlying sensitization. Of course, many years of experience with opiate addicts have already shown that the alleviation of withdrawal is not an effective long-term solution for addiction[363] and the drugs used in substitution 'therapies' usually are addictive themselves[363]. Furthermore, some drugs used to treat withdrawal also may induce sensitization[89,202,203,277].

An Incentive-Sensitization view of addiction suggests that to really 'cure' addiction agents need to be developed that directly target and reverse the neuroadaptations underlying sensitization. There are presently a number of agents known to prevent the development of sensitization, including dopamine antagonists (see above for references) and glutamate antagonists[161,164,369] (cf. ref. 342). Unfortunately, these compounds do not reverse the neuroadaptations underlying sensitization, but only prevent its development if they are given every time the addictive drug is given. This is not a practical approach for the treatment of addiction (see Note 1 in Ch. 6). The Incentive-Sensitization Theory of Addiction predicts that an especially effective pharmacotherapeutic agent would reverse sensitization-related neuroadaptations. However, to our knowledge, no one has identified such a compound. Of course, any rational drug design program will require that we know a lot more about the nature of sensitization-related neuroadaptations than we know at present.

5.8. Relationship between incentive sensitization and other views of addiction

In closing, we want to emphasize that the Incentive-Sensitization Theory of Addiction does not exclude other factors that contribute to drug-taking behavior. For example, the Incentive-Sensitization Theory does not address a number of features of drug use, including why people experiment with drugs in the first place (experimental drug use), casual (not addictive) patterns of drug use or why people often use drugs that do not usually lead to compulsive patterns of use (e.g., LSD; see also Note 7 in Ch. 6). The Incentive-Sensitization Theory of Addiction does not preclude a role for pleasure-seeking and withdrawal avoidance in drug-taking behavior. These different views of addiction are not mutually exclusive, unless they are taken as the sole explanations for addiction. There can be no doubt that addiction results from very complex interactions amongst social, cultural, economic, psychological and biological variables. These complex interactions determine whether experimentation with drugs first occurs, whether further drug use is sustained and whether drug use leads to addiction. Exactly which factors motivate behavior will vary over time and across different drugs. The Incentive-Sensitization view does not exclude the possibility, for example, that an explicit memory of drug pleasure or a conditioned 'high' could contribute to a desire to repeat the drug experience in some situations. This may be especially true early in the development of an addiction[363]. Early in the development of an addiction, before marked sensitization has occurred, the memory of the subjective pleasurable effects of drugs could be a major factor motivating drug-taking behavior. For example, it has been suggested that the initial subjective effects of drugs can predict later drug habits[120]. Also drug-taking behavior is influenced initially to a great extent by social factors, such as peer pressure.

Neither does the Incentive-Sensitization view of addiction deny that the unpleasant symptoms of withdrawal could motivate drug taking in some individuals, under some circumstances, in order to relieve symptoms. The role of withdrawal avoidance may vary greatly from drug-to-drug. In some respects drug taking motivated by pleasure-seeking or withdrawal avoidance seems 'normal'; that is, the reasons for drug taking are understandable to a non-addict. For example, recent suggestions that drug craving is caused by short-term dopamine depletion after drug use are based largely on the assumption that craving is merely a rational response to withdrawal symptoms[63,204,351]. But by our view this is not craving; nor is it the fundamental problem in addiction. Craving is obsessive, irrational, pathologically intense drug 'wanting' for no obvious reason, which leads to compulsive drug-seeking and drug-taking behavior. Craving is difficult for both the addict and the non-addict to understand and this is what we propose is primarily due to sensitization of incentive salience.

The Incentive-Sensitization Theory of Addiction is also compatible with the 'Psychomotor Stimulant Theory' of Wise and Bozarth[365]. Wise and Bozarth[365] argued that addictive drugs have in common the ability to induce 'psychomotor activation', which was proposed to be due to activation of a common biological mechanism associated with approach behavior and mediated by dopamine. This biological mechanism is thought to be fundamental in producing reinforcement[111,343]. The fact that the psychomotor-activating effects of addictive drugs are sensitized by repeated drug administration is certainly consistent with the 'sensitization' component of the Incentive-Sensitization Theory. But we further specify here that the psychological process responsible for 'reward-related' psychomotor activation is the attribution of incentive salience. Although incentive salience may lead to locomotion and approach, because this psychological process makes stimuli in the environment more salient, attractive and 'wanted', these functions may be separable[260]. For example, a brain manipulation could induce locomotion, perhaps by activating brainstem locomotor pattern generators, without producing incentive salience; and incentive salience could be attributed in the absence of locomotion (for example, in a rat rendered cataleptic by morphine, but who still acquires a conditioned place preference). Thus, in our view it is specifically the sensitization of incentive salience that makes drugs and drug-associated stimuli increasingly attractive and 'wanted'. Increased psychomotor activation is just a correlate of sensitized incentive salience.

In closing, the ability of the Incentive-Sensitization Theory of Addiction to capture the 'essence' of addictive behavior (compulsive drug seeking and drug taking) can be illustrated by a 'thought experiment'. For the sake of argument, imagine that our assumptions regarding the criteria for an adequate theory of addiction are correct and that the neural system involved in assigning incentive salience to drugs and drug-associated stimuli is indeed dissociable from those mediating the subjective pleasurable effects of drugs. Now imagine that repeated intermittent drug use causes gradual and incremental changes in the neural system responsible for incentive salience, such that this neural system becomes very hypersensitive (sensitized). Further imagine that the expression of this sensitized system is focussed expressly on stimuli that have become associated with its excessive activation, so drugs and drug-associated stimuli become irresistibly attractive ('wanted') and thus able to control behavior. But the neural system(s) responsible for the subjective pleasurable effects of drugs either does not change or else becomes hyposensitive (tolerant). Finally, imagine that incentive salience is attributed in the absence of conscious awareness. Now consider what a creature with this brain would be like. An addict, we think.

6. NOTES

6.1. Note 1. Role of control and intermittency of drug administration in sensitization

6.1.1. Control. Although there have been many reports of sensitization to addictive drugs, it is important to acknowledge that in nearly all of these studies sensitization was induced by non-contingent drug treatment. That is, the animal's behavior had no influence on whether it received a drug or not. It is known, however, that drugs can produce different effects depending on whether they are given in a response-contingent or response-non-contingent manner[309,310]. Also, the behavioral sensitization to amphetamine or cocaine induced by footshock stress is influenced by whether an animal has control in the situation. For example, MacLennan and Maier[200] reported that behavioral sensitization did not occur in rats who could control the duration of footshock, but did occur in rats receiving an identical amount of shock, but who had no control. It will be critical to determine, therefore, whether the response-contingent administration of drugs induces sensitization.

There have been very few studies directly addressing this issue. We are aware of one report of sensitization following experience with cocaine self-administration. Falk et al.[88] tested for behavioral sensitization by challenging animals with cocaine 7–10 days after the discontinuation of an oral cocaine self-administration regimen (involving a schedule-induced polydipsia paradigm). Cocaine-experienced animals showed a marked shift to the left in the dose-response curve for cocaine-induced locomotor activity. These data show that sensitization to cocaine can occur following response-contingent drug administration, as well as following non-contingent drug administration. It may also be relevant that in self-administration studies animals are often given non-contingent drug injections prior to training or during shaping, because this facilitates the acquisition of a self administration habit. It is possible the development of a drug self-administration habit is facilitated by these procedures because they produce the kinds of sensitization-related neuroadaptations under discussion here (although one also has to consider the possibility that prior non-contingent administration produces tolerance to the aversive properties of drugs).

6.1.2. Intermittency. On the other hand, sensitization was not found in a microdialysis experiment involving cocaine self-administration[143]. These researchers found that the ability of self-administered cocaine to elevate extracellular dopamine was actually decreased in drug experienced rats. However, in this experiment the dialysis test was given 24 h after the last self-administration session. Sensitization-related changes in dopamine neurotransmission often are not evident after such short periods of withdrawal, even following non-contingent drug administration[158,176,295,296,370]. This is probably because intermittency is a critical variable both in inducing sensitization and in its later expression[232,248,268,272]. If injections are given too close together in time tolerance, rather than sensitization, usually occurs. The development of sensitization is maximized by spacing injections far apart in time (2–3 days to a week). Similarly, if a challenge injection is given within the first few days after the discontinuation of escalating dose amphetamine treatment behavioral sensitization is not evident. But if a challenge injection is given after a longer period of withdrawal, from 1 week to 1 year, animals are markedly sensitized[232]. Thus, sensitization may not be apparent after self-administration regimens that allow animals to maintain elevated brain levels of a drug for prolonged periods of time, especially if animals are tested soon after the end of a bout of self-administration.

It is intriguing that intermittency is not only critical for inducing sensitization, but is thought to play an important role in the development of many persistent and habitual behaviors, including addictive behavior[86]. Of course, drug-taking behavior in human addicts is often characterized by intermittency. Drugs are frequently taken in 'runs' of self-administration, interspersed with 'crashes' lasting a few days. Intermittency may also be imposed because a considerable amount of time is required to obtain the money necessary to buy drugs. Falk and his colleagues[86,87] have argued that such intermittent schedules of drug administration may greatly enhance the reinforcing properties of drugs and catalyze "drug overindulgence in humans". They state "when life's crucial commodities are in short supply and available only on intermittent, marginal schedules... drugs can become all-powerful in reinforcing efficacy" (ref. 87, p. 1506). We would only add that the neural basis of this effect, in the context of Incentive-Sensitization, may involve a facilitation of sensitization-related neuroadaptations. We would expect that an intermittent pattern of drug self-administration, such as a cycle of 'runs' and 'crashes', would produce sensitization of dopamine neurotransmission and incentive salience[270].

6.2. Note 2. Specific motivational effects of dopamine blockade

The literature on the effects of dopamine antagonists on motivated behavior has been reviewed extensively and the reader is referred to papers cited in the text for comprehensive lists of citations. In brief, some of the most clearly motivational effects of dopamine antagonists include the following. (a) Mimicry of extinction by dopamine antagonists, in which instrumental responses for a food, drug or electrical brain stimulation decline only gradually after neuroleptic administration as though the reinforcer were no longer efficacious (the decline in response is not right away and does not occur unless the animal is allowed to perform the task)[99]. (b) The associative reinstatement of instrumental performance after a dopamine antagonist has suppressed instrumental responding, by transferring the animal to a separate task in which it has previously been reinforced, but in which it has not yet experienced the drug, and in which it responds again at a high level even though the drug is still in effect (i.e., it must learn to 'extinguish' again in the second task)[103]. (c) *Transfer between real extinction and extinction mimicry* in 'resistance to extinction' paradigms, as though a dopamine antagonist drug were perceived by the animal as being similar to 'no reinforcer'. (d) Reward†-specific 'curve shift' reductions in psychophysical paradigms that can distinguish between reductions in instrumental performance due to motor impairment versus reductions due to decreased reinforcement (refs. 78, 104 for example). (e) 'Reduced palatability' patterns of decrease in food consumption that mimic those produced by manipulations of the sensory pleasure of the food: for example, low doses of dopamine antagonists mimic the effects upon sucrose drinking that are produced by dilution of the sucrose solution[13,53,67,106,308,374].

6.3. Note 3. The neural substrate of drug 'liking' (pleasure)

We have argued that mesotelencephalic dopamine projections provide the neural substrate for drug 'wanting' (via attribution of incentive salience), but not for drug 'liking' (for the subjective pleasurable effects of drugs). This naturally raises the question: what is the neural substrate for drug 'liking'?; for the pleasurable affective states produced by addictive drugs? We cannot provide a definitive answer to this question, except to rule out dopamine, but we can point to other candidate neural systems. Chief among these are endogenous opioid neurotransmitter systems. Opioid agonists that increase motivated behavior towards food, such as morphine, do enhance the sensory pleasure of food as measured by the taste reactivity paradigm[75]. Similarly, activation of benzodiazepine-GABA systems within the brainstem enhances sensory pleasure by the taste reactivity measure, although it is not yet clear whether this depends on an interaction with brain opioid systems (ref. 340 for example). In summary, we do not know the neural substrate of drug pleasure, but these are a couple of candidate systems and future research may reveal others.

6.4. Note 4. Dopamine, sensitization and incentive salience

There are two issues regarding the neural system(s) responsible for sensitization of incentive salience that require further discussion. The first concerns elaboration of exactly which of the many different mesotelencephalic dopamine projection systems is likely to mediate incentive salience. We are well aware that there are multiple anatomically and functionally distinct mesotelencephalic dopamine projection systems. The extent to which the effects of manipulations of dopamine systems on incentive motivation are due to an action on any single one of these dopamine systems is not always clear. The contribution, for example, of dopamine projections to the frontal cortex, septum, caudate, accumbens (core vs. shell), olfactory tubercle or amygdala and the extent to which there may be interactions between these systems in the assignment of incentive salience, is, for the most part, unknown. We hesitate, therefore, to prematurely assign all responsibility for incentive salience or the sensitization of incentive salience, to a specific dopamine projection system. This is why we often use the broader term, mesotelencephalic dopamine systems. Nevertheless, we recognize that most of the evidence linking mesotelencephalic dopamine systems to incentive motivation primarily implicates the so-called mesolimbic dopamine projections to the ventral striatum (nucleus accumbens). Therefore, to the extent that the sensitization of incentive salience is mediated by a specific dopamine system it is probably the dopamine projection system to the ventral striatum. But we do not discount the possibility that other dopamine systems may play a role.

The second issue is whether only dopamine systems are involved in the sensitization of incentive salience. We have focused on dopamine systems as the site of sensitization-related neuroadaptations for the reasons described in the text. We acknowledge, however, that the neurobiology of drug craving involves much more than just a simple sensitization-related increase in dopamine neurotransmission and the neural substrate of incentive salience is surely much more complicated than this.

For example, Wise and Rompre[368] have cautioned that "while the evidence is strong that dopamine plays some fundamental and special role in the rewarding effects of brain stimulation, psychomotor stimulants, opiates and food, the exact nature of that role is not clear. One thing is clear: dopamine is not the only reward transmitter and dopaminergic neurons are not the final common path for all rewards" (p. 220). We agree with Wise's caution. To influence motivated behavior via the attribution of incentive salience, dopamine systems must interact with many other neural systems, especially those involved in hedonics and associative learning. It is also possible that some incentives may not directly activate dopamine systems at all[181] and it is conceivable that some behavior may be controlled by non-incentive based processes, such as Skinnerian S-R reinforcement, Hullian drive-reduction or goal-directed computational procedures (e.g., Test-Operate-Test-Exit procedures[216]) (see Toates[339] for a discussion of how to distinguish some of these alternatives).

The phenomenon of behavioral sensitization also surely involves more complex neuroadaptations than just an enhancement in dopamine release, although to date most studies of sensitization have focussed only on dopamine. There is already evidence that the induction of sensitization involves a different cellular site of drug action than the expression of sensitization[160,269], that cross-sensitization does not occur between all addictive drugs[160,269], that an action of drugs on neural systems other than dopamine is required to induce sensitization[54,161,164] and that there are sensitization-related changes in other neurotransmitter systems[122,235,313,314]. Similarly, Stewart[323] has argued that the conditioned stimulus control of sensitization may occur at different synaptic sites, depending on the specific actions of different drugs. All of this suggests that sensitization involves neuroadaptations at multiple sites and in multiple neurotransmitter systems.

Nevertheless, in our present state of ignorance it is a reasonable working hypothesis that the adaptations in dopamine systems described here, involving an enhancement in mesotelencephalic dopamine neurotransmission, form a critical link in a chain of events leading to drug craving in addicts. We readily acknowledge, however, that some addictive drugs could produce such incentive-sensitization effects by an action on other, as yet unidentified, neural systems, including, for example, output pathways from the ventral striatum to the ventral pallidum[180]. On the other hand, it is also possible that the dopamine-independent rewarding effects of some drug treatment regimens[181] involve the activation of this same dopamine-incentive salience circuitry, but at a later stage, 'downstream' from dopamine neurons. Regardless, we want to emphasize that the Incentive-Sensitization Theory of Addiction *does not require that the sole or even primary site of drug-induced neuroadaptations responsible for craving specifically be on dopamine neurons*. If it is not, then our assignment of sensitization of incentive salience to dopamine would be incorrect. Nevertheless, the concept that drug craving develops because of sensitization of incentive salience could still be fundamentally correct, but it would be mediated by another, as yet unidentified neural substrate.

6.5. Note 5. Tolerance to drug pleasure

The magnitude of the decrease in the subjective pleasurable effects of drugs is illustrated as being relatively small in Fig. 3 because, although the development of tolerance to the euphoric effects of drugs is widely accepted in the clinical literature, there is actually very little objective evidence for this. The evidence that is usually cited is that addicts tend to gradually escalate their dosage with repeated drug use. "One of the most insidious aspects of drug abuse is the seemingly inexorable tendency for addicts to increase their drug consumption over time" (ref. 86, p. 81). But Falk et al.[86] point out there is very little evidence linking escalation in dose with tolerance to the subjective pleasurable effects of drugs. They state: "It is commonly presumed that... as tolerance develops, more drug must be ingested to satiate the addict's need for the drug. It is fascinating that there is little experimental data relevant to this assumption and that which does exist does not support" (p. 81). Indeed, there are a number of reports that addicts continue to experience euphoria even after years of drug use[193,211,213]. Some studies have suggested there even may be an increase in the pleasurable effects of morphine in long-term addicts, because naive subjects usually rate the effects of morphine as unpleasant, whereas experienced users ('postaddicts') overwhelmingly rate morphine effects as pleasant[193]. This apparent increase in the subjective effects of morphine is probably not due, however, to sensitization to its euphoric effects, but to tolerance to its aversive effects; because 'postaddicts' also report a lower incidence of nausea and vomiting than naive subjects.

Why then do addicts typically escalate their dose? A possible alternative explanation to tolerance of euphoria is that addicts increase dose to achieve the more intense (and more desirable) subjective effects produced by larger doses. They are able to do this only because tolerance develops to the aversive 'side-effects' of drugs. That is, addicts increase their dose because they can, without the dire negative effects experienced by naive users. Doses that might be unpleasant or even life-threatening in inexperienced users, are 'tolerated' by experienced users, because of tolerance to many of the drug's negative effects, including effects on the autonomic nervous system.

On the other hand, short-term tolerance to the euphoric effects of drugs may play a role in the escalation of dose seen when drugs are administered in a 'run', as is often the case with amphetamine or cocaine. If a large supply of amphetamine or cocaine is readily available addicts often readminister the drug as soon as the effects of the previous dose begins to dissipate. However, if successive administrations are given too close together in time the positive effects of the drug may be 'masked' or suppressed by a transient depression of brain 'reward' systems[105,174,204]. As pointed out by Stewart[324]: "Tolerance to the rewarding effects of opiates has been found in experiments in which animals were exposed to the drugs continuously prior to place preference training[299]" (also see ref. 81) and in humans there is a "rapid within-session development of tolerance to the subjective mood effects of cocaine, but this dissipated completely within 24 h[97]" (also see ref. 95). Therefore, it may be that dose is escalated within a run to overcome this apparent short-term tolerance to the pleasurable effects of the drug. But this may not be relevant to the escalation of dose seen over the long-term, that is, between runs.

In summary, although we indicate in Fig. 3 that some tolerance develops to the subjective pleasurable effects of drugs we are aware that this is a complicated and largely unresolved issue. But whether the subjective pleasurable effects show some tolerance or no change with repeated drug administration, the development of an addiction is still characterized by an increasing dissociation between 'wanting' drugs and 'liking' drugs. As Fig. 3 illustrates, 'wanting' drugs, produced by the attribution of incentive salience to the act of drug taking and to drug-related stimuli and their mental representations, increases dramatically during addiction; 'wanting' evolves into craving. At the same time 'liking' drugs does not increase.

6.6. Note 6. The compulsive nature of addictive behavior

It is interesting to speculate that addictive behavior may be so compulsive in nature because the neuroadaptations underlying drug addiction are in some way related to other obsessive-compulsive disorders. It is well known that hyperactivity in dopamine systems results in behaviors with a highly stereotyped (compulsive?) structure. For example, relatively low doses of amphetamine or cocaine elicit high levels of locomotor activity and the pattern of locomotion is abnormally stereotyped[224,285]. At higher doses locomotor activity is diminished as animals engage in highly stereotyped, narrowly focussed, repetitive behaviors[254]. Similar patterns of stereotyped behavior ('punding') have been described extensively in human amphetamine users[254,286]. A number of compulsive behavioral disorders have been linked to dysfunction in the striatum, including obsessive-compulsive disorder itself, Tourette's syndrome, tic disorders[18,255,256] and Huntington's Disease (ref. 59 and N. Wexler, personal communication). Thus, there are a number of different disorders in which dysfunction in the striatum has been associated with compulsive, repetitive thoughts (obsessions) and actions (compulsions). It is interesting to speculate, therefore, that some of the neural changes underlying drug addiction may be, in some respects, similar to those responsible for other obsessive-compulsive disorders.

6.7. Note 7. Benzodiazepines and sedative-hypnotics

There are drugs of abuse that do not seem to fit this profile, namely the benzodiazepines (BZ) and barbiturates. These compounds have biphasic effects on behavior, producing mild psychomotor activation at low doses and a marked depression of motor activity at higher doses[365], but they may not increase dopamine neurotransmission. Although the psychomotor-activating effects of a low dose of diazepam (0.25 mg/kg) has been reported to require the activation of dopamine systems[311], microdialysis studies have found that diazepam and midazolam decrease extracellular dopamine in the nucleus accumbens[92,146] (although in these latter studies relatively high doses were used, > 0.5 mg/kg). It may be that the Incentive-Sensitization Theory does not account for why these particular drugs are used recreationally. It should be noted, however, the BZ's are not very addictive and in normal experimental subjects they have "little or virtually no reinforcing effects" (ref. 56, p. 142). They do not produce the compulsive pattern of drug-seeking and drug-taking behavior characteristic of amphetamine, cocaine or the opiates[371]. Whether the addictive potential of alcohol can be accounted for by Incentive-Sensitization remains to be seen. As cited in the text, there are reports that alcohol: (1) produces psychomotor activation, especially in alcohol-preferring strains; (2) increases extracellular dopamine; and (3) produces sensitization. But there have been very few studies, they are not all consistent and therefore, more work is needed to resolve the issue.

6.8. Note 8. The role of dopamine in mediating the effects of conditioned incentives

The view of how conditioned incentive stimuli evoke relapse proposed here is similar to that of Stewart et al.[326], except we hypothesize drug-associated stimuli evoke craving by activation of a sensitized neural system that specifically mediates incentive salience. Like Stewart et al.[326] we suggest that this neural system involves mesotelencephalic dopamine projections to the ventral striatum and that conditioned incentive stimuli act much like a 'priming' dose of a drug itself; producing a small increase in dopaminergic activity. The difference is that we specify the consequence of this enhanced dopamine activity to be conditioned incentive salience, not necessarily a conditioned affective state, a 'high'. We do not deny, however, that conditioned pleasure can be elicited seperately, presumably via associative activation of separate neural systems.

We need to acknowledge, however, that there has been relatively little research on the role of dopamine in mediating the effects of conditioned incentive stimuli, especially conditioned incentive stimuli established through their association with drugs. There is considerable evidence that activation of the ventral striatal dopamine system enhances responding for conditioned incentive stimuli established by pairing a neutral stimulus with a natural incentive, like food or water[44,127,168,169,262,333,334] (for reviews see refs. 85, 263). There is also a general consensus that dopamine systems are critical in the process by which stimuli acquire conditioned incentive properties through their association with natual incentives or drugs[2,20,21,32,74,77,113,129,219,222,344,352] (cf. refs. 207,260, 317). It has been suggested, however, that once acquired, conditioned incentive stimuli may activate behavior independently of dopamine. This conclusion is based on reports that dopamine receptor blockade with pimozide (or in one experiment, haloperidol) does not prevent the conditioned psychomotor activation evoked by a conditioned stimulus associated with food[139], or drugs[20,21,352]; although the absolute amount of psychomotor activation produced by a food-associated CS is reduced[139]. This idea is controversial, however, because others have reported that dopamine antagonism does attenuate the expression of conditioned 'preparatory behaviors' (including locomotor activity) produced by a conditioned stimulus signaling food[31,32,33] (also see ref. 353), as well as conditioned responses established by drugs[76,77,113,130,247]. Also, under some conditions dopamine antagonists may induce gradual extinction-like effects on conditioned responding[360,364]. Such effects may be interpreted by the hypothesis that low doses of dopamine antagonists impair the 'reboosting' of incentive salience to established conditioned stimuli, which could occur each time an incentive stimulus is encountered. This 'reboosting' may be essential for the maintainence of a conditioned response[27].

Direct measures of dopamine neurotransmission also support the hypothesis that this neural system mediates the incentive effects of conditioned stimuli[31]. Conditioned stimuli predictive of food have been reported to increase the discharge rate of dopamine neurons[183,199,287,289], to increase dopamine metabolism in the nucleus accumbens[34] and to increase a chronoamperometric signal thought to reflect extracellular dopamine[239]. Similarly, conditioned stimuli associated with psychomotor stimulants or opiates are reported to enhance dopamine metabolism[191,234,283], to elevate a dopamine-related electrochemical signal associated with cocaine[115] and in the presence of the unconditioned stimulus, to elevate dopamine in dialysate[252]. On the other hand, negative results have been reported as well[16,38,39,93,348] and therefore, more work is needed to resolve the discrepancies.

6.9. Note 9. Stress, aversive stimuli and stimulant-induced psychoses

Not only do pleasant natural incentives, such as food, water and access to a mate activate mesotelencephalic dopamine systems[51,66,126,214,246,376], but so do some presumably unpleasant aversive events, including classical stressors. Stressors are particularly effective in activating dopamine projections to the medial frontal cortex and to the shell of the nucleus accumbens[1,71,336]. Intense aversive stimuli may also activate the nigrostriatal dopamine system[1]. Conditioned stressors (previously neutral stimuli paired with an aversive event) can activate mesotelencephalic dopamine systems as well, increasing dopamine metabolism in the frontal cortex[125] and the concentration of dopamine in nucleus accumbens dialysate[377]. What does this mean for the hypothesis that dopamine mediates incentive salience and that dopaminergic activation makes stimuli salient, attractive and 'wanted'?

There are at least two alternative explanations that can reconcile stress-induced activation of dopamine and the incentive-sensitization hypothesis and until further data are available the incentive salience hypothesis does not commit to either one. First, it is possible that mesotelencephalic dopamine systems mediate the salience of stimuli that signal unpleasant consequences as well as those that signal pleasant ones. The rustling noise that signals an approaching tiger should grab the attention no less than the sight of delectable food. The salience of both tiger and food may be mediated by dopamine systems, whereas the valence of that salience (attractive incentive vs. frightening warning) may be determined by the coactivation of other neural systems. A second possibility is that moderate levels of dopamine activation, such as that produced by natural incentives and stressors (see above for references), always makes stimuli attractively salient, whereas even higher levels of dopamine activation makes stimuli frightening.

Is it non-sensical to say that stress can make stimuli more attractive? Not at all. Stressors are known to potentiate behavior that is ordinarily incentive-based. For example, stress-induced feeding is a phenomenon that has been well documented in both animals and humans[10,223]. Stress may cause mesotelencephalic dopamine systems to magnify the incentive salience attributed to known incentives such as familiar foods, thus leading to increased eating. Furthermore, stressors themselves may sometimes fascinate and elicit approach, rather than drive an individual away. For example, in a laboratory model of predator mobbing rats will repeatedly approach an electrified object that has in the past given them a shock and will attempt to bury the offending object by pushing sand, etc. upon it[245]. Also, under particular conditions animals will work (lever press) to deliver electric shocks to themselves, shocks that are known to be otherwise aversive (ref. 86 for review). Indeed, rats will even bar press to self-administer corticosterone i.v., in doses that produce a plasma concentration comparable to that seen during mild stress and this is associated with an increase in nucleus accumbens dopamine neurotransmission[244]. Furthermore, animals that are more prone to acquire a drug self-administration habit are more sensitive to the reinforcing effects of corticosterone than 'low risk' animals. Corticosterone also produces a larger increase in dopamine neurotransmission in 'high risk' animals than in 'low risk' animals[244]. These examples suggest that stress-induced dopamine activation may indeed activate incentive processes – quite separately from their activation of pain, aversion or discomfort. Which of these alternatives best describes the role of dopaminergic salience attribution during stress and in response to aversive stimuli will require further research to resolve.

In the examples above we suggest that the moderate level of dopamine activation produced by natural incentives and even stressors, may increase incentive salience. Likewise, we posit that a moderate level of dopamine activation produced by addictive drugs enhances incentive salience and the higher levels of dopamine activation produced by increasing doses of addictive drugs may progressively increase incentive salience. The ability of addictive drugs to elevate dopamine neurotransmission beyond that which normally occurs may be the feature of drugs that make them such potent incentives. However, this may be true only up to a point. Exceedingly high levels of dopamine activation may sometimes result in markedly aversive experiences. Although the attribution of incentive salience can make stimuli in the environment 'brighter' and more attractive, beyond a certain point the world may become too 'bright': stimuli may become confusing, distracting and potentially frightening. For example, the hallucinations and terror of amphetamine psychosis may reflect the excessive and indiscriminate attribution of salience to all stimuli in general, by a wildly hyperfunctioning dopamine system. The sensitization of dopamine neurotransmission may explain why the propensity to amphetamine or cocaine psychosis usually develops in a progressive, sensitization-like fashion and why the susceptibility to stimulant-induced (or stress-induced) psychosis persists for years after the discontinuation of drug use[279,280].

The symptoms of stimulant-induced psychosis are very similar to those seen in paranoid schizophrenia[292] and the suggestion that they are due to wildly excessive incentive salience is consistent with some current hypotheses regarding the nature of schizophrenia. It has been suggested[331], for example, that, "mesolimbic dopamine activation may regulate the extent to which particular types of environmental cues elicit or shape appetitive behavior"... and a loss of this 'gating' function by the overactivation of dopamine systems "may result in cognitive 'flooding', information overload and cognitive fragmentation in clinical states putatively associated with dopamine overactivity [such as schizophrenia][37,321,332]" (p. 419).

6.10. Note 10. Dopamine antagonists and therapy

At first sight, it might appear that an implication of the Incentive-Sensitization Theory is that an effective treatment for excessive craving would be to block dopamine receptors with a postsynaptic antagonist such as pimozide or haloperidol. However, it is not at all clear that such a treatment would be effective. In fact, there are several reasons for doubting the usefulness of dopamine antagonists as a treatment for addiction.

Even though the Incentive-Sensitization Theory proposes that excessive craving for drugs results directly from sensitization of dopamine neurotransmission, dopamine antagonists may not be as useful in reducing the expression of pre-established incentives (attribution of incentive salience that is directed by existing associations) as they are in blocking the *acquisition of new incentives* (attribution of incentive salience to previously neutral stimuli). An addict is already too late for a treatment that blocks the acquisition of incentive sensitization to work. Only a treatment that blocked the expression of sensitized incentive salience would be helpful.

A large body of evidence from animal studies of dopamine antagonist effects on incentive motivation indicates that while the acquisition of, for example, a conditioned preference for an environment paired with drug administration is nearly always blocked by a dopamine antagonist, the behavioral expression of a preference that was previously conditioned is only sometimes suppressed by the same drug (see the aforementioned Note 8). There are a number of possible explanations for the equivocal effects of dopamine antagonists on the expression of pre-existing incentives. First, it might be that dopamine antagonists actually do reduce the incentive salience of drug-paired conditioned stimuli, but that they also reduce the incentive salience of all other stimuli. This would produce an absolute reduction of all incentive motivation but would leave the relative incentive value of stimuli unchanged (ref. 139 for example). Although an addict might crave drugs less after taking a dopamine antagonist, drugs would still be wanted more than anything else and drug seeking would still dominate behavior. Second, it might be that the neural processes that mediate the expression of sensitized incentive salience truly are more resistant to the effects of dopamine antagonists than are the neural processes which mediate the establishment of sensitization. If so, only very high doses of neuroleptics, which might seriously disrupt many aspects of normal behavior, would be sufficient to suppress drug craving. We do not know why this should be true, but there are a number of possible mechanisms that could explain it. For example, once established sensitization might be associated with neuroadaptations that extend to systems 'downstream' from dopamine neurons themselves. These neural systems may continue to respond excessively even if dopamine neurotransmission is reduced. On the other hand, the acquisition of sensitization may depend more specifically upon dopamine activation alone.

Another possibility is that the acquisition vs. expression of sensitization are mediated by different dopamine subsystems that have, for example, different dopamine receptor subtypes, etc. Hiroi and White[130] noted that when a dopamine receptor antagonist failed to selectively decrease the expression of conditioned responding (see the aforementioned Note 8) "neuroleptics with a higher affinity for D2 than D1 receptors", were used and further noted that "a D1 antagonist, SCH23390 is equally effective in blocking acquisition and expression of an amphetamine conditioned place preference, whereas much higher doses of D2 antagonists are required to block expression than acquisition. Thus, some workers may have failed to observe blocking of the expression of learned behaviors because they used an inappropriate dose range of D2 antagonists" (pp. 40,41).

Finally, even if neuroleptic drugs were effective at suppressing drug craving at moderate doses, their usefulness could be compromised by the possibility that addicts would refuse to take them. Anecdotal evidence abounds to suggest that neuroleptics are unpopular drugs among patients who take them. Aside from their potential motor effects, it is not surprising that this should be so. By the incentive salience hypothesis, a drug that directly suppressed the attribution of incentive salience would make the world 'less bright'. Even though the neural substrates of pleasure would not be suppressed, such a drug could produce 'sham anhedonia' – that is, the conscious inference by the addict that pleasure was reduced via cognitive interpretation ("I don't want anything very much, therefore I must not like anything") – just as direct activation of incentive salience should produce 'sham reward'[27].

7. GLOSSARY

Addiction. There has been considerable debate regarding the appropriate definition of drug addiction. We will use the term here in the sense proposed by a World Health Organization Expert Committee in 1981[79,148]. Drug addiction is defined as "a syndrome in which the use of a drug is given a much higher priority than other behaviors that once had higher value."... "In its extreme form [addiction] is associated with compulsive drug-using behavior and it exhibits the characteristics of a chronic relapsing disorder" (ref. 148, p. 522). The phrase 'addictive behavior' is used to refer collectively to obsessive drug craving and to compulsive drug-seeking and drug-taking behavior.

Addictive behavior. (see Addiction)

Appetitive motivation. (see Incentive motivation)

Aversion. The subjective experience of a sensation as actively unpleasant or the underlying evaluative processes and neural mechanisms that directly produce this subjective experience. The opposite of pleasure or euphoria (see Pleasure). Aversion results from an active evaluation of a sensation carried out by brain systems. In the context of addiction, aversion can be synonymous with the symptoms associated with drug withdrawal, including physical distress and dysphoria. Aversion can also refer to direct subjective effects produced by a drug that can be discriminated from pleasure by the user.

Conditioned incentive stimuli. (see Incentives)

Craving and 'Wanting'. These are used in accordance with their usual English meaning, which for 'wanting' refers to the subjective experience of needing or desiring something ("to feel a need or desire for"; Random House Dictionary of the English Language, 2nd edn., 1987). We further propose, however, that this experience is produced by the psychological process of salience attribution (see incentive salience), that is, the attribution of incentive salience to an external event or its mental representation. The process of incentive salience attribution is pre-concious and only the result of this psychological process is accessible to consciousness. When this occurs it is interpreted[228] as a subjective feeling of 'wanting'. For our purposes craving and 'wanting' differ only in magnitude: craving equals intense 'wanting'[184]. In the addict, craving is the experience associated with excessive incentive salience, which results from drug-induced sensitization of the neural systems that attribute salience to incentives.

Dependence, drug. (see Addiction)

Euphoria. (see Pleasure)

Hedonics (see Pleasure)

Incentive motivation(al). A psychological theory (also see Fig. 2) of how goal-direction is controlled by the stimulus properties of the target[30,339]. Incentive motivation is one of a number of potential psychological mechanisms for controlling the direction of motivated behavior. Drive reduction and opponent processes are examples of other potential mechanisms that might control behavior independently of incentive processes (see Toates[339] for discussion and evidence).

Incentive motivation appears to be the chief mechanism that controls behavior directed towards natural incentives such as food, water and a potential mate and towards more artificial incentives, such as self-administered drugs and reinforcing electrical brain stimulation[30,339]. In the context of addiction, incentive motivation and appetitive motivation are synonymous: that is, appetitive motivation works primarily through incentive processes[339]. Incentive motivation directed towards particular stimuli results from the outcome of a three-stage process. First, the neural substrates for pleasure are activated by the consequences of a particular act or event. Second, pleasure is associated with the object, act, event or place in which pleasure occurs by the processes of classical associative learning. Third, salience is attributed to subsequent perceptions and mental representations of the associated object, act, event or place, by a separate neural system from those responsible for the first two processes. This third process of salience attribution (incentive salience) is proposed here to involve dopamine. The attribution of incentive salience causes the associated situation to become attractive and 'wanted' and it is this psychological process that produces the direct manifestation of incentive motivation: goal-directed seeking and instrumental behavior.

Incentive salience. Refers to the attractiveness of external stimuli, events, places and their mental representations; their ability to capture attention (also see Fig. 2). The term, incentive salience, applies always to the perception of external events and to internal representations of those events. Incentive salience must be actively generated (attributed) by the brain and assigned to particular perceptions and representations, based on their association with past activation of mesotelencephalic dopamine systems. For any given stimulus incentive salience will vary at different times depending upon changes in learned associations regarding the stimulus, the internal state of the perceiver and most specifically, the degree of activation of the dopamine systems that mediate incentive salience. Incentive salience is one of a number of psychological mechanisms that can produce direct behavior (other mechanisms include drive reduction and goal-directed computational algorithms that do not depend on modulated perception of the goal; see Toates[339]). Incentive salience constitutes one component of the complex process of incentive motivation. Although the assignment of incentive salience to an event normally is triggered by a pleasurable experience, manipulations of dopamine systems can disconnect incentive salience from pleasure and alter incentive salience independently. It is hypothesized that the attribution of incentive salience to an event or representation is an unconscious process; only the product of this process, the perception of the object as 'wanted', is interpreted and consciously experienced.

Incentive stimuli (incentives). Stimuli that have been attributed with incentive salience. The perception and mental representation of these stimuli are transformed as a consequence and as incentive stimuli they become salient, attractive, 'wanted', and approached. The terms *natural incentives* and *artificial incentives* are also used. The 3-stage process described for incentive motivation evolved to enable animals and humans to recognize and respond to 'natural' incentives. By natural incentives we mean stimuli such as food, water, social and sexual partners, thermal and tactile sensations, which have been endowed by evolution with the capacity to elicit pleasure and incentive salience under particular conditions (e.g., under certain hormonal conditions). Most natural incentives exert their effects via sensory receptors. 'Artificial' incentives, on the other hand, such as addictive drugs or electrical brain stimulation, bypass sensory receptors and activate the component processes of incentive motivation more directly. Most incentive stimuli are conditioned incentive stimuli: stimuli that have become incentives as a consequence of associative learning during the three-stage process described for incentive motivation. Conditioned incentive stimuli not only include the arbitrary lights and sounds used in laboratory experiments (e.g., an auditory tone that signals food delivery), but also the stimulus configurations that must be learned through experience that allow natural incentives to be recognized (e.g., the sight of a delectable food; the sound of a loved one's voice). Conditioned incentive stimuli are often referred to as conditioned rewards (see below), secondary rewards or secondary reinforcers (see below).

'Liking'. See Pleasure.

Negative reinforcement. See Reinforcement).

Pleasure and 'liking'. These are used in accordance with their usual English meaning, which refers to the subjective experience of a sensation as pleasurable or hedonic and the underlying evaluative and neural processes that directly produce this subjective experience. The opposite of aversion (see above). Pleasure is usually the first stage of the larger process of incentive motivation (together with incentive salience and associative learning) and serves as the normal trigger that activates components of associative learning and incentive salience. By itself, however, pleasure is not equivalent to either reward or 'wanting': it is merely a subjective experience or feeling. The evaluation of the sensation that produces pleasure is pre-conscious; only the product, the subjective pleasure, is experienced. In the present paper and in the context of addiction, the term pleasure is used synonymously with the terms euphoria, hedonia or positive affective state.

Positive affective state. (see Pleasure).
Positive reinforcement. (see Reinforcement).
Reinforcement. A purely behavioral and descriptive term for the relationship between the occurrence of a stimulus and changes in the subsequent probability of the behavior that preceded it. Reinforcement denotes a change in the probability of a behavior (increased or decreased) that is contingent on presentation of stimuli. Reinforcement does not offer either a psychological explanation or a physiological explanation of why the probability of a behavior is changed; it merely notes the existence of the change. Reinforcement can be positive or negative. Positive reinforcement refers to increases in the probability of emission of a behavior produced by subsequent presentation of a stimulus (the positive reinforcer). In the context of addiction the term positive reinforcement is sometimes used both in its proper descriptive sense and sometimes in the theoretical or explanatory sense of reward (see below), where the pleasure produced by a drug is implicitly assumed as a psychological explanation for the change in behavior. In order to avoid ambiguity in the present paper we use positive reinforcement only in its proper descriptive sense. Negative reinforcement refers to increases in the probability of emission of a behavior produced by subsequent omission or termination of a stimulus. For example, in the context of addiction, drugs may act as negative reinforcers by relieving the distress of drug withdrawal.
Reward. The word reward is used in the literature in many different ways and for the most part we avoid the term. For us, the process of reward is essentially equivalent to the process of incentive motivation; that is, reward refers to the process of creating incentives (or, as a noun, a stimulus that triggers this process). Rewards (or incentives) cause future behavior to be changed in a goal-directed fashion so as to obtain again the situation or stimulus that triggered the process. This process normally requires three separate stages. The first stage is the activation of pleasure by the consequences of a particular act or event. In the second stage pleasure is associated with a mental representation of the object, act, event or place in which pleasure occurred, by the process of classical (associative) conditioning. The third stage involves the attribution of incentive salience to subsequent perceptions and representations of the associated object, act, event or place, which causes them to become 'wanted'. Stimuli that signal the availability of the incentive become attractive. Acts that led to the situation in the past are likely to be repeated. New acts, which the animal or person can predict (cognitively) will lead to the incentive in the future, are likely to be produced. If the three stages of normal reward (pleasure, associative learning, incentive salience) are separated, the process remains incomplete. Some separations have been achieved by brain manipulations; others are useful simply as illustrative 'thought experiments'. If the first stage of pleasure is activated without associative learning or salience attribution, then it is merely an isolated hedonic experience that remains unconnected to other events in the world or to subsequent behavior. If the first two stages occur alone so that pleasure is activated in conjunction with associative learning only, then associative conditioning of pleasure will occur to the associated events, but they will not be attributed with incentive salience. The events will become 'liked', but they will not be 'wanted' (this separation may possibly be achieved by destruction of brain dopamine systems[28]). Conversely, if the third stage, incentive salience, is activated alone, then 'wanting' arises in isolation from other processes. This may be achieved, for example, by a stimulating electrode that directly activates brain dopamine systems[27]. If salience attribution is magnified abnormally in conjunction with associative learning, but pleasure is not, for example, by the process of drug-induced sensitization discussed here, then the attribution of incentive salience becomes intensified and focused narrowly on the stimuli and acts associated with drug administration and they become pathologically 'wanted' (craved). This may be considered a type of 'sham reward', which shapes instrumental behavior and creates craving, but is dissociated from pleasure. Viewed from the outside, the behavior produced by sham reward and natural reward is identical on all measures of 'wanting' or instrumental performance. Only behavioral measures that are specifically sensitive to pleasure – rather than wanting – will identify sham reward (without pleasure) as distinct from natural reward (triggered by pleasure).
Salience. A salient stimulus is a stimulus that has been (or is being) attributed with *incentive salience* (see above). Salience refers to the feature(s) of the percept or representation of a stimulus that makes it highly noticeable and difficult to ignore. A salient stimulus is not merely more obvious, but it also becomes 'wanted' and attractive because, according to our usage, it is incentive salience that is attributed to the percept or mental representation (but see Note 9 in Ch. 6 on aversive salience).
Salience attribution. (see Incentive salience; Incentive motivation).
Secondary reinforcers. (see Incentive stimuli)
'Wanting'. (see Craving/'wanting').

Acknowledgements. Preparation of this manuscript and research by the authors was supported by Grants from the National Institute on Drug Abuse (04294) to T.E.R. and from the National Institutes of Health to K.C.B. (NS23959). An earlier version of this theory was first presented at a UCLA/NIDA conference on The Biological Basis of Substance Abuse, Santa Monica, CA, January 9–12, 1991. We are grateful to Aldo Badiani, Jill Becker, Craig Berridge, Barry Everitt, Tim Schallert, Jane Stewart, Frederick Toates, Keith Trujillo, Elliot Valenstein, Derek van der Kooy, Ian Whishaw and Roy Wise for their helpful and thought-provoking comments on an earlier draft of this paper.

REFERENCES

1 Abercrombie, E.D., Keefe, K.A., Di Frischia, D.S. and Zigmond, M.J., Differential effect of stress on in vivo dopamine release in striatum, nucleus accumbens and medial frontal cortex, *J. Neurochem.*, 52 (1989) 1655–1658.

2 Acquas, E., Carboni, E., Leone, P. and Di Chiara, G., SCH 23390 blocks drug-conditioned place-preference and place-aversion: anhedonia (lack of reward) or apathy (lack of motivation) after dopamine-receptor blockade?, *Psychopharmacology*, 99 (1989) 151–155.

3 Aizenstein, M.L., Segal, D.S. and Kuczenski, R., Repeated amphetamine and fencamfamine: sensitization and reciprocal cross-sensitization, *Neuropsychopharmacology*, 3 (1990) 283–290.

4 Akimoto, K., Hamamura, T., Kazahaya, Y., Akiyama, K. and Otsuki, S., Enhanced extracellular dopamine level may be the fundamental neuropharmacological basis of cross-behavioral sensitization between methamphetamine and cocaine – an in vivo dialysis study in freely moving rats, *Brain Res.*, 507 (1990) 344–346.

5 Akimoto, K., Hamamura, T. and Otsuki, S., Subchronic cocaine treatment enhances cocaine-induced dopamine efflux, studied by in vivo intracerebral dialysis, *Brain Res.*, 490 (1989) 339–344.

6 Akiyama, K., Hamamura, T., Ujike, H., Kanzaki, A. and Otsuki, S., Methamphetamine psychosis as a model of relapse of schizophrenia – a behavioral and biochemical study in the animal model. In T. Nakazawa (Ed.), *Taniguchi Symposia on Brain Sciences, Vol. 14, Biological Basis of Schizophrenia*, Japan Scientific Societies Press, Tokyo, 1991, pp. 169–184.

7 Anonymous, *Alcoholics Anonymous*, Alcoholics Anonymous World Services, New York, 1976, 3rd edn.

8 Antelman, S.M. and Chiodo, L.A., Amphetamine as a stressor. In I. Creese (Ed.), *Stimulants: Neurochemical, Behavioral and Clinical Perspectives*, Raven Press, New York, 1983, pp. 269–299.

9 Antelman, S.M., Eichler, A.J., Black, C.A. and Kocan, D., Interchangeability of stress and amphetamine in sensitization, *Science*, 207 (1980) 329–331.

10 Antelman, S.M. and Szechtman, H., Tail pinch induces eating in sated rats which appears to depend on nigrostriatal dopamine, *Science*, 189 (1975) 731–733.

11 Babbini, M. and Davis, W.M., Time-dose relationships for locomotor activity effects of morphine after acute or repeated treatment, *Br. J. Pharmacol.*, 46 (1972) 213–224.

12 Babbini, M., Gaiardi, M. and Bartoletti, M., Persistence of chronic morphine effects upon activity in rats 8 months after ceasing the treatment, *Neuropharmacology*, 14 (1975) 611–6114.

13 Bailey, C.S., Hsiao, S. and King, J.E., Hedonic reactivity to sucrose in rats: modification by pimozide, *Physiol. Behav.*, 38 (1986) 447–452.

14 Baker, H., Joh, T.H. and Reis, D.J., Genetic control of number of midbrain dopaminergic neurons in inbred strains of mice: relationship to size and neuronal density of the striatum, *Proc. Natl. Acad. Sci. USA*, 77 (1980) 4369–4373.

15 Barnett, J.V., Segal, D.S. and Kuczenski, R., Repeated amphetamine pretreatment alters the responsiveness of striatal dopamine-stimulated adenylate cyclase to amphetamine-induced desensitization, *J. Pharmacol. Exp. Ther.*, 242 (1987) 40–47.

16 Barr, G.A., Sharpless, N.S., Cooper, S., Schiff, S.R., Paredes, W. and Bridger, W.H., Classical conditioning, decay and extinction of cocaine-induced hyperactivity and stereotypy, *Life Sci.*, 33 (1983) 1341–1351.

17 Bartoletti, M., Gaiardi, M., Gubellini, G., Bacchi, A. and Babbini, M., Long-term sensitization to the excitatory effects of morphine. A motility study in post-dependent rats, *Neuropharmacology*, 22 (1983) 1193–1196.

18 Baxter, L.R.J., Schwartz, J.M., Bergman, K.S., Szuba, M.P., Guze, B.H., Mazziotta, J.C., Alazraki, A., Selin, C.E., Ferng, H.K., Munford, P., et al., Caudate glucose metabolic rate changes with both drug and behavior therapy for obsessive-compulsive disorder, *Arch. Gen. Psychiatry*, 49 (1992) 681–689.

19 Beninger, R.J., The role of dopamine in locomotor activity and learning, *Brain Res. Rev.*, 287 (1983) 173–196.

20 Beninger, R.J. and Hahn, B.L., Pimozide blocks establishment but not expression of amphetamine-produced environment-specific conditioning, *Science*, 220 (1983) 1304–1306.

21 Beninger, R.J. and Herz, R.S., Pimozide blocks establishment but not expression of cocaine-produced environment-specific conditioning, *Life Sci.*, 38 (1986) 1425–1431.

22 Beninger, R.J., MacLennan, A.J. and Pinel, J.P., The use of conditioned defensive burying to test the the effects of pimozide on associative learning, *Pharmacol. Biochem. Behav.*, 12 (1980) 445–448.

23 Beninger, R.J., Mason, S.T., Phillips, A.G. and Fibiger, H.C., The use of conditioned suppression to evaluate the nature of neuroleptic-induced avoidance deficits, *J. Pharmacol. Exp. Ther.*, 213 (1980) 623–627.

24 Benjamin, D., Grant, E.R., Goldstein, K.R. and Pohorecky, L.A., Sensitization to the dopamine release-enhancing effects of ethanol demonstrated in male long-evans rats, *Soc. Neurosci. Abstr.*, 18 (1992) 1431.

25 Benwell, M.E.M. and Balfour, D.J.K., The effects of acute and repeated nicotine treatment on nucleus accumbens dopamine and locomotor activity, *Br. J. Pharmacol.*, 105 (1992) 849–856.

26 Berridge, K.C., Modulation of taste affect by hunger, caloric satiety and sensory-specific satiety in the rat, *Appetite*, 16 (1991) 103–120.

27 Berridge, K.C. and Valenstein, E.S., What psychological process mediates feeding evoked by electrical stimulation of the lateral hypothalamus?, *Behav. Neurosci.*, 105 (1991) 3–14.

28 Berridge, K.C., Venier, I.L. and Robinson, T.E., Taste reactivity analysis of 6-hydroxydopamine-induced aphagia: implications for arousal and anhedonia hypotheses of dopamine function, *Behav. Neurosci.*, 103 (1989) 36–45.

29 Bijerot, W., Addiction to pleasure: a biological and social-psychological theory of addiction. In D.J. Lettieri, M. Sayers and H.W. Pearson (Eds.), *Theories on Drug Abuse: Selected Contemporary Perspectives*, National Institute on Drug Abuse, Rockville, 1980, pp. 246–255.

30 Bindra, D., How adaptive behavior is produced: a perceptual-motivation alternative to response reinforcement, *Behav. Brain Sci.*, 1 (1978) 41–91.

31 Blackburn, J.R., Pfaus, J.G. and Phillips, A.G., Dopamine functions in appetitive and defensive behaviours, *Prog. Neurobiol.*, 39 (1992) 247–279.

32 Blackburn, J.R., Phillips, A.G. and Fibiger, H.C., Dopamine and preparatory behavior: I. Effects of pimozide, *Behav. Neurosci.*, 101 (1987) 352–360.

33 Blackburn, J.R., Phillips, A.G. and Fibiger, H.C., Dopamine and preparatory behavior: III. Effects of metoclopramide and thioridazine, *Behav. Neurosci.*, 103 (1989) 903–906.

34 Blackburn, J.R., Phillips, A.G., Jakubovic, A. and Fibiger, H.C., Dopamine and preparatory behavior: II. A neurochemical analysis, *Behav. Neurosci.*, 103 (1989) 15–23.

35 Borison, R.L., Havdala, H.S. and Diamond, B.I., Chronic phenylethylamine stereotypy in rats: a new animal model for schizophrenia?, *Life Sci.*, 21 (1977) 117–122.

36 Bradberry, C.W., Gruen, R.J., Berridge, C.W. and Roth, R.H., Individual differences in behavioral measures: correlations with nucleus accumbens dopamine measured by microdialysis, *Pharmacol. Biochem. Behav.*, 39 (1991) 877–882.

37 Braff, D.L. and Geyer, M.A., Sensorimotor gating and the

neurobiology of schizophrenia: human and animal model studies. In S.C. Schultz and C.A. Tamminga (Eds.), *Schizophrenia: Scientific Progress*, Oxford University Press, New York, 1989, pp. 124–136.
38 Brown, E.E. and Fibiger, H.C., Cocaine-induced conditioned locomotion: absence of associated increase in dopamine release, *Neuroscience*, 48 (1992) 621–629.
39 Brown, E.E., Robertson, G.S. and Fibiger, H.C., Evidence for conditional neuronal activation following exposure to a cocaine-paired environment: role of forebrain limbic structures, *J. Neurosci.*, 12 (1992) 4112–4121.
40 Browne, R.G. and Segal, D.S., Metabolic and experimental factors in the behavioral response to repeated amphetamine, *Pharmacol. Biochem. Behav.*, 6 (1977) 545–552.
41 Cabanac, M., Physiological role of pleasure, *Science*, 173 (1971) 1103–1107.
42 Cabanac, M., Sensory pleasure, *Q. Rev. Biol.*, 54 (1979) 1–29.
43 Cabanac, M. and Lafrance, L., Postingestive alliesthesia: the rat tells the same story, *Physiol. Behav.*, 47 (1990) 539–543.
44 Cador, M., Taylor, J.R. and Robbins, T.W., Potentiation of the effects of reward-related stimuli by dopaminergic-dependent mechanisms in the nucleus accumbens, *Psychopharmacology*, 104 (1991) 377–385.
45 Camp, D.M. and Robinson, T.E., Susceptibility to sensitization. I. Sex differences in the enduring effects of chronic D-amphetamine treatment on locomotion, stereotyped behavior and brain monoamines, *Behav. Brain Res.*, 30 (1988) 55–68.
46 Camp, D.M. and Robinson, T.E., Susceptibility to sensitization. II. The influence of gonadal hormones on enduring changes in brain monoamines and behavior produced by the repeated administration of D-amphetamine or restraint stress, *Behav. Brain Res.*, 30 (1988) 69–88.
47 Carlson, J.N. and Glick, S.D., Cerebral lateralization as a source of interindividual differences in behavior, *Experientia*, 45 (1989) 788–798.
48 Castañeda, E., Becker, J.B. and Robinson, T.E., The long-term effects of repeated amphetamine treatment in vivo on amphetamine, KCl and electrical stimulation evoked striatal dopamine release in vitro, *Life Sci.*, 42 (1988) 2447–2456.
49 Childress, A.R., Ehrman, R., McLellan, A.T., MacRae, J., Natale, M. and O'Brien, C.P., Negative mood states trigger conditioned drug craving and conditioned withdrawal in opiate abuse patients, *J. Subst. Abuse Treat*, in press.
50 Childress, A.R., McLellan, A.T., Ehrman, R. and O'Brien, C.P., Classically conditioned responses in opioid and cocaine dependence: a role in relapse?, *NIDA Res. Monogr.*, 84 (1988) 25–43.
51 Church, W.H., Justice Jr., J.B. and Neill, D.B., Detecting behaviorally relevant changes in extracellular dopamine with microdialysis, *Brain Res.*, 412 (1987) 397–399.
52 Clarke, P.B.S., Mesolimbic dopamine activation – the key to nicotine reinforcement? In *Ciba Foundation Symposium 152: The Biology of Nicotine Dependence*, Wiley, Chichester, 1990, pp. 153–168.
53 Clifton, P.G., Rusk, I.N. and Cooper, S.J., Stimulation and inhibition of food intake by the selective dopamine D2 agonist, N-0437: a meal pattern analysis, *Pharmacol. Biochem. Behav.*, 33 (1989) 21–26.
54 Cole, B.J., Cador, M., Stinus, L., Rivier, C., Rivier, J., Vale, W., Le Moal, M. and Koob, G.F., Critical role of the hypothalamic pituitary adrenal axis in amphetamine-induced sensitization of behavior, *Life Sci.*, 47 (1990) 1715–1720.
55 Cole, B.J., Cador, M., Stinus, L., Rivier, J., Vale, W., Koob, G.F. and Le Moal, M., Central administration of a CRF antagonist blocks the development of stress-induced behavioral sensitization, *Brain Res.*, 512 (1990) 343–346.
56 Cole, J.O. and Chiarello, R.J., The benzodiazepines as drugs of abuse, *J. Psychiat. Res.*, 24 (1990) 135–144.
57 Cools, A.R., Differential role of mineralocorticoid and glucocorticoid receptors in the genesis of dexamphetamine-induced sensitization of mesolimbic, alpha 1 adrenergic receptors in the ventral striatum, *Neuroscience*, 43 (1991) 419–428.
58 Crabbe, J.C., Johnson, N.A., Gray, D.K., Kosobud, A. and Young, E.R., Biphasic effects of ethanol on open-field activity: sensitivity and tolerance in C57BL/6N and DBA/2N mice, *J. Comp. Physiol Psychol.*, 96 (1982) 440–451.
59 Cummings, J.L. and Cunningham, K., Obsessive-compulsive disorder in Huntington's disease, *Biol. Psychiatry*, 31 (1992) 263–270.
60 Cunningham, C.L., Niehus, D.R., Malott, D.H. and Prather, L.K., Genetic differences in the rewarding and activating effects of morphine and ethanol, *Psychopharmacology*, 107 (1992) 385–393.
61 Cunningham, C.L. and Noble, D., Conditioned activation induced by ethanol: role in sensitization and conditioned place preference, *Pharmacol. Biochem. Behav.*, 43 (1992) 307–313.
62 Cunningham, S.T. and Kelley, A.E., Evidence for opiate-dopamine cross-sensitization in the nucleus accumbens: studies of conditioned reward, *Brain Res. Bull.*, 29 (1992) 675–680.
63 Dackis, C.A. and Gold, M.S., Bromocriptine as a treatment of cocaine abuse, *The Lancet*, May (1985) 1151–1152.
64 Dackis, C.A. and Gold, M.S., New concepts in cocaine addiction: the dopamine depletion hypothesis, *Neurosci. Biobehav. Rev.*, 9 (1985) 469–477.
65 Damsma, G., Day, J. and Fibiger, H.C., Lack of tolerance to nicotine-induced dopamine release in the nucleus accumbens, *Eur. J. Pharmacol.*, 168 (1989) 363–368.
66 Damsma, G., Pfaus, J.G., Wenkstern, D., Phillips, A.G. and Fibiger, H.C., Sexual behavior increases dopamine transmission in the nucleus accumbens and striatum of male rats: comparison with novelty and locomotion, *Behav. Neurosci.*, 106 (1992) 181–191.
67 Davis, J.D., The microstructure of ingestive behavior, *Ann. NY Acad. Sci.*, 575 (1989) 106–119.
68 Deminiere, J.M., Piazza, P.V., Guegan, G., Abrous, N., Maccari, S., Le Moal, M. and Simon, H., Increased locomotor response to novelty and propensity to intravenous amphetamine self-administration in adult offspring of stressed mothers, *Brain Res.*, 586 (1992) 135–139.
69 Deroche, V., Piazza, P.V., Casolini, P., Maccari, S., Le Moal, M. and Simon, H., Stress-induced sensitization to amphetamine and morphine psychomotor effects depend on stress-induced corticosterone secretion, *Brain Res.*, 598 (1992) 343–348.
70 Deroche, V., Piazza, P.V., Maccari, S., Le Moal, M. and Simon, H., Repeated corticosterone administration sensitizes the locomotor response to amphetamine, *Brain Res.*, 584 (1992) 309–313.
71 Deutch, A.Y. and Cameron, D.S., Pharmacological characterization of dopamine systems in the nucleus accumbens core and shell, *Neuroscience*, 46 (1992) 49–56.
72 Dews, P., Remarks. In T. Thompson and K.R. Unna (Eds.), *Predicting Dependence Liability of Stimulant and Depressant Drugs*, University Park Press, Baltimore, 1977, pp. 75–79.
73 Di Chiara, G. and Imperato, A., Drugs abused by humans preferentially increase synaptic dopamine concentrations in the mesolimbic system of freely moving rats, *Proc. Natl. Acad. Sci. USA*, 85 (1988) 5274–5278.
74 Di Lullo, S.L. and Martin-Iverson, M.T., Evidence for presynaptic dopamine mechanisms underlying amphetamine-conditioned locomotion, *Brain Res.*, 578 (1992) 161–167.
75 Doyle, T.J., Berridge, K.C. and Gosnell, B.A., Morphine enhances taste pleasure, *Pharmacol. Biochem. Behav.*, in press.
76 Drew, K.L. and Glick, S.D., Classical conditioning of amphetamine-induced lateralized and nonlateralized activity in rats, *Psychopharmacology*, 92 (1987) 52–57.
77 Drew, K.L. and Glick, S.D., Role of D-1 and D-2 receptor stimulation in sensitization to amphetamine-induced circling behavior and in expression and extinction of the Pavlovian conditioned response, *Psychopharmacology*, 101 (1990) 465–471.
78 Edmonds, D.E. and Gallistel, C.R., Reward versus performance in self-stimulation: electrode-specific effects of alpha-methyl-*p*-tyrosine on reward in the rat, *J. Comp. Physiol. Psychol.*, 91 (1977) 962–974.
79 Edwards, G., Nomenclature and classification of drug- and alcohol-related problems: a WHO memorandum, *Bull. World Health Org.*, 59 (1981) 225–242.

80 Ehrman, R., Ternes, J., O'Brien, C.P. and McLellan, A.T., Conditioned tolerance in human opiate addicts, *Psychopharmacology*, 108 (1992) 218–224.

81 Emmett-Oglesby, M.W. and Lane, J.D., Tolerance to the reinforcing effects of cocaine, *Behav. Pharmacol.*, 3 (1992) 193–200.

82 Ettenberg, A., Dopamine, neuroleptics and reinforced behavior, *Neurosci. Biobehav. Rev.*, 13 (1989) 105–111.

83 Ettenberg, A., Haloperidol prevents the reinstatement of amphetamine-rewarded runway responding in rats, *Pharmacol. Biochem. Behav.*, 36 (1990) 635–638.

84 Everitt, B.J., Sexual motivation: a neural and behavioural analysis of the mechanisms underlying appetitive and copulatory responses of male rats, *Neurosci. Biobehav. Rev.*, 14 (1990) 217–232.

85 Everitt, B.L. and Robbins, T.W., Amygdala-ventral striatal interactions and reward-related processes. In J.P. Aggleton (Ed.), *The Amygdala: Neurobiological Aspects of Emotion, Memory, and Mental Dysfunction*, Wiley-Liss, New York, 1992, pp. 401–429.

86 Falk, J.L., Dews, P.B. and Schuster, C.R., Commonalities in the environmental control of behavior. In P.K. Levison, D.R. Gerstein and D.R. Maloff (Eds.), *Commonalities in Substance Abuse and Habitual Behavior*, D.C. Heath and Co., Lexington, MA, 1983, pp. 47–110.

87 Falk, J.L. and Feingold, D.A., Environmental and cultural factors in the behavioral action of drugs. In H.Y. Meltzer (Ed.), *Psychopharmacology: The Third Generation of Progress*, Raven Press, New York, 1987, pp. 1503–1510.

88 Falk, J.L., Ma, F. and Lau, C.E., Chronic oral cocaine self-administration: pharmacokinetics and effects on spontaneous and discriminative motor functions, *J. Pharmacol. Exp. Ther.*, 257 (1991) 457–465.

89 Fibiger, H.C. and Phillips, A.G., Increased intracranial self-stimulation in rats after long-term administration of desipramine, *Science*, 214 (1981) 683–685.

90 Fibiger, H.C. and Phillips, A.G., Reward, motivation, cognition: psychobiology of mesotelencephalic dopamine systems. In *Handbook of Physiology, Vol. IV, Intrinsic Regulatory Systems of the Brain*, American Physiology Society, Bethesda, MD, 1986, pp. 647–675.

91 Fink, J.S. and Reis, D.J., Genetic variations in midbrain dopamine cell number: parallel with differences in responses to dopaminergic agonists and in naturalistic behaviors mediated by central dopaminergic systems, *Brain Res.*, 222 (1981) 335–349.

92 Finlay, J.M., Damsma, G. and Fibiger, H.C., Benzodiazepine-induced decreases in extracellular concentrations of dopamine in the nucleus accumbens after acute and repeated administration, *Psychopharmacology*, 106 (1992) 202–208.

93 Finlay, J.M., Jakubovic, A., Phillips, A.G. and Fibiger, H.C., Fentanyl-induced conditional place preference: lack of associated conditional neurochemical events, *Psychopharmacology*, 96 (1988) 534–540.

94 Fischman, M.W., Relationship between self-reported drug effects and their reinforcing effects: studies with stimulant drugs, *NIDA Res. Monogr.*, 92 (1989) 211–230.

95 Fischman, M.W. and Foltin, R.W., Self-administration of cocaine by humans: a laboratory perspective. In G.R. Bock and J. Whelan (Eds.), *Cocaine: Scientific and Social Dimensions. CIBA Foundation Symposium No. 166*, Wiley, Chichester, UK, 1992, pp. 165–180.

96 Fischman, M.W., Foltin, R.W., Nestadt, G. and Pearlson, G.D., Effects of desipramine maintenance on cocaine self-administration by humans, *J. Pharmacol. Exp. Ther.*, 253 (1990) 760–770.

97 Fischman, M.W., Schuster, C.R., Javaid, J., Hatano, Y. and Davis, J., Acute tolerance development to the cardiovascular and subjective effects of cocaine, *J. Pharmacol. Exp. Ther.*, 235 (1985) 677–682.

98 Foltin, R.W. and Fischman, M.W., Assessment of abuse liability of stimulant drugs in humans: a methodological survey, *Drug Alcohol Depend.*, 28 (1991) 3–48.

99 Fouriezos, G. and Wise, R.A., Pimozide-induced extinction of intracranial self-stimulation: response patterns rule out motor or performance deficits, *Brain Res.*, 103 (1976) 377–380.

100 Fujiwara, Y., Kazahaya, Y., Nakashima, M., Sato, M. and Otsuki, S., Behavioral sensitization to methamphetamine in the rat: an ontogenic study, *Psychopharmacology*, 91 (1987) 316–319.

101 Fung, Y.K., Effects of chronic nicotine pretreatment on (+)-amphetamine and nicotine-induced synthesis and release of [^{3}H]dopamine from [^{3}H]tyrosine in rat nucleus accumbens, *J. Pharm. Pharmacol.*, 41 (1989) 66–68.

102 Gaiardi, M., Bartoletti, M., Bacchi, A., Gubellini, C., Costa, M. and Babbini, M., Role of repeated exposure to morphine in determining its affective properties: Place and taste conditioning studies in rats, *Psychopharmacology*, 103 (1991) 183–186.

103 Gallistel, C.R., Boytim, M., Gomita, Y. and Klebanoff, L., Does pimozide block the reinforcing effect of brain stimulation?, *Pharmacol. Biochem. Behav.*, 17 (1982) 769–781.

104 Gallistel, C.R., Shizgal, P. and Yeomans, J.S., A portrait of the substrate for self-stimulation, *Psychol. Rev.*, 88 (1981) 228–273.

105 Gawin, F.H. and Ellinwood, E.J., Cocaine and other stimulants. Actions, abuse and treatment, *N. Engl. J. Med.*, 318 (1988) 1173–1182.

106 Geary, N. and Smith, G.P., Pimozide decreases the positive reinforcing effect of sham fed sucrose in the rat, *Pharmacol. Biochem. Behav.*, 22 (1985) 787–790.

107 Glick, S.D. and Hinds, P.A., Sex differences in sensitization to cocaine-induced rotation, *Eur. J. Pharmacol.*, 99 (1984) 119–121.

108 Glick, S.D. and Hinds, P.A., Differences in amphetamine and morphine sensitivity in lateralized and non-lateralized rats: locomotor activity and drug self-administration, *Eur. J. Pharmacol.*, 118 (1985) 239–244.

109 Glick, S.D., Merski, C., Steindorf, S., Wang, S., Keller, R.W. and Carlson, J.N., Neurochemical predisposition to self-administer morphine in rats, *Brain Res.*, 578 (1992) 215–220.

110 Glick, S.D., Shapiro, R.M., Drew, K.L., Hinds, P.A. and Carlson, J.N., Differences in spontaneous and amphetamine-induced rotational behavior and in sensitization to amphetamine, among Sprague-Dawley derived rats from different sources, *Physiol. Behav.*, 38 (1986) 67–70.

111 Glickman, S.E. and Schiff, B.B., A biological theory of reinforcement, *Psychol. Rev.*, 74 (1967) 81–109.

112 Gnegy, M.E., Hewlett, G.H.K., Yee, S.L. and Welsh, M.J., Alterations in calmodulin content and localization in areas of rat brain after repeated intermittent amphetamine, *Brain Res.*, 562 (1991) 6–12.

113 Gold, L.H., Swerdlow, N.R. and Koob, G.F., The role of mesolimbic dopamine in conditioned locomotion produced by amphetamine, *Behav. Neurosci.*, 102 (1988) 544–552.

114 Goldstein, K.R., Knapp, D.J., Saiff, E.I., Pohorecky, L.A. and Benjamin, D., Sensitization to ethanol demonstrated in place-preference and locomotor activation, *Soc Neurosci. Abstr.*, 18 (1992) 107.

115 Gratton, A., Wise, R.A. and Kiyatkin, E., Chronoamperometric measurements of dopamine levels in the rat nucleus accumbens during cocaine self-administration, *Soc Neurosci. Abstr.*, 18 (1992) 1076.

116 Greenberg, B.D. and Segal, D.S., Acute and chronic behavioral interactions between phencyclidine (PCP) and amphetamine: evidence for a dopaminergic role in some PCP-induced behaviors, *Pharmacol. Biochem. Behav.*, 23 (1985) 99–105.

117 Greenberg, B.D. and Segal, D.S., Evidence for multiple opiate receptor involvement in different phencyclidine-induced unconditioned behaviors in rats, *Psychopharmacology*, 88 (1986) 44–53.

118 Grill, H.J. and Norgren, R., Chronically decerebrate rats demonstrate satiation but not bait shyness, *Science*, 201 (1978) 267–269.

119 Grill, H.J. and Norgren, R., The taste reactivity test. I. Mimetic responses to gustatory stimuli in neurologically normal rats, *Brain Res.*, 143 (1978) 263–279.

120 Haertzen, C.A., Kocher, T.R. and Miyasato, K., Reinforcements from the first drug experience can predict later drug habits and/or addiction: results with coffee, cigarettes, alcohol, barbiturates, minor and major tranquilizers, stimulants, marijuana, hallucinogens, heroin, opiates and cocaine, *Drug Alcohol Depend.*, 11 (1983) 147–165.

121 Hamamura, T., Akiyama, K., Akimoto, K., Kashihara, K., Okumura, K., Ujike, H. and Otsuki, S., Co-administration of either a selective D1 or D2 dopamine antagonist with methamphetamine prevents methamphetamine-induced behavioral sensitization and neurochemical change, studied by in vivo intracerebral dialysis, *Brain Res.*, 546 (1991) 40–46.

122 Harris, G.C. and Williams, J.T., Sensitization of locus ceruleus neurons during withdrawal from chronic stimulants and antidepressants, *J. Pharmacol. Exp. Ther.*, 261 (1992) 476–483.

123 Harsing, L.G., Sershen, H. and Lajtha, A., Dopamine efflux from striatum after chronic nicotine: evidence for autoreceptor desensitization, *J. Neurochem.*, 59 (1992) 48–54.

124 Henry, D.J. and White, F.J., Repeated cocaine administration causes persistent enhancement of D1 dopamine receptor sensitivity within the rat nucleus accumbens, *J. Pharmacol. Exp. Ther.*, 258 (1991) 882–890.

125 Herman, J.P., Guillonneau, D., Dantzer, R., Scatton, B., Semerdjian-Rouquier, L. and Le Moal, M., Differential effects of inescapable footshocks and of stimuli previously paired with inescapable footshocks on dopamine turnover in cortical and limbic areas of the rat, *Life Sci.*, 30 (1982) 2207–2214.

126 Hernandez, L. and Hoebel, B.G., Food reward and cocaine increase extracellular dopamine in the nucleus accumbens as measured by microdialysis, *Life Sci.*, 42 (1988) 1705–1712.

127 Hill, R.T., Facilitation of conditioned reinforcement as a mechanism of psychomotor stimulation. In E. Costa and S. Garattini (Eds.), *Amphetamine and Related Compounds*, Raven Press, New York, 1970, pp. 781–795.

128 Hinson, R.E. and Poulos, C.X., Sensitization to the behavioral effects of cocaine: modification by Pavlovian conditioning, *Pharmacol. Biochem. Behav.*, 15 (1981) 559–562.

129 Hiroi, N. and White, N.M., Conditioned stereotypy: behavioral specification of the UCS and pharmacological investigation of the neural change, *Pharmacol. Biochem. Behav.*, 32 (1989) 249–258.

130 Hiroi, N. and White, N.M., The reserpine-sensitive dopamine pool mediates (+)-amphetamine-conditioned reward in the place preference paradigm, *Brain Res.*, 510 (1990) 33–42.

131 Hoebel, B.G., Neuroscience and motivation: pathways and peptides that define motivational systems. In R.C. Atkinson, R.J. Herrnstein, G. Lindzay and R.D. Lance (Eds.), *Steven's Handbook of Experimental Psychology, Vol. 1, Perception and Motivation*, John Wiley, New York, 1988, pp. 547–597.

132 Hooks, M.S., Colvin, A.C., Juncos, J.L. and Justice Jr., J.B., Individual differences in basal and cocaine-stimulated extracellualr dopamine in the nucleus accumbens using quantitative microdialysis, *Brain Res.*, 587 (1992) 306–312.

133 Hooks, M.S., Jones, G.H., Liem, B.J. and Justice Jr., J.B., Sensitization and individual differences to IP amphetamine, cocaine or caffeine following repeated intracranial amphetamine infusions, *Pharmacol. Biochem. Behav.*, 43 (1992) 815–823.

134 Hooks, M.S., Jones, G.H., Neill, D.B. and Justice Jr., J.B., Individual differences in amphetamine sensitization: dose-dependent effects, *Pharmacol. Biochem. Behav.*, 41 (1992) 203–210.

135 Hooks, M.S., Jones, G.H., Smith, A.D., Neill, D.B. and Justice Jr., J.B., Individual differences in locomotor activity and sensitization, *Pharmacol. Biochem. Behav.*, 38 (1991) 467–470.

136 Horger, B.A., Giles, M.K. and Schenk, S., Preexposure to amphetamine and nicotine predisposes rats to self-administer a low dose of cocaine, *Psychopharmacology*, 107 (1992) 271–276.

137 Horger, B.A., Shelton, K. and Schenk, S., Preexposure sensitizes rats to the rewarding effects of cocaine, *Pharm. Biochem. Behav.*, 37 (1990) 707–711.

138 Horger, B.A., Wellman, P.J., Morien, A., Davies, B.T. and Schenk, S., Caffeine exposure sensitizes rats to the reinforcing effects of cocaine, *Neuroreport*, 2 (1991) 53–56.

139 Horvitz, J.C. and Ettenberg, A., Conditioned incentive properties of a food-paired conditioned stimulus remain intact during dopamine receptor blockade, *Behav. Neurosci.*, 105 (1991) 536–541.

140 Hu, X.-T., Brooderson, R.J. and White, F.J., Repeated stimulation of D1 dopamine receptors causes time-dependent alterations in the sensitivity of both D1 and D2 dopamine receptors within the rat striatum, *Neuroscience*, 50 (1992) 137–147.

141 Hunt, H.F., Some effects of drugs on classical (type s) conditioning, *Ann. NY Acad. Sci.*, 65 (1956) 258–267.

142 Hunt, W.A. and Lands, W.E., A role for behavioral sensitization in uncontrolled ethanol intake, *Alcohol*, 9 (1992) 327–328.

143 Hurd, Y.L., Weiss, F., Koob, G.F., And, N.E. and Ungerstedt, U., Cocaine reinforcement and extracellular dopamine overflow in rat nucleus accumbens: an in vivo microdialysis study, *Brain Res.*, 498 (1989) 199–203.

144 Ichikawa, J., Changes in behavior and central monoaminergic systems in the rat after repeated methamphetamine pretreatment: presynaptic regulatory mechanism, *Yakubutsu Seishin Kodo*, 8 (1988) 389–403.

145 Ingram, D.K. and Corfman, T.P., An overview of neurobiological comparisons in mouse strains, *Neurosci. Biobehav. Rev.*, 4 (1980) 421–435.

146 Invernizzi, R., Pozzi, L. and Samanin, R., Release of dopamine is reduced by diazepam more in the nucleus accumbens than in the caudate nucleus of conscious rats, *Neuropharmacology*, 30 (1991) 575–578.

147 Iwamoto, E.T., Comparison of the pharmacologic effects of *N*-allylnormetazocine and phencyclidine: sensitization, cross-sensitization and opioid antagonist activity, *Psychopharmacology*, 89 (1986) 221–229.

148 Jaffe, J.H., Drug addiction and drug abuse. In A.G. Gilman, T.W. Rall, A.S. Nies and P. Taylor (Eds.), *The Pharmacological Basis of Therapeutics*, Pergamon Press, New York, 1990, pp. 522–573.

149 Jaffe, J.H., Current concepts of addiction. In C.P. O'Brien and J.H. Jaffe (Eds.), *Addictive States*, Raven Press, New York, 1992, pp. 1–21.

150 Jaffe, J.H., Cascella, N.G., Kumor, K.M. and Sherer, M.A., Cocaine-induced cocaine craving, *Psychopharmacology*, 97 (1989) 59–64.

151 Jones, B.E. and Prada, J.A., Drug-seeking behavior during methadone maintenance, *Psychopharmacologia*, 41 (1975) 7–10.

152 Jones, G.H., Marsden, C.A. and Robbins, T.W., Increased sensitivity to amphetamine and reward-related stimuli following social isolation in rats: possible disruption of dopamine-dependent mechanisms of the nucleus accumbens, *Psychopharmacology*, 102 (1990) 364–372.

153 Joyce, E.M. and Iversen, S.D., The effect of morphine applied locally to mesencephalic dopamine cell bodies on spontaneous motor activity in the rat, *Neurosci. Lett.*, 14 (1979) 207–212.

154 Kalivas, P.W., Sensitization to repeated enkephalin administration into the ventral tegmental area of the rat. II. Involvement of the mesolimbic dopamine system, *J. Pharmacol. Exp. Ther.*, 235 (1985) 544–550.

155 Kalivas, P.W. and Duffy, P., Effects of daily cocaine and morphine treatment on somatodendritic and terminal field dopamine release, *J. Neurochem.*, 50 (1988) 1498–1504.

156 Kalivas, P.W. and Duffy, P., Similar effects of daily cocaine and stress on mesocorticolimbic dopamine neurotransmission in the rat, *Biol. Psychiatry*, 25 (1989) 913–928.

157 Kalivas, P.W. and Duffy, P., Effect of acute and daily cocaine treatment on extracellular dopamine in the nucleus accumbens, *Synapse*, 5 (1990) 48–58.

158 Kalivas, P.W. and Duffy, P., Time course of extracellular dopamine and behavioral sensitization to cocaine: I. Dopamine axon terminals, *J. Neurosci.*, 13 (1993) 266–275.

159 Kalivas, P.W., Duffy, P., Abhold, R. and Dilts, R.P., Sensitization of mesolimbic dopamine neurons by neuropeptides and stress. In P.W. Kalivas and C.D. Barnes (Eds.), *Sensitization in the Nervous System*, Telford Press, Caldwell, NJ, 1988, pp. 119–143.

160 Kalivas, P.W. and Stewart, J., Dopamine transmission in the initiation and expression of drug- and stress-induced sensitization of motor activity, *Brain Res. Rev.*, 16 (1991) 223–244.

161 Karler, R., Calder, L.D., Chaudhry, I.A. and Turkanis, S.A., Blockade of "reverse tolerance" to cocaine and amphetamine by MK-801, *Life Sci.*, 45 (1989) 599–606.

162 Karler, R., Calder, L.D. and Turkanis, S.A., Changes in CNS sensitivity to cannabinoids with repeated treatment: tolerance and auxoesthesia, *NIDA Res. Monogr.*, 54 (1984) 312–322.
163 Karler, R., Calder, L.D. and Turkanis, S.A., DNQX blockade of amphetamine behavioral sensitization, *Brain Res.*, 552 (1991) 295–300.
164 Karler, R., Chaudhry, I.A., Calder, L.D. and Turkanis, S.A., Amphetamine behavioral sensitization and the excitatory amino acids, *Brain Res.*, 537 (1990) 76–82.
165 Katz, J.L. and Goldberg, S.R., Preclinical assessment of abuse liability of drugs, *Agents and Actions*, 23 (1988) 18–26.
166 Kazahaya, Y., Akimoto, K. and Otsuki, S., Subchronic methamphetamine treatment enhances methamphetamine- or cocaine-induced dopamine efflux in vivo., *Biol. Psychiatry*, 25 (1989) 903–912.
167 Keller, R.W., Maisonneuve, I.M., Carlson, J.N. and Glick, S.D., Within-subject sensitization of striatal dopamine release after a single injection of cocaine: an in vivo microdialysis study, *Synapse*, 11 (1992) 28–34.
168 Kelley, A.E. and Delfs, J.M., Dopamine and conditioned reinforcement. I. Differential effects of amphetamine microinjections into striatal subregions, *Psychopharmacology*, 103 (1991) 187–196.
169 Kelley, A.E. and Delfs, J.M., Dopamine and conditioned reinforcement. II. Contrasting effects of amphetamine microinjection into the nucleus accumbens with peptide microinjection into the ventral tegmental area, *Psychopharmacology*, 103 (1991) 197–203.
170 Khantzian, E.J., The self-medication hypothesis of addictive disorders: focus on heroin and cocaine dependence, *Am. J. Psychiatry*, 142 (1985) 1259–1264.
171 Kita, T., Okamoto, M. and Nakashima, T., Nicotine-induced sensitization to ambulatory stimulant effect produced by daily administration into the ventral tegmental area and the nucleus accumbens in rats, *Life Sci.*, 50 (1992) 583–590.
172 Kiyatkin, E., Wise, R.A. and Gratton, A., Chronamperometic measurements of dopamine levels in the rat nucleus accumbens, *Soc. Neurosci. Abstr.*, 18 (1992) 374.
173 Knoblich, G., Curtis, D., Faustman, W.O., Zarcone, V., Stewart, S., Mefford, I. and King, R., Increased CSF HVA with craving in long-term abstinent cocaine abusers, *Biol. Psychiatry*, 32 (1992) 96–100.
174 Kokkinidis, L., Zacharko, R.M. and Anisman, H., Amphetamine withdrawal: a behavioral evaluation, *Life Sci.*, 38 (1986) 1617–1623.
175 Kolta, M.G., Scalzo, F.M., Ali, S.F. and Holson, R.R., Ontogeny of the enhanced behavioral response to amphetamine in amphetamine-pretreated rats, *Psychopharmacology*, 100 (1990) 377–382.
176 Kolta, M.G., Shreve, P., De Souza, V. and Uretsky, N.J., Time course of the development of the enhanced behavioral and biochemical responses to amphetamine after pretreatment with amphetamine, *Neuropharmacology*, 24 (1985) 823–829.
177 Kolta, M.G., Shreve, P. and Uretsky, N.J., Effect of methylphenidate pretreatment on the behavioral and biochemical responses to amphetamine, *Eur. J. Pharmacol.*, 117 (1985) 279–282.
178 Kolta, M.G., Shreve, P. and Uretsky, N.J., Effect of pretreatment with amphetamine on the interaction between amphetamine and dopamine neurons in the nucleus accumbens, *Neuropharmacology*, 28 (1989) 9–14.
179 Koob, G.F., Dopamine, addiction and reward, *Sem. Neurosci.*, 4 (1992) 139–148.
180 Koob, G.F. and Bloom, F.E., Cellular and molecular mechanisms of drug dependence, *Science*, 242 (1988) 715–723.
181 Koob, G.F. and Goeders, N.E., Neuroanatomical substrates of drug self-administration. In J.M. Liebman and S.J. Cooper (Eds.), *The Neuropharmacological Basis of Reward*, Oxford University Press, New York, 1989, pp. 214–263.
182 Koob, G.F., Stinus, L., Le Moal, M. and Bloom, F.E., Opponent process theory of motivation: neurobiological evidence from studies of opiate dependence, *Neurosci. Biobehav. Rev.*, 13 (1989) 135–140.
183 Kosobud, A.E., Harris, A.E. and Chapin, J.K., Actions of drugs of abuse on reward-related activity in neurons of the ventral tegmental area and prefrontal cortex in the rat, *Soc. Neurosci. Abstr.*, 18 (1992) 900.
184 Kozlowski, L.T. and Wilkinson, D.A., Use and misuse of the concept of craving by alcohol, tobacco and drug researchers, *Br. J. Addict.*, 82 (1987) 31–36.
185 Krieckhaus, E.E. and Wolf, G., Acquisition of sodium by rats: interactions of innate mechanisms and latent learning, *J. Comp. Physiol. Psychol.*, 65 (1968) 197–201.
186 Ksir, C., Hakan, R., Hall, D.P. and Kellar, K.J., Exposure to nicotine enhances the behavioral stimulant effect of nicotine and increases binding of [^{3}H]acetylcholine to nicotinic receptors, *Neuropharmacology*, 24 (1985) 527–531.
187 Kuczenski, R. and Leith, N.J., Chronic amphetamine: is dopamine a link in or mediator of the development of tolerance or reverse tolerance?, *Pharmacol. Biochem. Behav.*, 15 (1981) 405–413.
188 Kuczenski, R. and Segal, D.S., Psychomotor stimulant-induced sensitization: behavioral and neurochemical correlates. In P.W. Kalivas and C.D. Barnes (Eds.), *Sensitization in the Nervous System*, Telford Press, Caldwell, NJ, 1988, pp. 175–205.
189 Kuroki, T., Tsutsumi, T., Hirano, M., Matsumoto, T., Tatebayashi, Y., Nishiyama, K., Uchimura, H., Shiraishi, A., Nakahara, T. and Nakamura, K., Behavioral sensitization to beta-phenylethylamine (PEA): enduring modifications of specific dopaminergic neuron systems in the rat, *Psychopharmacology*, 102 (1990) 5–10.
190 La Hoste, G.J., Mormede, P., Rivet, J.M. and Le Moal, M., Differential sensitization to amphetamine and stress responsivity as a function of inherent laterality, *Brain Res.*, 453 (1988) 381–384.
191 Lal, H., Miksic, S., Drawbaugh, R., Numan, R. and Smith, N., Alleviation of narcotic withdrawal syndrome by conditional stimuli, *Pavlov J. Biol. Sci.*, 11 (1976) 251–262.
192 Lamb, R.J., Preston, K.L., Schindler, C., Meisch, R.A., Davis, F., Katz, J.L., Henningfield, J.E. and Goldberg, S.R., The reinforcing and subjective effects of morphine in post-addicts: a dose-response study, *J. Pharmacol. Exp. Ther.*, 259 (1991) 1165–1173.
193 Lasagna, L., von Felsinger, J.M. and Beecher, H.K., Drug-induced mood changes in man. 1. Observations on healthy subjects, chronically ill patients and "postaddicts", *JAMA*, 157 (1955) 1006–1020.
194 Leith, N.J. and Kuczenski, R., Two dissociable components of behavioral sensitization following repeated amphetamine administration, *Psychopharmacology*, 76 (1982) 310–5.
195 Lett, B.T., Repeated exposures intensify rather than diminish the rewarding effects of amphetamine, morphine and cocaine, *Psychopharmacology*, 98 (1989) 357–362.
196 Leyton, M. and Stewart, J., Preexposure to foot-shock sensitizes the locomotor response to subsequent systemic morphine and intra-nucleus accumbens amphetamine, *Pharmacol. Biochem. Behav.*, 37 (1990) 303–310.
197 Lin-Chu, G., Robinson, T.E. and Becker, J.B., Sensitization of rotational behavior produced by a single exposure to cocaine, *Pharmacol. Biochem. Behav.*, 22 (1985) 901–903.
198 Ljungberg, T., Apicella, P. and Schultz, W., Responses of monkey midbrain dopamine neurons during delayed alternation performance, *Brain Res.*, 567 (1991) 337–341.
199 Ljungberg, T., Apicella, P. and Schultz, W., Responses of monkey dopamine neurons during learning of behavioral reactions, *J. Neurophysiol.*, 67 (1992) 145–163.
200 MacLennan, A.J. and Maier, S.F., Coping and the stress-induced potentiation of stimulant stereotypy in the rat, *Science*, 219 (1983) 1091–1093.
201 Magos, L., Persistence of the effect of amphetamine on stereotyped activity on rats, *Eur. J. Pharmacol.*, 6 (1969) 200–201.
202 Maj, J. and Wedzony, K., Repeated treatment with imipramine

or amitriptyline increases the locomotor response of rats to (+)-amphetamine given into the nucleus accumbens, *J. Pharm. Pharmacol.*, 37 (1985) 362–364.

203 Maj, J., Wedzony, K. and Klimek, V., Desipramine given repeatedly enhances behavioural effects of dopamine and *d*-amphetamine injected into the nucleus accumbens, *Eur. J. Pharmacol.*, 140 (1987) 179–185.

204 Markou, A. and Koob, G.F., Postcocaine anhedonia: an animal model of cocaine withdrawal, *Neuropsychopharmacology*, 4 (1991) 17–26.

205 Martin, G.M., Bechara, A. and van der Kooy, D., The perception of emotion: parallel neural processing of the affective and discriminative properties of opiates, *Psychobiology*, 19 (1991) 147–152.

206 Martin, S.D., Yeragani, V.K., Lodhi, R. and Galloway, M.P., Clinical ratings and plasma HVA during cocaine abstinence, *Biol. Psychiatry*, 26 (1989) 356–362.

207 Martin-Iverson, M.T., Ortmann, R. and Fibiger, H.C., Place preference conditioning with methylphenidate and nomifensine, *Brain Res.*, 332 (1985) 59–67.

208 Masur, J. and Boerngen, R., The excitatory component of ethanol in mice: a chronic study, *Pharmacol. Biochem. Behav.*, 13 (1980) 777–780.

209 Masur, J., Oliveira de Souza, M.L. and Zwicker, A.P., The excitatory effect of ethanol: absence in rats, no tolerance and increased sensitivity in mice, *Pharmacol. Biochem. Behav.*, 24 (1986) 1225–1228.

210 Mazurski, E.J. and Beninger, R.J., Environment-specific conditioning and sensitization with (+)-amphetamine, *Pharmacol. Biochem. Behav.*, 27 (1987) 61–65.

211 McAuliffe, W.E., A second look at first effects: the subjective effects of opiates on nonaddicts, *J. Drug Issues*, 5 (1975) 369–399.

212 McAuliffe, W.E., A test of Wikler's theory of relapse: the frequency of relapse due to conditioned withdrawal sickness, *Int. J. Addict*, 17 (1982) 19–33.

213 McAuliffe, W.E. and Gordon, R.A., A test of Lindesmith's theory of addiction: the frequency of euphoria among long-term addicts, *Am. J. Sociol.*, 79 (1974) 795–840.

214 Meisel, R.L., Camp, D.M. and Robinson, T.E., A microdialysis study of ventral striatal dopamine during sexual behavior in female Syrian hamsters, *Behav. Brain Res.*, in press.

215 Meyer, R.E., Conditioning phenomena and the problem of relapse in opioid addicts and alcoholics, *NIDA Res. Monogr.*, 84 (1988) 161–179.

216 Miller, G.A., Galanter, E. and Pribram, K.H., *Plans and the Structure of Behavior*, Holt, Rinehart & Winston, New York, 1965.

217 Miller, J.D., Sanghera, M.K. and German, D.C., Mesencephalic dopaminergic unit activity in the behaviorally conditioned rat, *Life Sci.*, 29 (1981) 1255–1263.

218 Mitchell, J.B. and Stewart, J., Facilitation of sexual behaviors in the male rat associated with intra-VTA injections of opiates, *Pharmacol. Biochem. Behav.*, 35 (1990) 643–650.

219 Mithani, S., Martin-Iverson, M.T., Phillips, A.G. and Fibiger, H.C., The effects of haloperidol on amphetamine- and methylphenidate-induced conditioned place preferences and locomotor activity, *Psychopharmacology*, 90 (1986) 247–252.

220 Mittleman, G., Castañeda, E., Robinson, T.E. and Valenstein, E.S., The propensity for nonregulatory ingestive behavior is related to differences in dopamine systems: behavioral and biochemical evidence, *Behav. Neurosci.*, 100 (1986) 213–220.

221 Mittleman, G. and Valenstein, E.S., Individual differences in non-regulatory ingestive behavior and catecholamine systems, *Brain Res.*, 348 (1985) 112–117.

222 Morency, M.A. and Beninger, R.J., Dopaminergic substrates of cocaine-induced place conditioning, *Brain Res.*, 399 (1986) 33–41.

223 Morley, J.E., Levine, A.S. and Rowland, N.E., Stress induced eating, *Life Sci.*, 32 (1983) 2169–2182.

224 Mueller, K., Kunko, P.M., Whiteside, D. and Haskett, C., Time course of amphetamine-induced locomotor stereotypy in an open field, *Psychopharmacology*, 99 (1989) 501–507.

225 Nabeshima, T., Fukaya, H., Yamaguchi, K., Ishikawa, K., Furukawa, H. and Kameyama, T., Development of tolerance and supersensitivity to phencyclidine in rats after repeated administration of phencyclidine, *Eur. J. Pharmacol.*, 135 (1987) 23–33.

226 Nakayama, M., Koyama, T. and Yamashita, I., Long-lasting decrease in dopamine uptake sites following repeated administration of methamphetamine in the rat striatum, *Brain Res.*, 601 (1993) 209–212.

227 Nestler, E.J., Molecular mechanisms of drug addiction, *J. Neurosci.*, 12 (1992) 2439–2450.

228 Nisbett, R.E. and Wilson, T.D., Telling more than we can know: verbal reports on mental processes, *Psychol. Rev.*, 84 (1977) 231–259.

229 O'Brien, C.P., Childress, A.R., McLellan, A.T. and Ehrman, R., A learning model of addiction. In C.P. O'Brien and J.H. Jaffe (Eds.), *Addictive States*, Raven Press, New York, 1992, pp. 157–177.

230 Parker, L.A., Taste reactivity responses elicited by reinforcing drugs: a dose–response analysis, *Behav. Neurosci.*, 105 (1991) 955–964.

231 Patrick, S.L., Thompson, T.L., Walker, J.M. and Patrick, R.L., Concomitant sensitization of amphetamine-induced behavioral stimulation and in vivo dopamine release from the rat caudate nucleus, *Brain Res.*, 538 (1991) 343–346.

232 Paulson, P.E., Camp, D.M. and Robinson, T.E., The time course of transient behavioral depression and persistent behavioral sensitization in relation to regional brain monoamine concentrations during amphetamine withdrawal in rats, *Psychopharmacology*, 103 (1991) 480–492.

233 Paulson, P.E. and Robinson, T.E., Sensitization to systemic amphetamine produces an enhanced locomotor reoponse to a subsequent intra-accumbens amphetamine in rats, *Psychopharmacology*, 104 (1991) 140–141.

234 Pérez-Cruet, J., Conditioning of striatal dopamine metabolism with methadone, morphine or bulbocapnine as an unconditioned stimulus, *Pavlov J. Biol. Sci.*, 11 (1976) 237–250.

235 Pérez-de la Mora, M., López-Quiroz, D., Méndez-Franco, J. and Drucker-Colin, R., Chronic administration of amphetamine increases glutamic acid decarboxylase activity in the rat substantia nigra, *Neurosci. Lett.*, 109 (1990) 315–320.

236 Peris, J. and Zahniser, N.R., One injection of cocaine produces a long-lasting increase in [^{3}H]-dopamine release, *Pharmacol. Biochem. Behav.*, 27 (1987) 533–535.

237 Peris, J. and Zahniser, N.R., Persistent augmented dopamine release after acute cocaine requires dopamine receptor activation, *Pharmacol. Biochem. Behav.*, 32 (1989) 71–76.

238 Pettit, H.O., Pan, H.T., Parsons, L.H. and Justice Jr., J.B., Extracellular concentrations of cocaine and dopamine are enhanced during chronic cocaine administration, *J. Neurochem.*, 55 (1990) 798–804.

239 Phillips, A.G., Pfaus, J.G. and Blaha, C.D., Dopamine and motivated behavior: insights provided by in vivo analyses. In P. Willner and J. Scheel-Kruger (Eds.), *The Mesolimbic Dopamine System: from Motivation to Action*, John Wiley, New York, 1991, pp. 199–224.

240 Phillips, T.J. and Crabbe, J.C., Behavioral studies of genetic differences in alcohol action. In J.C. Crabbe and R.A. Harris (Eds.), *The Genetic Basis of Alcohol and Drug Actions*, Plenum Press, New York, 1991, pp. 25–104.

241 Piazza, P.V., Deminière, J.-M., Maccari, S., Le Moal, M., Mormède, P. and Simon, H., Individual vulnerability to drug self-administration: action of corticosterone on dopaminergic systems as a possible pathophysiological mechanism. In P. Willner and J. Scheel-Krüger (Eds.), *The Mesolimbic Dopamine System: From Motivation to Action*, John Wiley, New York, 1991, pp. 473–495.

242 Piazza, P.V., Deminière, J.M., Le Moal, M. and Simon, H., Factors that predict individual vulnerability to amphetamine self-administration, *Science*, 245 (1989) 1511–1513.

243 Piazza, P.V., Deminière, J.M., Le Moal, M. and Simon, H., Stress- and pharmacologically induced behavioral sensitization

increases vulnerability to acquisition of amphetamine self-administration, *Brain Res.*, 514 (1990) 22–26.

244 Piazza, P.V., Deroche, V., Rougé-Pont, F., Deminière, J.M., Maccari, S., Le Moal, M. and Simon, H., Individual differences in the sensitivity to corticosterone's reinforcing effects and in corticosterone-induced dopamine release may be a biological basis for sensation-seeking, *Soc. Neurosci. Abstr.*, 18 (1992) 1076.

245 Pinel, J.P.J. and Mana, M.J., Adaptive interactions of rats with dangerous inanimate objects: support for a cognitive theory of defensive behavior. In R.J. Blanchard, P.F. Brain, D.C. Blanchard and S. Parmigiani (Eds.), *Ethoexperimental Approaches to the Study of Behavior*, Kluwer Academic Publishers, Dordrecht, The Netherlands, 1989, pp. 137–150.

246 Pleim, E.T., Matochik, J.A., Barfield, R.J. and Auerbach, S.B., Correlation of dopamine release in the nucleus accumbens with masculine sexual behavior in rats, *Brain Res.*, 524 (1990) 160–163.

247 Poncelet, M., Dangoumau, L., Soubrie, P. and Simon, P., Effects of neuroleptic drugs, clonidine and lithium on the expression of conditioned behavioral excitation in rats, *Psychopharmacology*, 92 (1987) 393–397.

248 Post, R., Intermittent versus continuous stimulation: effect of time interval on the development of sensitization or tolerance, *Life Sci.*, 26 (1980) 1275–1282.

249 Post, R.M., Cocaine psychoses: a continuum model, *Am. J. Psychiatry*, 132 (1975) 225–231.

250 Post, R.M. and Contel, N.R., Human and animal studies of cocaine: implications for development of behavioral pathology. In I. Creese (Ed.), *Stimulants: Neurochemical, Behavioral and Clinical Perspectives*, Raven Press, New York, 1983, pp. 169–203.

251 Post, R.M., Lockfeld, A., Squillace, K.M. and Contel, N.R., Drug-environment interaction: context dependency of cocaine-induced behavioral sensitization, *Life Sci.*, 28 (1981) 755–760.

252 Post, R.M., Weiss, S.R., Fontana, D. and Pert, A., Conditioned sensitization to the psychomotor stimulant cocaine. In P.W. Kalivas and H.H. Samson (Eds.), *Annals of the New York Academy of Sciences: The Neurobiology of Drug and Alcohol Addiction*, The New York Academy of Sciences, New York, 1992, pp. 386–399.

253 Powell, J., Bradley, B. and Gray, J., Classical conditioning and cognitive determinants of subjective craving for opiates: an investigation of their relative contributions, *Br. J. Addict.*, 87 (1992) 1133–1144.

254 Randrup, A. and Munkvad, I., Stereotyped activities produced by amphetamine in several animal species and man, *Psychopharmacologia*, 11 (1967) 300–310.

255 Rapoport, J.L., The biology of obsessions and compulsions, *Sci. Am.*, 260 (1989) 82–89.

256 Rapoport, J.L., Obsessive compulsive disorder and basal ganglia dysfunction, *Psychol. Med.*, 20 (1990) 465–469.

257 Rebec, G.V., Changes in brain and behavior produced by amphetamine: a perspective based on microdialysis, voltammery and single-unit electrophysiology in freely moving animals. In R.R. Watson (Ed.), *Biochemistry and Physiology of Substance Abuse*, CRC Press, Boca Raton, FL, 1991, pp. 93–115.

258 Rebec, G.V. and Segal, D.S., Enhanced responsiveness to intraventricular infusion of amphetamine following its repeated systemic administration, *Psychopharmacology*, 62 (1979) 101–102.

259 Rescorla, R.A., Hierarchical associative relations in Pavlovian conditioning and instrumental training, *Curr. Direct Psychol. Sci.*, 1 (1992) 66–70.

260 Risinger, F.O., Dickinson, S.D. and Cunningham, C.L., Haloperidol reduces ethanol-induced motor activity stimulation but not conditioned place preference, *Psychopharmacology*, 107 (1992) 453–456.

261 Rivet, J.M., Stinus, L., Le Moal, M. and Mormede, P., Behavioral sensitization to amphetamine is dependent on corticosteroid receptor activation, *Brain Res.*, 498 (1989) 149–153.

262 Robbins, T.W., Cador, M., Taylor, J.R. and Everitt, B.J., Limbic-striatal interactions in reward-related processes, *Neurosci. Biobehav. Rev.*, 13 (1989) 155–162.

263 Robbins, T.W. and Everitt, B.J., Functions of dopamine in the dorsal and ventral striatum, *Sem. Neurosci.*, 4 (1992) 119–127.

264 Robbins, T.W., Watson, B.A., Gaskin, M. and Ennis, C., Contrasting interactions of pipradrol, *d*-amphetamine, cocaine, cocaine analogues, apomorphine and other drugs with conditioned reinforcement, *Psychopharmacology*, 80 (1983) 113–119.

265 Roberts-Lewis, J.M., Roseboom, P.H., Iwaniec, L.M. and Gnegy, M.E., Differential down-regulation of D1-stimulated adenylate cyclase activity in rat forebrain after in vivo amphetamine treatments, *J. Neurosci.*, 6 (1986) 2245–2251.

266 Robinson, J.H. and Pritchard, W.S., The meaning of addiction: reply to West, *Psychopharmacology*, 108 (1992) 411–416.

267 Robinson, T.E., Behavioral sensitization: characterization of enduring changes in rotational behavior produced by intermittent injections of amphetamine in male and female rats, *Psychopharmacology*, 84 (1984) 466–475.

268 Robinson, T.E., Stimulant drugs and stress: factors influencing individual differences in the susceptibility to sensitization. In P.W. Kalivas and C. Barnes (Eds.), *Sensitization of the Nervous System*, Telford Press, Caldwell, N.J., 1988, pp. 145–173.

269 Robinson, T.E., The neurobiology of amphetamine psychosis: evidence from studies with an animal model. In T. Nakazawa (Ed.), *Taniguchi Symposia on Brain Sciences, Vol. 14, Biological Basis of Schizophrenia*, Japan Scientific Societies Press, Tokyo, 1991, pp. 185–201.

270 Robinson, T.E., Persistent sensitizing effects of drugs on brain dopamine systems and behavior: implications for addiction and relapse. In S.G. Korenman and J.D. Barchas (Eds.), *The Biological Basis of Substance Abuse*, Oxford University Press, New York, in press.

271 Robinson, T.E. and Becker, J.B., Behavioral sensitization is accompanied by an enhancement in amphetamine-stimulated dopamine release from striatal tissue in vitro, *Eur. J. Pharmacol.*, 85 (1982) 253–254.

272 Robinson, T.E. and Becker, J.B., Enduring changes in brain and behavior produced by chronic amphetamine administration: a review and evaluation of animal models of amphetamine psychosis, *Brain Res. Rev.*, 396 (1986) 157–198.

273 Robinson, T.E., Becker, J.B. and Presty, S.K., Long-term facilitation of amphetamine-induced rotational behavior and striatal dopamine release produced by a single exposure to amphetamine: sex differences, *Brain Res.*, 253 (1982) 231–241.

274 Robinson, T.E., Jurson, P.A., Bennett, J.A. and Bentgen, K.M., Persistent sensitization of dopamine neurotransmission in ventral striatum (nucleus accumbens) produced by past experience with (+)-amphetamine: a microdialysis study in freely moving rats, *Br. Res.*, 462 (1988) 211–222.

275 Romo, R. and Schultz, W., Dopamine neurons of the monkey midbrain: contingencies of responses to active touch during self-initiated arm movements, *J. Neurophysiol.*, 63 (1990) 592–606.

276 Roseboom, P.H. and Gnegy, M.E., Acute in vivo amphetamine produces a homolgous desensitization of dopamine receptor-coupled adenylate cyclase activities and decreases agonist binding to the D1 site, *Mol. Pharmacol.*, 34 (1989) 148–156.

277 Rossetti, Z.L., D'Aquila, P.S., Hmaidan, Y., Gessa, G.L. and Serra, G., Repeated treatment with imipramine potentiates cocaine-induced dopamine release and motor stimulation, *Eur. J. Pharmacol.*, 201 (1991) 243–245.

278 Rozin, P. and Fallon, A.E., A perspective on disgust, *Psychol. Rev.*, 94 (1987) 23–41.

279 Sato, M., Acute exacerbation of methamphetamine psychosis and lasting dopaminergic supersensitivity – a clinical survey, *Psychopharmacol. Bull.*, 22 (1986) 751–756.

280 Sato, M., Chen, C.C., Akiyama, K. and Otsuki, S., Acute exacerbation of paranoid psychotic state after long-term abstinence in patients with previous methamphetamine psychosis, *Biol. Psychiatry*, 18 (1983) 429–440.

281 Schenk, S., Lacelle, G., Gorman, K. and Amit, Z., Cocaine self-administration in rats influenced by environmental conditions: implications for the etiology of drug abuse, *Neurosci. Lett.*, 81 (1987) 227–231.

282 Schenk, S., Valadez, A., McNamara, C. and Horger, B.A., Blockade of sensitizing effects of amphetamine preexposure on

cocaine self-administration by the NMDA antagonist MK-801, *Soc. Neurosci. Abstr.*, 18 (1992) 1237.

283 Schiff, S.R., Conditioned dopaminergic activity, *Biol. Psychiatry*, 17 (1982) 135–154.

284 Schiorring, E., Amphetamine induced selective stimulation of certain behaviour items with concurrent inhibition of others in an open-field test with rats, *Behaviour*, 39 (1971) 1–17.

285 Schiorring, E., An open field study of stereotyped locomotor activity in amphetamine-treated rats, *Psychopharmacology*, 66 (1979) 281–287.

286 Schiorring, E., Psychopathology induced by "speed drugs", *Pharmacol. Biochem. Behav.*, 1 (1981) 109–122.

287 Schultz, W., Responses of midbrain dopamine neurons to behavioral trigger stimuli in the monkey, *J. Neurophysiol.*, 56 (1986) 1439–1461.

288 Schultz, W., Activity of dopamine neurons in the behaving primate, *Sem. Neurosci.*, 4 (1992) 129–138.

289 Schultz, W. and Romo, R., Dopamine neurons of the monkey midbrain: contingencies of responses to stimuli eliciting immediate behavioral reactions, *J. Neurophysiol.*, 63 (1990) 607–624.

290 Schuster, C., Drug-seeking behaviour: implications for theories of drug dependence. In G. Edwards and M. Lader (Eds.), *The Nature of Drug Dependence*, Oxford, New York, 1990, pp. 171–193.

291 Segal, D.S., Behavioral and neurochemical correlates of repeated *d*-amphetamine administration, *Adv. Biochem. Psychopharmacol.*, 13 (1975) 247–262.

292 Segal, D.S., Geyer, M.A. and Schuckit, M.A., Stimulant-induced psychosis: an evaluation of animal models, *Essays Neurochem. Neuropharmacol.*, 5 (1981) 95–129.

293 Segal, D.S., Kelly, P.H., Koob, G. and Roberts, D.C.S., Nonstriatal dopamine mechanisms in the response to repeated *d*-amphetamine administration. In E. Usdin, I. Kopin and J. Barchas (Eds.), *Catecholamines: Basic and Clinical Frontiers, Vol. 2*, Pergamon Press, New York, 1979, pp. 1672–1674.

294 Segal, D.S. and Kuczenski, R., Individual differences in responsiveness to single and repeated amphetamine administration: behavioral characteristics and neurochemical correlates, *J. Pharmacol. Exp. Ther.*, 242 (1987) 917–926.

295 Segal, D.S. and Kuczenski, R., In vivo microdialysis reveals a diminished amphetamine-induced DA response corresponding to behavioral sensitization produced by repeated amphetamine pretreatment, *Brain Res.*, 571 (1992) 330–337.

296 Segal, D.S. and Kuczenski, R., Repeated cocaine administration induces behavioral sensitization and corresponding decreased extracellular dopamine responses in caudate and accumbens, *Brain Res.*, 577 (1992) 351–355.

297 Segal, D.S. and Schuckit, M.A., Animal models of stimulant-induced psychosis. In I. Creese (Ed.), *Stimulants: Neurochemical, Behavioral and Clinical Perspectives*, Raven Press, New York, 1983, pp. 131–167.

298 Sherer, M.A., Intravenous cocaine: psychiatric effects, biological mechanisms, *Biol. Psychiatry*, 24 (1988) 865–885.

299 Shippenberg, T.S., Emmett-Oglesby, M.W., Ayesta, F.J. and Herz, A., Tolerance and selective cross-tolerance to the motivational effects of opioids, *Psychopharmacology*, 96 (1988) 110–115.

300 Short, P.H. and Shuster, L., Changes in brain norepinephrine associated with sensitization to *d*-amphetamine, *Psychopharmacology*, 48 (1976) 59–67.

301 Shuster, L., Hudson, J., Anton, M. and Righi, D., Sensitization of mice to methylphenidate, *Psychopharmacology*, 77 (1982) 31–36.

302 Shuster, L., Webster, G.W. and Yu, G., Increased running response to morphine in morphine-pretreated mice, *J. Pharmacol. Exp. Ther.*, 192 (1975) 64–67.

303 Shuster, L., Webster, G.W. and Yu, G., Perinatal narcotic addiction in mice: sensitization to morphine stimulation, *Addict. Dis.*, 2 (1975) 277–292.

304 Shuster, L., Yu, G. and Bates, A., Sensitization to cocaine stimulation in mice, *Psychopharmacology*, 52 (1977) 185–190.

305 Siegel, S., Learning and psychopharmacology. In M.E. Jarvik (Ed.), *Psychopharmacology in the Practice of Medicine*, Appleton-Century-Crofts, New York, 1977.

306 Siegel, S., Drug anticipation and drug tolerance. In M. Lader (Ed.), *The Psychopharmacology of Addiction*, Oxford University Press, New York, 1988, pp. 73–97.

307 Skinner, B.F., Are theories of learning necessary?, *Psychol. Rev.*, 57 (1950) 193–216.

308 Smith, G.P. and Schneider, L.H., Relationships between mesolimbic dopamine function and eating behavior, *Ann. NY Acad. Sci.*, 537 (1988) 254–261.

309 Smith, J.E., Co, C., Freeman, M.E. and Lane, J.D., Brain neurotransmitter turnover correlated with morphine seeking behavior of rats, *Pharmacol. Biochem. Behav.*, 16 (1982) 509–519.

310 Smith, J.E. and Dworkin, S.I., Behavioral contingencies determine changes in drug-induced transmitter turnover, *Drug Dev. Res.*, 20 (1990) 337–348.

311 Söderpalm, B., Svensson, L., Hulthe, P., Johannessen, K. and Engel, J.A., Evidence for a role for dopamine in the diazepam locomotor stimulating effect, *Psychopharmacology*, 104 (1991) 97–102.

312 Solomon, R.L., Acquired motivation and affective opponent-processes. In J. Madden (Ed.), *Neurobiology of Learning, Emotion and Affect*, Raven Press, New York, 1991, pp. 307–348.

313 Sorensen, S.M., Hattox, S., Johnson, S.W., Bickford, P., Murphy, R. and Freedman, R., Norepinephrine-dependent and independent mechanisms of persistent effects of amphetamine in rat cerebellum, *Life Sci.*, 36 (1985) 2383–2389.

314 Sorensen, S.M., Johnson, S.W. and Freedman, R., Persistent effects of amphetamine on cerebellar Purkinje neurons following chronic administration, *Brain Res.*, 247 (1982) 365–371.

315 Sorg, B.A. and Kalivas, P.W., Effects of cocaine and footshock stress on extracellular dopamine levels in the ventral striatum, *Brain Res.*, 559 (1991) 29–36.

316 Spanos, L.J. and Yamamoto, B.K., Acute and subchronic effects of methylenedioxy-methamphetamine [(+/-)MDMA] on locomotion and serotonin syndrome behavior in the rat, *Pharmacol. Biochem. Behav.*, 32 (1989) 835–840 [published erratum appears in Pharmacol. Biochem. Behav. 1989, 34:679].

317 Spyraki, C., Fibiger, H.C. and Phillips, A.G., Cocaine-induced place preference conditioning: lack of effects of neuroleptics and 6-hydroxydopamine lesions, *Brain Res.*, 253 (1982) 195–203.

318 Squire, L.R. and Zola-Morgan, S., The medial temporal lobe memory system, *Science*, 253 (1991) 1380–1386.

319 Steiner, J.E., Human facial expressions in response to taste and smell stimulation, *Adv. Child Dev. Behav.*, 13 (1979) 257–295.

320 Steketee, J.D., Sorg, B.A. and Kalivas, P.W., The role of the nucleus accumbens in sensitization to drugs of abuse, *Prog. Neuropsychopharmacol. Biol. Psychiatry*, 16 (1992) 237–246.

321 Stevens, J.R., An anatomy of schizophrenia?, *Arch. Gen. Psychiatry*, 29 (1973) 177–189.

322 Stewart, J., Reinstatement of heroin and cocaine self-administration behavior in the rat by intracerebral application of morphine in the ventral tegmental area, *Pharmacol. Biochem. Behav.*, 20 (1984) 917–923.

323 Stewart, J., Conditioned stimulus control of the expression of sensitization of the behavioral activating effects of opiate and stimulant drugs. In I. Gormezano and E.A. Wasserman (Eds.), *Learning and Memory: The Behavioral and Biological Substrates*, Erlbaum, Hillsdale, NJ, 1992, pp. 129–151.

324 Stewart, J., Tolerance and sensitization to the behavioral effects of drugs. In P. Nencini (Ed.), *Controllo Farmacologico del Comportamento*, Unione Tipografico, Torino, Italy, 1992, pp. 161–183.

325 Stewart, J. and De Wit, H., Reinstatement of drug-taking behavior as a method of assessing incentive motivational properties of drugs. In M.A. Bozarth (Ed.), *Methods of Assessing the Reinforcing Properties of Abused Drugs*, Springer-Verlag, New York, 1987, pp. 211–227.

326 Stewart, J., de Wit, H. and Eikelboom, R., Role of unconditioned and conditioned drug effects in the self-administration of opiates and stimulants, *Psychol. Rev.*, 91 (1984) 251–268.

327 Stewart, J. and Vezina, P., A comparison of the effects of intra-accumbens injections of amphetamine and morphine on reinstatement of heroin intravenous self-administration behavior, *Brain Res.*, 457 (1988) 287–294.

328 Stewart, J. and Vezina, P., Extinction procedures abolish conditioned stimulus control but spare sensitized responding to amphetamine, *Behav. Pharmacol.*, 2 (1991) 65–71.

329 Stewart, J. and Wise, R.A., Reinstatement of heroin self-administration habits: morphine prompts and naltrexone discourages renewed responding after extinction, *Psychopharmacology*, 108 (1992) 79–84.

330 Strecker, R.E., Steinfels, G.F. and Jacobs, B.L., Dopaminergic unit activity in freely moving cats: lack of relationship to feeding, satiety and glucose injections, *Brain Res.*, 260 (1983) 317–321.

331 Swerdlow, N.R., Braff, D.L., Masten, V.L. and Geyer, M.A., Schizophrenic-like sensorimotor gating abnormalities in rats following dopamine infusion into the nucleus accumbens, *Psychopharmacology*, 101 (1990) 414–420.

332 Swerdlow, N.R. and Koob, G.F., Dopamine, schizophrenia, mania and depression: toward a unified hypothesis of cortico-striato-pallido-thalamic function, *Behav. Brain Sci.*, 10 (1987) 197–245.

333 Taylor, J.R. and Robbins, T.W., Enhanced behavioural control by conditioned reinforcers following microinjections of *d*-amphetamine into the nucleus accumbens, *Psychopharmacology*, 84 (1984) 405–412.

334 Taylor, J.R. and Robbins, T.W., 6-Hydroxydopamine lesions of the nucleus accumbens, but not of the caudate nucleus, attenuate enhanced responding with reward-related stimuli produced by intra-accumbens *d*-amphetamine, *Psychopharmacology*, 90 (1986) 390–397.

335 Ternes, J.W., Ehrman, R.N. and O'Brien, C.P., Nondependent monkeys self-administer hydromorphone, *Behav. Neurosci.*, 99 (1985) 583–588.

336 Thierry, A.M., Tassin, J.P., Blanc, G. and Glowinski, J., Selective activation of the mesocortical DA system by stress, *Nature*, 263 (1976) 242–243.

337 Tiffany, S.T., A cognitive model of drug urges and drug-use behavior: role of automatic and nonautomatic processes, *Psychol. Rev.*, 97 (1990) 147–168.

338 Tilson, H.A. and Rech, R.A., Conditioned drug effects and absence of tolerance to *d*-amphetamine induced motor activity, *Pharmacol. Biochem. Behav.*, 1 (1973) 149–153.

339 Toates, F., *Motivational Systems*, Cambridge University Press, Cambridge, 1986.

340 Treit, D. and Berridge, K.C., A comparison of benzodiazepine, serotonin and dopamine agents in the taste-reactivity paradigm, *Pharmacol. Biochem. Behav.*, 37 (1990) 451–456.

341 Trulson, M.E. and Preussler, D.W., Dopamine-containing ventral tegmental area neurons in freely moving cats: activity during the sleep-waking cycle and effects of stress, *Exp. Neurol.*, 83 (1984) 367–377.

342 Ujike, H., Tsuchida, H., Kanzaki, A., Akiyama, K. and Otsuki, S., Competitive and non-competitive *N*-methyl-D-aspartate antagonists fail to prevent the induction of methamphetamine-induced sensitization, *Life Sci.*, 50 (1992) 1673–1681.

343 Vaccarino, F.J., Schiff, B.B. and Glickman, S.E., Biological view of reinforcement. In S.B. Klein and R.R. Mowrer (Eds.), *Contempory Learning Theories*, Erlbaum, Hillsdale, NJ, 1989, pp. 111–142.

344 Vezina, P. and Stewart, J., Conditioning and place-specific sensitization of increases in activity induced by morphine in the VTA, *Pharmacol. Biochem. Behav.*, 20 (1984) 925–934.

345 Vezina, P. and Stewart, J., The effect of dopamine receptor blockade on the development of sensitization to the locomotor activating effects of amphetamine and morphine, *Brain Res.*, 499 (1989) 108–120.

346 Vezina, P. and Stewart, J., Amphetamine administered to the ventral tegmental area but not to the nucleus accumbens sensitizes rats to systemic morphine: lack of conditioned effects, *Brain Res.*, 516 (1990) 99–106.

347 Vezina, P. and Zurakowski, B., Prior exposure to intra-VTA amphetamine sensitizes the nucleus accumbens dopaminergic response to systemic amphetamine as measured by invivo microdialysis, *Soc. Neurosci. Abstr.*, 18 (1992) 720.

348 Walter, S. and Kuschinsky, K., Conditioning of morphine-induced locomotor activity and stereotyped behaviour in rats, *J. Neural Transm. Gen. Sect.*, 78 (1989) 231–247.

349 Watson, S.J., Trujillo, K.A., Herman, J.P. and Akil, H., Neuroanatomical and neurochemical substrates of drug-seeking behavior: overview and future directions. In A. Goldstein (Ed.), *Molecular and Cellular Aspects of the Drug Addictions*, Springer-Verlag, New York, 1989, pp. 29–91.

350 Weiskrantz, L., Warrington, E.K., Sanders, M.D. and Marshall, J., Visual capacity in the hemianopic field following a restricted occipital ablation, *Brain*, 97 (1974) 709–728.

351 Weiss, F., Markou, A., Lorang, M.T. and Koob, G.F., Basal extracellular dopamine levels in the nucleus accumbens are decreased during cocaine withdrawal after unlimited-access self-administration, *Brain Res.*, 593 (1992) 314–318.

352 Weiss, S.R., Post, R.M., Pert, A., Woodward, R. and Murman, D., Context-dependent cocaine sensitization: differential effect of haloperidol on development versus expression, *Pharmacol. Biochem. Behav.*, 34 (1989) 655–661.

353 Whishaw, I.Q. and Kornelsen, R.A., Two types of action revealed by ibotenic acid nucleus accumbens lesions: dissociation of food carrying and hoarding and the role of primary incentive motivation, *Behav. Brain Res.*, in press.

354 White, F.J. and Wolf, M.E., Psychomotor stimulants. In J. Pratt (Ed.), *The Biological Bases of Drug Tolerance and Dependence*, Academic Press, New York, 1991, pp. 153–197.

355 White, N., Sklar, L. and Amit, Z., The reinforcing action of morphine and its paradoxical side effect, *Psychopharmacology*, 52 (1977) 63–66.

356 White, N.M. and Milner, P.M., The psychobiology of reinforcers, *Annu. Rev. Psychol.*, 43 (1992) 443–471.

357 Wikler, A., Recent progress in research on the neurophysiological basis of morphine addiction, *Am. J. Psychiatry*, 105 (1948) 329–338.

358 Wilcox, R.A., Robinson, T.E. and Becker, J.B., Enduring enhancement in amphetamine-stimulated striatal dopamine release in vitro produced by prior exposure to amphetamine or stress in vivo, *Eur. J. Pharmacol.*, 124 (1986) 375–376.

359 Wise, R.A., Catecholamine theories of reward: a critical review, *Brain Res.*, 152 (1978) 215–247.

360 Wise, R.A., Neuroleptics and operant behavior: the anhedonia hypothesis, *Behav. Brain Sci.*, 5 (1982) 39–87.

361 Wise, R.A., The anhedonia hypothesis: Mark III, *Behav. Brain Sci.*, 8 (1985) 178–186.

362 Wise, R.A., The role of reward pathways in the development of drug dependence, *Pharmacol. Ther.*, 35 (1987) 227–263.

363 Wise, R.A., The neurobiology of craving: implications for the understanding and treatment of addiction, *J. Abnorm. Psychol.*, 97 (1988) 118–132.

364 Wise, R.A. and Bozarth, M.A., Brain mechanisms of drug reward and euphoria, *Psychiatry Med.*, 3 (1985) 445–460.

365 Wise, R.A. and Bozarth, M.A., A psychomotor stimulant theory of addiction, *Psychol. Rev.*, 94 (1987) 469–492.

366 Wise, R.A. and Hoffman, D.C., Localization of drug reward mechanisms by intracranial injections, *Synapse*, 10 (1992) 247–263.

367 Wise, R.A., Murray, A. and Bozarth, M.A., Bromocriptine self-administration and bromocriptine-reinstatement of cocaine-trained and heroin-trained lever pressing in rats, *Psychopharmacology*, 100 (1990) 355–360.

368 Wise, R.A. and Rompre, P.-P., Brain dopamine and reward, *Annu. Rev. Psychol.*, 40 (1989) 191–225.

369 Wolf, M.E. and Khansa, M.R., Repeated administration of MK-801 produces sensitization to its own locomotor stimulant effects but blocks sensitization to amphetamine, *Brain Res.*, 562 (1991) 164–168.

370 Wolf, M.E., White, F.J., Nassar, R., Brooderson, R.J. and

Khansa, M.R., Differential development of autoreceptor subsensitivity and enhanced dopamine release during amphetamine sensitization, *J. Pharmacol. Exp. Ther.*, 264 (1993) 249–1255.

371 Woods, J.H., Katz, J.L. and Winger, G., Use and abuse of benzodiazepines, *J. Am. Med. Assoc.*, 260 (1988) 3476–3480.

372 Woods, J.H. and Schuster, C.R., Reinforcement properties of morphine, cocaine and SPA as a function of unit dose, *Int. J. Addict.*, 3 (1968) 231–237.

373 Woolverton, W.L., Cervo, L. and Johanson, C.E., Effects of repeated methamphetamine administration on methamphetamine self-administration in rhesus monkeys, *Pharmacol. Biochem. Behav.*, 21 (1984) 737–741.

374 Xenakis, S. and Sclafani, A., The dopaminergic mediation of a sweet reward in normal and VMH hyperphagic rats, *Pharmacol. Biochem. Behav.*, 16 (1982) 293–302.

375 Yamada, S., Kojima, H., Yokoo, H., Tsutsumi, T., Takamuki, K., Anraku, S., Nishi, S. and Inanaga, K., Enhancement of dopamine release from striatal slices of rats that were subchronically treated with methamphetamine, *Biol. Psychiatry*, 24 (1988) 399–408.

376 Young, A.M., Joseph, M.H. and Gray, J.A., Increased dopamine release in vivo in nucleus accumbens and caudate nucleus of the rat during drinking: a microdialysis study, *Neuroscience*, 48 (1992) 871–876.

377 Young, A.M.J., Gray, J.A. and Joseph, M.H., Dopamine function in the nucleus accumbens in conditioning studied by microdialysis, *Abstracts of the 7th International Catecholamine Symposium in Amsterdam*, (1992) 360.

Psychological Review
1990, Vol. 97, No. 2, 147-168

0033-295X/90/$00.75

A Cognitive Model of Drug Urges and Drug-Use Behavior: Role of Automatic and Nonautomatic Processes

Stephen T. Tiffany
Purdue University

Contemporary urge models assume that urges are necessary but not sufficient for the production of drug use in ongoing addicts, are responsible for the initiation of relapse in abstinent addicts, and can be indexed across 3 classes of behavior: verbal report, overt behavior, and somatovisceral response. A review of available data does not provide strong support for these assumptions. An alternative cognitive model of drug use and drug urges is proposed that hypothesizes that drug use in the addict is controlled by automatized action schemata. Urges are conceptualized as responses supported by nonautomatic cognitive processes activated in parallel with drug-use action schemata either in support of the schema or in support of attempts to block the execution of the schema. The implications of this model for the assessment of urge responding and drug-use behavior are presented.

The construct of urge has occupied an important position in many conceptualizations of addictive behavior from the outset of scientific studies of addictions. The use of urges and cravings as key explanatory concepts in models of addiction reached a peak in the 1950s and early 1960s, supported largely by Jellinek's (1955, 1960) writings on the etiology of alcoholism. Jellinek (1955, 1960) argued that craving was the essential defining characteristic of alcohol addiction or alcoholism and could be used to explain the initiation and maintenance of compulsive alcohol consumption as well as relapse to alcohol use after a period of abstinence.

Urges and cravings as explanatory constructs fell out of favor in the late 1960s and early 1970s as a result of two factors. First, several studies indicated that in laboratory settings, Jellinek's (1955, 1960) model of alcohol addiction did not adequately characterize the drinking behavior of alcoholics (e.g., Marlatt, Demming, & Reid, 1973; Mello and Mendelson, 1972; Nathan, Titler, Lowenstein, Solomon, & Rossi, 1970). Specifically damaging to Jellinek's (1955, 1960) concept of craving was the finding that abstinent alcoholics did not necessarily engage in loss-of-control drinking when they consumed small doses of alcohol (e.g., Engle & Williams, 1972; Marlatt et al., 1973; Paredes, Hood, Seymour, & Gollob, 1973). Because Jellinek (1955, 1960) assumed that craving mediates between initial consumption and subsequent loss of control, the absence of such a pattern of drinking cast doubt upon this conceptualization of craving (e.g., Mello, 1972, 1978). A second factor contributing to the demise of urges and cravings in models of addiction was the rise of behavioral approaches to the study of addiction that eschewed the use of mentalistic concepts, such as craving, as explanatory constructs (e.g., Mello, 1972, 1978; Mello & Mendelson, 1978).

Over the past 10 years, there has been a resurgence of interest in the role of urges and cravings in addictive behavior. Several factors have promoted this revival. One has been the decline in the influence of radical behavioral theories in the study of addictive behavior with a corresponding ascendancy of social cognitive models (e.g., Marlatt, 1978; Wilson, 1978). These newer approaches are more accepting of the possibility that hypothetical entities such as urges may be of some use in conceptualizations of addictive processes (e.g., Wilson, 1987).

The past decade has also seen a considerable amount of basic research investigating the role of conditioning processes in drug tolerance and drug dependence (e.g., Baker & Tiffany, 1985; Goudie & Demellweek, 1986; Siegel, 1983; Tiffany & Baker, 1986). This research has provided an impetus for the suggestion that conditioned drug effects form the substrate of drug urges and cravings (e.g., Ludwig & Wikler, 1974; Poulos, Hinson, & Siegel, 1981). Urges and cravings have also been found to be useful diagnostically. For example, urges and cravings are listed in *DSM-III-R* (American Psychiatric Association, 1987) as part of the symptom characteristics of certain drug dependencies. The diagnostic usefulness of urges and cravings reflects a simple fact. In spite of theoretical disputes regarding the adequacy of various conceptualizations of urges and cravings, the behavioral manifestations of these constructs continue to be important features of addictive disorders (Baker, Morse, & Sherman, 1987). Some researchers, in their rejection of particular conceptualizations of urges and cravings, have also rejected or ignored the data base on which these conceptualizations rest (e.g., Mello, 1978). Given the ubiquity of urge responding among addicts (particularly during periods of abstinence), a truly comprehensive theory of addictive disorders can ill afford to overlook this salient feature of addictive behavior.

I thank the members of my research laboratory—Antonio Cepeda, Susan Burton, David Drobes, Denise Hakenewerth, and Peg Maude-Griffin—who helped me shape and refine the ideas presented in this article. I also thank Tim Baker, Gordon Logan, Kristine Tiffany, Saul Shiffman, Roelof Eikelboom, and two anonymous reviewers for their helpful comments on drafts of this article. I wish to acknowledge the assistance of Cris Pecknold and Peggy Treece in the preparation of the manuscript.

Correspondence concerning this article should be addressed to Stephen T. Tiffany, Department of Psychological Sciences, Purdue University, West Lafayette, Indiana 47907.

In the following sections of this article, I provide an overview of current conceptualizations of drug urges and cravings and then review some data relevant to general assumptions shared by most contemporary models of drug urges. These sections are followed by a presentation of a new model of drug urges and drug-use behavior derived from recent cognitive theories of automatic and nonautomatic cognitive processes. In the final section, I outline some of the implications of this model for research on drug-use behavior and on drug urges and cravings.

Models of Drug Urges

Across almost all theories, drug urges are assumed to be subjective, emotional–motivational states. They are viewed as subjective in the sense that they refer to the phenomenological experience of the individual, emotional in that the subjective experience of urge has some hedonic quality, and motivational in the sense that the subjective urge state presumably activates drug-seeking behavior (e.g., Baker et al., 1987; Jellinek, 1955; Kozlowski & Wilkinson, 1987b; Ludwig & Wikler, 1974; Marlatt, 1985; West & Schneider, 1987; Wikler, 1972). There is a general presumption that urges should be associated with concordant changes in overt behavior (e.g., the pursuit and consumption of drugs), verbal responses, and somatovisceral responses (e.g., Baker et al., 1987; Kozlowski & Wilkinson, 1987a, 1987b; Ludwig, Wikler, & Stark, 1974; Niaura et al., 1988; Rickard-Figueroa & Zeichner, 1985); that is, these response classes represent the behavioral manifestations of the subjective urge state.

Models of drug urges can be classified loosely as attributing the genesis of urges and cravings to one of two sources: drug withdrawal or the positive reinforcing effects of drugs. These two classes of theories reflect the two sources of reinforcement, negative and positive, that have often been proposed as being fundamental to the initiation and maintenance of addictive behavior (Wise, 1988).

Withdrawal-Based Models of Urges

Most drugs that support compulsive self-administration will produce a physiological dependence syndrome when the drug is withdrawn. Although dependence syndromes differ across classes of drugs (e.g., Hughes & Hatsukami, 1986; Jones, 1980, 1984; Kalant, 1977; Kalant, LeBlanc, & Gibbons, 1971; Shiffman, 1979), the presence of withdrawal signs is seen as a pathognomonic sign of addiction in many definitions of addictive behavior (e.g., American Psychiatric Association, 1980, 1987; Edwards, Arif, & Hodgson, 1981). Given the important role assigned to withdrawal signs and symptoms across various conceptualizations of addictive behavior, it is not surprising that many theorists have proposed that urges and cravings are intimately related to drug withdrawal.

Some models propose that urges and cravings are merely a component of drug withdrawal. Such approaches are purely descriptive in that they recognize that people withdrawing from drugs often report urges and cravings. This can be seen in *DSM-III-R*'s (American Psychiatric Association, 1987) description of the nicotine and opioid withdrawal syndrome, where craving for nicotine or an opioid is included in the list of symptoms of withdrawal. (In fact, they occupy the first position in the symptom lists for these two disorders—presumably an indication of the importance assigned by the authors of *DSM-III-R* to this aspect of withdrawal.) Another example of the idea that urges and cravings are a component of withdrawal can be observed in the research of Shiffman and Jarvik (1976) on the nicotine withdrawal syndrome. They developed a 27-item questionnaire that was broken down into five subscales on the basis of a factor analysis conducted on the responses of 40 smokers who were attempting to quit smoking. The authors identified a craving subscale as accounting for the largest share of the variance, suggesting that self-reports of craving and urges are the primary manifestation of nicotine withdrawal in abstinent smokers.

Other approaches assume that rather than being components of withdrawal syndromes, urges and cravings are distinct states that are caused by the physiological symptoms of drug withdrawal. For instance, Jellinek (1955) proposed that cravings for alcohol represented the anticipation of relief from withdrawal, and it was this type of craving that led to compulsive or loss-of-control drinking during a drinking bout. The belief that craving represents the anticipation of, and desire for, the relief of withdrawal has been a popular conceptualization of the role of craving in drug addiction (e.g., Eddy, 1973; Isbell, 1955; Lindesmith, 1968; Marlatt, 1978).

One major feature of addictive disorders is clearly inconsistent with the hypothesis that craving is directly elicited by the physical symptoms of withdrawal: People often report urges and cravings long after their acute withdrawal has abated (e.g., Flaherty, McGuire, & Gatski, 1955; Fletcher & Doll, 1969; Mathew, Claghorn, & Largen, 1979). For example, Fletcher and Doll (1969) found that upward of 20% of ex-smokers report experiencing desires to smoke 10–14 years after quitting. One way to explain the presence of urges that persist beyond acute withdrawal is to posit that some sort of learning process is responsible for the production of conditioned withdrawal effects. There are two kinds of theories that embody this approach. The first was Wikler's (1948) classical conditioning model of drug withdrawal. This theory stated that situations reliably paired with drug withdrawal become conditioned stimuli that elicit conditioned withdrawal responses. Abstinent addicts exposed to situations that had been associated with drug withdrawal should experience some conditioned withdrawal responses that, in turn, engender craving and urges. Across various expositions of his model, Wikler presented several versions of how conditioned withdrawal might produce urges and cravings. In some of his writings, Wikler (e.g., 1948, 1972; Wikler & Pescor, 1967) described craving simply as one component of the unconditioned withdrawal syndrome that, like other features of withdrawal, could become conditioned to environmental stimuli. More recently, Ludwig and Wikler (1974) described craving as a "psychological or cognitive correlate of a subclinical, conditioned withdrawal syndrome" (p. 114). In that same article, they described craving as a desire for relief of withdrawal that was a necessary, but not a sufficient, condition for relapse in abstinent addicts.

A related conditioning model with relevance to urges to use drug is Siegel's (1975) theory of drug tolerance. This theory states that stimuli or situations reliably paired with administration of a drug become conditioned stimuli that elicit behavioral responses opposite in direction to the direct effects of drug. For example, stimuli paired repeatedly with injections of morphine, which unconditionally produces analgesia, should elicit a compensatory response of hyperalgesia (i.e., hyperresponsivity to a painful stimulus) if they are presented in the absence of actual drug administrations (e.g., Krank, 1987; Krank, Hinson, & Siegel, 1981; Siegel, 1975; cf. Maude-Griffin & Tiffany, 1989a, 1989b; Tiffany, Petrie, Baker, & Dahl, 1983). These compensatory responses summate with direct drug effects and produce a net reduction in the overall drug response, that is, tolerance. These hypothesized compensatory responses are also thought to play a critical role in drug relapse (e.g., Poulos et al., 1981; Siegel, 1983). According to this theory, an abstinent addict exposed to cues previously associated with drug administration will have conditioned compensatory responses that are experienced as withdrawal and craving. These reactions would, in turn, increase the probability of relapse. The process by which conditioned compensatory responses become translated into urges or cravings has not been clearly specified by Siegel and his colleagues. In virtually all of their (Hinson & Siegel, 1982; MacRae, Scoles, & Siegel, 1987; Poulos et al., 1981; Siegel, 1979, 1983) discussions of this topic, urges and cravings are described as major components of the drug withdrawal syndrome, a view identical to Wikler's (1948, 1972) initial conceptualization of drug urges.

Although the compensatory response model (Poulos et al., 1981; Siegel, 1983) and the conditioned withdrawal model (Wikler, 1948) are quite similar in their approach to drug urges and relapse, a comparison of the two theories reveals one clear difference. The conditioned withdrawal model predicts that urges and cravings should be most strongly associated with situations paired with drug withdrawal, whereas the compensatory response model predicts that situations paired with drug administration should be the most consistent elicitors of urges. This distinction, although theoretically viable, may not be useful in distinguishing these models in practice because these two sets of cues often overlap in the natural history of addictions.

More recent models of withdrawal-based urges have integrated some social cognitive concepts with conditioning theories of drug withdrawal or drug tolerance. These models are essentially an extension of Schachter and Singer's (1962) cognition-arousal theory of emotion to the problem of drug urges. These theories state that urges represent the operation of an attributional process whereby physiological responses produced by conditioned withdrawal or conditioned compensatory responses are interpreted by the addict as desires to use drug (Melchior & Tabakoff, 1984; West & Schneider, 1987). Thus, the combination of conditioned physiological arousal with a particular attribution regarding the source of that arousal is necessary for the production of the urge state. One implication of this model is that physiological sensations other than withdrawal might be misattributed to a desire to use drug, or withdrawal sensations, under some circumstances, may not be identified by the addict as urges and cravings (West & Schneider, 1987; also, see Ludwig, 1988; Ludwig & Wikler, 1974).

Appetitively Based Models of Urges

Another distinguishing feature of drugs of abuse is that they appear to have appetitive, positive reinforcing effects. For example, experimental paradigms can be established such that animals self-administer opiates, alcohol, cocaine, or amphetamine at high rates, sometimes to the point of intoxication or even dependence (for reviews, see Stewart, de Wit, & Eikelboom, 1984; Wise & Bozarth, 1987; Young & Herling, 1986). Most drugs of abuse appear to have stimulating or excitatory effects; this is obviously characteristic of drugs classified as stimulants (e.g., amphetamine, cocaine, and nicotine) but is equally true of drugs often classified as depressants. For example, striking excitatory effects can be obtained on several response measures with opiates (e.g., Gunne, 1960; Mucha, Volkovskis, & Kalant, 1981; Schwarz & Cunningham, 1989; Seevers & Deneau, 1963; Zelman, Tiffany, & Baker, 1985) and alcohol (e.g., Pohorecky, 1977; Tabakoff & Kiianmaa, 1982). Recently, Wise and Bozarth (1987) equated many of the stimulating effects of abused drugs with their appetitive or positively reinforcing properties and argued that these are all mediated by a common neural pathway located in the medial forebrain bundle.

Various theorists have associated urges and cravings with the appetitive, positively reinforcing, or excitatory effects of abused drugs. For instance, McAuliffe and Gordon (1974) argued that craving among opiate addicts represents the desire for, and anticipation of, the euphoria produced by drug use. Similarly, Wise (1988) hypothesized that memory for the positive reinforcing effect of a drug represents a major source of drug craving (see Stewart et al., 1984, for a similar depiction of drug craving).

Marlatt (1985) has presented a social learning model of addictive behavior in which craving is defined as a subjective state motivated by the incentive properties of positive-outcome expectancies. Although positive-outcome expectancies may reflect anticipation of withdrawal relief, Marlatt's (1985) model emphasizes the anticipation of euphoria, excitation, or stimulation as the primary determinant of craving in addicts. Marlatt (1985) also suggested a distinction should be drawn between urges and cravings, stating that urges reflect intention to use a drug that is motivated by the anticipation of positive outcome from drug use (i.e., craving).

In presenting a recent model of drug urges, Baker et al. (1987) described urges as affective states and posited that there are two kinds of urge systems, positive-affect urges and negative-affect urges. The hypothesis of the model is that these two types of urges are mutually inhibitory; that is, activation of one urge system will increase the threshold for the activation of the other. Positive-affect urges represent the activation of a general appetitive–motivational system (e.g., Fowles, 1980; Gray, 1982; Panksepp, 1982). This motivational system is directly stimulated by addictive drugs and is hypothesized to support compulsive drug use (Stewart et al., 1984). Its activation is characterized by increased behavioral and physiological activity, a strong tendency to pursue previously rewarded behaviors, and positive affect.

Baker et al. (1987) used a bioinformation-processing paradigm (e.g., Lang, 1984) to model the cognitive structure of urges. Thus, urges (like other affective systems) are assumed to be organized at a cognitive level within a propositional network that encodes information on eliciting stimuli, drug-related responses (e.g., verbal reports, physiological adjustments, and pursuit of drugs), and the meaning or interpretation of stimuli and responses. Baker et al. (1987) proposed that when the prevailing stimulus conditions provide a sufficient match for the encoded eliciting stimuli, the positive-affect urge network will be activated en masse, and the response information within the urge network will be enacted; for example, the person will report that he or she is experiencing urges and positive affect and will seek out and self-administer drugs. Several stimuli may activate this system, including information that drug is available, a small priming dose of the drug, stimuli previously associated with drug use, and positive affect.

Although positive-affect urges are assumed to be closely tied to the appetitive effects of drugs, Baker et al. (1987) proposed that negative-affect urges are strongly associated with drug withdrawal. Thus, stimulus information encoded within this type of urge network would include actual drug withdrawal, stimuli previously associated with withdrawal, negative affect, and aversive stimuli. The responses produced by the activation of this network should promote drug seeking and descriptions of urges, as well as negative affect and signs of withdrawal.

Models of Drug Urges: Evaluation of Common Assumptions

Most urge theories differ primarily in their description of the stimulus conditions that give rise to the urge state. Surprisingly, there is little disagreement regarding the impact of urge on drug-use behavior. An assumption of all of the theories is that urges are necessary but probably not sufficient for the production of drug seeking and drug consumption. That is, the theorists assume a causal link between an urge and drug use and acknowledge that the translation of urge into action can be modified by variables such as drug availability or social constraints on drug use. In all of the theories, urges and cravings are seen as the primary determinants of ongoing drug-use behavior in addicts and as the principal cause of relapse in addicts attempting abstinence. Shiffman's (1979) statement that "The urge to smoke, when it becomes stronger than the ex-smoker's determination to quit, leads to relapse" (p. 160) summarizes the prevalent view of most theories of drug urges with regard to drug relapse.

Models of drug urges generally propose the following chain of events: Some sort of stimulus condition activates an urge state that then elicits drug use. A further assumption of most models is that the subjective urge state can be indexed by self-report. Therefore, self-report of urges and actual drug use should be strongly associated. Some models also predict that particular patterns of physiological responses should accompany subjective urge states (e.g., Baker et al., 1987; Ludwig et al., 1974; Melchior & Tabakoff, 1984; Poulos et al., 1981; Stewart et al., 1984; West & Schneider, 1987; Wikler, 1972). Consequently, physiological responses, self-report, and actual drug use should covary.

I have recently reviewed studies in which correlations have been reported between physiological variables and self-reported urges or between measures of drug consumption and self-reported urges (Tiffany, 1988). In all of these studies, the subjects, either alcoholics or cigarette smokers, were exposed to drug-related or neutral stimuli while their physiological responses and self-reported urges were monitored. Various stimulus exposure conditions were used in these studies, including having alcoholics sniff partially filled bottles of alcohol (Cooney, Baker, Pomerleau, & Josephy, 1984; Kaplan et al., 1985; Monti et al., 1987), having alcoholics drink alcohol or placebo beverages (Hodgson, Rankin, & Stockwell, 1979; Kaplan, Meyer, & Stroebel, 1983; Laberg & Ellertsen, 1987; Ludwig et al., 1974; Rankin, Hodgson, & Stockwell, 1979; Stockwell, Hodgson, Rankin, & Taylor, 1982), having cigarette smokers watch other smokers light a cigarette (Abrams, Monti, Carey, Pinto, & Jacobus, 1988; Niaura, Abrams, DeMuth, Pinto, & Monti, 1989; Rickard-Figueroa & Zeichner, 1985), or having a smoker take a puff on a cigarette (Baker et al., 1987). Several physiological variables were monitored in these studies, including (but not limited to) heart rate, skin conductance, blood pressure, tremor, salivation, and temperature.

One notable feature of these studies was that many of the correlations between physiological responses and self-report urges were not reported. For example, across the 13 studies I've described, only 17 of the approximately 48 coefficients that could have been calculated were reported. In some cases, this was because the authors explicitly stated that the correlations were not significant. Most of the reported correlations were positive (e.g., 13 of 17 of all correlations and 8 of 10 of the significant correlations), suggesting that self-reported urges tended to be generally associated with increased arousal or physiological activation. The overall magnitude of these correlations was not impressive. The average of all correlations, regardless of sign, was .38, accounting for less than 15% of the variance. Even when the analysis was restricted to the 10 significant correlations, the average of the absolute values of the coefficients was .52, accounting for only approximately 27% of the variance. Because the nonreported correlation coefficients across these studies were probably of low magnitude, the cumulative message of these studies is that physiological variables may at best be only modestly related to self-report of urges. These low correlations would seem to be particularly troublesome for urge theories that claim that conditioned physiological responses provide the substrate for drug urges and cravings (e.g., Ludwig & Wikler, 1974; Poulos et al., 1981; Siegel, 1983; Wikler, 1972).

Although these data indicate that physiological responses and self-report of urges are not highly concordant, it seems reasonable to believe, based on theoretical assumptions noted previously, that self-report of urges and actual drug-use behavior are strongly associated. Six of the studies described reported correlations between self-report urges or craving and actual drug-use behavior: five of them used alcoholics as subjects, and the sixth used cigarette smokers. The behavioral measures for the studies with alcoholics were amount of work (lever presses) for an alcohol reward (Ludwig et al., 1974), speed of drinking (Hodgson et al., 1979; Rankin et al., 1979; Stockwell et al., 1982), or choice of alcohol versus nonalcoholic beverage (Kaplan et al., 1983). The study with cigarette smokers measured the speed with which one cigarette was smoked during a free smoking period (Rickard-Figueroa & Zeichner, 1985). The correlations between these measures and self-reported urges or cravings collected just prior to the behavioral consumption tests are shown in Table 1. As with physiological measures, the correlations between self-reported urges and drug-use behavior are not exceptionally strong. The average correlation across all nine coefficients was .40, accounting for approximately 16% of the

Table 1
Correlations of Urge Report With Consumption Measures

Study	Correlation
Ludwig, Wikler, & Stark (1974)	.83*
	.56
Hodgson, Rankin, & Stockwell (1979)	.44*
Rankin, Hodgson, & Stockwell (1979)	.59*
Stockwell, Hodgson, Rankin, & Taylor (1982)	.30*
	−.04
Kaplan, Meyer, & Stroebel (1983)	.52*
Rickard-Figueroa & Zeichner (1985)	.31*
	.07
Overall mean correlation	.40
Mean significant correlation	.50*

Note. Studies showing two correlation coefficients used two exposure conditions.
* $p < .05$.

variance. Even if only the significant correlations are examined, the average coefficient is .50, indicating only 25% shared variance between self-reported urges and actual drug-use behavior.[1]

Of course, there are many reasons for why the correlations between self-reported urges and drug-use behavior shown in Table 1 might be attenuated. These range from poor reliability of one or both variables to situational constraints on self-report or drug consumption. Nonetheless, the data as they currently stand do not provide much support for the assumption that self-report of urges and drug consumption are necessarily strongly related. Indeed, the data permit the hypothesis that the psychological processes that support drug-use behavior may be only loosely coupled to the processes that control verbal reports of drug urges and cravings. Or perhaps urges and cravings may not be necessary for the initiation or maintenance of drug-use behavior.

Data from follow-up studies of addicts who have gone through a treatment program and have relapsed also support the notion that drug use is not necessarily preceded by urges or cravings (e.g., Ludwig, 1972; Marlatt & Gordon, 1980; O'Connell & Martin, 1987). For instance, Marlatt and Gordon (1980) examined the characteristics of relapse situations for 70 alcoholics, 35 smokers, and 32 heroin addicts. They found that only 7% of these addicts (11% alcoholics, 6% smokers, 0% heroin addicts) described urges and temptations as major factors in their relapse to drug use. Similarly, Shiffman (1986) reported that only 23% of smokers in a relapse crisis identified cravings to smoke as a component of their cognitions regarding the crisis situation. The data from these studies are somewhat misleading because the subjects were not asked specifically about urges or cravings; for example, only 7% of the subjects in Marlatt and Gordon's (1980) study volunteered that urges or cravings were major precipitants of their relapse. In spite of this limitation, these data are revealing in that they indicate that addicts typically do not spontaneously identify urges and cravings as an important component of their relapse. In a follow-up of smokers who have completed a smoking-treatment program, Maude-Griffin and I (1989b) have frequently encountered smokers who have relapsed yet state categorically that they had no urge or craving to smoke just prior to their relapse. These observations, in combination with the data I have reviewed thus far, permit the hypothesis that the psychological processes supporting drug-use behavior can operate independently of those that control urge responding. A view of cognitive functioning that would provide for the operation of drug-use behavior independent of urge responding can be derived from the cognitive conceptions of automatic and nonautomatic processes.

Automaticity and Drug-Use Behavior

Repeated practice of a cognitive or motor task under fixed-stimulus conditions typically leads to the development of a level of skilled behavior that is qualitatively different from the performance level observed when the task was originally undertaken. A person learning to drive a car initially pays a great deal of attention to each component action, and his or her performance is slow, hesitant, and filled with error. With extended practice, this task can become virtually effortless, and what once demanded considerable attention and concentration can be carried out rapidly and accurately, with little or no awareness of the component actions. This transformation of performance with practice has been described by many cognitive psychologists as the development of automaticity, and considerable research has been conducted over the past decade in an attempt to elucidate essential features and cognitive processes underlying automatic and nonautomatic functioning.

[1] Although not explicitly labeled as such, Siegel's (1983) depiction of the relapse process could be conceptualized as a version of a two-process motivational model (e.g., Rescorla & Solomon, 1967) in which the instrumental behavior of drug consumption is mediated by a reduction in aversive, classically conditioned withdrawal reactions. This view would suggest that drug consumption is controlled more directly by conditioned physiological responses than by urges; the latter perhaps representing cognitive manifestations of the anticipation of withdrawal relief. According to this interpretation, relapse and urges, although both produced by conditioned compensatory responses, may be imperfectly associated with each other, thus accounting for low correlations between self-reported urges and drug self-administration. Of course this approach would mandate a strong relationship between physiological measures and drug-use behavior, but across seven studies allowing for an evaluation of this association (including all the studies listed in Table 1 as well as Ludwig, Cain, Wikler, Taylor, & Bendfeldt, 1977), only 3 of a possible 37 correlation coefficients were reported as significant. Even in these three instances, there was no clear evidence of a strong, direct relationship between conditioned physiological responses and drug use. For example, Kaplan, Meyer, and Stroebel (1983) performed a multiple regression analysis of the variables predictive of whether alcoholics would choose a beer reward at the completion of their laboratory session. Heart rate acceleration to an alcohol stimulus emerged as one of the significant predictors ($sR^2 = .13$), although, notably, a measure of self-reported alcohol urges was a better predictor ($sR^2 = .27$), and the zero-order, point-biserial correlation of heart rate with choice behavior was nonsignificant, $r(14) = .38, p > .10$. Ludwig et al. (1977) described several multiple regression analyses of their data in which tonic blood pressure levels (systolic and diastolic) produced significant increments in prediction of work for alcohol in alcoholics in some of their regression models. Interpreting these results is difficult because the unique contributions of the physiological variables to the prediction model were not reported and because all the analyses were confounded with a subject variable (i.e., steady vs. binge drinkers) that had significant associations with both the physiological and drug-use measures.

A theme recurrent throughout most theorizing on automaticity is that this type of cognitive functioning is characteristic of most of the daily activities of humans, the notion being that with sufficient practice, performance on any task, from tooth brushing to piano playing, can become automatic. The thesis presented in this article is that drug-use behavior in the addict represents one such activity, controlled largely by automatic processes. Furthermore, urge responding is assumed to be controlled largely by nonautomatic cognitive processes. I believe that the application of the automatic–nonautomatic distinction to addictive behavior has important implications for understanding the cognitive processes subserving drug-use behavior, and it suggests a view of the concept of drug urges distinctly different from that offered by current models. Before this approach is detailed, I briefly review current conceptualizations of the features and processes of automatic and nonautomatic cognitive functioning. This review is not comprehensive, and I assert generalizations that focus on commonalities rather than differences across theories. There are theoretical disputes regarding the fundamental manifestations of automatic and nonautomatic functioning, but there appears to be sufficient agreement across theoretical approaches to warrant an application of general ideas distilled from cognitive research on automaticity to certain aspects of addictive behavior.

Theories of Automaticity

Although discussion of a distinction between automatic and nonautomatic cognitive processing dates back nearly 100 years to William James (1890), this distinction was not formally introduced into cognitive models of human performance until the mid-1970s. A predominant view through the 1970s was that the distinction between automatic and nonautomatic functioning arose as a function of capacity or resource limitations in some sort of general-purpose central processor (e.g., Hasher & Zacks, 1979; LaBerge & Samuels, 1974; Logan, 1978; Posner & Snyder, 1975; Shiffrin & Schneider, 1977). The most influential account of automaticity along these lines was Shiffrin and Schneider's (1977) model of automatic and controlled processes. In this theory, an *automatic process* was defined as a relatively permanent sequence of tightly integrated associative connections stored in long-term memory that always became active in response to a particular input configuration. When activated, this set of nodes entered short-term memory, and responses encoded within the sequence were generated. In contrast, controlled processes represented a sequence of nodes activated temporarily in short-term memory through attention by the individual. Because the activation of these nodes required the active attention of the subject, only one sequence at a time could be controlled. Thus, the capacity of attention set a limit on the processing accomplished by this mode of functioning. Controlled processing in this model was seen as dependent on attention, relatively slow, flexible, subject controlled, and serial. Automatic processing was considered to be independent of attention, fast, stimulus bound, somewhat beyond subject control, and parallel (i.e., automatic processes could be activated in parallel with one another and in parallel with a controlled process).

The idea that nonautomatic functions were limited primarily because they were controlled by one type of cognitive resource (e.g., attention) was challenged by some theorists claiming that many cognitive resources might be critical for task performance and that limits on these could constrain task performance (e.g., Navon & Gopher, 1979; Wickens, 1984). Cognitive resources involved in task performance may differ as a function of the modality of input, the processing code, the stages of processing, or the form of the response (Wickens, 1984). This perspective also suggested that because different tasks might rely on different resources, interference between tasks would occur to the extent that there was overlap among the resources demanded by the tasks. In these theories, automaticity was characterized by a change in the utilization of resources; that is, with practice, resources were used less or were used more efficiently. With regard to the development of automatic processes, this view was similar to the theory of Shiffrin and Schneider (1977), with the focus being on multiple resources rather than a single, limited resource of attention.

An alternative conceptualization of automaticity that does not invoke the idea of limitations in single or multiple resources has been offered by Logan (1988), who hypothesized that lack of knowledge limits nonautomatic processing (see also Neumann, 1984). In his approach, task performance is automatic when it is based on retrieval from long-term memory. So, for instance, in most adults, the solution to the problem $2 + 2 = ?$ is generated automatically from long-term memory. In contrast, children learning single-digit addition will solve the problem in a nonautomatic fashion, applying some algorithm to generate a solution. To the extent that particular solutions are always associated with a certain configuration of stimuli, those stimuli will, with practice, produce an obligatory retrieval of the solution from memory. Logan (1988) assumed that in many circumstances, memory retrieval and algorithm-based processing operate in parallel; on any given trial, the process that produces the appropriate solution first will control responding. (A model developed by Schneider, 1985, makes similar predictions regarding the development of automaticity.)

Across most of the theoretical conceptualizations of automaticity there are some shared assumptions.[2] First, theories of automaticity generally assert that the differences in the performance of unpracticed and practiced subjects on the same task arise from fundamental differences in the cognitive processes subserving task performance. Although automatic and nonautomatic processes may produce a similar outcome, they are assumed to arrive at the same point through the operation of distinct cognitive mechanisms. A second assumption is that automaticity develops through practice. Initially, some theorists indicated that massive bouts of extended practice were necessary for the development of fully automatized performance

[2] The general application of the concepts of automatic and nonautomatic processing to drug use and urge responding need not await the resolution of theoretical disputes about the best way to conceptualize these modes of cognitive function. Indeed, if a marriage between cognitive psychology and psychopathology depended on the complete resolution of theoretical conflict within the former, then the researcher could be left standing forever at the altar. In fact, the study of these issues within the context of drug addiction may provide an enriched understanding of the generality and limitations of current conceptualizations of automaticity.

(e.g., Shiffrin & Schneider, 1977), but more recent approaches have suggested that certain aspects of automaticity may be detectable after more limited training (e.g., Logan, 1985c, 1988; Schneider, 1985).

A third assumption is that automaticity develops most rapidly when stimulus conditions are consistently and uniquely associated with response. In their early experiments, Schneider and Shiffrin (1977; Shiffrin & Schneider, 1977) used visual-search tasks in which subjects had to indicate when a particular target stimulus, embedded among distractors, was encountered. When training was consistent (i.e., targets were always targets and never distractors), performance at an automatic level was established easily. In contrast, inconsistent training (i.e., when distractors and targets varied randomly over trials) produced little or no automaticity. Although absolute inconsistency between stimuli and responses will not support automaticity, the development of automatic processes does not depend on perfect consistency (e.g., Schneider & Fisk, 1982).

A final assumption regarding automatic and nonautomatic functioning is that complex behavioral sequences can rarely be regarded as fully or completely automatic. Most theorists have noted that skilled performance on complex tasks is likely to be controlled by an ensemble of automatic and nonautomatic processes (e.g., Allport, 1980; Jonides, Naveh-Benjamin, & Palmer, 1985; Logan, 1985c; Shiffrin & Dumais, 1981; Shiffrin & Schneider, 1977). Thus, performance on a task may be more or less automatic as a function of the extent to which component processes have been automatized. With extended practice under consistent training conditions, more and more components may become automatized, and subordinate components may become integrated into higher order automatized structures.

Characteristics of Automatic Processes

Several properties have been proposed as key features of automatic processing. Although lists of essential features have varied across authors (Logan, 1979; Neumann, 1984; cf. Posner & Snyder, 1975; Shiffrin & Dumais, 1981; Shiffrin & Schneider, 1977), the following characteristics have been cited as important manifestations of automaticity by most or all researchers in the area. This list is intended to be descriptive, not definitive. It focuses on characteristics of automaticity, with the greatest potential relevance for addictive behavior.

1. *Speed.* A considerable number of laboratory studies indicate that with practice, task performance speeds up, with a corresponding decline in performance variability (Logan, 1988; Newell & Rosenbloom, 1981). Across tasks that can be affected by practice, there is a remarkable similarity in the form of the function relating the time to complete the task to the number of practice trials; that is, the speedup conforms to a power function (Logan, 1988; Newell & Rosenbloom, 1981). Furthermore, the reduction in variability in task performance across practice trials also follows a power function (Logan, 1988). Most current theories of automaticity assume that reduction in variability and increased speed in task performance over practice represent a transition from nonautomatic to automatic processes in the control of task performance (e.g., Logan, 1985c, 1988; Posner & Snyder, 1975; Schneider & Shiffrin, 1977; Shiffrin & Schneider, 1977).

2. *Autonomy.* Many authors have noted that an automatized act can be carried out without initiation through intention (James, 1890; Kahneman & Treisman, 1984; Norman & Shallice, 1985; Reason, 1984; Underwood, 1982). The implication is that under proper stimulus conditions, an automatized action may be initiated involuntarily. Another way to describe this property of automaticity while avoiding the theoretically troubling concept of intentionality (e.g., Neumann, 1984) is to describe performance as *stimulus bound;* in other words, the presentation of a stimulus may be sufficient to cause the enactment of an automatized action sequence.

Reason (1979, 1984) suggested that many action slips (i.e., absentminded behaviors or behavioral sequences that are not consistent with the intentions of the individual) occur when the immediate stimulus conditions automatically elicit well-practiced action schemata that run counter to the current plans of the individual (see also, Norman, 1981). For example, Reason (1979) provided the following description from one of his subjects: "I had decided to cut down my sugar consumption and wanted to have my cornflakes without it. However, I sprinkled sugar on my cereal just as I have always done" (p. 538). Reason (1984) suggested that this kind of error occurs when the intention system is captured by some internal preoccupation or by some unexpected external event. Concurrently, the action system is captured by the motor program that is most strongly associated with the current stimulus conditions. Reason labeled these types of absentminded behaviors *double-capture slips,* and his explanation for these may be relevant to instances of drug relapses that occur in the absence of a precipitating urge.

3. *Lack of control.* Related to the notion that automatic actions may be enacted without intention is the idea that with appropriate eliciting stimuli, it may be difficult to inhibit the elicitation of an automatic process, and once initiated, the process may be difficult to impede or curtail (Posner & Snyder, 1975; Shiffrin & Schneider, 1977). The notion behind this aspect of automaticity is that automatic processes are easily triggered by external stimulus conditions and somewhat less penetrable by executive cognitive processes (e.g., strategies, decisions, intentions, heuristics, and plans). Moreover, once initiated, an automatized process may have a ballistic quality, in that it is difficult to impede and tends to run on to completion (Hasher & Zacks, 1979; Shiffrin & Dumais, 1981; cf. Logan & Cowan, 1984).

4. *Effortlessness.* The fast, coherent, and consistent performance of well-practiced individuals on certain tasks is generally described by participants as being easy and nondemanding. For instance, Shiffrin and Dumais (1981) reported that, after extended practice on a consistently mapped visual-search task, their subjects described the task as relatively simple, requiring little attention or cognitive effort. In fact, subjects would often carry on conversations while performing the tasks. Similar effects are clearly manifested in more complex, yet everyday skills. For example, driving a car in traffic while concentrating on a conversation with a passenger is not a difficult feat for an experienced driver.

Many have suggested that because nonautomatic processing might be restricted by general capacity or cognitive resource limitations (e.g., Logan, 1979; Posner & Snyder, 1975; Shiffrin & Schneider, 1977) and automatic processing is not, the latter demands less cognitive effort than the former. Results from dual-task experiments showing little or no interference between tasks when subjects had extensive practice on one or both of the component tasks (e.g., Allport, Antonis, & Reynolds, 1972; Logan, 1978; Schneider & Fisk, 1982) provide experimental support for this interpretation.

5. *Conscious awareness.* Many theorists either describe automatic processing as occurring without awareness or suggest that awareness is not a necessary aspect of automatic performance (e.g., Posner & Snyder, 1975). Common experience suggests that people can engage in complex acts without awareness (e.g., Neisser, 1967; Reason, 1979), and there are numerous laboratory examples of complex cognitive processing that occur in the absence of awareness (Kihlstrom, 1987). Of course, awareness, or its absence, can only be inferred by the verbal report of the individual. Perhaps a better way to characterize this aspect of automaticity is to say that these processes can be enacted without concurrent activation of cognitive structures that permit an accurate or veridical description of the mechanics of the automatized functioning. That is, with regard to automatized performance, people may be made aware of and will be able to describe what they are doing, but they may not be able to explain how they are doing it. Moreover, even if they can describe accurately what they are doing, they may not be able to provide a clear statement of the stimulus conditions that evoked the behavioral sequence (Nisbett & Wilson, 1977).

Characteristics of Nonautomatic Processes

Nonautomatic processing is typically described as having characteristics opposite those assigned to automatic processes. So, for instance, where automatic processing is seen as fast, autonomous, obligatory, and effortless, nonautomatic processing is defined as slow, dependent on attention and intention, and effortful (e.g., Hasher & Zacks, 1979; LaBerge & Samuels, 1974; Logan, 1978; Posner & Snyder, 1975; Shiffrin & Schneider, 1977). The cognitive processes subsumed under the descriptor *nonautomatic* vary across authors. Posner and Snyder (1975) described nonautomatic processes as strategic operations under the conscious control of the subject. Shiffrin and Schneider (1977) stated that control (i.e., nonautomatic) processes included "maintenance or rote rehearsal, coding rehearsal, serial search, long-term memory search, and decisions and strategies of all kinds" (p. 160). Others have noted that nonautomatic processes could be described as executive systems that function to coordinate activities in circumstances in which automatic processes are not adequately developed to control responding (e.g., Logan, 1985a; Sternberg, 1985). For example, Sternberg (1985) identified seven metacomponents operating within executive systems. These include decisions regarding the nature of the problem and allocation of resources, selection of lower order processing components, selection of strategies for combining lower order components, and monitoring of task performance. Similarly, Logan (1985a) described four executive functions: choice among possible strategies, construction of the strategy, execution and maintenance of the strategy, and inhibition or disablement of the strategy in response to relevant environmental changes.

One theme that emerges from these conceptualizations of nonautomatic processing is that this type of processing is required in situations in which automatic processes either have not or cannot be invoked to produce appropriate responses. These may include novel situations or tasks in which the relationships between stimuli and responses are sufficiently variable to prevent the development of automatic processes. Another situation that may demand considerable nonautomatic processing is one in which the individual is attempting to impede or inhibit automatic processing (Norman & Shallice, 1985; Schneider, Dumais, & Shiffrin, 1984).

Automatic Action Schemata and Drug-Use Behavior

I contend that drug-use behavior in the addict represents a constellation of specific skills involving drug acquisition and drug consumption. Over a history of repeated practice, the cognitive systems controlling many aspects of drug procurement and consumption take on the character of automatic processes. That is, much of the drug-use behavior of the addict may become largely automatized. Thus, drug-use behaviors tend to be relatively fast and efficient, readily enabled by particular stimulus configurations (i.e., stimulus bound), initiated and completed without intention, difficult to impede in the presence of triggering stimuli, effortless, and enacted in the absence of awareness. I propose that the procedures for carrying out these skills are stored in memory in the form of automatized action schemata (Norman & Shallice, 1985; Schmidt, 1976; Shallice, 1972) or action plans (Allport, 1980; Newell, 1978). These are conceived of as unitized memory systems that are somewhat self-sufficient in that they contain adequate information for the initiation and coordination of complex sequences of drug-use behavior. Encoded within these memory systems will be information specifying the following.

1. *Stimulus configurations necessary for the elicitation of component actions.* These critical stimulus configurations may be external events or internal events or both. Examples of external events would be particular environmental locations (e.g., a barroom), isolated stimuli (e.g., the smell of a burning cigarette or the sight of a hypodermic syringe), or even a particular time of day (e.g., a break from work). Examples of internal events might include activation of emotional networks (e.g., being in a celebratory or angry mood), physical states (e.g., fatigue or drug withdrawal), or stimulating effects of drugs. These examples may be particularly important for the initiation of a drug-use action plan. Other kinds of stimuli may be more important in the coordinated execution of the sequence. So, for instance, in the act of smoking a cigarette, certain sensory experiences, such as the sensation of warm air in the back of the throat (Rose, Zinser, Tashkin, Newcomb, & Ertle, 1984), may be critical in guiding some components of the action plan.

2. *Procedures for the enactment of specific actions.* This model makes the relatively noncontroversial assumption that drug-use action plans or schemata must incorporate many different actions or goals, each of which has some sort of representation in the action plan. An example of a particular action might be finding a vein for an injection of heroin. (Of course, this action may be composed of several lower level actions that have, over repeated practice, become fully integrated into the superordinate action.)

3. *Coordination of specific actions into action sequences.* Even a relatively simple sequence involving drug use comprises many actions that require a substantial degree of organization across actions for the sequence to be executed coherently. Consider the act of smoking a cigarette. The smoker must remove a cigarette from the pack, place it to his or her lips, light a match or a lighter, place the flame to the end of the cigarette, inhale, remove the cigarette from his or her mouth, exhale, and then extinguish the flame. This process is followed by a series of behaviors wherein the smoker places the cigarette to his or her lips, inhales, takes the cigarette away from his or her lips, and exhales. These behaviors continue until the cigarette is gone, at which point the smoker extinguishes the butt. Each of these component actions has several subcomponents, and the entire sequence in well-practiced smokers is highly stereotyped and ritualized (e.g., Nil, Buzzi, & Bättig, 1984). The coordination of these actions into integrated sequences can be accomplished within the action plan.

4. *Alternative action sequences in the event of minor obstacles.* Encoded within drug-use action schemata may be contingency plans for the execution of alternative actions in case a particular sequence is blocked or impeded by unexpected environmental conditions. These would be present in the action plan only to the extent that these obstacles have been encountered relatively frequently in the past and their solution is somewhat easy (i.e., does not require extensive problem-solving activity). For instance, the experienced heroin addict who misses his or her vein on the first attempt can withdraw the needle and insert it again, with the entire sequence being controlled within the action plan. (In this example, the alternative sequence would merely be a repeat of one of the component actions.)

5. *Support physiology for action components.* The model assumes that patterns of somatovisceral responding are encoded within the action plan. These physiological responses (e.g., increased cardiac output and changes in respiration) are coupled to, and are in support of, particular components of the drug-use action plan. The timing, patterning, and magnitude of responses across physiological channels will vary as a function of the behavioral or metabolic demands of component actions (e.g., Elliott, 1974; Obrist, Webb, Sutterer, & Howard, 1970). Over an extended history of drug use, this physiology could become less pronounced, primarily as a result of the acquisition of more coordinated and less behaviorally demanding movement patterns in the well-practiced user.

This conceptualization of the somatovisceral response elements encoded within drug-use action schemata draws heavily from Lang's (Lang, 1979, 1984, 1985; Lang, Kozak, Miller, Levin, & McLean, 1980) bioinformational model of emotion. In that analysis, emotion is described as an action disposition encoded within an associative, propositional network. A primary part of this network is response information including self-referent verbal statements, overt behavioral acts, and physiology supportive of those acts. In the application of these ideas to the construct of drug-use action plans, I emphasize the latter two categories of response information (i.e., overt acts and support physiology) but downplay the first. I do not believe that self-referent statements regarding the desirability of drug use (e.g., "I need a drink") are integral components of drug-use action plans in highly practiced addicts. As discussed later, this model posits that these types of responses are more likely to be generated when the drug-use action plan is disrupted.

6. *Generation of physiological adjustments in anticipation of drug intake.* Considerable evidence indicates that drug tolerance can readily come under the associative control of stimuli reliably paired with drug administration (e.g., Baker & Tiffany, 1985; Goudie & Demellweek, 1986; Siegel, 1975, 1983; Tiffany & Baker, 1986). Although there is considerable controversy regarding the exact nature of the conditioned responses subserving associative tolerance (Baker & Tiffany, 1985; Eikelboom & Stewart, 1982; Maude-Griffin & Tiffany, 1989a; Siegel, 1983; Tiffany et al., 1983), there is no question that physiological adjustments responsible for reductions in certain drug effects are easily conditioned. The stimuli that evoke these conditioned tolerance effects should be the same as those that trigger certain components of the drug-use sequence. In particular, stimuli that immediately precede and overlap with drug intake may be strongly associated with conditioned tolerance responses.

The physiology supporting drug tolerance may be distinctly different from that supporting particular action components in the drug-use sequence. The physiology of conditioned tolerance should be relatively specific to the drug that is being used. For example, tolerance to the effects of opiates would demand a pattern of physiological adjustments that is different from that required for tolerance to the effects of alcohol (Baker & Tiffany, 1985; Tiffany & Baker, 1986). In contrast, the support physiology for component actions of the drug-use sequence should be specific to the behavioral demands of the particular action. This suggests that physiological changes in a given response channel (e.g., cardiac responding) at a particular point in the drug-use sequence may reflect the influence of two different response demands. Thus, the functional significance of a particular physiological change in the presence of a configuration of stimuli that have been strongly associated with drug intake may be difficult to determine unless these different influences are taken into account.

Development of Drug-Use Action Plans

The scope and coherence of any action plan should depend on the previous learning history of the individual. Consistent practice of the component actions involved in drug acquisition and drug consumption, under relatively fixed stimulus configurations, would lead to the development of more integrated and efficient drug-use action plans. They would be integrated in the sense that the subcomponents of the skill sequence would be combined within the same action plan and efficient in the sense that the components of the action plan could be coordinated locally (i.e., within the action schema), with a corresponding decrease in the processing time in the execution of skill sequences.

Several factors should promote the development of coherent action plans supportive of drug-use behavior. First is the extent to which drug is readily available and easily procured over an addict's history of involvement with that drug. When a drug demands extensive planning and problem solving for its procurement, that cognitive activity would require nonautomatic processing. A street addict who daily must find a new way of obtaining heroin would never be able to fully automatize those components of his or her drug-use behavior. (Of course, such a situation might not prevent other aspects of the drug-use sequence, such as actual consumption once the drug is obtained, from becoming automatized.) In contrast, cigarette smokers or successful heroin pushers who happen to be addicted usually have no difficulty getting their drugs. As a consequence, this portion of their drug-use sequence might be enacted automatically.

A related factor that might moderate the extent to which aspects of drug-use sequences become automatized could be the degree to which drug consumption is constrained by social, legal, situational, or interpersonal factors. For instance, in some settings, certain drugs may be relatively inexpensive and easy to procure, but, because of their illegality, an addict must be fairly cautious about where he or she decides to use it. To the degree that "safe use" of a drug continually requires careful planning, that section of the drug-use sequence may not become automatic, although sequences leading up to that point (e.g., procurement) and sequences that ensue when the planning is completed (e.g., consumption) may become automatized.

Finally, certain characteristics of abused drugs may affect the development of drug-use action schemata. Drugs of abuse appear to have powerfully reinforcing properties capable of supporting stable rates of self-administration as a generally positive function of dose (Henningfield, Lukas, & Bigelow, 1986; Young & Herling, 1986). A high rate of self-administration would itself allow for the development of automaticity, merely as a result of practice. Moreover, the primary reinforcing effects of abused drugs may have a more direct influence on the acquisition of automatized sequences, perhaps promoting the more rapid development of coherent and integrated drug-use action schemata. This last proposal is purely speculative, because the influence of reinforcement as a direct factor in the development of automaticity or acquisition of skills has received virtually no attention in the literature on cognition.

Drug Urges and Nonautomatic Processes

The characterization of action plans I have outlined suggests that the cognitive processes subserving drug-use behavior in well-established addictions are distinct from, and operate independently of, those responsible for the generation of responses identified as urges and cravings. In particular, I argue that the cognitive processes responsible for urge responding do not typically lead to the activation of action plans subserving drug pursuit and consumption; that is, urges may not be necessary for drug use. Indeed, an implication of this model is that the causal sequence may generally work in the opposite direction: The activation of memory structures that support drug use may be a necessary, but not a sufficient, condition for the generation of urge responding.

It may be useful to conceptualize urges and cravings as responses supported by nonautomatic cognitive processes that are activated in parallel with drug-use action schemata. There are two situations under which this nonautomatic processing might be invoked: (a) Some environmental condition impedes or blocks the drug-use action plan in an individual not attempting to avoid drug use, or (b) nonautomatic cognitive processes are invoked in an explicit attempt to impede or block a drug-use action plan.

There should be a fundamental difference in the nonautomatic processing elicited by these two types of situations. In the first situation, nonautomatic processing will be activated in support of the drug-use action plan: The addict will attempt to avoid abstinence. In the second situation, the addict is trying to maintain abstinence. Therefore, nonautomatic processing will be activated to counteract or prevent the drug-use action plan from going through to completion. The different types of nonautomatic processing elicited by these two situations may give rise to different constellations of verbal, behavioral, and (perhaps) somatovisceral responses. In this model, these behavioral manifestations of nonautomatic processing are identified as urge responses.[3]

Abstinence-Avoidance Urges

When drug-use action plans are blocked or impeded in individuals not attempting abstinence, nonautomatic forms of cognitive processing would be brought to bear on the problem situation. There may be some limited flexibility in action plans when minor obstacles are encountered (e.g., the smoker's match doesn't light on the first strike) that allows many problems to be handled locally, within the action plan. The solution to certain problems (e.g., problems that are infrequent or demand the application of some higher order algorithm) would not be encoded within the action plan. For example, the cigarette smoker discovers that he or she has run out of cigarettes in the middle of the night, the alcoholic's spouse comes home unexpectedly and the alcoholic has to figure out a way to sneak a drink, or the heroin addict goes to a pick-up spot to score drug only to find out that the regular supplier has been arrested. The drug-use action plan would rarely be sufficiently flexible to deal adequately with these exigencies. Obviously, more intensive, effortful, focused, and resource-demanding processing would be called for in these circumstances.

The manifestations of this type of processing can be indexed across three broad classes of behavior: overt behavioral acts, somatovisceral responses, and verbal report. Overt behavior would probably be characterized by actions to overcome or neutralize the obstacle blocking the execution of the action plan. Of course, the particular action would depend on the specific nature of the problem. Going out at midnight to buy a pack of cigarettes demands a different set of actions than searching through the house to find some matches.

The somatovisceral responses activated during attempts at abstinence avoidance might reflect the demands of two kinds of effort required by the situation. First, to the extent that the problem impeding the drug-use action plan is particularly difficult, the individual may have to engage in a considerable degree of cognitive effort to produce an adequate solution.

[3] These classifications of urge situations are separated here only for descriptive purposes. Many types of urge situations may represent an admixture of both kinds of processing. For instance, in relapse situations, nonautomatic processing that is initially invoked to avoid drug use might be abandoned, and the addict may then need to engage in problem-solving activity in support of the drug-use action plan.

There is evidence that cognitively challenging tasks or active coping elicit somatovisceral adjustments in excess of the metabolic demands of the task setting (e.g., Cacioppo, Petty, & Morris, 1985; Gliner, Bunnell, & Horvath, 1982; Obrist, 1976; Obrist et al., 1978; Turner & Carroll, 1985). Recently, Carroll, Turner, and Hellawell (1986) showed that subjects engaging in two cognitively challenging tasks, mental arithmetic and Raven's matrices, displayed increases in heart rate that were sensitive to manipulations in the difficulty level of each task. If the problems encountered by the addict in his or her attempt to complete a drug-use action plan demand considerable nonautomatic processing (i.e., are cognitively challenging), this cognitive effort may be associated with corresponding changes in somatovisceral activity (e.g., heart rate increases).

Effort of another sort might also have an impact on somatovisceral responses elicited in an abstinence-avoidance situation. The solutions generated by the addict to surmount obstacles to the drug-use action plan may demand some amount of physical effort. The somatovisceral responses, in anticipation of or during the execution of the actions required by the solution, will reflect to some degree the energy demands of the solution (e.g., Obrist et al., 1970). For instance, I would expect that the alcoholic who decides that he or she has to run to the corner bar to buy a six-pack of beer before the bar closes will show a different pattern of somatovisceral responses in anticipation of that activity than the alcoholic who realizes a full hour before bar closing time that he or she is out of beer. In general, the types of physiological adjustments demanded by these behavioral acts are identical in concept to the support physiology that I have already proposed is encoded within drug-use action plans.

The verbal responses emitted in abstinence-avoidance situations would, in general, be characterized by reports of frustration, annoyance, and irritation. (This should not be surprising because the situation as I have described it represents a frustrative, nonreward paradigm, e.g., Gray, 1982.) These responses may be particularly pronounced when the solution to the problem situation is not readily apparent or the solution requires actions that are inconvenient or disruptive of other, strongly motivated activities. The individual should also report a desire to use the drug ("I want to drink"; "I crave heroin"; "I have an urge") and should express a clear intention to obtain or use the drug (e.g., "I'm going to smoke as soon as possible"). Additionally, the addict should, if prompted, be able to describe certain aspects of any planning or problem solving that has been engaged to overcome obstacles to his or her drug use. This last aspect of verbal report might not provide a complete account of the nonautomatic processes that are activated in this situation (Nisbett & Wilson, 1977), but it would almost certainly capture more aspects of the components of this processing than would be provided by a verbal description of the automatic processes encoded within the drug-use action plan.

In addition to changes in the three general classes of behavior described above, other indications of the operation of nonautomatic cognitive processing in abstinence-avoidance situations might be obtained. One manifestation of the activation of these processes would be a disruption of performance on concurrent tasks that also require some degree of nonautomatic processing for their successful completion. As noted earlier, dual-task interference should be characteristic of situations in which both tasks require nonautomatic processing (e.g., Logan, 1978; Schneider & Fisk, 1982). To provide a simple example, an addict preoccupied with the problem of how to get drugs would probably not perform very well on a mental-arithmetic task.

Abstinence-Promotion Urges

Urge responding in this situation is produced by nonautomatic cognitive processes invoked in an explicit attempt to avoid drug consumption. In essence, this situation represents an approach–avoidance conflict, with approach behavior subserved by the automatic action plan and avoidance supported by nonautomatic cognitive processing. Addicts attempting to remain abstinent in the presence of stimuli that enable automatic action plans supportive of drug-use behavior face a particularly difficult task. Nonautomatic processing must be brought to bear on cognitive functions that with a history of repeated practice are not easily altered by a straightforward decision or plan to simply not engage in that behavior anymore.

The task facing the addict is much like that of subjects in an experiment (Shiffrin & Schneider, 1977, Experiment 1) who were initially trained to respond to target letters from the first half of the alphabet with distractors from the second half. After extensive training, the target and distractor sets were reversed, and the subjects' performance (hit rate) dropped well below that seen at the start of training, when subjects were unpracticed. In fact, only after 2,400 trials of reversal training was the hit rate comparable with the level of performance obtained with 900 trials of original training. Apparently, people can inhibit or counteract automatic processing, but a considerable commitment from nonautomatic functions will be demanded to achieve this result. As noted by Schneider et al. (1984), "Once the appropriate enabling stimuli occur (both internal and external), the automatic process may take place without additional control or effort by the subject. Subjects have difficulty ignoring or excluding automatic processes if the appropriate internal conditions are met and the stimuli elicit competing automatic responses" (p. 11).

Addicts attempting abstinence not only have to learn to inhibit old responses in the presence of enabling stimuli, but they also face an additional dilemma: The reinforcement contingencies that supported the old action plan are most likely still in effect. For instance, if positive-incentive effects of drugs are critical factors in the establishment and maintenance of an automatized drug-use action plan (e.g., Baker et al., 1987; Stewart et al., 1984; Wise, 1988; Wise & Bozarth, 1987), they should continue to operate in support of the action plan if the behavioral sequence were allowed to go through to completion. Thus, the addict attempting abstinence has to learn to inhibit automatized actions that would be reinforced if they were enacted.

The behavioral manifestations of nonautomatic processing invoked by the addict in an attempt to avoid drug use should be similar, but not identical, to urge responses produced in abstinence-avoidance situations. Overt behavior may or may not be instigated in these situations. If it is, the behavior will neutralize or impede the enactment of the drug-use action plan. Perhaps the most effective behaviors would be actions that eliminate or change the stimulus conditions that are triggering the drug-use action plan. Logan (1983, 1985b) has shown that one of the most effective means of inhibiting cognitive processing that is initiated by particular stimulus configurations is to disrupt the stimuli driving the cognitive activity.

There is evidence that abstinent addicts who engage in behavioral activities in an effort to avoid relapsing may be less likely to use drugs. Shiffman's (1984, 1986) studies of abstinent cigarette smokers suggest that ex-smokers who reported that they engaged in behavioral coping responses when faced with high-risk situations (e.g., situations in which smoking was highly likely) were less likely to relapse than smokers who did nothing in these situations. Examples of behavioral coping identified by Shiffman (1984) include physical activity, relaxation, distracting activity, or escape from the situation. Interestingly, subjects who stated that they used willpower (i.e., they did not report engaging in any specific cognitive or behavioral activity) were much less likely to avoid relapse than were subjects who instigated some sort of specific coping strategy.

Not all addicts attempting to avoid relapse will engage in behavioral activities to circumvent their drug-use action plans. Some may use what Shiffman (1984) has labeled *cognitive coping* in an effort to delay or inhibit drug use. For example, the individual may focus on the potential negative consequences of drug use or may remember the benefits of continued abstinence. These strategies, too, appear to be moderately successful in preventing relapse (Bliss, Garvey, Heinhold, & Hitchcock, 1989; Shiffman, 1984, 1986).

The patterning and magnitude of somatovisceral responses evident in situations in which the addict is attempting to maintain abstinence should be determined by at least two factors: the metabolic demands of behavioral acts undertaken to resist the drug-use action plan (i.e., support physiology) and physiology associated with the cognitive effort required to establish an effective strategy to avoid drug use. These two forms of physiology have already been described in the discussion of the somatovisceral responses characteristic of abstinence-avoidance urges. Physiological adjustments encoded within the activated action schema might also be evident in any urge situation. Consequently, physiological changes in a given urge situation may derive from four sources: support physiology for behavioral acts within the action schema, physiological adjustments in anticipation of drug intake, physiology associated with strategic planning to avoid drug use, and support physiology for behavioral acts undertaken to avoid drug use. If the physiological responses elicited in urge situations are multiply determined, then identifying a single, general pattern of somatovisceral responses associated with drug urges would not be possible. In particular, this theory suggests that the constellation of physiological responses activated in urge situations may not reflect a straightforward somatovisceral readout of the motivational states supporting compulsive drug-use behavior (cf. Baker et al., 1987). This apparent lack of clarity does not mean that assessment of physiological responses would not provide valuable insight into the cognitive structure of urge processing. Rather, this theory provides guidelines on what factors may need to be controlled in research evaluating the relationship between input information and somatovisceral responses in urge situations.

The verbal reports of individuals attempting to maintain abstinence in the face of activated drug-use action plans will, in general, reflect the approach–avoidance character of the situation. Individuals in these circumstances will be likely to describe a desire to use drugs but should express considerably more ambivalence (relative to abstinence-avoidance situations) about their intention to use drugs (e.g., "If this urge doesn't go away, maybe I'll drink"). Furthermore, if addicts were prompted, they might be able to provide some descriptions regarding the cognitive processing they are undertaking to avoid drug use (e.g., "I'm thinking that I should leave here, before I give in and have a drink").

As with urge responding in abstinence-avoidance situations, the activation of nonautomatic processing to stop automatic action plans should interfere with performance on concurrent tasks that also demand nonautomatic processing. In the clinic setting, it is not unusual to hear abstinent addicts complain that their urges and cravings disrupt their daily activities. Abstinent addicts often describe their battle with urges as an exhausting and effortful undertaking that demands concentration and vigilance. Ludwig (1988) provided vivid descriptions from alcoholics of the disruptive effect of bouts of craving on general functioning. Also, it is interesting that abstinent smokers who say their urges to smoke are affecting their lives relapse sooner than other ex-smokers (Brandon, Tiffany, & Baker, 1987). More than 70% of smokers in the Brandon et al. (1987) study who reported that urges were affecting their lives stated specifically that these urges were disrupting their thinking or functioning. This finding is entirely consistent with the conceptualization of urge responding proposed in this article: In addicts attempting abstinence, urges represent the operation of nonautomatic cognitive processes that serve to prevent the initiation or completion of drug-use action plans, but they operate at the cost of disruption of other activities that also demand nonautomatic processing.

Urge Responding and Drug Relapse

Although most models of drug urges have the assumption that urges and cravings are responsible for drug relapse, there have been surprisingly few studies on the role of drug urges in relapse (cf., Brandon et al., 1987; Ludwig, 1972; Marlatt & Gordon, 1980). Most investigators appear to accept as a given that urges always precede relapse, so evidence of relapse is generally interpreted as obviously indicative of the presence of urges (e.g., Shiffman, 1982; West & Schneider, 1987). For example, in a recent study of the factors that promote relapse to smoking, Baer and Lichtenstein (1988) followed up on 176 subjects for 1 year after the subjects completed a smoking-cessation program. As part of the follow-up interview, subjects who had relapsed were asked the following questions: "Were there any circumstances or sets of events which triggered off the desire to smoke?" and "Were there any inner thoughts or emotional feelings that triggered off the desire to smoke?" (Baer & Lichtenstein, 1988, p. 105). Subjects were never asked if they had any urge just before smoking, or, if they had, how strong that urge might have been.

I have already reviewed evidence that drug relapses can occur in the absence of self-reported urges. My interpretation of these data is that, given the right circumstances, the automatic action plans subserving drug use may be engaged and completed without activation of nonautomatic processes that generate urge responding. Abstinent addicts may be particularly prone to this kind of relapse episode if their nonautomatic processing is devoted to some other task (e.g., they are distracted) and the current environmental circumstances are completely supportive of the drug-use action plan (e.g., stimuli that trigger the plan are present, and the drug is readily available). These absentminded relapses may be an example of double-capture slips described by Reason (1979, 1984) as characteristic of much absentminded behavior.

Certainly many relapses are preceded by urge responding, and the contiguity of these two types of behaviors gives rise to the popular belief that urges are necessary for, and indeed cause, drug use. This analysis suggests an alternative version of the relationship between urge responding and drug relapse. Relapse occurs when the nonautomatic processing that gives rise to abstinence-promotion urge responding does not adequately impede the execution of the drug-use action plan. An examination of some factors that seem to be strongly associated with relapse may provide some suggestions for why nonautomatic processing may sometimes fail.

Relapsed addicts frequently report that stress and negative emotional states often immediately preceded their return to drug use (e.g., Baer & Lichtenstein, 1988; Bliss et al., 1989; Brandon et al., 1987; Condiotte & Lichtenstein, 1981; Marlatt & Gordon, 1980; O'Connell & Martin, 1987; Shiffman, 1982). A common interpretation of the apparent relationship between stress (negative affect) and relapse is that the former serves as a cue that elicits drug urges as a consequence of a history of using drugs in the presence of negative affect (e.g., Baker et al., 1987; Niaura et al., 1988; Poulos et al., 1981). A related explanation for this relationship is provided by Marlatt (1985), who proposed that negative affect elicits an expectation that drug use will relieve the individual's negative hedonic state. These expectations, manifested subjectively as cravings, motivate actual drug use. My analysis acknowledges that negative affect may provide stimulus conditions for the triggering of drug-use action schemata, although unlike the other theories, it does not posit that negative affect promotes drug use because it directly stimulates some urge state. Recent data by Payne, Schare, Levis, and Colletti (1987), showing that induction of negative mood increased cigarette consumption in smokers with no concomitant increase in self-reported urge to smoke, support this interpretation.

My theory suggests that negative affect may also promote relapse in one other way. Negative emotional states, or the situations that give rise to them, may invoke some degree of nonautomatic processing and, as a consequence, may compete with the nonautomatic processing required to prevent the execution of automatic drug-use action plans. Moreover, these emotional states might tend to inhibit the allocation of nonautomatic cognitive resources to the task of maintaining drug abstinence. For example, a person who is mildly depressed may not be able to maintain his or her motivation to fight off drug use (e.g., Shiffman, 1982; Shiffman & Jarvik, 1987).

Another factor that appears to be strongly associated with relapse, particularly in cigarette smokers, is the consumption of alcohol (Brandon et al., 1987; Shiffman, 1982, 1984). Baker et al. (1987) argued that alcohol may promote relapse because it serves to prime positive-affect urge structures that, as part of their activation, motivate further drug use (see Wise, 1988, for a similar argument regarding the possibility that nicotine may prime relapse in alcoholics). The model of drug-use action plans could accommodate the hypothesis that alcohol consumption may be one of the stimulus conditions that might be encoded within the action schema for some smokers. Certainly, alcohol consumption and smoking are frequently associated activities in many cigarette smokers (e.g., Adesso, 1979; Istvan & Matarazzo, 1984; Mello, Mendelson, Sellers, & Kuehnle, 1980). Recently, Nil et al. (1984) showed that alcohol consumption in nondeprived smokers intensified cigarette consumption with no concordant changes in self-reported desire to smoke. These data support the hypothesis that alcohol may promote increased cigarette consumption without mediation by urge processing. Consumption of alcohol might provide another type of trigger condition for the elicitation of automatized drug-use action plans, thus partially accounting for the strong association between alcohol use and smoking relapse.

Another possibility is that alcohol consumption may reduce the efficiency of nonautomatic processes that might be applied to deter the execution of a drug-use action plan. Schneider et al. (1984) have reviewed data suggesting that alcohol tends to have substantial deleterious effects on controlled (i.e., nonautomatic) processing, whereas automatic skills tend to be resistant to the effects of alcohol. Data collected by Shiffman (1982) indicate that smokers in a relapse crisis who had consumed alcohol were less likely to engage in behavioral coping in an attempt to avoid smoking. Furthermore, Shiffman's (1982) results indicate that the efficacy of coping in preventing relapse was reduced when the smoker had consumed alcohol. If, as I assume, coping responses during abstinence-promotion situations are the product of nonautomatic processes, then my interpretation of these data would be that alcohol consumption may increase the probability of relapse to the extent that it disrupts this cognitive activity.

Proposed Tests of the Model

With the model presented in this article, I attempt to provide a comprehensive account of the cognitive organization of drug-use behavior and urge processing in the addict. My theory furnishes predictions for several domains of addictive behavior that are either not anticipated by any other formal conceptualization or are in direct contravention to predictions derived from selected models of drug urges and drug-use behavior. These predictions are outlined in the following sections.

Urge Elicitation and Manifestations of Nonautomatic Processing

According to this model, drug urges represent the operation of nonautomatic cognitive processes activated to facilitate or impede the execution of automatized drug-use action schemata. The operation of nonautomatic processes that give rise to urge responding could be revealed through various indexes. For example, urge responding should be associated with interference on concurrent tasks that require nonautomatic processing for their successful completion. The dual-task procedure has been used extensively in cognitive research to demonstrate the extent to which performance on a primary task uses some limited processing capacity (Kerr, 1973; Posner, 1978, 1982). In a typical application of this procedure, subjects are instructed to respond quickly to a probe stimulus (e.g., to press a button when a tone is presented) concurrent with the presentation of a primary task that presumably requires some degree of cognitive effort (e.g., anagram solution). Reaction times to the probe stimulus are assumed to be related positively to the amount of cognitive effort required by the primary task (e.g., Tyler, Hertel, McCallum, & Ellis, 1979).

The dual-task paradigm could be used in studies of the cognitive processes subserving urge responding by requiring addicts to respond quickly to a probe stimulus while urge responding is concurrently activated. Response times to the probe should increase to the extent that urge-related nonautomatic processing has been simultaneously engaged. This result could be compared with a dual-task situation in which the primary task involved actual drug-use behavior. To the extent that drug consumption is controlled by relatively automatized processes, such performance should have a less deleterious impact on probe-task performance. Furthermore, the magnitude of disruption on the secondary task should be related negatively to the degree to which the drug-use sequence has been automated. Consequently, estimates of previous practice of the drug-use sequence, such as frequency and duration of previous drug use, would be correlated negatively with reaction times to the probe stimulus. These predictions, consistent with considerations of the impact of automatic and nonautomatic processing on secondary task performance, would seem to be anticipated uniquely by the theory proposed in this article.

The processing demands of nonautomatic activity subserving urge responding should also be evident in certain physiological indexes of problem-solving activity. For example, increases in heart rate and decreases in heart rate variability during urge processing should reflect, in part, the cognitive difficulty of the eliciting task (e.g., Boyce, 1974; Carroll et al., 1986; Luczak, 1979; Obrist, 1976). Thus, researchers should be able to manipulate systematically the difficulty level of urge-eliciting situations and to observe corresponding changes in the magnitude and variability of cardiac responses. Furthermore, physiological responding during urge-producing situations should be more strongly associated with reports of the difficulty of the problem presented by the eliciting task, estimates of the cognitive effort required by the task, and descriptions of the anticipated behavioral demands of acts necessary to impede or facilitate drug-use schemata than with self-report of urges. This is in direct contrast to urge theories that view certain patterns of physiological responses and urge reports as parallel manifestations of drug-motivational states (e.g., Baker et al., 1987) or that argue that conditioned physiological responses provide a substrate necessary for the production of urges and cravings (e.g., Ludwig & Wikler, 1974; Poulos et al., 1981; West & Schneider, 1987).

I have proposed that physiological responding manifested during urge activation is indicative primarily of effortful cognitive processing and somatovisceral adjustments in support of anticipated or implemented situation-specific motor responses. This interpretation of the physiology observed during urge responding can be contrasted with two different conceptualizations. Baker et al. (1987) have hypothesized the existence of two urge states and have argued that the patterns of physiology associated with urge states elicited by negative mood should mimic the physiology of drug withdrawal, whereas urges generated by positive mood should be characterized by physiological responses that parallel the activating or stimulant effects of drugs. Alternatively, theories that emphasize a conditioned withdrawal or conditioned compensatory response origin of drug urges (Ludwig & Wikler, 1974; Melchior & Tabakoff, 1984; Pomerleau, 1981; Poulos et al., 1981; Wikler, 1948) posit that withdrawallike physiology should distinguish urge responding regardless of the eliciting stimulus conditions. These conceptualizations of urge physiology can be translated directly into experimental tests that offer straightforward evaluations of the differential predictions generated by the three approaches. For example, as is well documented, one of the stimulant effects of nicotine is a pronounced tachycardia (Benowitz, Jacob, Jones, & Rosenberg, 1982; Benowitz, Kuyt, & Jacob, 1984; Porchet, Benowitz, & Steiner, 1988), and nicotine withdrawal is characterized by bradycardia (American Psychiatric Association, 1987; Gilbert & Pope, 1982; West, Russell, Jarvis, & Feyerabend, 1984). Consequently, the Baker et al. (1987) model mandates that smoking urges produced by positive or negative mood inductions be associated with increases or decreases, respectively, in heart rate, whereas conditioned withdrawal models require that urges produced through either a negative or positive mood manipulation be associated with a withdrawallike decrease in heart rate. Finally, the theory described in this article would predict that smoking urges generated through positive and negative mood inductions will display patterns of cardiac responding indicative of cognitive effort and support physiology, that is, a tendency toward increased heart rate and decreased cardiac variability.

An evaluation of the predictions outlined thus far is predicated on the assumption that drug urges can be manipulated in a controlled laboratory setting. Most urge research has been restricted to an examination of the natural variability of self-reported urges in abstinent subjects participating in some sort of treatment program (e.g., Erickson, Tiffany, Martin, & Baker, 1983; Shiffman & Jarvik, 1987; West, Hajek, & Belcher, 1987) or in subjects instructed to remain abstinent for some period of time (e.g., Baker et al., 1987; Glassman, Jackson, Walsh, Roose, & Rosenfeld, 1984; Rankin et al., 1979; West & Russell, 1985). Another strategy for studying urges and cravings has been to present subjects with stimuli that presumably have been strongly associated with drug use over the history of the addictive disorder. This exposure paradigm has been moderately successful in the production of self-reported urges in cigarette smokers, alcoholics, and heroin addicts (for reviews of this methodology, see Baker et al., 1987; Niaura et al., 1988; Sherman, Jorenby, & Baker, in press). Unfortunately, these stimulus-presentation procedures are somewhat limited for my purposes in that they do not lend themselves to a convenient manipulation of theoretically relevant stimulus content. In most of these studies, the stimuli (e.g., the sight of another smoker smoking, the smell of an alcoholic beverage, and videotapes of heroin addicts shooting up) are merely present or absent on a given trial. According to the perspective outlined in this article, urge responding requires the concurrent activation of drug-use action schemata along with nonautomatic processing in service of the facilitation or impedance of the automatized drug-use sequence. The cue-exposure paradigm as it is typically used may be more or less successful in activating portions of a drug-use action schema, but the extent and the content of the nonautomatic processing concurrently activated will depend on factors that are generally not explicitly controlled in these studies. So, for instance, the intentions of the addicts regarding abstinence (i.e., are they attempting to avoid or promote abstinence) and the availability of drug or the difficulty in obtaining drug (either within the exposure session or outside of it) should influence the nature and magnitude of the nonautomatic processing activated in the situation.

I have begun evaluating an imagery manipulation as an alternative to the in vivo cue-exposure procedure for the production of urge responses in a laboratory setting. My approach, patterned after the paradigm used by Lang et al. (1980) in studies of fear behavior, provides an excellent method for manipulating urge-relevant information with concurrent monitoring of verbal and psychophysiological output. In my research, smokers are presented with audiotaped imagery scripts and instructed to vividly imagine the scene being described. A colleague and I (Hakenewerth & Tiffany, 1988) have determined that scripts containing descriptions of smoking-urge situations (urge scripts) elicit substantially stronger reports of smoking urges than do scripts devoid of explicit urge content (neutral scripts). Furthermore, relative to neutral scripts, urge scripts produce significant increases in heart rate and significantly higher levels of tonic skin conductance during imagery trials. Thus, this procedure shows excellent promise as an effective method for manipulating urge responding in a laboratory setting.

The advantage of the imagery procedure over an in vivo cue-exposure paradigm is the ease with which stimulus content can be manipulated simply by encoding different material within imagery scripts. For instance, a colleague and I (Tiffany & Drobes, in press) recently investigated the impact of affect on urge responding in cigarette smokers by adding descriptors of positive and negative affect to imagery scripts (both neutral and urge scripts) and assessing self-report of smoking urges and cravings. Our data showed clearly that scripts containing descriptions of smoking urges elicited strong reports of smoking urges and cravings that were comparable in magnitude across positive and negative affective content. Among scripts that did not explicitly describe smoking urges, negative-affect scripts were more effective in generating urges and cravings than positive-affect scripts, although positive-affect scripts produced significantly stronger urges and cravings than did neutral-affect scripts.

In future research, I will be incorporating physiological assessments into this imagery manipulation to evaluate predictions regarding the patterning and directionality of physiological responding associated with urges produced through imagery scripts containing descriptions of negative or positive affect. These imagery procedures could also be combined with an auditory probe task to assess the extent to which urge processing interferes with other forms of nonautomatized cognitive activity. Thus, subjects could be instructed to vividly imagine abstinence-avoidance or abstinence-promotion scenarios of varying degrees of intractability while engaging in a secondary, auditory probe task. To the extent that urge processing interferes with the cognitive operations required by the probe task, reaction times to the probes should increase as a function of the difficulty level of the urge scenario.

The Structure of Urge Report and Its Relationship to Drug Use

A clear implication of the present model is that the verbal manifestations of urge responding should differ as a function of whether nonautomatic processing is engaged in an effort to impede or facilitate the execution of an automatized drug-use action schema. Both circumstances will invoke descriptions of desire to consume drug, but an intention to actually engage in drug-use behavior should be a more prominent component of urge report in abstinence-avoidance situations than in abstinence-promotion situations. Moreover, the focus of any problem-solving or planning activities described by the individual should differ across these two situations: Cognitive activity during abstinence promotion will be directed against drug use; cognitive activity during abstinence avoidance will be in service of the action schema.

A core assumption of the model I have presented is that urge responding is not necessary for the initiation or maintenance of automatized drug-use sequences. This is not to suggest that under some circumstances there could not be a fairly strong association between selected components of urge report and certain aspects of drug-use behavior. The model specifies that in abstinence-avoidance situations, urge report in general and intention to use drug in particular would be most strongly correlated with latency to initial drug use and the degree of effort expended to obtain drug. These are components of drug-use behavior that, in situations in which the action schema is interrupted, would tend to be under the control of nonautomatic processing. The model suggests further that general urge report or stated intention to use drug would display only a modest association, if any, with the amount of drug that is self-administered or the pattern of administration once use is initiated. This prediction is derived from the contention that these aspects of drug use are controlled by automatized action schemata rather than the nonautomatic processes that give rise to the urge report. Because all other models of drug urges tend to view urge report as an index of a drug-motivational state that, in turn, influences the initiation and magnitude of drug consumption in the addict, it is not clear that any other theory would, a priori, predict a lower association between urge report and amount or pattern of drug administration than between urge report and latency to initial administration.

Current strategies in the assessment of verbal reports of urges may be inadequate for evaluating these hypotheses regarding the verbal manifestations of urge processing. Most researchers rely on only one or two face-valid items of unknown reliability when asking subjects about drug urges (e.g., Childress, McLellan, & O'Brien, 1986; Cooney et al., 1984; Ikard & Tomkins, 1973; Mirin, Meyer, & McNamee, 1976; Nil et al., 1984; West et al., 1987; West & Russell, 1985). Although in the case of cigarette smoking some researchers have developed longer (e.g., five or six items) questionnaires of smoking urges (Shiffman & Jarvik, 1976; West, Jarvis, Russell, Carruthers, & Feyerabend, 1984), the usefulness of these is limited by the small sample sizes used to evaluate item characteristics and their theoretically limiting assumption that smoking urges are unidimensional subjective states directly representative of drug-motivational processes. The model I have proposed suggests that the verbal structure of drug urges may be more complex than can be captured by current urge assessments. For example, it is unfortunate from the perspective of this model that no current urge assessments directly evaluate an addict's intentions or plans to use drug. Questionnaires with more diverse item content may need to be developed to allow multidimensional aspects of the verbal report of urges to emerge.[4]

Organization of Drug-Use Behavior

Over the course of an addictive disorder, drug-use behavior should take on the general characteristics of automatized functioning. These should be manifest as patterns of stimulus-bound drug acquisition and administration that are stereotyped, effortless, difficult to impede, initiated and completed without intention, and enacted in the absence of awareness. There are several ways that these features of automaticity might be assessed. For example, an examination of the behavioral sequences in support of the acquisition and consumption of drug should show that they become increasingly stereotyped or less variable over time. Stereotyped alcohol consumption is a commonly accepted hallmark of alcoholism (e.g., Edwards, Gross, Keller, & Moser, 1976) and has been observed in laboratory studies of chronic alcoholics (Sobell, Schaefer, & Mills, 1972). Similarly, heavy cigarette smokers are remarkably consistent in their smoking behavior, not only with regard to the regularity of their smoking across days (e.g., Griffiths & Henningfield, 1982; Griffiths, Henningfield, & Bigelow, 1982) but also with respect to patterns of smoking behavior across cigarettes (e.g., Bättig, Buzzi, & Nil, 1982; Nil et al., 1984). In general, stereotyped drug-use behavior should be characteristic of all drug-abuse disorders to the extent that the user has had consistent practice under relatively fixed stimulus conditions of the actions subserving drug acquisition and drug administration.

Another method of assessing the automaticity of drug-use sequences would be to have addicts report the extent to which their drug-use behavior displays major features of automaticity. An automaticity factor has emerged consistently in factor analyses of questionnaires designed to evaluate reasons for smoking (Costa, MacCrae, & Bossé, 1980; Ikard, Green, & Horn, 1969; Russell, Peto, & Patel, 1974). The automaticity scale that can be derived from these questionnaires may be of limited usefulness because it consists of only four items that tend to address a single facet of automaticity, that is, absence of conscious control.[5] A comprehensive evaluation of self-described automated drug-use behaviors would require the development of an instrument that includes all core features of the automaticity concept as described by this theory.

Researchers should be able to find evidence of automatic processes controlling drug-use behaviors by studying the effects of disruption of self-administration sequences in experienced drug users. A relevant manipulation would be to require addicts to administer drug in a fashion that is close but not identical to their usual pattern of consumption. For example, smokers could be instructed to smoke with their nonpreferred hand and hold their cigarette differently than they typically would. Drug administration under these conditions, relative to normal consumption behaviors, should lead to a decline in secondary task performance (e.g., slowed auditory probe reaction time), increased urge report, and physiological reactivity associated with nonautomatic processing allocated to the inhibition of selected portions of the drug-use action schema. (Enhanced somatovisceral responding may also reflect the increased behavioral demands of the alternative administration actions.) There might even be indications of electromyographic activity in muscle groups generally involved in drug self-administration to the extent that the drug user was not completely successful in gating out automatized motor sequences.

All indexes of automatization, whether they be direct, such as stereotyped drug use, or indirect, such as the sequelae of schemata disruption, should be related strongly to the amount of practice the user has had with the drug-use pattern. Indeed, researchers should be able to predict a more exact relationship between practice of drug-use sequences and certain manifestations of automaticity. If drug-use behaviors are conceptualized as skills that become increasingly automatized with consistent practice, then, like nearly all other forms of skill acquisition (Lane, 1987; Logan, 1988; Newell & Rosenbloom, 1981), the relationship between previous trials of drug administration under fixed-stimulus conditions and selected indexes of automaticity (e.g., the reduction in variability in patterns of administration) should conform to a power function. That is, plotting the logarithm of a measure of automaticity against the logarithm of practice trials of drug administration should yield a straight line. This prediction could be evaluated in longitudinal studies of individuals over the course of their drug-use careers,

[4] As an example of this strategy, I and my colleagues are currently evaluating a 32-item questionnaire developed in our laboratory in order to assess urges and cravings in cigarette smokers (Questionnaire of Smoking Urges, QSU). Four theoretically distinct conceptualizations of drug urges are represented in this questionnaire: desire to smoke, intention to smoke, anticipation of positive outcome from smoking, and anticipation of relief from nicotine withdrawal or negative emotion. The diversity of item content should provide a clearer picture of the semantic structure of urge report in cigarette smokers. Our initial factor analysis of the questionnaire indicates that self-reports of smoking urges in ongoing smokers are multifactorial and that intentions and plans to smoke are major components of one of the most prominent factors.

[5] The Automaticity factor on the Ikard, Green, and Horn (1969) questionnaire consists of the following items: "I've found a cigarette in my mouth and didn't remember putting it there," "I light up a cigarette without realizing I still have one burning in the ashtray," "I smoke cigarettes automatically without even being aware of it," and "I smoke cigarettes just from habit, without even really wanting the one I'm smoking." The Automatic factor scores consistently show moderate to strong correlations with the Addict factor scores derived from the same questionnaires (Costa, MacCrae, & Bossé, 1980; Ikard et al., 1969; Leventhal & Avis, 1976; Russell, Peto, & Patel, 1974). The Addict factor consists of items that indicate the extent to which the smoker feels uncomfortable or experiences desires to smoke when cigarettes are unavailable. According to the terminology of the theory presented in this article, this factor could be interpreted easily as one describing abstinence-avoidance urge situations. Consequently, it would not be surprising that the extent to which a smoker reports abstinence-avoidance urges is related to the degree to which smoking behavior is automatized.

or in cross-sectional studies of large groups of subjects having various levels of drug usage. A complete evaluation of this proposal would require accurate estimates of previous drug-use practice trials, examinations of manifestations of automaticity under eliciting stimulus conditions similar to those that prevailed during previous practice, and use of automaticity indexes with ratio or interval scale properties. (This last requirement would probably exclude the use of self-report measures of automaticity.)

Absentminded Relapse

Although relapses in the absence of self-reported urges or other indexes of urge processing may constitute a substantial portion of relapse episodes, no systematic research has been conducted on this phenomenon. This is not surprising, because the general concept of relapses without precipitating urges or cravings is antithetical to basic premises of most models of drug urges and drug-use behavior. Examples of urgeless relapse represent a serious challenge to theories of addiction that assume that urges are a necessary component of the relapse process. The theory advanced in this article would characterize many of these relapse episodes as variants of absentminded behavior, that is, relapses that occur when the action schemata controlling drug use are fully engaged with little or no concurrent activation of nonautomatic processing directed toward impeding the action schemata. Relapses of this sort may display degrees of absentmindedness. At one extreme would be the situation in which the abstinent addict is not even aware that he or she is engaging in drug use until the sequence is already well under way. Less dramatic, but perhaps more common, would be the situation in which addicts are more or less cognizant of the unfolding of their drug-use behavior and may also be fully aware of some previous intention to remain abstinent, but simply fail to deploy nonautomatic processes to stop the action schema. In such relapses executive systems seem to be merely along for the ride, monitoring the progress of the automatic sequences but not intervening.

A consideration of the role of automatic and nonautomatic cognitive processing in drug relapse leads to the prediction that the likelihood of absentminded relapse should increase as a function of four factors. First, such relapse should be more common in long-term, heavy users who tend to consume drug under fixed-stimulus conditions. In general, addicts whose drug-use behavior is controlled strongly by highly automatized action schemata should be more prone to absentminded relapse. Second, the setting in which the relapse occurs would probably be one that is strongly associated with previous drug use but that has not been encountered frequently over the course of the current abstinence attempt. These settings would contain stimulus configurations that clearly match those encoded within the action schemata, but their ability to trigger the action schema would not have declined as a consequence of nonreinforced exposures. Third, the situation would be characterized by ready availability of drug with limited constraints on its use. In the absence of these conditions, nonautomatic processing would have to be invoked to facilitate the execution of the action plan. Finally, absentminded relapse, like many other forms of action slips (e.g., Norman, 1981; Reason, 1979, 1984), should be more likely when nonautomatic cognitive resour are otherwise engaged. For example, the individual might concentrating on a difficult task, preoccupied with some otl activity, or experiencing intense negative affect, any of whi would decrease the availability of cognitive resources direct toward inhibiting a drug-use action schema. Nonautoma processes may also not be directed against the execution of t action schema if the coordination of executive processes we disrupted, or the total pool of available cognitive processes we restricted, as a result of other drug use (such as alcohol) or b cause of fatigue.

Summary and Conclusions

A review of contemporary models of drug urges suggests th they can be categorized according to whether they emphasi drug withdrawal or the positive, appetitive effects of drugs i the genesis of drug urges and cravings. An assumption commo to all of these theories is that urges represent subjective, motiva tional–emotional states that are necessary but not sufficient fo the production of drug-use behavior in ongoing addicts and ar responsible for the initiation of relapse in abstinent addicts Most theories also assume that the operation of urges and crav ings can be indexed across three classes of behavior: verbal re port, overt behavior, and somatovisceral response. The available data do not provide strong support for the assumption that responses across these classes of behavior are necessarily strongly associated. One implication of the lack of coherence across these putative manifestations of drug urges may be that the processes that control drug-use behavior might operate independently of those responsible for urge responding.

I have drawn from the cognitive concepts of automatic and nonautomatic processing to develop an alternative model of drug use and drug urges. This model proposes that drug-use behavior in the addict represents activity controlled largely by automatic processes. Thus, drug-use behaviors represent skills that are relatively fast and efficient, stimulus bound, initiated and completed without intention, difficult to impede, cognitively effortless, and capable of being enacted in the absence of awareness. I hypothesized that the procedures for enacting these automatized skills are organized in unitized memory structures in the form of action schemata that contain adequate information for the initiation and coordination of complex sequences of drug-use behavior. Urges and cravings are conceptualized as responses supported by nonautomatic cognitive processes. These are activated in parallel with drug-use action schemata either in support of the action schema (abstinence-avoidance urges) or in support of attempts to block or impede the execution of a drug-use action schema (abstinence-promotion urges). The manifestations of nonautomatic processing in urge situations can be indexed across three broad classes of behavior: overt behavioral acts, somatovisceral responses, and verbal report. The implications of this model for the assessment of urge responding have been outlined, and several studies designed to evaluate hypotheses derived from this conceptualization of urge processing and drug-use behavior have been proposed.

The data derived from the study of drug urges and cravings are of insufficient quality and too loosely tied to theory for evaluation of any of the contemporary models of drug urges. Certainly the model presented in this article is generally consistent with extant data on drug urges and the relationships between urge responding and drug-use behavior. There are very little new data from studies that provide critical tests of hypotheses generated from the theory. The results of studies proposed in this article would indicate the extent to which this conceptualization provides a viable model of drug urges and drug-use behavior and would also indicate where the model needs revision and clarification. At the very least, I believe that this approach provides a distinct alternative to other contemporary models of drug urges.

References

Abrams, D. B., Monti, P. M., Carey, K. B., Pinto, R. P., & Jacobus, S. I. (1988). Reactivity to smoking cues and relapse: Two studies of discriminant validity. *Behaviour Research and Therapy, 26,* 225–233.

Adesso, V. J. (1979). Some correlates between cigarette smoking and alcohol use. *Addictive Behaviors, 4,* 269–273.

Allport, D. A. (1980). Attention and performance. In G. Claxton (Ed.), *Cognitive psychology: New directions* (pp. 112–153). London: Routledge & Kegan Paul.

Allport, D. A., Antonis, B., & Reynolds, P. (1972). On the division of attention: A disproof of the single channel hypothesis. *Quarterly Journal of Experimental Psychology, 24,* 225–235.

American Psychiatric Association (1980). *Diagnostic and statistical manual of mental disorders* (3rd ed.). Washington, DC: Author.

American Psychiatric Association (1987). *Diagnostic and statistical manual of mental disorders* (3rd ed., rev.). Washington, DC: Author.

Baer, J. S., & Lichtenstein, E. (1988). Classification and prediction of smoking relapse episodes: An exploration of individual differences. *Journal of Consulting and Clinical Psychology, 56,* 104–110.

Baker, T. B., Morse, E., & Sherman, J. E. (1987). The motivation to use drugs: A psychobiological analysis of urges. In P. C. Rivers (Ed.), *The Nebraska symposium on motivation: Alcohol use and abuse* (pp. 257–323). Lincoln: University of Nebraska Press.

Baker, T. B., & Tiffany, S. T. (1985). Morphine tolerance as habituation. *Psychological Review, 92,* 78–108.

Bättig, K., Buzzi, R., & Nil, R. (1982). Smoke yield of cigarettes and puffing behavior in men and women. *Psychopharmacology, 76,* 139–148.

Benowitz, N. L., Jacob, P., Jones, R. T., & Rosenberg, J. (1982). Interindividual variability in the metabolism and cardiovascular effects of nicotine in man. *Journal of Pharmacology and Experimental Therapeutics, 221,* 368–372.

Benowitz, N. L., Kuyt, F., & Jacob, P. (1984). Influence of nicotine on cardiovascular and hormonal effects of cigarette smoking. *Clinical Pharmacology and Therapeutics, 36,* 74–81.

Bliss, R. E., Garvey, A. J., Heinhold, J. W., & Hitchcock, J. L. (1989). The influence of situation and coping on relapse crisis outcomes after smoking cessation. *Journal of Consulting and Clinical Psychology, 57,* 443–449.

Boyce, P. R. (1974). Sinus arrhythmia as a measure of mental load. *Ergonomics, 17,* 177–183.

Brandon, T. H., Tiffany, S. T., & Baker, T. B. (1987). Characterization of the process of smoking relapse. In F. Tims & C. Leukefeld (Eds.), *Relapse and recovery in drug abuse* (National Institute on Drug Abuse Research Monograph No. 72, pp. 104–117). Washington, DC: U.S. Government Printing Office.

Cacioppo, J. T., Petty, R. E., & Morris, K. T. (1985). Semantic, evaluative, and self-referent processing: Memory, cognitive effort, and somatovisceral activity. *Psychophysiology, 22,* 371–384.

Carroll, D., Turner, J. R., & Hellawell, J. C. (1986). Heart rate and oxygen consumption during active psychological challenge: The effects of level of difficulty. *Psychophysiology, 23,* 174–181.

Childress, A. R., McLellan, A. T., & O'Brien, C. P. (1986). Abstinent opiate abusers exhibit conditioned craving, conditioned withdrawal and reductions in both through extinction. *British Journal of Addiction, 81,* 655–660.

Condiotte, M. M., & Lichtenstein, E. (1981). Self-efficacy and relapse in smoking cessation programs. *Journal of Consulting and Clinical Psychology, 49,* 648–658.

Cooney, N. L., Baker, L. H., Pomerleau, O. F., & Josephy, B. (1984). Salivation to drinking cues in alcohol abusers: Toward the validation of a physiological measure of craving. *Addictive Behaviors, 9,* 91–94.

Costa, P. T., MacCrae, R. R., & Bossé, R. (1980). Smoking motive factors: A review and replication. *The International Journal of the Addictions, 15,* 537–549.

Eddy, N. B. (1973). Prediction of drug dependence and abuse liability. In L. Goldberg & F. Hoffmeister (Eds.), *Bayer Symposium IV, psychic dependence: Definition, assessment in animals and man. Theoretical and clinical implications* (pp. 192–198). New York: Springer-Verlag.

Edwards, O., Arif, A., & Hodgson, R. (1981). Nomenclature and classification of drug- and alcohol-related problems: A WHO memorandum. *Bulletin of the World Health Organization, 59,* 225–242.

Edwards, G., Gross, M. M., Keller, M., & Moser, J. (1976). Alcohol-related problems in the disability perspective. *Journal of Studies on Alcohol, 37,* 1360–1382.

Eikelboom, R., & Stewart, J. (1982). Conditioning of drug-induced physiological responses. *Psychological Review, 89,* 507–528.

Elliott, R. (1974). The motivational significance of heart rate. In P. A. Obrist, A. H. Black, J. Brener, & L. V. DiCara (Eds.), *Cardiovascular psychophysiology: Current issues in response mechanisms, biofeedback and methodology* (pp. 505–537). Chicago: Aldine.

Engle, K. B., & Williams, T. K. (1972). Effect of an ounce of vodka on alcoholics' desire for alcohol. *Quarterly Journal of Studies on Alcohol, 33,* 1099–1105.

Erickson, L. M., Tiffany, S. T., Martin, E. M., & Baker, T. B. (1983). Aversive smoking therapies: Conditioning analysis of therapeutic effectiveness. *Behaviour Research and Therapy, 21,* 595–611.

Flaherty, J. A., McGuire, H. T., & Gatski, R. L. (1955). The psychodynamics of the "dry drunk." *American Journal of Psychiatry, 112,* 460–464.

Fletcher, C., & Doll, R. (1969). A survey of doctors' attitudes to smoking. *British Journal of Preventive and Social Medicine, 23,* 145–153.

Fowles, D. C. (1980). The three arousal model: Implications of Gray's two-factor learning theory for heart rate, electrodermal activity, and psychopathy. *Psychophysiology, 17,* 87–104.

Gilbert, R. M., & Pope, M. A. (1982). Early effects of quitting smoking. *Psychopharmacology, 285,* 537–540.

Glassman, A. H., Jackson, W. K., Walsh, B. T., Roose, S. P., & Rosenfeld, B. (1984). Cigarette craving, smoking withdrawal, and clonidine. *Science, 226,* 864–866.

Gliner, J. A., Bunnell, D. E., & Horvath, S. M. (1982). Hemodynamic and metabolic changes prior to speech performance. *Physiological Psychology, 10,* 108–113.

Goudie, A. J., & Demellweek, C. (1986). Conditioning factors in drug tolerance. In S. R. Goldberg & I. P. Stolerman (Eds.), *Behavioral analysis of drug dependence* (pp. 225–285). New York: Academic Press.

Gray, J. A. (1982). *The neurophysiology of anxiety.* New York: Oxford University Press.

Griffiths, R. R., & Henningfield, J. E. (1982). Experimental analysis of human cigarette smoking behavior. *Federation Proceedings, 41,* 234–240.

Griffiths, R. R., Henningfield, J. E., & Bigelow, G. E. (1982). Human cigarette smoking: Manipulation of number of puffs per bout, inter-bout interval and nicotine dose. *Journal of Pharmacology and Experimental Therapeutics, 220,* 256–265.

Gunne, L. M., (1960). The temperature response in rats during acute and chronic morphine administration: A study of morphine tolerance. *Archives Internationales de Pharmacodynamie et Therapie, 129,* 416–428.

Hakenewerth, D. M., & Tiffany, S. T. (1988, March). *The production of smoking urges through an imagery manipulation: Preliminary data.* Paper presented at the Conference on Theory and Research in Psychopathology, Performance, and Cognition, Gainesville, FL.

Hasher, L., & Zacks, R. T. (1979). Automatic and effortful processes in memory. *Journal of Experimental Psychology: General, 108,* 356–388.

Henningfield, J. E., Lukas, S. E., & Bigelow, G. E. (1986). Human studies of drugs as reinforcers. In S. R. Goldberg, & I. P. Stolerman (Eds.), *Behavioral analysis of drug dependence* (pp. 69–122). New York: Academic Press.

Hinson, R. E., & Siegel, S. (1982). Nonpharmacological bases of drug tolerance and dependence. *Journal of Psychosomatic Research, 26,* 495–503.

Hodgson, R., Rankin, H., & Stockwell, T. (1979). Alcohol dependence and the priming effect. *Behaviour Research and Therapy, 17,* 379–387.

Hughes, J. R., & Hatsukami, D. K. (1986). Signs and symptoms of tobacco withdrawal. *Archives of General Psychiatry, 43,* 289–294.

Ikard, F. F., Green, D., & Horn, D. (1969). A scale to differentiate between types of smoking as related to the management of affect. *The International Journal of the Addictions, 4,* 649–659.

Ikard, F. F., & Tomkins, S. (1973). The experience of affect as a determinant of smoking behavior: A series of validity studies. *Journal of Abnormal Psychology, 81,* 172–181.

Isbell, H. (1955). Craving for alcohol. *Quarterly Journal of Studies on Alcohol, 16,* 38–42.

Istvan, J., & Matarazzo, J. D. (1984). Tobacco, alcohol and caffeine use: A review of their interrelationships. *Psychological Bulletin, 95,* 301–326.

James, W. (1890). *Principles of psychology* (Vol. 1). New York: Holt.

Jellinek, E. M. (1955). The "craving" for alcohol. *Quarterly Journal of Studies on Alcohol, 16,* 35–38.

Jellinek, E. M. (1960). *The disease concept of alcoholism.* New Brunswick, NJ: Hillhouse Press.

Jones, R. T. (1980). Human effects: An overview. In R. C. Peterson (Ed.), *Marijuana research findings: 1980* (pp. 54–80). Washington, DC: National Institute on Drug Abuse.

Jones, R. T. (1984). The pharmacology of cocaine. In J. Grabowski (Ed.), *Cocaine: Pharmacology, effects, and treatment of abuse* (pp. 34–53). Washington, DC: National Institute on Drug Abuse.

Jonides, J., Naveh-Benjamin, M., & Palmer, J. (1985). Assessing automaticity. *Acta Psychologica, 60,* 157–171.

Kahneman, D., & Treisman, A. M. (1984). Changing views of attention and automaticity. In R. Parasuraman & R. Davies (Eds.), *Varieties of attention* (pp. 29–61). New York: Academic Press.

Kalant, H. (1977). Comparative aspects of tolerance to, and dependence on, alcohol, barbiturates, and opiates. In M. M. Gross (Ed.), *Alcohol intoxication and withdrawal III* (pp. 169–186). New York: Plenum Press.

Kalant, H., LeBlanc, A. E., & Gibbons, R. J. (1971). Tolerance to, and dependence on, some nonopiate psychotropic drugs. *Pharmacological Reviews, 23,* 135–191.

Kaplan, R. F., Cooney, N. L., Baker, L. H., Gillespie, R. A., Meyer, R. E., & Pomerleau, O. F. (1985). Reactivity to alcohol-related cues: Physiological and subjective responses in alcoholics and nonproblem drinkers. *Journal of Studies on Alcohol, 46,* 267–272.

Kaplan, R. F., Meyer, R. E., & Stroebel, C. F. (1983). Alcohol dependence and responsivity to an ethanol stimulus as predictors of alcohol consumption. *British Journal of Addiction, 78,* 259–267.

Kerr, B. (1973). Processing demands during mental operations. *Memory & Cognition, 1,* 401–412.

Kihlstrom, J. F. (1987). The cognitive unconscious. *Science, 237,* 1445–1451.

Kozlowski, L. T., & Wilkinson, D. A. (1987a). Comments on Kozlowski and Wilkinson's 'use and misuse of the concept of craving by alcohol, tobacco, and drug researchers': A reply from the authors. *British Journal of Addiction, 82,* 489–492.

Kozlowski, L. T., & Wilkinson, D. A. (1987b). Use and misuse of the concept of craving by alcohol, tobacco, and drug researchers. *British Journal of Addiction, 82,* 31–36.

Krank, M. D. (1987). Conditioned hyperalgesia depends on the pain sensitivity measure. *Behavioral Neuroscience, 101,* 854–857.

Krank, M. D., Hinson, R. E., & Siegel, S. (1981). Conditioned hyperalgesia is elicited by environmental signals of morphine. *Behavioral and Neural Biology, 32,* 148–157.

Laberg, J. C., & Ellertsen, B. (1987). Psychophysiological indicators of craving in alcoholics: Effects of cue exposure. *British Journal of Addiction, 82,* 1341–1348.

LaBerge, D., & Samuels, S. J. (1974). Toward a theory of automatic information processing in reading. *Cognitive Psychology, 6,* 293–323.

Lane, N. E. (1987). *Skill acquisition rates and patterns: Issues and training applications.* New York: Springer-Verlag.

Lang, P. J. (1979). A bioinformational theory of emotional imagery. *Psychophysiology, 16,* 495–512.

Lang, P. J. (1984). Cognition in emotion: Concept and action. In C. Izard, J. Kagan, & R. Zajonc (Eds.), *Emotion, cognition, and behavior* (pp. 192–226). New York: Cambridge University Press.

Lang, P. J. (1985). The cognitive psychophysiology of emotion: Fear and anxiety. In A. H. Tuma & J. D. Mazer (Eds.), *Anxiety and the anxiety disorders* (pp. 131–170). Hillsdale, NJ: Erlbaum.

Lang, P. J., Kozak, M. J., Miller, G. A., Levin, D. N., & McLean, A., Jr. (1980). Emotional imagery: Conceptual structure and pattern of somatovisceral response. *Psychophysiology, 17,* 179–192.

Leventhal, H., & Avis, N. (1976). Pleasure, addiction and habit: Factors in verbal report or factors in smoking behavior? *Journal of Abnormal Psychology, 85,* 478–488.

Lindesmith, A. R. (1968). *Addiction and opiates.* Chicago: Aldine.

Logan, G. D. (1978). Attention in character classification tasks: Evidence for the automaticity of component stages. *Journal of Experimental Psychology: General, 107,* 32–63.

Logan, G. D. (1979). On the use of a concurrent memory load to measure attention and automaticity. *Journal of Experimental Psychology: Human Perception and Performance, 5,* 189–207.

Logan, G. D. (1983). On the ability to inhibit simple thoughts and actions: I. Stop-signal studies of decision and memory. *Journal of Experimental Psychology: Learning, Memory, and Cognition, 9,* 585–606.

Logan, G. D. (1985a). Executive control of thought and action. *Acta Psychologica, 60,* 193–210.

Logan, G. D. (1985b). On the ability to inhibit simple thoughts and actions: II. Stop-signal studies of repetition priming. *Journal of Experimental Psychology: Learning, Memory and Cognition, 11,* 675–691.

Logan, G. D. (1985c). Skill and automaticity: Relations, implications, and future directions. *Canadian Journal of Psychology, 39,* 367–386.

Logan, G. D. (1988). Toward an instance theory of automatization. *Psychological Review, 95,* 492–527.

Logan, G. D., & Cowan, W. B. (1984). On the ability to inhibit thought and action: A theory of an act of control. *Psychological Review, 91,* 295–327.

Luczak, H. (1979). Fractioned heart rate variability. Part II: Experiments on superimposition of components of stress. *Ergonomics, 22,* 1315–1323.

Ludwig, A. M. (1972). On and off the wagon: Reasons for drinking and abstaining by alcoholics. *Quarterly Journal of Studies on Alcohol, 33,* 91–96.

Ludwig, A. M. (1988). *Understanding the alcoholic's mind: The nature of craving and how to control it.* New York: Oxford University Press.

Ludwig, A. M., Cain, R. B., Wikler, A., Taylor, R. M., & Bendfeldt, F. (1977). Physiological and situational determinants of drinking behavior. In M. M. Gross (Ed.), *Alcohol intoxication and withdrawal: Vol. B. Studies in alcohol dependence* (pp. 589–600). New York: Plenum Press.

Ludwig, A. M., & Wikler, A. (1974). "Craving" and relapse to drink. *Quarterly Journal of Studies on Alcohol, 35,* 108–130.

Ludwig, A. M., Wikler, A., & Stark, L. H. (1974). The first drink: Psychobiological aspects of craving. *Archives of General Psychiatry, 30,* 539–547.

MacRae, J. R., Scoles, M. T., & Siegel, S. (1987). The contribution of Pavlovian conditioning to drug tolerance and dependence. *British Journal of Addiction, 82,* 371–380.

Marlatt, G. A. (1978). Craving for alcohol, loss of control, and relapse: Cognitive-behavioral analysis. In P. E. Nathan, G. A. Marlatt, & T. Loberg (Eds.), *Alcoholism: New directions in behavioral research and treatment* (pp. 271–314). New York: Plenum Press.

Marlatt, G. A. (1985). Cognitive factors in the relapse process. In G. A. Marlatt & J. R. Gordon, (Eds.), *Relapse prevention* (pp. 128–200). New York: Guilford Press.

Marlatt, G. A., Demming, B., & Reid, J. B. (1973). Loss of control drinking in alcoholics: An experimental analogue. *Journal of Abnormal Psychology, 81,* 233–241.

Marlatt, G. A., & Gordon, J. R. (1980). Determinants of relapse: Implications for the maintenance of behavior change. In P. O. Davidson & S. M. Davidson (Eds.), *Behavioral medicine: Changing health lifestyles* (pp. 410–452). New York: Brunner/Mazel.

Mathew, R. J., Claghorn, J. L., & Largen, J. (1979). Craving for alcohol in sober alcoholics. *American Journal of Psychiatry, 136,* 603–606.

Maude-Griffin, P. M., & Tiffany, S. T. (1989a). Associative morphine tolerance in the rat: Examinations of compensatory responding and cross-tolerance with stress-induced analgesia. *Behavioral and Neural Biology, 51,* 11–33.

Maude-Griffin, P. M., & Tiffany, S. T. (1989b). *An evaluation of situational and affective correlates of smoking relapse.* Unpublished manuscript.

McAuliffe, W. E., & Gordon, R. A. (1974). A test of Lindesmith's theory of addiction: The frequency of euphoria among long-term addicts. *American Journal of Sociology, 79,* 795–840.

Melchior, C. L., & Tabakoff, B. (1984). A conditioning model of alcohol tolerance. In M. Galanter (Ed.), *Recent developments in alcoholism* (Vol. 2, pp. 5–16). New York: Plenum Press.

Mello, N. K. (1972). Behavioral studies of alcoholism. In B. Kissin & H. Begleiter (Eds.), *Biology of alcoholism* (Vol. 2, pp. 219–291). New York: Plenum Press.

Mello, N. K. (1978). A semantic aspect of alcoholism. In H. D. Cappell & A. E. LeBlanc (Eds.), *Biological and behavioral approaches to drug dependence* (pp. 73–87). Toronto, Ontario, Canada: Addiction Research Foundation.

Mello, N. K., & Mendelson, J. H. (1972). Drinking patterns during work-contingent and non-contingent alcohol acquisition. *Psychosomatic Medicine, 34,* 139–164.

Mello, N. K., & Mendelson, J. H. (1978). Alcohol and human behavior. In L. L. Iversen, S. D. Iversen, & S. H. Snyder (Eds.), *Handbook of psychopharmacology* (Vol. 12, pp. 235–317). New York: Plenum Press.

Mello, N. K., Mendelson, J. H., Sellers, M. L., & Kuehnle, J. C. (1980). Effect of alcohol and marijuana on tobacco smoking. *Clinical Pharmacology and Therapeutics, 27,* 202–209.

Mirin, S. M., Meyer, R. E., & McNamee, H. B. (1976). Psychopathology, craving, and mood during heroin acquisition: An experimental study. *The International Journal of the Addictions, 11,* 525–544.

Monti, P. M., Binkoff, J. A., Abrams, D. B., Zwick, W. R., Nirenberg, T. D., & Liepman, M. R. (1987). Reactivity of alcoholics and nonalcoholics to drinking cures. *Journal of Abnormal Psychology, 96,* 122–126.

Mucha, R. F., Volkovskis, C., & Kalant, H. (1981). Conditioned increases in locomotor activity produced with morphine as unconditioned stimulus, and the relation of conditioning to acute morphine effects and tolerance. *Journal of Comparative and Physiological Psychology, 95,* 357–362.

Nathan, P. E., Titler, N. A., Lowenstein, L. M., Solomon, P., & Rossi, A. M. (1970). Behavioral analysis of chronic alcoholism. *Archives of General Psychiatry, 22,* 419–430.

Navon, D., & Gopher, D. (1979). On the economy of the human-processing system. *Psychological Review, 86,* 214–255.

Neisser, U. (1967). *Cognitive psychology.* New York: Appleton-Century-Crofts.

Neumann, O. (1984). Automatic processing: A review of recent findings and a plea for an old theory. In W. Prinz & A. F. Sanders (Eds.), *Cognition and motor processes* (pp. 255–293). Berlin, Federal Republic of Germany: Springer-Verlag.

Newell, K. M. (1978). Some issues on action plans. In G. E. Stelmach (Ed.), *Information processing in motor control and learning* (pp. 41–54). New York: Academic Press.

Newell, A., & Rosenbloom, P. S. (1981). Mechanisms of skill acquisition and the law of practice. In J. R. Anderson (Ed.), *Cognitive skills and their acquisition* (pp. 1–55). Hillsdale, NJ: Erlbaum.

Niaura, R. S., Abrams, D., DeMuth, B., Pinto, R., & Monti, D. (1989). Responses to smoking-related stimuli and early relapse to smoking. *Addictive Behaviors, 14,* 419–428.

Niaura, R. S., Rohsenow, D. J., Binkoff, J. A., Monti, P. M., Pedraza, M., & Abrams, D. B. (1988). Relevance of cue reactivity to understanding alcohol and smoking relapse. *Journal of Abnormal Psychology, 97,* 133–152.

Nil, R., Buzzi, R., & Bättig, K. (1984). Effects of single doses of alcohol and caffeine on cigarette smoke puffing behavior. *Pharmacology, Biochemistry and Behavior, 20,* 583–590.

Nisbett, R. E., & Wilson, T. D. (1977). Telling more than we can know: Verbal reports on mental processes. *Psychological Review, 84,* 231–259.

Norman, D. A. (1981). Categorization of action slips. *Psychological Review, 88,* 1–15.

Norman, D. A., & Shallice, T. (1985). Attention to action: Willed and automatic control of behavior. In R. J. Davidson, G. E. Schwartz, & D. Shapiro (Eds.), *Consciousness and self-regulation: Vol. 4. Advances in research and theory* (pp. 2–18). New York: Plenum Press.

Obrist, P. A. (1976). The cardiovascular-behavioral interaction—As it appears today. *Psychophysiology, 13,* 85–107.

Obrist, P. A., Gaebelein, C. J., Teller, E. S., Langer, A. W., Grignolo, A., Light, K. C., & McCubbin, J. A. (1978). The relationship among heart rate, carotid dP/dt, and blood pressure in humans as a function of the type of stress. *Psychophysiology, 15,* 102–115.

Obrist, P. A., Webb, R. A., Sutterer, J. R., & Howard, J. L. (1970). The cardia-somatic relationship: Some reformulations. *Psychophysiology, 6,* 569–587.

O'Connell, K. A., & Martin, E. J. (1987). Highly tempting situations associated with abstinence, temporary lapse, and relapse among participants in smoking cessation programs. *Journal of Consulting and Clinical Psychology, 55,* 367–371.

Panksepp, J. (1982). Toward a general psychobiological theory of emotions. *Behavioral Brain Science, 5,* 407–467.

Paredes, A., Hood, W. R., Seymour, H., & Gollob, M. (1973). Loss of control in alcoholism: An investigation of the hypothesis with experimental findings. *Quarterly Journal of Studies on Alcohol, 34,* 1146–1161.

Payne, T. J., Schare, M. L., Levis, D. J., & Colletti, G. (1987, March). *Cue responsivity in smokers: The effects of environmental stimuli and negative affective state on topographical changes in smoking behavior.* Paper presented at the Eighth Annual Convention of the Society of Behavioral Medicine, Washington, DC.

Pohorecky, L. A. (1977). Biphasic action of ethanol. *Behavioral Reviews, 1,* 231–240.

Pomerleau, O. F. (1981). Underlying mechanisms in substance abuse. Examples from research on smoking. *Addictive Behaviors, 6,* 187–196.

Porchet, H. C., Benowitz, N. L., & Steiner, L. B. (1988). Pharmacodynamic model of tolerance: Application to nicotine. *Journal of Pharmacology and Experimental Therapeutics, 244,* 231–236.

Posner, M. I. (1978). *Chronometric explorations of mind.* Hillsdale, NJ: Erlbaum.

Posner, M. I. (1982). Cumulative development of attentional theory. *American Psychologist, 37,* 168–178.

Posner, M. I., & Snyder, C. R. R. (1975). Attention and cognitive control. In R. L. Solso (Ed.), *Information processing and cognition: The Loyala symposium* (pp. 55–85). New York: Wiley.

Poulos, C. W., Hinson, R., & Siegel, S. (1981). The role of Pavlovian processes in drug tolerance and dependence: Implications for treatment. *Addictive Behaviors, 6,* 205–211.

Rankin, H., Hodgson, R., & Stockwell, T. (1979). The concept of craving and its measurement. *Behaviour Research and Therapy, 17,* 389–396.

Reason, J. (1979). Actions not as planned: The price of automatization. In G. Underwood & R. Stevens (Eds.), *Aspects of consciousness: Vol. 1. Psychological issues* (pp. 67–89). London: Academic Press.

Reason, J. (1984). Lapses of attention in everyday life. In R. Parasuraman & D. R. Davis (Eds.), *Varieties of attention* (pp. 515–549). New York: Academic Press.

Rescorla, R. A., & Solomon, R. A. (1967). Two-process learning theory: Relationships between Pavlovian conditioning and instrumental learning. *Psychological Review, 74,* 151–182.

Rickard-Figueroa, K., & Zeichner, A. (1985). Assessment of smoking urge and its concomitants under an environmental smoking cue manipulation. *Addictive Behaviors, 10,* 249–256.

Rose, J. E., Zinser, M. C., Tashkin, D. P., Newcomb, R., & Ertle, A. (1984). Subjective response to cigarette smoking following airway anesthetization. *Addictive Behaviors, 9,* 211–215.

Russell, M. A. H., Peto, J., & Patel, U. A. (1974). The classification of smoking by factorial structure of motives. *Journal of the Royal Statistical Society, 137,* 313–333.

Schachter, S., & Singer, J. E. (1962). Cognitive, social, and physiological determinants of emotional state. *Psychological Review, 69,* 379–399.

Schmidt, R. A. (1976). The schema as a solution to some persistent problems in motor learning theory. In G. E. Stelmach (Ed.), *Motor control: Issues and trends* (pp. 41–65). New York: Academic Press.

Schneider, W. (1985). Toward a model of attention and the development of automatic processing. In M. E. Posner & O. S. M. Martin (Eds.), *Attention and performance* (Vol. 11, pp. 475–492). Hillsdale, NJ: Erlbaum.

Schneider, W., Dumais, S. T., & Shiffrin, R. M. (1984). Automatic and control processing and attention. In R. Parasuraman & D. R. Davies (Eds.), *Varieties of attention* (pp. 1–25). New York: Academic Press.

Schneider, W., & Fisk, A. D. (1982). Degree of consistent training: Improvements in search performance and automatic process development. *Perception and Psychophysics, 31,* 160–168.

Schneider, W., & Shiffrin, R. M. (1977). Controlled and automatic human information processing: I. Detection, search, and attention. *Psychological Review, 84,* 1–66.

Schwarz, K. S., & Cunningham, C. L. (1989). Tolerance and sensitization to the heart-rate effects of morphine. *Pharmacology, Biochemistry and Behavior, 31,* 561–566.

Seevers, M. H., & Deneau, G. A. (1963). Physiological aspects of tolerance and physiological dependence. In W. S. Root & F. G. Hofmann (Eds.), *Physiological pharmacology* (Vol. 1, pp. 565–640). New York: Academic Press.

Shallice, T. (1972). Dual functions of consciousness. *Psychological Review, 79,* 383–393.

Sherman, J. E., Jorenby, M. S., & Baker, T. B. (in press). Classical conditioning with alcohol: Acquired preferences and aversions, tolerance and urges/craving. In D. A. Wilkinson & D. Chaudron (Eds.), *Theories of alcoholism.* Toronto, Ontario, Canada: Addiction Research Foundation.

Shiffman, S. (1979). The tobacco withdrawal syndrome. In N. W. Krasnegor (Ed.), *Cigarette smoking as a dependence process* (pp. 158–184). Washington, DC: National Institute on Drug Abuse.

Shiffman, S. (1982). Relapse following smoking cessation: A situational analysis. *Journal of Consulting and Clinical Psychology, 50,* 71–86.

Shiffman, S. (1984). Coping with temptations to smoke. *Journal of Consulting and Clinical Psychology, 52,* 261–267.

Shiffman, S. (1986). A cluster-analytic classification of smoking relapse episodes. *Addictive Behaviors, 11,* 295–307.

Shiffman, S., & Jarvik, M. E. (1976). Smoking withdrawal symptoms in two weeks of abstinence. *Psychopharmacology, 50,* 35–39.

Shiffman, S., & Jarvik, M. E. (1987). Situational determinants of coping in smoking relapse crises. *Journal of Applied Social Psychology, 17,* 3–15.

Shiffrin, R. M., & Dumais, S. T. (1981). The development of automatism. In J. R. Anderson (Ed.), *Cognitive skills and their acquisition* (pp. 111–140). Hillsdale, NJ: Erlbaum.

Shiffrin, R. M., & Schneider, W. (1977). Controlled and automatic human information processing: II. Perceptual learning, automatic attending, and a general theory. *Psychological Review, 84,* 127–190.

Siegel, S. (1975). Evidence from rats the morphine tolerance is a learned response. *Journal of Comparative and Physiological Psychology, 89,* 498–506.

Siegel, S. (1979). The role of conditioning in drug tolerance and addiction. In J. D. Keehn (Ed.), *Psychopathology in animals: Research and treatment implications.* New York: Academic Press.

Siegel, S. (1983). Classical conditioning, drug tolerance and drug dependence. In Y. Israel, F. B. Glaser, H. Kalant, R. E. Popham, W. Schmidt, & R. G. Smart (Eds.), *Research advances in alcohol and drug problems* (Vol. 7, pp. 207–246). New York: Plenum Press.

Sobell, M. B., Schaefer, H. H., & Mills, K. C. (1972). Differences in baseline drinking behavior between alcoholics and normal drinkers. *Behaviour Research and Therapy, 10,* 257–267.

Sternberg, R. J. (1985). *Beyond IQ: A triarchic theory of human intelligence.* New York: Cambridge University Press.

Stewart, J., de Wit, H., Eikelboom, R. (1984). Role of unconditioned and conditioned drug effects in self-administration of opiates and stimulants. *Psychological Review, 91,* 251–268.

Stockwell, T. R., Hodgson, R. J., Rankin, H. J., & Taylor, C. (1982). Alcohol dependence, beliefs and the priming effect. *Behaviour Research and Therapy, 20,* 513–522.

Tabakoff, B., & Kiianmaa, K. (1982). Does tolerance develop to the activating, as well as the depressant, effects of ethanol? *Pharmacology, Biochemistry and Behavior, 17,* 1073–1076.

Tiffany, S. T. (1988, March). *Contemporary theories of drug urges, con-*

flicting data, and an alternative cognitive framework. Paper presented at the Conference on Theory and Research in Psychopathology, Performance, and Cognition, Gainesville, FL.

Tiffany, S. T., & Baker, T. B. (1986). Tolerance to alcohol: Psychological models and their application to alcoholism. *Annals of Behavioral Medicine, 8,* 2–3, 7–12.

Tiffany, S. T., & Drobes, D. J. (in press). Imagery and smoking urges: The manipulation of affective content. *Addictive Behaviors.*

Tiffany, S. T., Petrie, E. C., Baker, T. B., & Dahl, J. (1983). Conditioned morphine tolerance in the rat: Absence of a compensatory response and cross-tolerance with stress. *Behavioral Neuroscience, 97,* 335–353.

Turner, J. R., & Carroll, D. (1985). Heart rate and oxygen consumption during mental arithmetic, a video game and graded exercise: Further evidence of metabolically-exaggerated cardiac adjustments? *Psychophysiology, 22,* 261–267.

Tyler, S. W., Hertel, P. T., McCallum, M. C., & Ellis, H. C. (1979). Cognitive effort and memory. *Journal of Experimental Psychology: Human Learning and Memory, 5,* 607–617.

Underwood, G. (1982). Attention and awareness in cognitive and motor skills. In G. Underwood (Ed.), *Aspects of consciousness: Vol. 3. Awareness and self-awareness* (pp. 111–145). New York: Academic Press.

West, R. J., Hajek, P., & Belcher, M. (1987). Time course of cigarette withdrawal symptoms during four weeks of treatment with nicotine chewing gum. *Addictive Behaviors, 12,* 199–203.

West, R. J., Jarvis, M. J., Russell, M. A. H., Carruthers, M. E., & Feyerabend, C. (1984). Effect of nicotine replacement on the cigarette withdrawal syndrome. *British Journal of Addiction, 79,* 215–219.

West, R. J., & Russell, M. A. H. (1985). Pre-abstinence smoke intake and smoking motivation as predictors of severity of cigarette withdrawal symptoms. *Psychopharmacology, 87,* 334–336.

West, R. J., Russell, M. A. H., Jarvis, M. J., & Feyerabend, C. (1984). Does switching to an ultra-low nicotine cigarette induce nicotine withdrawal effects? *Psychopharmacology, 84,* 120–123.

West, R., & Schneider, N. (1987). Craving for cigarettes. *British Journal of Addiction, 82,* 407–415.

Wickens, C. D. (1984). Processing resources in attention. In R. Parasuraman & R. Davies (Eds.), *Varieties of attention* (pp. 63–102). New York: Academic Press.

Wikler, A. (1948). Recent progress in research on the neurophysiological basis of morphine addiction. *American Journal of Psychiatry, 105,* 329–338.

Wikler, A. (1972). Sources of reinforcement for drug using behavior—a theoretical formulation. *Pharmacology and the Future of Man. Proceedings of 5th International Congress of Pharmacology, 1,* 18–30.

Wikler, A., & Pescor, F. T. (1967). Classical conditioning of a morphine abstinence phenomenon, reinforcement of opioid-drinking behavior and "relapse" in morphine-addicted rats. *Psychopharmacologia, 10,* 255–284.

Wilson, G. T. (1978). Booze, beliefs, and behavior: Cognitive processes in alcohol use and abuse. In P. E. Nathan, G. A. Marlatt, & T. Loberg (Eds.), *Alcoholism: New directions in behavioral research and treatment* (pp. 315–339). New York: Plenum Press.

Wilson, G. T. (1987). Cognitive studies in alcoholism. *Journal of Consulting and Clinical Psychology, 55,* 325–331.

Wise, R. A. (1988). The neurobiology of craving: Implications for understanding and treatment of addiction. *Journal of Abnormal Psychology, 97,* 118–132.

Wise, R. A., & Bozarth, M. A. (1987). A psychomotor stimulant theory of addiction. *Psychological Review, 94,* 469–492.

Young, A. M., & Herling, S. (1986). Drugs as reinforcers: Studies in laboratory animals. In S. R. Goldberg, & I. P. Stolerman (Eds.), *Behavioral analysis of drug dependence* (pp. 9–67). New York: Academic Press.

Zelman, D. C., Tiffany, S. T., & Baker, T. B. (1985). Influence of stress on morphine-induced hyperthermia: Relevance to drug conditioning and tolerance development. *Behavioral Neuroscience, 99,* 122–144.

Received November 4, 1988
Revision received June 26, 1989
Accepted September 25, 1989 ■

Decreased striatal dopaminergic responsiveness in detoxified cocaine-dependent subjects

N. D. Volkow*†, G.-J. Wang*, J. S. Fowler‡, J. Logan†, S. J. Gatley*, R. Hitzemann†, A. D. Chen*, S. L. Dewey‡ & N. Pappas*

** Medical and ‡ Chemistry Departments, Brookhaven National Laboratory, Upton, New York 11973, USA*
† Department of Psychiatry, State University of New York at Stony Brook, Stony Brook, New York, 11794, USA

Cocaine blocks the reuptake of dopamine, a neurotransmitter involved in the control of movement, cognition, motivation and reward. This leads to an increase in extracellular dopamine; the reinforcing effect of cocaine is associated with elevated dopamine levels in the nucleus accumbens[1,2]. But addiction to cocaine involves other effects, such as craving, loss of control and compulsive drug intake; the role of the dopamine system in these effects is less well-understood. We therefore used positron emission tomography (PET) to compare the responses of cocaine addicts and normal controls to intravenous methylphenidate, a drug that, like cocaine, causes an increase in synaptic dopamine[3]. Addicts showed reduced dopamine release in the striatum, the brain region where the nucleus accumbens is located, and also had a reduced 'high' relative to controls. In contrast, addicts showed an increased response to methylphenidate in the thalamus (a region that conveys sensory input to the cortex). This thalamic response was associated with cocaine craving and was not seen in control subjects. Thus, our findings challenge the notion that addiction involves an enhanced striatal dopamine response to cocaine and/or an enhanced induction of euphoria. Moreover, they suggest a participation of thalamic dopamine pathways in cocaine addiction, a possibility that merits further investigation.

It has been hypothesized that cocaine addiction could result from decreased function of dopamine in the brain[4]. Hence we compared the function of the brain dopamine system of 20 cocaine-dependent subjects with 23 controls using positron emission tomography (PET) and [^{11}C]raclopride, a dopamine D2 receptor ligand sensitive to competition with endogenous dopamine[5], by measuring the relative changes in extracellular dopamine induced by intravenous methylphenidate (MP)[6]. MP, like cocaine, increases synaptic dopamine by inhibiting dopamine reuptake[3], it has equivalent reinforcing effects to those of cocaine[7], and its intravenous administration induces a 'high' similar to that of cocaine[8]. Because [^{11}C]raclopride binding is highly reproducible[9], differences in binding between placebo and MP predominantly reflect MP-induced changes in extracellular dopamine[10,11]. Dopamine responses to MP (0.5 mg kg^{-1} intravenously (i.v.)) were measured in striatum and thalamus[12], brain regions where binding of D2 PET radioligands is inhibited by D2 antagonists[13].

Parallel assessment of the behavioural effects of MP revealed significant differences between the groups; whereas MP-induced 'high' and 'restlessness' was more intense in controls MP-induced 'cocaine craving' was more intense in cocaine-dependent subjects (Table 1). There were no differences between the groups in MP-induced cardiovascular changes (not shown), or in plasma MP concentration (controls, 119 s.d. 36 ng ml^{-1}; dependent subjects, 107 s.d. 36 ng ml^{-1}).

Figure 1 shows representative [^{11}C]raclopride images at the level of striatum obtained after placebo and after MP in a control and in a cocaine-dependent subject. Although MP did not affect the transport of [^{11}C]raclopride from blood to brain (rate, K_1) for any of the brain regions it induced a significant reduction in the distribution volume (DV) in all brain regions as well as in the estimates for dopamine D2 receptor availability (B_{max}/K_d) in striatum (Table 2). The DV in cerebellum, which is used to normalize the receptor measures for global changes in DV, was decreased by MP. The magnitude of this decrease, which reflects a global change in the relative distribution of raclopride between tissue and plasma with MP[14], did not differ between groups (ANOVA diagnosis by drug interaction effect $F = 0.19$; d.f. 1,41; $P = 0.67$). In contrast, MP-induced decreases in DV in striatum were significantly larger in controls than in dependent subjects (interaction effect $F = 5.6$, $P = 0.02$). Similarly, MP-induced changes in B_{max}/K_d in striatum were significantly larger in controls (21 s.d. 13% change from baseline) than in cocaine-dependent subjects (9 s.d. 13%) (interaction effect $F = 9.3$, $P < 0.004$) (Fig. 2). There were also significant differences between the groups in the response to MP in thalamus; the DV decreases in thalamus were significantly larger in the cocaine-dependent subjects ($F = 5.4$, $P = 0.03$) and in cocaine-dependent subjects,but not in controls, MP decreased B_{max}/K_d values in thalamus (29 s.d. 35%) (interaction effect $F = 11.0$, $P < 0.002$) (Fig. 2).

In striatum, MP-induced changes in B_{max}/K_d were significantly correlated with MP-induced changes in self reports of 'restlessness' (correlation for the two groups: $r = 0.49$, d.f. 42; $P < 0.002$; correlation for cocaine-dependent subjects only: $r = 0.52$, d.f. 19; $P < 0.05$). In thalamus, MP-induced changes in B_{max}/K_d were significantly correlated with MP-induced changes in 'cocaine craving' (correlation for the two groups: $r = 0.57$, d.f. 42; $P < 0.0001$; correlation for cocaine-dependent subjects only: $r = 0.61$, d.f. 19; $P < 0.005$) (Fig. 3). B_{max}/K_d changes were not correlated with the high or with plasma MP concentration (not shown).

Because MP increases dopamine by blocking dopamine transporters, the blunted response to MP in striatum may reflect decreased outflow of dopamine in the baseline state as well as changes in dopamine in anticipation of receiving a psychostimulant drug. These results are compatible with a decrease in striatal dopamine brain function in cocaine-dependent subjects. Decreased striatal dopamine responsiveness would make cocaine, in principle, less reinforcing because it would be the equivalent of administering smaller doses. One could also predict that decreased dopamine responsiveness would result in a blunted response to behaviours resulting from increases in striatal dopamine. In this respect MP-induced restlessness was more intense in normals than in dependent subjects and was correlated with changes in striatal dopamine. Similarly the high from MP in the dependent subjects was of a lower intensity than in controls and although it was not associated

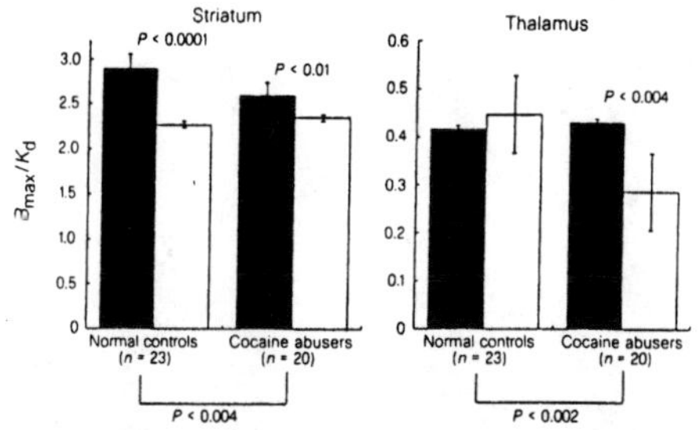

Figure 2 Mean and standard error for the B_{max}/K_d estimates in striatum and in thalamus after placebo (filled bar) and after methylphenidate (MP) administration (empty bar) in normals and in cocaine-dependent subjects. In striatum, results for the ANOVA reveal a significant drug effect ($F = 51$, d.f. 1; $P < 0.0001$) as well as a significant drug by diagnosis interaction effect ($F = 9.3$, d.f. 1,41; $P < 0.004$). Cocaine-dependent subject's response to MP was significantly smaller than that of controls (baseline-MP). In thalamus, MP significantly decrease B_{max}/K_d only in cocaine-dependent subjects ($P < 0.004$). At baseline, B_{max}/K_d in striatum was significantly lower in cocaine-dependent subjects than in controls ($P < 0.01$).

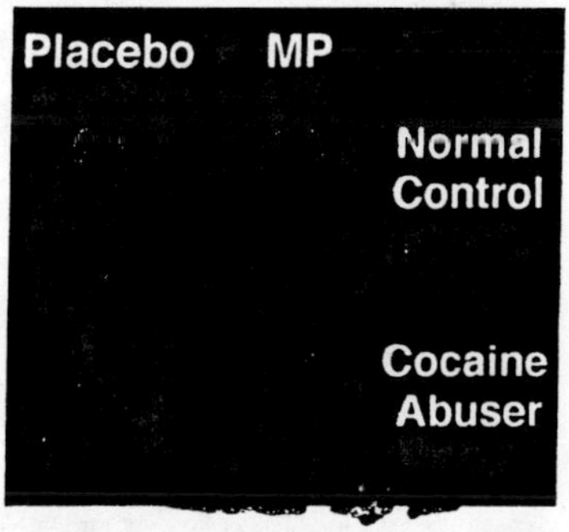

Figure 1 Distribution volume images of [^{11}C]raclopride at the level of the striatum in a normal control and in a cocaine-dependent subject tested after placebo (baseline) and after methylphenidate (MP) administration. Baseline binding for [^{11}C]raclopride in striatum and the reductions in striatal binding with MP were lower in the cocaine-dependent subject than in the control.

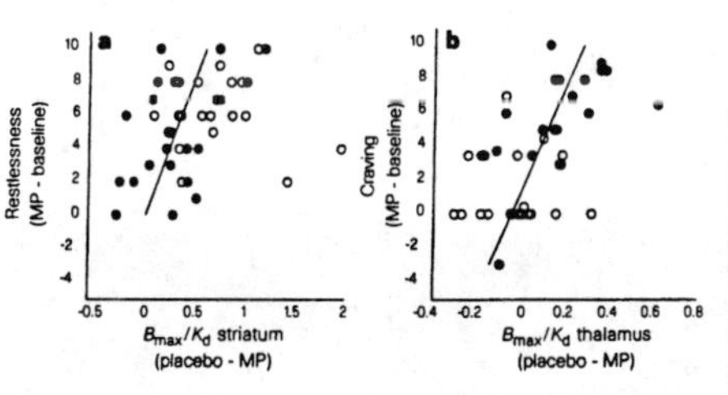

Figure 3 a, Regression slopes for the correlation between methylphenidate (MP)-induced changes in dopamine D2 receptor availability in striatum and MP-induced changes in self-reports of restlessness. **b**, Regression slopes for the correlation between MP-induced changes in dopamine receptor availability in thalamus and MP-induced changes in self-reports of cocaine craving. Normal controls are shown as empty circles and cocaine-dependent subjects as filled circles.

Table 1 Mean and standard deviations (±) for self reports of drug-induced (placebo or methylphenidate) behavioural effects in controls and in cocaine-dependent subjects

	Normal controls Placebo	Normal controls MP	Cocaine dependent Placebo	Cocaine dependent MP	MP effect P
Alert	7 ± 1	9 ± 1	8 ± 1	9 ± 2	NS
Anxiety	2 ± 2	4 ± 3	4 ± 3	6 ± 4	NS
Distrustful	0	1 ± 2	1 ± 1	2 ± 3	NS
High*	1 ± 1	6 ± 3	0	4 ± 3	$P < 0.005$
Restlessness**	2 ± 2	7 ± 2	2 ± 2	5 ± 4	$P < 0.0001$
Craving***	0	1 ± 2	3 ± 3	8 ± 3	$P < 0.001$

Self reports were recorded 27 min after administration of placebo or of methylphenidate (MP). MP significantly increased self reports for high, restlessness and cocaine craving. Behavioural responses to MP were significantly larger in controls for restlessness and high whereas for cocaine craving responses were larger in the cocaine-dependent subjects. ANOVA interaction effect (diagnosis × drug): *$P < 0.05$, **$P < 0.005$, ***$P < 0.001$. NS, not significant.

Table 2

	Normal controls Placebo	Normal controls MP	Cocaine dependent Placebo	Cocaine dependent MP	MP effect P
K_1					
Striatum	0.10 ± 0.02	0.10 ± 0.02	0.10 ± 0.02	0.10 ± 0.02	NS
Thalamus	0.09 ± 0.08	0.10 ± 0.03	0.13 ± 0.07	0.17 ± 0.13	NS
Cerebellum	0.06 ± 0.02	0.07 ± 0.02	0.08 ± 0.03	0.08 ± 0.03	NS
DV					
Striatum*	1.62 ± 0.3	1.24 ± 0.2**	1.62 ± 0.2	1.43 ± 0.2*	0.0001
Thalamus*	0.59 ± 0.08	0.55 ± 0.09	0.65 ± 0.10	0.55 ± 0.11	0.0001
Cerebellum	0.42 ± 0.06	0.38 ± 0.08	0.45 ± 0.06	0.43 ± 0.06	0.001
B_{max}/K_d					
Striatum**	2.90 ± 0.34	2.27 ± 0.37	2.59 ± 0.34	2.35 ± 0.41	0.0001
Thalamus**	0.42 ± 0.10	0.45 ± 0.15	0.43 ± 0.15	0.29 ± 0.15	0.04

MP did not change K_1 but it decreased the DV and the B_{max}/K_d. MP-induced changes in DV and B_{max}/K_d in striatum were significantly smaller in cocaine-dependent subjects whereas MP-induced changes in DV and B_{max}/K_d in thalamus were significantly larger in cocaine-dependent subjects than in controls. ANOVA interaction effect (diagnosis × drug): *$P < 0.02$, **$P < 0.005$. Striatal B_{max}/K_d measures for the placebo condition were significantly lower ($P < 0.01$) in cocaine-dependent subjects than in controls.

with changes in striatal dopamine, this could have been due to the fact that measurements were done in dorsal striatum and not in nucleus accumbens, the brain structure associated with drug reinforcement in laboratory animals[15], and that measurements were recorded at 27 min when peak effects for the high had subsided. In laboratory animals, prior exposure to psychostimulants results in accentuated drug responses and this phenomenon of sensitization, which in some studies but not in others has been associated with enhanced dopamine responses, has been implicated in cocaine addiction[16]. The blunted response to MP in cocaine-dependent subjects does not support an enhancement of dopamine release and/or of the reinforcing effects of cocaine as one of the mechanisms underlying human addiction. The discrepancies with some of the laboratory animal data are likely to reflect differences between species, patterns of psychostimulant administration[16], and/or conditions of drug administration[17].

Addicted subjects were distinguished from controls by the cocaine craving induced by MP. Under appropriate conditions, the craving would have most likely led to compulsive cocaine intake ('bingeing'). The abnormal activation of the thalamus in dependent subjects, but not in controls, and its significant association with MP-induced cocaine craving suggests that abnormal activation of thalamic dopamine pathways may participate in the expression of this unique behaviour of the addicted subject. The thalamus has a relatively high uptake of cocaine[18,19] and it is sensitive to D2 receptor-mediated effects of cocaine[20]. Although current PET scanners lack the spatial resolution to distinguish individual thalamic nuclei, one could speculate that MP-induced dopamine changes in the dependent subjects involve the mediodorsal nucleus (MD), which receives dopamine projections[21] and is a relay between accumbens and orbitofrontal cortex[22]. MD lesions disrupt conditioned reinforcement behaviours[23]. Because pathology in orbitofrontal cortex is associated with the emergence of repetitive behaviours in laboratory animals[24], and with compulsive disorders in humans[25], it is possible that abnormal MD activation in cocaine-dependent subjects activates the orbitofrontal cortex, which enables the compulsive drug intake. In this respect it is interesting to note that decreases in D2 receptors in cocaine-dependent subjects are associated with metabolic abnormalities in orbitofrontal cortex[26] and that the striato-thalamic-orbitofrontal circuit has been postulated as a common mechanism underlying drug and alcohol addiction[26,27]. However, because the specific to nonspecific binding ratio of [^{11}C]raclopride in thalamus is quite low and MP decreased the nonspecific binding of raclopride (DV in cerebellum) we cannot exclude the possibility that MP-induced changes in thalamus in cocaine-dependent subjects reflects nonspecific effects and further studies are required to replicate these findings.

Baseline striatal D2 B_{max}/K_d values were lower in cocaine-dependent subjects (2.59 s.d. 0.3) than in controls (2.90 s.d. 0.3) ($P < 0.01$) and agree with previous findings of D2 receptor reductions in cocaine-dependent subjects[26]. Striatal D2 receptor measurements with PET predominantly reflect postsynaptic receptors[28] and thus indicate involvement of GABA and/or acetylcholine cells. The decreased response to MP in striatum, on the other hand, indicates that there are also functional changes in DA cells in cocaine-addicted subjects.

Although unlikely, we cannot exclude the possibility that the decreased response to MP in cocaine-dependent subjects could also result from affinity changes in dopamine receptors and/or from changes in dopamine transporters. Although raclopride binds both to D2 and to D3 receptors, the striatal concentration of D3 receptors is very low so that the PET measurements mainly reflect binding to D2 receptors[28]. Also, although this study evaluated subjects 3–6 weeks after drug discontinuation and the findings may not generalize to periods of more protracted withdrawal, it represents a period when addictive behaviours rapidly emerge[29] and in this respect directly pertains to the investigation of cocaine addiction.

This study provides evidence of decreased striatal dopamine brain function in cocaine-dependent subjects. It also shows an abnormal response in thalamus in cocaine-dependent subjects which was associated with cocaine craving. Further studies are required to determine if MP-induced changes in thalamic raclopride binding in cocaine-dependent subjects reflect competition with dopamine and to assess its role in the loss of control and the compulsive drug intake in the cocaine addict. □

Methods

Subjects. Cocaine-dependent subjects were 20 male right-handed subjects (age 36 s.d. 4 years) studied 3–6 weeks after drug discontinuation. Subjects were inpatients who fulfilled DSM IV diagnostic criteria for cocaine dependence and had used cocaine (free-base or crack) for at least the prior 6 months (at least 'four grams' a week) but were otherwise medically healthy. Exclusion criteria were current or past psychiatric (other than cocaine dependence), neurological, cardiovascular or endocrinological disease, dependence on any substance other than cocaine, nicotine or caffeine and more than moderate (12 ounces per week) use of ethanol. Controls were 23 male right-handed healthy subjects (age 34 s.d. 7 years) who were screened for a lack of history of drug or alcohol abuse (excluding nicotine/caffeine). Exclusion criteria were otherwise as for cocaine-dependent subjects. None of the subjects was taking medications at the time of the study. Toxicological drug screens were performed before each PET scan. Informed consent was obtained for all subjects after procedures were explained.

Scans. Subjects had two scans done with [^{11}C]raclopride, the first scan after placebo and the second after 0.5 mg kg^{-1} i.v. MP, performed on separate days at the same time of day. Subjects were blind to whether placebo or MP was administered, which were injected 6–9 min before [^{11}C]raclopride. Scans were done using a CTI 931 tomography (6 × 6 × 6.5 mm full width half maximum) after i.v. injection of 4–10 mCi of [^{11}C]raclopride (specific activity 0.5–1.5 Ci μM^{-1} at end of bombardment) as described[9].

Drug effect ratings. Behavioural effects were evaluated using analogue scales that assessed self reports of alertness, anxiety, distrustfulness, high, restlessness and cocaine craving from 0 (felt nothing) to 10 (felt intensely)[8] recorded 5 min before and 27 min after MP or placebo. Cocaine craving was scored both as the desire for cocaine and the perception of loss of control for drug intake if the drug were to be available. Vital signs were obtained periodically.

Image analysis. Regions of interest (ROI) were outlined for striatum (ST), thalamus (TH) and cerebellum (CB) by an investigator blind to the subject's diagnosis using procedures previously described[9]. Briefly, ROI were initially outlined on the individual's summed baseline [^{11}C]raclopride image (images obtained between 15 and 54 min) and were then projected into the subject's corresponding coregistered MRI to ensure adequate anatomical localization. ROI were then projected into the dynamic [^{11}C]raclopride images for the baseline and MP studies to generate time activity curves for ST, Th and CB. These time activity curves for tissue concentration along with the time activity curves for unchanged tracer in plasma were used to calculate [^{11}C]raclopride's transfer constant from plasma to brain (K_1) and the distribution volumes (DV), which correspond to the equilibrium measurement of the ratio of tissue concentration to plasma concentration in ST, TH and CB using a graphical analysis technique for reversible systems[30]. The ratios of DV in ST and DV in TH to those of DV in CB correspond to $(B_{max}/K_d) + 1$ and are insensitive to changes in cerebral blood flow[14]. The response to MP was quantified as the difference in B_{max}/K_d between placebo and MP.

B_{max}/K_d can be related to the DV as follows

$$DV = (K_1/k_2)(1 + NS + (B_{max} - RL)/K_d)$$

K_1 and k_2 are plasma to tissue and tissue to plasma transport constants, respectively. B_{max} is the total D2 receptor concentration and RL is concentration of receptors occupied with endogenous dopamine. NS is the ratio of binding constants for nonspecific binding, which is considered to be essentially instantaneous (compared to receptor binding) and therefore in an equilibrium state. In a non-receptor region the DV is given by

$$DV = K_1/k_2(1 + NS)$$

Assuming that the ratio K_1/k_2 is the same for receptor and nonreceptor regions, the ratio of DV for ST to CB is

$$DV(ST)/DV(CB) = (B_{max} - RL)/(K_d(1 + NS)) + 1$$

Although the DV is an equilibrium quantity it can be easily determined from nonequilibrium data by graphical analysis. The free receptor concentration $(B_{max} - RL)$ is therefore a linear function of the DV ratio. We have designated B_{max}/K_d as the quantity $(B_{max} - RL)/K_d$ where we have replaced $K_d(1 + NS)$ with K_d, which is the K_d that comes out of PET measurements without having to measure the quantity NS separately.

Data analysis. Differences in B_{max}/K_d between groups were compared using ANOVA. Pearson correlations were used to assess the relationship between MP-induced changes in B_{max}/K_d and its behavioural effects. Differences in the behavioural and cardiovascular response to MP between groups were tested with nonparametric tests (Mann–Whitney U-test) using score differences between placebo and MP. Values of $P < 0.01$ were considered significant and P values between 0.01 and 0.05 are reported as trends.

Received 3 December 1996; accepted 26 February 1997.

1. Koob, G. F. & Bloom, F. E. Cellular and molecular mechanism of drug dependence. *Science* **242**, 715–723 (1988).
2. Di Chiara, G. & Imperato, A. Drugs abused by humans preferentially increase synaptic dopamine concentrations in the mesolimbic system of freely moving rats. *Proc. Natl Acad. Sci. USA* **85**, 5274–5278 (1988).
3. Volkow, N. D. *et al.* Is methylphenidate like cocaine? Studies on their pharmacokinetics and distribution in human brain. *Arch. Gen. Psychiatry* **52**, 456–463 (1995).
4. Dackis, C. A. & Gold, M. S. New concepts in cocaine addiction: the dopamine depletion hypothesis. *Neurosci. Biobehav.* **9**, 469–477 (1985).
5. Seeman, P., Guan, H. C. & Niznik, H. B. Endogenous dopamine lowers the dopamine D2 receptor density as measured by 3H raclopride: implications for positron emission tomography of the human brain. *Synapse* **3**, 96–97 (1996).
6. Volkow, N. D. *et al.* Imaging endogenous dopamine competition with [^{11}C]raclopride in the human brain. *Synapse* **16**, 255–262 (1994).
7. Bergman, J., Madras, B. K., Johnson, S. E. & Spealman, R. D. Effects of cocaine and related drugs in nonhuman primates: III, Self administration by squirrel monkeys. *J. Pharmacol. Exp. Ther.* **251**, 150–155 (1989).
8. Wang, G.-J. *et al.* Behavioral and cardiovascular effects of intravenous methylphenidate in normal subjects and cocaine abusers. *Eur. Addiction Res.* **3**, 49–54 (1997).
9. Volkow, N. D. *et al.* Reproductibility of repeated measures of ^{11}C raclopride binding in the human brain. *J. Nucl. Med.* **34**, 609–613 (1993).
10. Dewey, S. L. *et al.* Striatal binding of the PET ligand ^{11}C-raclopride is altered by drugs that modify synaptic dopamine levels. *Synapse* **13**, 350–356 (1993).
11. Gifford, A., Gatley, S. J. & Ashby, C. R. Endogenously released dopamine inhibits the binding of dopaminergic PET and SPECT ligands in superfused rat striatal slices. *Synapse* **22**, 232–238 (1996).
12. Wang, G.-J. *et al.* Comparison of two PET radioligands for imaging extrastriatal dopamine receptors in human brain. *Synapse* **15**, 246–249 (1993).
13. Youssef, K. *et al.* Inhibition of extrastriatal dopamine receptors by haloperidol. *Synapse* **19**, 14–17 (1995).
14. Logan, J. *et al.* Effects of blood flow on [^{11}C]raclopride binding in the brain: model simulations and kinetic analysis of PET data. *J. Cereb. Blood Flow Metab.* **14**, 995–1010 (1994).
15. Pontieri, F. E., Tanda, G., Orzi, F. & Di Chiara, G. Effects of nicotine on the nucleus accumbens and similarity to those of addictive drugs. *Nature* **382** 255–257 (1996).
16. Robinson, T. E. & Berridge, K. C. The neural basis of drug craving: an incentive-sensitization theory of addiction. *Brain Res. Rev.* **18**, 247–291 (1993).
17. Brown, E. E., Robertson, G. S. & Fibiger, H. C. Evidence for conditioned neuronal activation following exposure to a cocaine paired environment: role of forebrain limbic structures. *J. Neurosci.* **12**, 4112–4121 (1992).
18. Wang, G.-J. *et al.* Comparison of two PET radioligands for imaging extrastriatal dopamine transporters in human brain. *Life Sci.* **57**, 187–191 (1995).
19. Madras, B. K. & Kaufman, M. J. Cocaine accumulates in dopamine-rich regions of primate brain after iv administration: comparison with mazindol distribution. *Synapse* **18**, 261–275 (1994).
20. Shyu, B. C., Kiritsy-Roy, J. A., Morrow, T. J. & Casey, K. L. Neurophysiological and behavioral evidence for medial thalamic mediation of cocaine-induced dopaminergic analgesia. *Brain Res.* **572**, 216–223 (1992).
21. Groenewegen, H. J. Organization of the afferent connections of the mediodorsal thalamic nucleus in the rat, related to the mediodorsal-prefrontal topography. *Neuroscience* **24**, 379–431 (1988).
22. Nauta, W. J. H. The problem of the frontal lobe: a reinterpretation. *J. Psychiatric Res.* **8**, 167–189 (1971).
23. McAlonan, G. M., Robbins, T. W. & Everitt, B. J. Effects of medial dorsal thalamic and ventral pallidal lesions on the acquisition of a conditioned place preference: further evidence for the involvement of the ventral striatopallidal system in reward-related processes. *Neuroscience* **52**, 605–620 (1993).
24. Kolb, B. Studies on the caudate putamen and the dorsomedial thalamic nucleus: implications for mammalian frontal lobe function. *Physiol. Behav.* **18**, 237–244 (1977).
25. Insel, T. R. Towards a neuroanatomy of obsessive-compulsive disorder. *Arch. Gen. Psychiatry* **49**, 739–744 (1992).
26. Volkow, N. D. *et al.* Decreased dopamine D2 receptor availability is associated with reduced frontal metabolism in cocaine abusers. *Synapse* **14**, 169–177 (1993).
27. Modell, J. G., Mountz, J. M. & Beresford, T. P. Basal ganglia/limbic striatal and thalamocortical involvement in craving and loss of control in alcoholism. *J. Neuropsychiatry* **2**, 123–144 (1990).
28. Volkow, N. D. *et al.* Evaluation of the human brain dopamine system with PET. *J. Nucl. Med.* **37**, 1242–1256 (1996).
29. Gawin, F. & Kleber, H. D. Abstinence symptomatology and psychiatric diagnosis in cocaine abusers. *Arch. Gen. Psychiatry* **43**, 107–113 (1986).
30. Logan, J. *et al.* Graphical analysis of reversible radioligand binding from time-activity measurements applied to [N-^{11}C-methyl]-(-)-cocaine: PET studies in human subjects. *J. Cereb. Blood Flow Metab.* **10**, 740–747 (1990).

Acknowledgements. We thank D. Schlyer and R. Carciello for Cyclotron operations; P. King, A. Levy, D. Warner and C. Wong for PET operations; C. Shea, R. Ferrieri and R. MacGregor for radiotracer preparation; N. Netusil and K. Piscani for patient care; C. Redvanly for organization and C. Springer and A. Wolf for thoughtful discussions. This research was supported by the US Department of Energy and the National Institutes of Drug Abuse.

Correspondence and requests for materials should be addressed to N.D.V. (email: volkow@bnl.gov).

ELSEVIER

Brain Research Reviews 28 (1998) 309–369

BRAIN RESEARCH REVIEWS

Full-length review

What is the role of dopamine in reward: hedonic impact, reward learning, or incentive salience?

Kent C. Berridge *, Terry E. Robinson [1]

Department of Psychology, University of Michigan, Ann Arbor, MI 48109-1109, USA

Accepted 23 June 1998

Abstract

What roles do mesolimbic and neostriatal dopamine systems play in reward? Do they mediate the *hedonic impact* of rewarding stimuli? Do they mediate hedonic *reward learning* and *associative prediction?* Our review of the literature, together with results of a new study of residual reward capacity after dopamine depletion, indicates the answer to both questions is 'no'. Rather, dopamine systems may mediate the *incentive salience* of rewards, modulating their motivational value in a manner *separable from hedonia and reward learning*. In a study of the consequences of dopamine loss, rats were depleted of dopamine in the nucleus accumbens and neostriatum by up to 99% using 6-hydroxydopamine. In a series of experiments, we applied the 'taste reactivity' measure of affective reactions (gapes, etc.) to assess the capacity of dopamine-depleted rats for: 1) normal affect (hedonic and aversive reactions), 2) modulation of hedonic affect by associative learning (taste aversion conditioning), and 3) hedonic enhancement of affect by non-dopaminergic pharmacological manipulation of palatability (benzodiazepine administration). We found normal hedonic reaction patterns to sucrose vs. quinine, normal learning of new hedonic stimulus values (a change in palatability based on predictive relations), and normal pharmacological hedonic enhancement of palatability. We discuss these results in the context of hypotheses and data concerning the role of dopamine in reward. We review neurochemical, electrophysiological, and other behavioral evidence. We conclude that dopamine systems are not needed either to mediate the hedonic pleasure of reinforcers or to mediate predictive associations involved in hedonic reward learning. We conclude instead that dopamine may be more important to *incentive salience attributions* to the neural representations of reward-related stimuli. Incentive salience, we suggest, is a distinct component of motivation and reward. In other words, dopamine systems are necessary for *'wanting' incentives*, but not for 'liking' them or for learning new 'likes' and 'dislikes'. © 1998 Elsevier Science B.V. All rights reserved.

Keywords: Neostriatum; Nucleus accumbens; Substantia nigra; Tegmentum; Mesolimbic; Nigrostriatal; Mesotelencephalic mesostriatal; Dopamine; 6-hydroxydopamine; Lateral hypothalamus; Brain; Reinforcement; Motivation; Self-administration; Conditioning; Reward; Emotion; Palatability; Pleasure; Feeding; Food intake appetitive behavior; Consummatory behavior; Affect; Anhedonia; Hedonic; Diazepam; Conditioned taste aversion; Taste reactivity; Aphagia; Aversion; Appetite; Ingestion; Neurotransmitters; Substance-related disorders; Addiction

Contents

1. Introduction 311

2. Evidence for a role of dopamine in reward 311
   2.1. Nature of dopamine's role in reward: hedonia, incentive salience or reward learning? 312

3. Brain manipulations of behavior for revealing dopamine's function in reward 315
   3.1. Traditional measures of reward: instrumental behavior and choice ('wanting') 316

* Corresponding author. Fax: +1-734-763-7480; E-mail: berridge@umich.edu
[1] E-mail: ter@umich.edu.

0165-0173/98/$ - see front matter © 1998 Elsevier Science B.V. All rights reserved.
PII: S0165-0173(98)00019-8

3.2. Measures of reward based on affective reactions ('liking') . . . 316
3.3. Dopamine manipulations dissociate 'wanting' vs. 'liking' . . . 317

4. Effects of mesolimbic and neostriatal dopamine depletion on subcomponents of reward . . . 317
4.1. General experimental approach . . . 318

5. Experiment 1: Unconditioned affective reactions to sucrose or quinine . . . 318
5.1. Methods . . . 318
5.2. Results . . . 320
5.3. Discussion of Experiment 1 . . . 321

6. Experiment 2: Modulation of affective reactions by taste aversion conditioning . . . 323
6.1. Methods . . . 323
6.2. Results . . . 324
6.3. Discussion of Experiment 2 . . . 324

7. Experiment 3: enhancement of hedonic reaction patterns by diazepam . . . 324
7.1. Methods . . . 326
7.2. Results . . . 326
7.3. Discussion of Experiment 3 . . . 327

8. General discussion . . . 328
8.1. Unconditioned hedonic reactivity . . . 328
8.2. Palatability modulation . . . 328

9. Dopamine and reward: choosing among competing explanations . . . 328
9.1. Not motor deficits . . . 328
9.2. Not anhedonia . . . 328
9.3. Not reward learning? . . . 330
9.4. Loss of incentive salience? . . . 332

10. Conditioned dopamine activity: re-examination of implications for incentive salience and reward learning hypotheses . . . 335
10.1. Predictions of 'reward learning' vs. 'incentive salience' hypotheses of dopamine function . . . 335

11. Effects of dopamine antagonists: a re-examination of anhedonia, incentive salience or anergia explanations . . . 338
11.1. Comparing dopamine antagonist effects on hedonic activation . . . 338
11.2. Affective taste reactivity and dopamine antagonists: sensorimotor anergia but not anhedonia . . . 339
11.3. Subjective hedonic ratings by humans and dopamine antagonists: conscious pleasure persists . . . 339

12. Phenomena that don't fit: problems for the incentive salience model? . . . 340
12.1. Euphorigenic dopaminergic drugs . . . 340
12.2. Paradoxical effects of dopamine antagonists . . . 341
12.3. The 'Two Motivational Systems' hypothesis (Bechara et al.) . . . 345

13. Caveats to the 'Incentive Salience' hypothesis . . . 348
13.1. Beyond reward to aversion . . . 348
13.2. Beyond the dopamine synapse . . . 349

14. General conclusion . . . 350

15. Addendum 1: Taste reactivity patterns as a measure of 'liking' . . . 350
15.1. Insufficiency of alternative interpretations of affective taste reactivity . . . 351
15.2. Conclusion: Affective reaction patterns reflect hedonic impact of 'liked' stimulus . . . 354

16. Addendum 2: Measuring cognitive expectations of reward in animals (studies of incentive learning by Dickinson and Balleine) . . . 355

17. Note added in proof . . . 356

Acknowledgements . . . 356

References . . . 356

Appearances to the mind are of four kinds. Things either are what they appear to be; or they neither are, nor appear to be; or they are, and do not appear to be; or they are not, and yet appear to be. Rightly to aim in all these cases is the wise man's task.

Epictetus (60 A.D. Translation: Elizabeth Carter [142] — Thomas Higginson [143])

1. Introduction

Among the most thoroughly studied of all brain substrates for reward are dopamine projections from the substantia nigra and ventral tegmentum to forebrain structures such as the nucleus accumbens and neostriatum. It is generally recognized that mesolimbic and neostriatal dopamine projections are crucial to *sensorimotor* function, and so the sensorimotor consequences of dopamine manipulations complicate understanding the role of dopamine in reward [66,202,216,286,303,378,379,381,383,391,392, 456,487]. Nevertheless, many investigators have concluded that dopamine projections play a role in mediating the *reward* value of food, drink, sex, social reinforcers, drugs of abuse, and brain stimulation, above and beyond sensorimotor contributions [13,17,19,26,52,115,117,145,152,155, 158,225,254,259,266,268,310,325,345,347,362,363,401, 423,429,505,513,518]. The focus of this paper is on the *nature* of the contribution of mesolimbic and mesostriatal dopamine systems to reward.

Reward is often conceptualized as if it were a single psychological process or a unitary feature of a reinforcing stimulus. It is sometimes identified with the pleasure or hedonic impact of a stimulus, and is viewed by some as necessarily subjective in nature. We will argue that reward is *not a unitary process*, but instead a constellation of multiple processes many of which can be separately identified in behavior, especially after the component processes are dissociated by brain manipulations. Nor is reward a necessarily subjective event. Evidence for the proposition that reward and motivational processes are not necessarily subjective has been presented and reviewed elsewhere [34,35,161,271,273,316,366] (for discussion see Berridge, in press [35]). Here we will be concerned solely with the separation of component processes of reward, and with the particular component mediated by dopamine-related brain systems.

2. Evidence for a role of dopamine in reward

Mesolimbic and neostriatal dopamine projections have been suggested to serve as a 'common neural currency' for rewards of most kinds sought by animals and humans [268,325,347,421,505]. Activation of dopamine systems, as quantified by electrophysiological, microdialysis, or voltammetric measures, is triggered in animals by encounters with food, sex, drugs of abuse, electrical stimulation at brain sites that support self-stimulation, and by secondary reinforcers for these incentives [5,52,159,233,259,260,263, 283,300,301,344–346,359,401,403–405,425,478]. In humans, presentation of rewards such as cocaine, drug-associated stimuli, and even a video game ('tank combat'), has similarly been reported in PET and fMRI imaging studies to modulate activity in dopamine target sites such as the nucleus accumbens, neostriatum, or prefrontal cortex [62,160,265,477].

Much of the causal evidence that dopamine systems mediate reward comes from studies of pharmacological blockade of dopamine receptors in animals. [2] Many studies show that dopamine antagonists reduce reward-directed instrumental and consummatory behavior in subtle but definite ways—ways that cannot be explained by sensorimotor impairments alone [7,50,145,146,182,234,236,325, 395,429,448,499,500,514,517,518]. Even more dramatic effects are produced by extensive dopamine depletion caused by intracranial application of dopamine-selective neurotoxins such as 6-hydroxydopamine (6-OHDA). After extensive destruction of ascending dopamine neurons, animals become oblivious to food and many other rewards. Rats typically are aphagic and adipsic after 6-OHDA lesions, and will starve to death unless nourished artificially, even though food may be readily available

[2] Regarding *subtypes* of dopamine receptors, a great deal of evidence has implicated the D1 family of dopamine receptor subtypes (containing D1 and D5 receptors) in food and drug reward [13,26,94,457,458,490]. Considerable evidence also suggests that the D2 family of dopamine receptors (containing D2, D3, and D4 receptor subtypes) plays a role in reward [13,83,88,415,429,457,458,490]. To the degree that individual receptor subtypes can be separately manipulated by selective drugs, D1, D2, D3, and D4 dopamine receptor subtypes have all been suggested to participate in at least some aspect of food, drug, or brain stimulation reward [13,27,77,185,228,312,457,458]. Indeed among the dopamine receptors subtypes so far known, it may be safe to say that no subtype has been conclusively ruled out as involved in reward. The proliferation of dopamine receptor subtypes greatly multiplies the complexity of identifying the role of dopamine systems in reward. If individual subtypes are considered separately, the question of 'does dopamine mediate hedonic pleasure', for example, is converted into at least five questions: "does the D1 dopamine receptor subtype mediate hedonic pleasure?, does the D2...?" and so on. Given that the specific roles of different dopamine receptor subtypes in reward are not yet clear [13,457,458], we decline to address the roles of subtypes here. Rather we will be concerned with mesostriatal dopamine projections in general, as dopamine is the endogenous ligand for all subtypes of dopamine receptors. Our approach is based on the logic that *if dopamine systems do not mediate the hedonic impact of reinforcers*, then it is unlikely that the *D3 or any other particular dopamine receptor subtype* will be found to do so. The question if answered negatively for dopamine in general, is answered for each dopamine receptor subtype in turn. Our aim is to identify the *particular reward functions* that are most likely mediated by mesolimbic and mesostriatal dopamine systems. Once that is done, future analyses may answer the important question of which receptor subtypes mediate particular functions. That lies beyond our present scope.

[287,394,407,451,471,531]. Such rats retain the motor capacity to walk, chew, swallow, perform other movements, and to generate many other movement components required for eating, at least under certain conditions, but fail to employ those movements to gain food even if it is available literally under their noses [32,45,111,352,353, 456].

2.1. Nature of dopamine's role in reward: hedonia, incentive salience or reward learning?

Although most investigators would agree that mesolimbic and mesostriatal dopamine systems are crucial to reward in some sense, they disagree about the exact nature of the psychological reward function mediated by dopamine. Perhaps the most influential interpretation has been the *anhedonia* hypothesis, developed by Wise et al. [174,175,499,500,514] to explain the effect of dopamine receptor blockade on behavior. The anhedonia hypothesis (or, regarding normal dopamine function, the *hedonia hypothesis* [181]) suggests that brain dopamine systems mediate the *pleasure* produced by food and other unconditioned incentives such as sex or drugs of abuse, and also the conditioned pleasure elicited by secondary reinforcers. After the administration of dopamine antagonists, according to the anhedonia hypothesis, "all of life's pleasures—the pleasures of primary reinforcement and the pleasures of their associated stimuli—lose their ability to arouse the animal" (Wise, p. 52) [499]. Wise himself has subsequently retracted the hypothesis that dopamine blockade reduces pleasure [504]. However, the anhedonia hypothesis has become so widely accepted that even contemporary media reports often refer to dopamine as the 'brain's pleasure neurotransmitter' [314,491].

The wide acceptance of the hedonia hypothesis has extended to neuroscience investigators as well as to the lay public. This is illustrated by repeated suggestions that suppression of dopaminergic neurotransmission mediates the *anhedonia* of drug withdrawal in addiction [107,268,284,373,477,480,491]. For example, Koob et al. [267,268] suggested that suppression of dopamine neurotransmission in withdrawal produces 'hedonic homeostatic dysregulation', and that addicts seek drugs that activate dopamine systems in order to re-establish 'hedonic homeostasis'. Changes in dopamine neurotransmission appear to move an individual up and down along a 'hedonic scale', according to a recent account by Koob and Le Moal (Fig. 4, p. 56 [268]), in a fashion that follows opponent-process rules [434,435]. Similarly, when Gardner (p. 69 [180]) asks the question "What, then, is the actual role of the ascending DA reward-relevant neuron and the seemingly crucial DA synapse to which it feeds?", he replies (while noting that hedonic encoding by dopamine systems is complex) that, "Even after more than a decade and a half, no suggestion appears to have bettered Wise's hypothesis that "the dopamine junctions represent a synaptic way station... (where) sensory inputs are translated into the hedonic messages we experience as pleasure, euphoria or 'yumminess'"" (quotation from Wise [497], p. 94). A recent commentary by Di Chiara and Tanda "proposes as a biochemical test for anhedonia... the blunting of reactivity of DA neurotransmission in the NAc 'shell'" (p. 353) [119], going so far as to equate anhedonia with a reduction in measured dopamine. Many other investigators have suggested that dopamine specifically mediates the *reinforcing* properties of food, drugs, and other rewards, often using the term 'reinforcement' in a way difficult to distinguish conceptually from hedonic impact [17,148, 234,236,291,310,421,422,429]. [3]

There are, however, alternatives to the an-hedonia/hedonia hypothesis to explain the role of brain dopamine systems in reward. They sprang from the realization that dopamine function in reward often appears linked to *anticipatory, preparatory, appetitive*, or *approach phases* of motivated behavior (as opposed to the consummatory

[3] The term 'reinforcement' can be used in a purely behaviorist sense instead: to mean either *strengthening a stimulus–response habit* (Hull's sense of reinforcement [237,238] or to *increase the rate (probability) of response emission* (Skinner's sense of reinforcement [427,428]). Used in those ways, it is purely descriptive (describing an environment-behavior relation). It applies only to responses that have actually been reinforced, and is equivalent to the measured strength or rate of a behavioral response. White has suggested a distinction between 'reinforcement' (strengthening of stimulus–response tendencies, equivalent to the meaning of non-Skinnerian behaviorists [237,333,459]) and 'reward' (conferring ability to elicit approach, more similar to incentive motivation) [488]. However, these meanings are often combined, and the term 'reinforcement' is typically used by behavioral neuroscientists in ways that differ from the original behaviorist meaning of increased habit strength (quite reasonably, since the behaviorist meaning is inadequate to account for many effects [356,460,502]). For example, place preference measures are sometimes used to assess 'reinforcement' even when no response has been 'reinforced' (as when the animal is trained by putting it passively in the 'reinforced place'). Or, as another example, some have inferred a *decrease* in reinforcement from an *increase* in drug self-administration responses after neuroleptic treatment (e.g., [13,112,267]), a direct contradiction of the behaviorist definition that reinforcement is proportional to the change in response strength. Or, as a final example, 'reinforcement' has been used to refer to a *neural* event elicited by a food or drug *stimulus*, independent of whether any behavioral response is strengthened (e.g., [215,301,359]). Reinforcement always carries additional non-behaviorist connotations whenever it is used in these and many other ways to refer to a psychological or neural property other than response strength. When used in such ways, 'reinforcement' becomes at least implicitly a synonym for a hidden psychological process—typically equivalent to hedonic impact—and often is used as a way of invoking this psychological process without naming it and without giving any other clear definition of what is meant. As Kiyatkin (p. 582 [259]) puts it, "Although it has not been clearly stated, implicit in much of the current literature is the hypothesis that phasic activation of VTA DA cells with subsequent increase in DA release, particularly in NAcc, is the principal neurochemical event associated with natural and drug reinforcement." Dopamine hypotheses of 'reinforcement' that are not restricted to behaviorist S–R habit strengthening will be treated here as implicit equivalents of the hedonia hypothesis (see Wise [502] for more discussion of meanings of 'reinforcement', and Berridge [35] for discussion of meanings of 'hedonic impact').

phase, when hedonic activation is maximal) [51,157,322, 325,378,381,400,401,405,508]. This has led to the proposal of alternative hypotheses regarding the psychological function mediated by mesolimbic dopamine systems in reward.

First, a number of behavioral neuroscientists have suggested that dopamine mediates some aspect of reward learning, or the capacity to predict rewarding events based upon associative correlations [3,4,23,24,89,116,117,304, 400,405,416,488].

Second, we have previously suggested that dopamine-related neural systems mediate a different psychological component of reward, the attribution of incentive salience to otherwise neutral events [34,44,45,347,366].

The incentive salience hypothesis in particular is built on earlier incentive theory formulations of motivation and of dopamine's role [52,157,322,460,508]. It goes further in that it suggests the process of reward can be dissociated into separate components of 'wanting' and 'liking', and that these two psychological processes are mediated by different neural systems. It suggests that dopamine mediates the 'wanting' but not the 'liking' component of rewards. [4] The two words combined in the phrase 'incentive salience' are jointly crucial to its meaning. Incentive salience has both perceptual and motivational features. According to our hypothesis, it transforms the brain's neural representations of conditioned stimuli, converting an event or stimulus from a neutral 'cold' representation (mere information) into an attractive and 'wanted' incentive that can 'grab attention'. But incentive salience is not merely perceptual salience. It is also motivational, and is an essential component of the larger process of reward. Its attribution transforms the neural representation of a stimulus into an object of attraction that animals will work to acquire. It can also make a rewarded response the thing rewarded. By the incentive salience hypothesis, dopamine-related neural systems that mediate 'wanting' interact with hedonic and associative learning components (but is separable from them) to produce the larger composite process of reward. Although incentive salience attribution ordinarily is coordinated by associative learning and hedonic activation, it can be triggered independently of them by some neural and pharmacological manipulations [44,366]. Further,—as will be shown here—incentive salience can be stripped away by other neural manipulations, which leave the hedonic and predictive learning components of reward able to occur normally, but by themselves, and unable to be translated into goal directed behavior.

In principle, 'liking' and 'wanting' are separate psychological components of reward, corresponding to the hedonic impact of a reward vs. its attributed incentive salience [34,366]. In practice, the two processes can be distinguished by comparing appropriate behavioral measures of reward. Traditional methods directly measure reward value by the degree to which the reward is 'wanted': *consumption tests, choice tests, place preference, instrumental performance*. Such behavioral measures require an animal to seek the reinforcer, and infer 'liking' only indirectly from 'wanting', on the assumption that something is 'wanted' if and only if it is 'liked'. By contrast, measures based on *affective reactions*, such as described originally by Darwin [109], provide a more direct measure of whether a stimulus is 'liked'. Affective reactions more specifically reflect the hedonic or aversive affect evoked by a stimulus [34,35,144,241,273] (for discussion of the use of affective reactions to study motivation in animals, see Berridge [35], Epstein [144], or LeDoux [273]). Affective reactions can be used to assess 'liking' for a stimulus independently of 'wanting' it—a fact that will be exploited and discussed below.

The purpose of this paper is to explicitly compare various formulations of hedonia, reward learning, and incentive salience hypotheses of dopamine function. We will present evidence from the literature, and new data, to indicate that dopamine systems contribute to reward by mediating incentive salience attributions to neural representations of stimuli associated with primary hedonic rewards. This evidence indicates that dopamine systems do not mediate the hedonic impact of a stimulus, nor are they necessary for learning new associative relationships involving hedonic stimuli.

2.1.1. Anticipatory dopamine activation: implications for the hedonia hypothesis

One source of data that has been taken as evidence against a hedonia interpretation comes from correlational studies of the *timing* of dopamine activation. Neurochemical studies using microdialysis or in vivo electrochemistry indicate that dopamine systems are often activated *before* animals actually receive a pleasurable incentive such as food or a drug. The hedonia hypothesis predicts dopamine systems to be *maximally* aroused during *maximal* pleasure, that is, during physical commerce with a hedonic reward. Although dopamine systems may indeed be activated during a palatable meal [225,289,290], they are often activated before the meal, *prior* to the taste of food, to the same or even to a greater extent than during food con-

[4] We will place 'liking' and 'wanting' in quotation marks because our use differs in an important way from the ordinary use of these words. By their ordinary meaning, these words typically refer to the subjective experience of conscious pleasure or conscious desire. However, evidence reviewed elsewhere indicates that the conscious experience of these and similar states is separable from the underlying core processes that normally constitute them: the core psychological processes can exist and control human and animal behavior even in the absence of the subjective states [35,273,366]. By 'liking', we refer to the underlying core process of hedonic evaluation that typically produces conscious pleasure, but that can occur without it. By 'wanting', we refer to the underlying core process that instigates goal-directed behavior, attraction to an incentive stimulus, and consumption of the goal object. For a recent review of evidence for 'unconscious core processes' of reward, see Berridge [35].

sumption. For example, Simansky et al. [425] found that hypothalamic DOPAC/dopamine ratios were increased by conditioned stimuli that ordinarily preceded a meal as much as by the meal itself. Blackburn et al. [52] showed that nucleus accumbens DOPAC/dopamine ratios were more highly elevated by *conditioned stimuli* for food presented alone, without food itself, than by the unexpected opportunity to eat. Using in vivo voltammetry, Phillips et al. found that, during the course of a meal, dopamine release was triggered *before* the meal by conditioned stimuli, and remained high until after the end of the meal [345–347]. Richardson and Gratton similarly reported that, as rats became experienced with the associative relationship between cues and food, dopamine release in the nucleus accumbens shifted forward in time from the presentation of food itself to presentation of conditioned stimuli that had been paired with food [359]. Using voltammetry, Kiyatkin and Gratton [260] found that a dopamine-related signal increased in *anticipation* of a food reward as trained rats performed a bar press response, and that increments in dopamine activity were time-locked to the goal-directed response in advance of food delivery.

Electrophysiological studies by Schultz and colleagues also have shown that dopamine neurons discharge in response to conditioned stimuli predictive of food rewards to a greater extent than when animals actually eat the food (i.e., before they presumably experience the pleasurable taste of food). In *inexperienced* monkeys mesolimbic and mesostriatal dopamine neurons discharged only when a palatable liquid was delivered to their mouth or when they were allowed to touch food with their hand [5,278,398,403]. But after a neutral conditioned stimulus (e.g., light) was repeatedly paired with food, dopamine neurons *stopped* responding to food itself and instead fired vigorously in response to the newly established *conditioned incentive* stimulus [5,278,398,403]. In direct contradiction of a 'hedonia prediction' the neurons often failed to discharge when an experienced animal actually obtained the sensory pleasure of food in the mouth [450]. Nor was dopaminergic discharge, according to the investigators, coupled to "mnemonic or preparatory representational task components" [277] (p. 337), to the execution of reaching movements to obtain and retrieve food, or to sensory properties of a light unrelated to food [5,278,398,401–404,450,467]. Similarly, Kosobud et al. [269] reported that in rats trained to bar press for sucrose, ventral tegmental area (VTA) unit activity increased *prior* to the presentation of sucrose. The discharge of VTA neurons was not correlated with the moment when sucrose actually was in the mouth, when presumably the animal would experience the greatest sensory pleasure produced by the taste of sucrose, but rather preceded it [269]. Based on findings such as those described above, Schultz (1992, p. 134) concluded "that dopamine neurons respond specifically to salient stimuli that have alerting, arousing and attention-grabbing properties".

A similar pattern of anticipatory dopamine activation has been reported for drug rewards such as cocaine and heroin [194,263]. The mere presentation of conditioned stimuli for cocaine or amphetamine may trigger dopamine activation [120,262]. In some cases, dopamine neurons may even be more active when an animal 'wants' a drug reward than when it receives and presumably 'likes' it. For example, Kiyatkin and Rebec (p. 2583 [261]) recorded the electrophysiological activity of presumed dopamine neurons in the VTA, and found that the neurons increased their discharge rate as a rat approached and began to press the lever that would earn heroin delivery, but then decreased their discharge rate once the heroin was on board. As those authors put it, their analysis "revealed a frank neuronal activation that began and amplified during approximately the last 40 s before the lever-press at a time when searching behavior was most intense. After the lever-press, neuronal activity declined and this change (decline) became statistically significant at 36–38 s after the onset of drug injection at a time when the rat completely froze."

2.1.2. Failures to find conditioned anticipatory dopamine activation

By contrast, several microdialysis studies have failed to find anticipatory dopamine activation, instead finding it only when the food or heroin reward was actually obtained [493,511]. For example, Wilson et al. reported that dopamine in dialysate increased during the act of eating, but not following mere placement in a location predictive of food [493]. [5] In that study, however, it is not clear whether the training procedure (10 exposures for 10 min) sufficed to give strong *incentive* properties to the conditioning location. Wise et al. found a good relationship between dopamine overflow in the nucleus accumbens and the timing of a bar press for heroin, but dopamine levels in dialysate typically declined slightly before each new bar press, and then rose again after the drug was delivered [510,511]. This contrasts with the voltammetric and electrophysiological studies discussed above [5,120,194,260,262,263,269,278,345–347,359,398,403,425]. Furthermore, once the first heroin reinforcer was administered, dopamine levels were 2 to 8 times higher than baseline throughout the entire session. It is important to remember that in drug self-administration studies, after the first reinforcer is delivered, small bar press-related 'peaks' take place on a 'mountain range' of already-elevated dopamine overflow. Still, Hemby et al. [224] reported that dopamine overflow in the nucleus accumbens (the average height of the mountain range) was higher for rats that

[5] It is interesting that Wilson et al. [493] also found that prior food deprivation increased the dopamine overflow triggered by actual eating. Greater dopamine activation when hungry is consistent with both a hedonia and incentive salience view, since hunger increases both the hedonic palatability and the incentive value of food [33,70,71,73,212].

self-administered cocaine than for rats that passively received cocaine on a yoked schedule. It is difficult to choose among possible explanations for an enhancement of dopamine by response contingency, but the effect suggests that dopamine overflow is influenced by more than the pharmacological properties of cocaine itself. Finally, Bassareo and Di Chiara [14] found that a conditioned stimulus that predicted a palatable food elicited an anticipatory dopamine response in the prefrontal cortex but not in the nucleus accumbens.

These negative microdialysis results (also Wilson et al. [493]) are difficult to interpret. One major problem in making strong inferences from negative microdialysis results concerns the inherent insensitivity of the microdialysis method for detecting small transient events in vivo [279,342] (of the sort to be expected in response to a conditioned stimulus). Lu et al. [279] and Peters and Michael [342] have provided a powerful illustration of these limitations. Negative results must be considered, therefore, in light of the positive results from the voltammetric and electrophysiological studies reviewed above. It remains unclear what experimental factors determine a positive vs. negative outcome. In conclusion, although the literature remains a little mixed, there is ample evidence to support the contention that mesolimbic and mesostriatal dopamine systems often are activated in advance by conditioned stimuli for hedonic incentives.

2.1.3. Anticipatory dopamine activation: multiple interpretations

Anticipatory responses by dopamine neurons to conditioned incentive stimuli have provided the grounds for various 'reward learning' hypotheses of dopamine function. These anticipatory dopamine responses have often been interpreted to reflect a form of 'neural expectation', a prediction of subsequent reward value, a correlational error detector, a teaching signal, or similar component of an associative mechanism that is dedicated to learning about rewards [3,4,23,24,61,89,116,304,400,405,416,488]. However, anticipatory responses to salient stimuli that have alerting, arousing and attention-grabbing properties are equally compatible with the incentive salience hypothesis. If the conditioned stimulus itself is attractive to the animal, and serves as a conditioned reinforcer, then it has acquired incentive salience of its own. The difference between the two views is that a learning hypothesis posits that dopamine neurons mediate *associative learning* and expectations *based on previous experience* with a stimulus. It ascribes conditioned dopamine activity chiefly to the *predictive* value of the conditioned stimulus: what has been in the past is predicted for the future. The incentive salience hypothesis, by contrast, ascribes conditioned dopamine activity to its *incentive* value: whether it is 'wanted'. This difference will be elaborated below.

But even the hedonia hypothesis of dopamine function could be reconciled with anticipatory neural activity if one interpreted early neural activity to reflect *conditioned hedonic activation*. Conditioned stimuli that have been paired with hedonic stimuli can sometimes evoke a conditioned hedonic response on their own [42,49,63,113,377,460,463,499,500]. Conditioned stimuli for pleasant tastes or unpleasant shocks, for example, do indeed evoke a variety of hedonic or fearful affective reactions [42,113,273,358].

As mentioned above, however, it is difficult for the hedonia hypothesis to explain why a conditioned hedonic response should sometimes be of *greater magnitude* than the unconditioned hedonic response to food itself. It is also difficult for the hedonia hypothesis to explain why with training neurons should *stop responding to the unconditioned reward itself*, and respond only to a conditioned stimulus, as described by Schultz et al. [5,278,398,403,450]. However, it should be noted that some of these experiments involved overtraining of a rewarded response (10,000 to 30,000 trials). Extensive overtraining has been shown to detach motivational properties from conditioned responses, leaving the response relatively automatic and habitual in nature, devoid of hedonic/incentive features that characterized it earlier (see Dickinson [124,125]).

A further defense of the hedonia hypothesis could be mounted if the activation of dopamine neurons turns out to have *self-limiting* properties, which shut the neurons off after they have fired. There may be some grounds for this defense. Depolarization inactivation may inhibit dopamine neurons from subsequent activation under some circumstances [192,502]. For example, phasic bursts of firing may produce post-burst inhibition of dopamine neurons [192,193], and post-burst inhibition of subsequent neural firing is especially strong for dopamine neurons that project to the nucleus accumbens [84]. A 'burst pattern' of firing seems to be a strong feature of dopamine neurons [321]. The phenomenon of post-burst inhibition of dopamine neurons means that a robust response to a conditioned hedonic stimulus could conceivably inhibit the response to the unconditioned event that follows, at least under some conditions.

3. Brain manipulations of behavior for revealing dopamine's function in reward

The electrophysiological and neurochemical studies of dopamine activity discussed above do not allow us to conclusively exclude any hypothesis of dopamine function in reward. At best, these studies provide *correlational* evidence for a particular functional hypothesis, and at worst, the evidence is compatible with more than one hypothesis, perhaps with all. Thus, the results of electrophysiological and neurochemical studies so far do not by themselves justify rejection of the anhedonia hypothesis, or permit a choice between reward prediction and incentive salience alternatives.

A different approach to the question is to *manipulate neural systems* by drugs, electrical stimulation, or lesions, and to apply *behavioral measures* designed to choose among competing hypotheses. Of special interest to our discussion are behavioral measures of *affective reactions* designed specifically to detect the hedonic impact of a reinforcer. A behavioral measure that separates *hedonic impact* ('liking') from incentive value ('wanting') or reward prediction (expected reward) could potentially distinguish between the effects of dopamine manipulations on hedonia, incentive salience or reward learning.

3.1. Traditional measures of reward: instrumental behavior and choice ('wanting')

Traditional behavioral methods for measuring reward typically quantify preference (choice), consumption of a goal (intake), or instrumental behavior (bar press, runway, or approach). Whether an incentive stimulus is 'liked' is then *inferred* based on behavioral evidence that it is 'wanted' (i.e., whether an animal will choose it, consume it, or work to acquire it). The inference is grounded on the assumption that rewards are always 'wanted' to the same degree as they are 'liked'. With these traditional methods 'wanting' cannot be discriminated from 'liking', because both are viewed through the same lens (measured by the same dependent variable). Direct evidence that dopamine mediates 'wanting' specifically or 'liking' specifically would require that changes in reward '*liking*' be measured *separately* from reward '*wanting*'.

3.2. Measures of reward based on affective reactions ('liking')

An entirely different approach to studying brain mechanisms of reward (especially food reward) is to use a measure of hedonic impact such as behavioral affective reactions [35,144,273]. Unlike measures of instrumental behavior, affective expressions do not assess the 'wanting' for a reward in advance of obtaining it. Instead, as pointed out over a century ago by Darwin [109] and James [241], affective reactions typically reflect the *emotional impact* of a motivational event once the event is actually encountered. Regarding reward, emotional or hedonic impact corresponds more closely to 'liking' than to 'wanting'.

Most familiar to readers are human *affective facial expressions* as a measure of emotional impact. Affective facial expressions often reflect emotional states, but have the potential limitation (in socially competent individuals) of being feigned or suppressed in the service of social intentions [109,140,141,177]. The human ability to voluntarily control affective expressions to pleasant or unpleasant tastes and odors appears in childhood [184,436]. But newborn humans show distinct facial affective reactions to sweet or bitter tastes *even on the day of birth*, before they are subject to social control. Thus, in newborns, facial affective reactions are thought to reflect relatively directly the infant brain's hedonic or aversive evaluation of the taste [441,442,445]. Human infants, and both infant and adult apes and monkeys, show similar hedonic and aversive expressions to sweet and bitter, and the expressions become increasingly different in pattern from humans' as phylogenetic distance grows [443–445]. Related patterns of hedonic and aversive affective reactions are found even in rats: patterns of tongue protrusion by rats to sweet sucrose, and of gapes and headshakes to bitter quinine (described originally by Grill and Norgren [210]).

3.2.1. Taste reactivity patterns as a measure of 'liking'

The taste reactivity test is a method that can be used to assess the hedonic impact of tastes ('liking' or perceived palatability) by quantifying behavioral affective reaction patterns elicited by tastes [34,206,210]. Rats, which are generalized omnivores, prefer sweet foods and avoid bitter ones, as do many primates [377], and these preferences are reflected in their affective reactions to tastes. Some affective reactions of rats to food overlap with those of primates (including gapes to quinine and rhythmic tongue protrusions to sucrose [445]), whereas others are different [210,445]. The taste reactivity test measures the immediate 'liking' reaction of a rat to a taste reward after it is received, even if delivered by an intra-oral cannula. *(The rationale and evidence for this proposition are summarized in Addendum 1).* Thus, with the taste reactivity test affective 'liking' evaluations of a taste can be quantified independently of whether a taste stimulus is 'wanted' (i.e., of whether an animal will work for it or choose it). Indeed, taste reactivity can be measured even in animals incapable of any instrumental action or voluntary eating [211].

There is now considerable evidence that measures of taste reactivity reflect core evaluations of a taste's hedonic and aversive impact [34,206]. That is, taste reactivity patterns are true affective expressions, connoting core processes of 'liking' and 'disliking' (see Addendum 1). Thus, the taste reactivity test provides a means to explore the neural substrates for hedonic 'liking', and can complement studies of human hedonic affect. Of course, data for human subjective reports are available for only a few selective manipulations, usually pharmacological (which will be discussed later). By comparison, an important strength of the taste reactivity technique is that it can be applied to many diverse brain systems using animal subjects. Hedonic and aversive reaction patterns have been used in neurobehavioral studies to identify brain substrates of food 'liking'.

- The opioid agonist, morphine, administered systemically, intraventricularly, or directly into the shell region of the nucleus accumbens enhances hedonic reactions to sweet and other tastes under conditions similar to those in which it elicits feeding [131,336,338]. Aversive reactions, by contrast, are not enhanced, but instead inhibited by morphine [86,131,332]. In other words, an accumbens opioid neural circuit is involved in hedonic activation or 'liking'.

This is consistent with suggestions that opioid systems mediate food palatability [87,98,186,226,227,276,481], a hypothesis that receives some support from human subjective rating studies [133,520].

• Benzodiazepines, such as diazepam, chlordiazepoxide, or midazolam, promote feeding in animals and humans [92,97,257,509]. This has been argued by Cooper et al. [92,93] to be driven by a drug-induced increase in the hedonic palatability of food. Taste reactivity studies confirm this hypothesis. When administered to rats systemically, into the cerebral ventricles, or directly to the hindbrain, benzodiazepines enhance hedonic reaction patterns just as morphine does [40,43,95,328,337,431,465]. Aversive reaction patterns are never enhanced by benzodiazepines. In other words, a brainstem benzodiazepine/GABA circuit contributes to hedonic taste processing [40].

• Conversely, blanket 'disliking' for food is produced by several forms of brain damage that result in aphagia. After electrolytic lesions of the lateral hypothalamus, circumscribed excitotoxic lesions of the ventral pallidum, or ablation of the ventral forebrain even sweet foods elicit aversive reactions, and hedonic reactions are suppressed or abolished [36,106,211,446,455]. These lesions overlap each other in their pattern of neuronal destruction, and have been suggested to involve the loss of a common 'liking' circuit in the ventral pallidum, resulting in disinhibition of aversion [34].

3.3. *Dopamine manipulations dissociate 'wanting' vs. 'liking'*

Manipulations of mesolimbic/neostriatal dopamine systems also potently modify the motivation to eat ('wanting' measured by voluntary intake, preference tests, or instrumental behavior for food). However, dopamine-related manipulations *fail to alter 'liking'* (measured by hedonic or aversive reaction patterns).

3.3.1. *Pharmacological manipulations*

Haloperidol, pimozide, and other dopamine receptor blockers decrease the incentive or reward value of food, as measured by intake, preference, or instrumental measures [429,499,500,514]. But dopamine antagonists do not shift the hedonic palatability of tastes toward aversion, as measured by taste reactivity [339,465]. [6] Conversely, dopamine agonists do not increase hedonic reactions to tastes [34,465], although they can alter their incentive value [150,151,424], and produce sensorimotor disruption of elicited reactions [326,379,382,386,391,392,452].

3.3.2. *Electrical stimulation of the lateral hypothalamus*

Electrical stimulation of the lateral hypothalamus (LH) can elicit robust eating and is typically rewarding in its own right [231,474]. LH stimulation involves many neural systems, but activation of ascending dopamine projections appears to be one crucial link in the chain of neural events important to feeding and reward [157,348,375,472,519]. A stimulation-induced increase in perceived palatability has been suggested as one way by which LH stimulation might increase feeding [232]. The hedonia hypothesis also predicts LH stimulation would increase food hedonics, if dopamine activation mediates the effect of stimulation. But Berridge and Valenstein found that electrical stimulation of the lateral hypothalamus *fails to enhance hedonic taste reactivity patterns* in rats even though they eat avidly when the stimulation is on [44]. If anything, electrical stimulation increases *aversive* reactions to palatable tastes. That is, LH electrical stimulation apparently elicits eating not because it makes food 'taste better', but despite making it 'taste worse' [44]. The feeding induced by LH stimulation is strikingly unlike that produced by opioids or benzodiazepines, and unlike natural hunger or specific appetites such as salt hunger. All of these other manipulations make the eaten food both 'liked' and 'wanted'—that is, they enhance both feeding and hedonic reaction patterns [38,40,73,131]. The paradoxical 'wanting' without 'liking' produced by LH stimulation can be explained by hypothesizing that the electrode activates dopamine substrates of incentive salience selectively, but bypasses hedonic neural systems of food reward [34,44] (see Fig. 6).

3.3.3. *6-Hydroxydopamine (6-OHDA) lesions*

The massive destruction of ascending dopamine neurons with 6-OHDA causes profound aphagia [470,471]. But an earlier study by us of whether dopamine depletion diminishes the *hedonic impact* of foods found that intranigral 6-OHDA lesions, which produced both aphagia and adipsia, *failed to suppress hedonic reaction patterns or to increase aversive reaction patterns* [45]. Instead, hedonic and aversive taste reactivity patterns to sweet, sour or bitter tastes remained normal after 6-OHDA lesions. From those results, we concluded that the nigrostriatal dopamine pathway was not necessary for a normal hedonic response to food rewards, and that dopamine depletion did not induce anhedonia [45].

4. Effects of mesolimbic and neostriatal dopamine depletion on subcomponents of reward

This brings us to our current study, which was intended to deal with short-comings in our previous study, and to determine if any aspects of reward remain intact after the

[6] The conclusion that dopamine antagonists do not shift 'liking' was the focus of an earlier controversy, because several studies by Parker and colleagues had indicated that pimozide might gradually reduce hedonic 'liking' and increase aversive 'disliking' if the taste stimulus was sustained continuously for more than a few minutes [274,331]. However, crucial evidence for anhedonia has failed to replicate in a recent collaborative re-examination of those data by Peciña et al. (discussed below) [339]. It can be stated as a general conclusion, now shared among all laboratories that have studied the effect of neuroleptics on affective taste reactivity, that dopamine antagonists do not produce anhedonic palatability shifts in taste reactivity patterns.

brain is depleted of mesolimbic and mesostriatal dopamine. First, several objections can be raised to our earlier conclusion that dopamine loss fails to produce anhedonia.

· The average dopamine depletion in our earlier 6-OHDA study was only 85% [45]. Our animals were aphagic, but some have argued that dopamine depletion above 90% to 95% may be required in order for 6-OHDA lesions to produce their full behavioral impact [451,452].

· Dopamine concentrations in the nucleus accumbens were not measured in our earlier study [45]. Residual accumbens dopamine probably exceeded 15% because 6-OHDA lesions in the substantia nigra would have spared substantial projections from the ventral tegmentum to the nucleus accumbens. Therefore, the normal hedonic reactions could have been mediated by residual dopamine in the nucleus accumbens.

· Only *unconditioned* affective reactions to novel tastes were investigated in our earlier study [45]. This leaves open an alternative interpretation: namely, that dopamine depletion may have *decoupled control of taste reactivity patterns from forebrain control* rather than preserving normal hedonic evaluations (an alternative originally suggested to us by Jane Stewart) [449]. That interpretation hinges on the following logic. The evidence that taste reactivity patterns ordinarily reflect forebrain hedonic evaluations comes from demonstrations that associative experience alters affective taste reactivity patterns [30,42,63,209,330,530]. This effect is eliminated after decerebration or certain forebrain lesions [206,207,209,426]. The capacity of decerebration to block modulations of affective reactions indicates that the modulation normally reflects forebrain hierarchical control of brainstem circuitry [206]. The possibility arises, therefore, that 6-OHDA lesions might also eliminate the forebrain's capacity for *hierarchical control* of affective reactivity patterns based on forebrain hedonic evaluations, even though they spare unconditioned taste reactivity reflexes mediated by the brainstem. If the 'forebrain decoupling' hypothesis were true, then it would be possible for dopamine depletion to have rendered the forebrain anhedonic without any evidence appearing in behavioral taste reactivity patterns. It is possible to test this hypothesis. If it is true, then effects such as conditioned aversion shifts in taste reactivity patterns, induced by associative taste-LiCl pairing, would no longer be possible in animals that had extensive 6-OHDA lesions.

· Finally, no attempt has been made in previous taste reactivity studies to examine the *reward learning hypothesis* of dopamine function. There is evidence that dopamine systems are not needed for all types of associative learning [23]. However, dopamine might still be required to mediate *learning of reward associations*, which would be needed to give new hedonic reward properties to a stimulus, for example, as has been suggested by Di Chiara [116,117] and by Beninger and Miller [26]. Can hedonic reactions to a stimulus be transformed by new learning after dopamine depletion, based on conditioned relations that predict later consequences of that stimulus?

4.1. General experimental approach

The present experimental study was undertaken in order to deal with these issues. It aimed to test more adequately whether mesolimbic and neostriatal dopamine systems are needed for normal hedonic reactions to food reward, or for modulation of hedonic reward properties. In this study 6-OHDA lesions were placed in the lateral hypothalamus at a point where fibers from both the substantia nigra and the ventral tegmentum pass closely together. This produced, in some animals, a 98% to 99% depletion of dopamine in the nucleus accumbens and neostriatum (caudate/putamen).

In Experiment 1, we assessed unconditioned hedonic and aversive taste reactivity patterns to sucrose and quinine in aphagic rats that had extensive dopamine depletion.

In Experiment 2, we assessed the capacity of dopamine-depleted rats to *change the hedonic reward value* of a stimulus by *forebrain-mediated associative learning*, using a taste-aversion conditioning procedure. A novel preferred taste was associatively paired with systemic administration of LiCl. The affective reactions emitted by 6-OHDA rats were monitored to determine whether their reactions switched from hedonic patterns to aversive patterns as a consequence of associative learning.

In Experiment 3, we assessed the capacity of dopamine-depleted rats to show *enhancement of hedonic reactions* after administration of a benzodiazepine agonist, diazepam, that normally induces hyperphagia and that increases hedonic palatability.

In every experiment, the affective taste reactivity patterns of 6-OHDA rats were similar to those of control rats. The elimination of dopamine from the nucleus accumbens and neostriatum does not appear to produce anhedonia for food rewards, nor to block the pharmacological modulation of food 'liking', nor to block the learning or expression of new likes and dislikes.

5. Experiment 1: Unconditioned affective reactions to sucrose or quinine

5.1. Methods

5.1.1. Surgery

Thirty-eight female and male Sprague–Dawley rats (260–310 g at surgery) were housed individually in plastic tub cages with wood shaving bedding.

Rats were anesthetized with ketamine (87 mg/kg. i.p.) and Rompun (13 mg/kg, i.p.). Each was pretreated with atropine methyl nitrate (5 mg/kg, i.p.) to prevent respiratory distress, bicillin (30,000 units, i.m.) to prevent infection, and desipramine (15 mg/kg, i.p.) and pargyline (50 mg/kg) to protect norepinephrine terminals and maximize dopamine depletion. Thirty min after drug pretreatment, a midline incision was made, the dorsal skull was exposed, skull screws were placed, and bilateral holes were drilled for microinjections. The dura was opened, and a 30-gauge injection cannula was lowered to intercept ascending dopamine projections (AP = −4.0 mm from bregma; L = +1.8 mm from midline; V = −8.3 mm from skull surface). Twenty-eight rats received bilateral infusions of 8 μg of 6-hydroxydopamine HBr (6-OHDA) dissolved in 4 μl of vehicle (0.9% NaCl solution containing 0.1 mg/ml ascorbic acid). Ten control rats received microinjections of the vehicle solution alone. Infusions were delivered over an 8 min period using an infusion pump, and the injection cannula was left in place for 5 min after the infusion.

In the same surgery, bilateral chronic oral cannulae to permit taste reactivity testing were implanted. The PE-100 cannulae, heat flared at the oral end, entered the mouth lateral to the first maxillary molars, where they were anchored with a Teflon washer. Oral cannulae ascended lateral to the skull, beneath the zygomatic arch, and exited the head dorsally where they were attached to 19-gauge. steel tubing and anchored to the skull screws with dental acrylic cement.

5.1.2. Postsurgical maintenance and recovery

Rats that received lesions were artificially fed and watered by intragastric intubation as follows. On the day after surgery, each rat was intubated twice with 10 ml of water to prevent dehydration. Each day a palatable cereal mash (moistened Gerber's baby cereal) and fresh Purina rat chow pellets were provided on a free access basis. Food and water intake and body weight were monitored daily. Beginning on the second day after surgery, rats that lost weight were intubated with a liquid diet. For every 5 g body weight loss, the rat was intubated with 12 ml of a liquid diet (made of equal parts of sweetened condensed milk and water, with a multivitamin supplement added), up to a maximum of three intubations per day.

Rats were classified as *aphagic* on a given day if they ate neither cereal mash nor chow. Aphagic rats received all of their nourishment by intubation of liquid diet. If rats ate *any* cereal mash or chow pellets on a given day, they were classified as *not aphagic* and were excluded from the study. Rats that were aphagic for at least one week were used in this study, and *only data collected during their period of aphagia* were used for the analysis presented below. Non-aphagic rats were excluded because for this study it was of interest to determine if 'liking' remained only if 'wanting' was abolished.

Of the twenty-eight rats that received 6-OHDA lesions, two died during the 7-day recovery period before testing began. Four 6-OHDA rats began to eat cereal mash or chow during this time, and were dropped from the study. Twenty-two 6-OHDA rats remained aphagic on the 8th day after surgery, and proceeded to taste reactivity testing. Of these, 12 remained aphagic throughout the entire test series (17 days after surgery), and data are presented only for these long-term aphagic rats.

5.1.3. Behavioral taste reactivity testing

Behavioral testing began on the eighth day after surgery. A single taste reactivity trial was given each day, using one of three stimulus solutions: Sucrose (either 0.3 M or 1.0 M), or Quinine HCl (3×10^{-4} M). Each stimulus solution was administered three times, in counter-balanced order, over a period of nine days.

On each trial, a rat's oral cannula was connected to an infusion line (PE-50 tubing with a PE-10 nozzle). The rat was placed in a transparent test chamber and allowed to habituate for 5 min. A 1 ml volume of the stimulus solution was infused into the rat's mouth over a period of 1 min. A mirror positioned beneath the transparent floor of the chamber reflected the image of the rat's face and mouth into the close-up lens of a video camera. Videotaped records were saved for later slow-motion analysis of taste reactivity.

Taste reactivity components were scored in slow-motion, ranging from frame-by-frame to 1/10th actual speed [210]. Three classes of affective taste reactivity patterns were scored: hedonic, aversive, and neutral (for discussion of hedonic/aversive classification of taste reactivity patterns, see [34,40,206]. *Hedonic* reaction patterns were considered to be: lateral tongue protrusions, rhythmic tongue protrusions, and paw licks. *Aversive* reaction patterns were considered to be: gapes, chin rubs, face washing, forelimb flails, paw tread, and locomotion (see [210] for descriptions). Several reaction patterns are less reliable as indicators of an acceptability evaluation, and were classified here as *Neutral*: rhythmic mouth movements, passive drip of the solution, and sequential alternation between face washing and paw licks with less than 1 s transition (a sequential combination which is typical of self-grooming, and which when combined in sequential alternation is not associated with other hedonic or aversive reactions; for hedonic/neutral/aversive classification of taste reactivity patterns, see [40]). Each lateral tongue protrusion, gape, and chin rub were counted as individual events. Each *instance* of face washing, forelimb flailing, and locomotion (in which several rapid movements are typically chained in a brief bout) was counted as a separate event. Rhythmic midline tongue protrusions, which may be emitted in continuous bouts of several seconds, were counted in 2-s bins (one tongue protrusion or a continuous series of up to 2 s duration were counted as 1 bin; 3–4 continuous seconds of tongue protrusions were counted as 2 bins, etc.). Rhythmic mouth movements and paw licks, which often are emitted in even longer bouts, were counted similarly in 5-s bins. This scoring system helps equalize the contribution of different reaction types to the final hedonic or aversive scores, by preventing actions that occur more frequently from dominating the affective category [39].

5.1.4. Neurochemistry

At the end of the experiments 7 control rats and 12 6-OHDA lesion rats that had remained aphagic for at least 2 weeks were killed humanely by instantaneous decapitation, and their brains were removed and placed in iced saline within 40 s of death. Each brain was cooled for 1 min, placed on a cutting block, and sliced [222]. The left and right neostriatum (caudate-putamen) and the left and right nucleus accumbens were extracted by micropunch. Each tissue core was weighed, and the left and right sides from each structure were placed together in separate tubes containing 400 ml $HClO_4$ (0.05 N), to which 250 ng dihydroxybenzylamine was added. The tissue was homogenized, and the suspension was centrifuged for 45 min ($5000 \times g$). The supernatant was filtered through 0.45-mm pore filters, and the samples were frozen at −20°C. Within two weeks, the samples were assayed by HPLC with electrochemical detection, using procedures similar to those described previously [368]. Dopamine concentrations in the neostriatum and nucleus accumbens were ascertained for each rat, and the *percentage of dopamine depletion* for each 6-OHDA brain was calculated based on the mean concentrations of dopamine in the neostriatum and the nucleus accumbens of control rats.

5.2. Results

5.2.1. Neurochemistry

The mean concentration of neostriatal dopamine in control rats was 10.36 ± 0.51 ng per mg wet tissue weight, and was 8.50 ± 0.31 ng/mg in the nucleus accumbens (Fig. 1). Rats that had received 6-OHDA lesions had reduced concentrations of dopamine: 1.09 ± 0.58 ng/mg in the neostriatum, and 2.19 ± 0.49 ng/mg in the nucleus accumbens. Overall, the group of 12 rats with 6-OHDA lesions had dopamine depletion of 90% in the neostriatum and 74% in the nucleus accumbens.

Many of the 6-OHDA lesion rats, however, had more severe dopamine depletion. Eight of the 12 were depleted of neostriatal dopamine by more than 98%. In this group of 8 rats, *neostriatal dopamine was depleted by 98.8 ± 0.5%, and nucleus accumbens dopamine was depleted by 85.0 ± 4.8%* (Fig. 1). A further subgroup of 3 rats from this group were depleted of dopamine by over 99% in *both* the neostriatum and the nucleus accumbens (*99.8 ± 0.1% in the neostriatum and 99.0 ± 0.2% in the nucleus accumbens;* Fig. 1).

Since the purpose of this study was to assess the consequences of the most severe dopamine depletion on affective reaction patterns, separate analyses were conducted for each group and subgroup in every experiment described below: a) aphagic 6-OHDA group as a whole

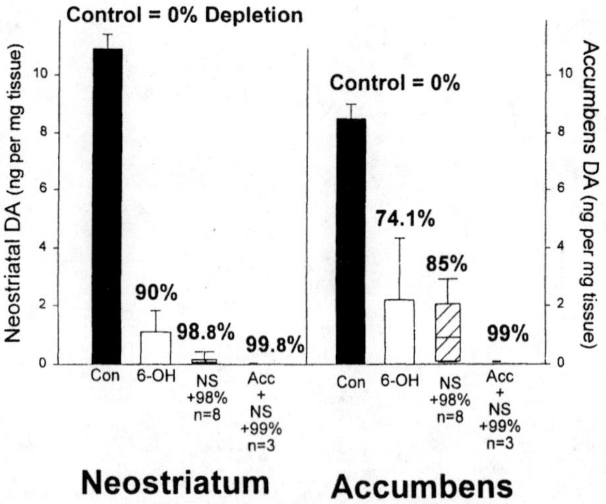

Fig. 1. Dopamine concentrations in the neostriatum and nucleus accumbens of control and 6-OHDA lesion groups. Absolute concentrations shown by bars and boxes (ng/mg tissue). Relative percent depletion of each group compared to controls is listed at top of each plot. Control and aphagic 6-OHDA groups are shown by filled and open bars (mean ± S.E.M.). The 6-OHDA subgroup with neostriatal depletion > 98% is depicted by hatched box plot (box = 25th to 75th percentile range, line shows median, error bar shows 90th percentile). The 6-OHDA subgroup with accumbens and neostriatal depletion > 99% had values too low to be graphed.

($n = 12$); b) confirmed > *98% dopamine depletion in neostriatum* ($n = 8$); and c) confirmed > *99% depletion in both neostriatum and accumbens* ($n = 3$).

5.2.2. Hedonic taste reactivity patterns to sucrose

Hedonic reactions. Sucrose elicited hedonic reaction patterns (rhythmic tongue protrusions, lateral tongue protrusions, paw licks) from both aphagic 6-OHDA rats and control rats; the groups did not differ in total number of hedonic reactions (Fig. 2; two-factor analysis of variance (lesion condition × sucrose concentration) $F(1,40) = 2.66$, n.s.). Concentrated 1.0 M solution elicited more hedonic reactions than did 0.3 M sucrose in both control and 6-OHDA lesion groups ($F(1,40) = 10.15$, $p < 0.01$; in this and subsequent analyses, interaction effects between lesion/control groups and other factors were never significant). In other words, aphagic 6-OHDA rats emitted the same number of hedonic reactions to sucrose as did controls, and they modulated their number of reactions appropriately to sucrose concentration.

The group of rats with > 98% neostriatal dopamine depletion ($n = 8$) similarly showed a concentration-dependent increase in hedonic reactions when compared with controls ($F(1,34) = 20.24$, $p < 0.001$). This group of severely depleted rats actually appeared to emit *more* hedonic reactions overall than did controls (mean ± S.E.M. = 5.9 + 0.9 for the neostriatum depletion > 98% group compared to 3.3 + 0.8 for the control group; $F(1,34) = 4.79$, $p < 0.05$; Fig. 2). The hedonic elevation disappeared for the subgroup of lesion rats with > 99% depletion from both accumbens and neostriatum ($n = 3$; Fig. 2). There were no significant interaction effects between dopamine group and stimulus concentration. Taken together, these data demonstrate that extensive dopamine depletion in the neostriatum and nucleus accumbens fails to impair the emission of hedonic reactions to sweet stimuli.

5.2.3. Taste reactivity component distribution

There were no differences between the control group and 6-OHDA lesion groups in the *distribution* of motor components *within* the hedonic category. For example, the groups did not differ in terms of the relative number of rhythmic tongue protrusions vs. of lateral tongue protrusions or other reactions elicited by sucrose (compared by the Mann–Whitney test). Nor did the groups differ in the *incidence* or proportion of rats that emitted each particular reaction (compared by the z test of proportion).

5.2.4. Few aversive reactions to sucrose

Sucrose elicited relatively few aversive reaction patterns from either group. The 0.3 M solution elicited slightly more aversive reactions than the concentrated 1.0 M solution ($F(1,40) = 6.12$, $p < 0.02$), but the aphagic 6-OHDA lesion rats did not differ from the control group, ($F(1,40) = 0.76$, n.s.), nor did the group of 6-OHDA rats with neostriatal depletion > 98% ($F(1,34) = 1.82$, n.s.). When the analysis was restricted to rats that were confirmed to have both accumbens and neostriatal dopamine depletion > 99%, 6-OHDA rats emitted slightly more aversive reactions to 0.3 M sucrose (3.0 + 0.5) than did control rats (1.4 + 0.3). However, neither group emitted any aversive reactions at all to more concentrated 1.0 M sucrose.

5.2.5. Aversive taste reactivity patterns to quinine

Quinine HCl elicited predominantly aversive reactions, and few hedonic reactions, from both 6-OHDA lesion rats and from control rats (Fig. 3). There was no difference between the aphagic 6-OHDA and control groups in the number of (few) hedonic reactions ($F(1,18) = 2.0$, n.s.) or aversive reactions ($F(1,18) = 0.01$, n.s.). Separate analyses restricted to the 6-OHDA 'neostriatal depletion > 98% group' or 'both accumbens and neostriatal depletion > 99% group' produced identical outcomes: in each case, 6-OHDA reactions to quinine were not different from control group reactions.

These data suggest that although some 6-OHDA rats may occasionally be more responsive than controls in both hedonic and aversive reaction patterns, dopamine depletion did not shift reactions consistently toward aversive patterns, nor did it shift reactions away from hedonic patterns. No consistent difference in hedonic/aversive reaction patterns to sucrose or quinine was produced by severe dopamine depletion.

5.3. Discussion of Experiment 1

The results of Experiment 1 confirm our earlier report that unconditioned affective reaction patterns elicited by sucrose and quinine solutions are essentially normal in rats after 6-OHDA lesions of the striatal/accumbens dopamine system [45]. They extend our earlier results to show that affective reaction patterns remain normal even after essentially complete depletion of dopamine from these structures, at levels exceeding 99% depletion from both nucleus accumbens and neostriatum.

The loss of dopamine from the neostriatum and accumbens does not appear to lead to anhedonia or a motor inability to emit affective reactions. Rats with nearly complete dopamine depletion showed no suppression of unconditioned hedonic reaction patterns to sucrose.

But the possibility remains that dopamine depletion might disrupt the expression in taste reactivity patterns of *learned hedonic shifts* induced by manipulations that depend on the forebrain. If that were true, it would raise the possibility that hedonic reaction patterns might no longer provide evidence of forebrain evaluation of hedonic events. After all, decerebration or other forebrain lesions that isolate the brainstem from forebrain control leave basic unconditioned taste reactivity motor patterns intact—but only as simpler reflexes, no longer modifiable by associative or neural manipulations that change forebrain affective

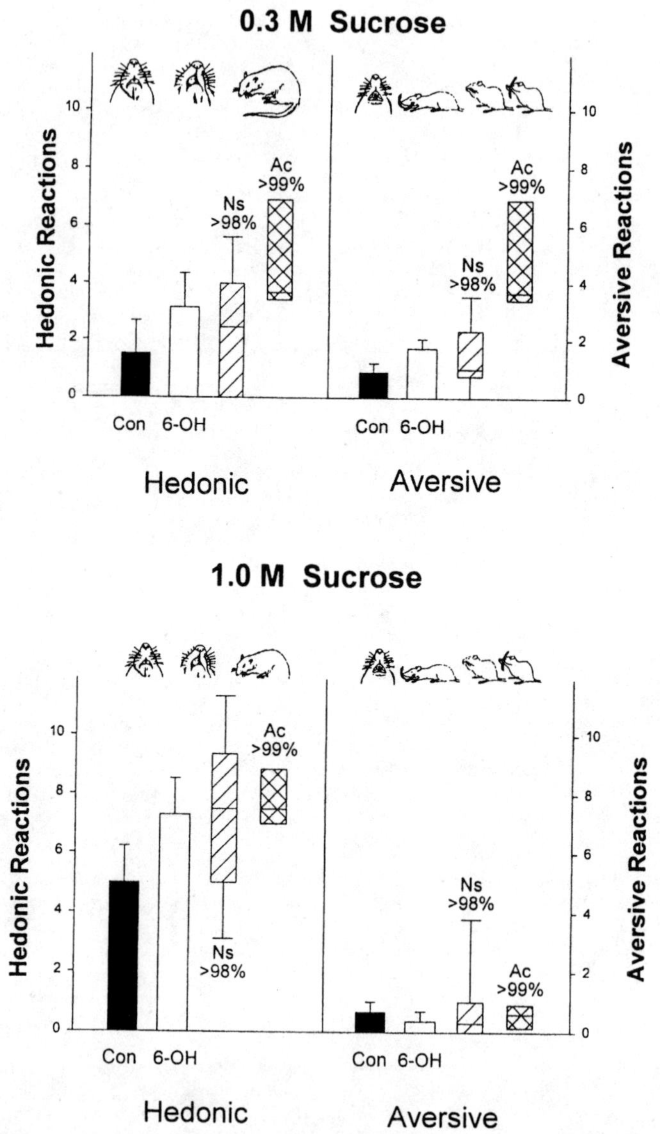

Fig. 2. Hedonic reaction patterns of control and 6-OHDA groups to oral infusions of 0.3 M (top) and 1.0 M (bottom) sucrose. Hedonic reactions are on the left half and aversive reactions on the right half of each graph. Each shows the reactions of the control group (solid bar), aphagic 6-OHDA group (open bar), 6-OHDA group with neostriatum depletion > 98% (hatched box), and 6-OHDA subgroup with accumbens + neostriatal depletion > 99% (double hatched box). Bars for control and aphagic 6-OHDA groups depict mean ± S.E.M. Hatched box plot shows affective reactions for neostriatum depletion > 98% group ($n = 8$; median shown by horizontal line, box ends show 25th to 75th percentile range, and error bars show 10th to 90th percentile range). Double hatched box plot shows entire range of affective reactions for accumbens/neostriatum depletion > 99% group ($n = 3$; horizontal line shows middle member; box end shows extreme members).

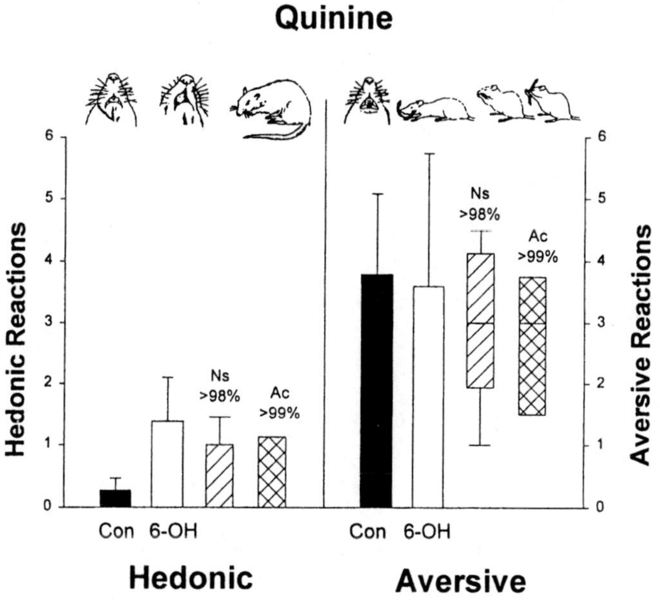

Fig. 3. Aversive taste reaction patterns of 6-OHDA and control groups to oral quinine infusion (3×10^{-5} M quinine HCl). Symbols as in Fig. 2.

evaluations [206–209,258]. On the other hand, if associative taste aversion learning still produced a normal shift from hedonic to aversive reaction patterns after dopamine depletion, it would imply that taste reactivity patterns still reflect palatability evaluations that require the forebrain.

The role of dopamine in *reward learning* is another issue that hinges importantly on whether associative conditioning can alter affective taste reactivity patterns after dopamine depletion. If 6-OHDA lesions disrupted the capacity of taste aversion conditioning to shift affective reactions, it would support the hypothesis that dopamine is especially important in order for a stimulus *to acquire new hedonic value via associative learning*, and that this is its major role in reward. But if severe dopamine depletion does not prevent the shift from hedonic to aversive reaction patterns after taste aversion learning, it indicates that dopamine is not needed to mediate associatively-acquired shifts in hedonic value.

6. Experiment 2: Modulation of affective reactions by taste aversion conditioning

6.1. Methods

6.1.1. Subjects

Eight 6-OHDA lesion rats that remained aphagic 20 days after surgery but were otherwise in good health, and 7 control rats, were used in this Experiment. The 6-OHDA group included 7 rats that had > 98% neostriatal dopamine depletion, and the 3 rats that had > 99% depletion in both nucleus accumbens and neostriatum.

6.1.2. Taste CS +

A palatable and novel saccharin/polycose solution (0.2% w/v sodium saccharin and 32% w/v polycose) was used as the conditioned stimulus [408]. Polycose by itself does not taste sweet to humans, but is a preferred solution for rats, and behavioral short term intake and electrophysiological studies indicate it to be recognized as a distinct taste by rats [156,187,313,409]. Adding saccharin to polycose increases its attractiveness to rats in preference tests [408]. Since our rats had never tasted either polycose or saccharin before, we expected this mixture to be palatable yet novel to them, suitable as a conditioned stimulus for aversion conditioning.

6.1.3. Associative conditioning and behavioral analysis

Three associative pairings were arranged of the CS + saccharin/polycose solution with a LiCl injection (unconditioned stimulus). On the first day, the oral cannula of a rat was connected to a stimulus delivery tube, and the rat was allowed to habituate in the taste reactivity test chamber for 5 min. Then a 1-ml volume of saccharin/polycose solution was infused into the rat's mouth via the cannula at a constant rate over 1 min. Taste reactivity was videotaped during the infusion as in Experiment 1 for subsequent analysis. Immediately after the oral infusion, the rat was injected with 1.5 mEq/kg LiCl (1 ml per 100 g body weight of isotonic LiCl, i.p.), and returned to its home cage. This pairing was repeated two days later, and a third pairing was administered two days after that. A test infu-

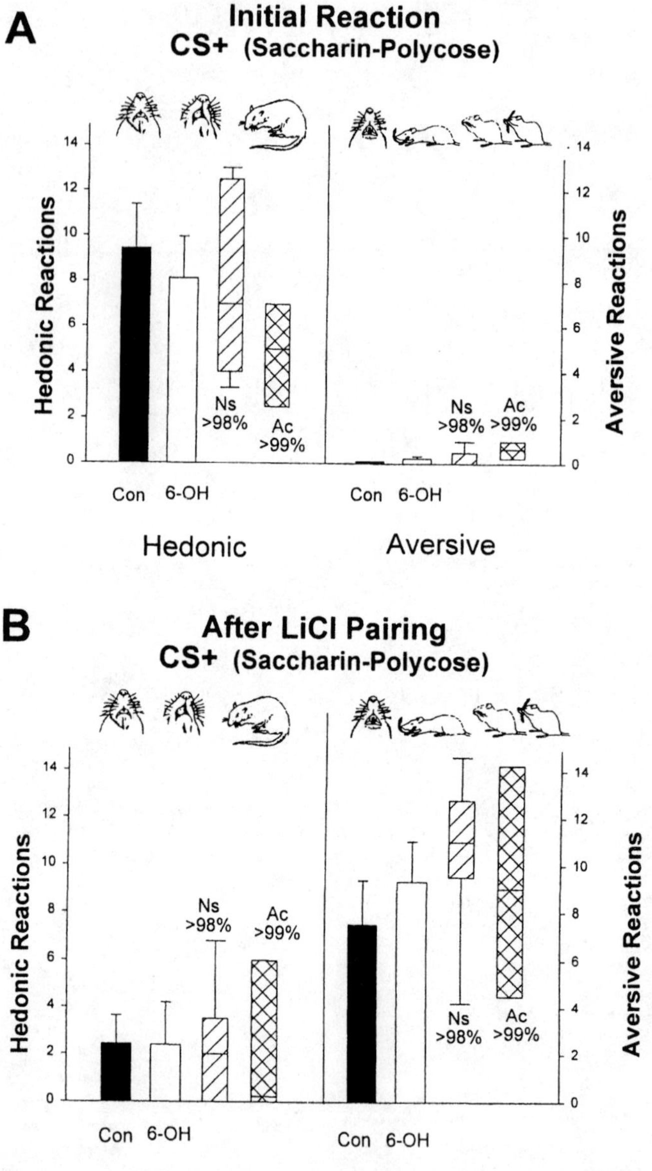

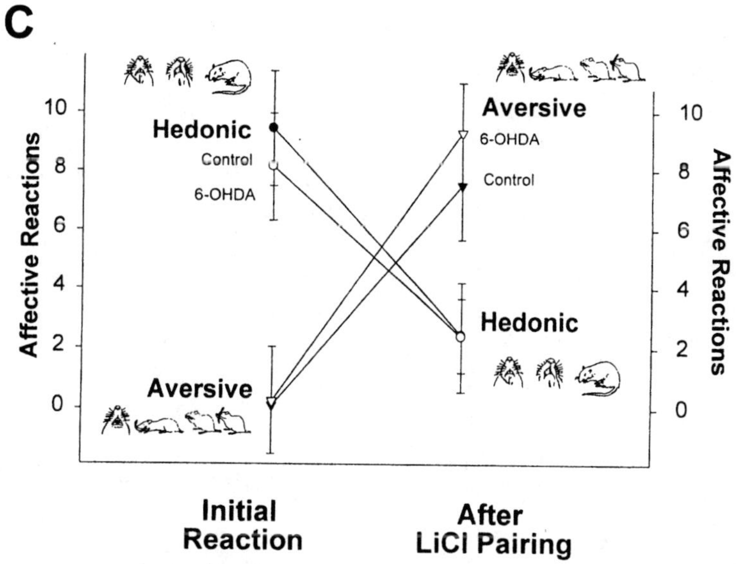

Fig. 4. Associative learning changes hedonic impact of gustatory reward. A. Initial hedonic and aversive taste reactivity patterns to saccharin/polycose solution by 6-OHDA and control groups. B. After associative pairings of saccharin/polycose taste (as CS +) with LiCl (as UCS). The relatively high hedonic reaction rate for the accumbens > 99% depletion subgroup after aversion conditioning reflects the response of 1 rat (Bar shows entire range of subgroup). The other 2 rats in this subgroup had zero hedonic reactions after LiCl pairing. Symbols as for Fig. 2. C. Summary of 'before and after effects' of associative aversion learning on hedonic and aversive reactions produced by the entire 6-OHDA group and the control group. The change in hedonic impact of the CS + taste is equivalent for the two groups.

sion of saccharin/polycose was administered a fourth time two days after the third pairing, and taste reactivity was recorded. A slow-motion videoanalysis of behavioral taste reactivity patterns was conducted as in Experiment 1.

6.2. Results

Strongly hedonic reaction patterns were emitted by both the aphagic 6-OHDA lesion and control groups to the saccharin/polycose infusion the first time it was delivered (Fig. 4). After 3 associative pairings, however, a marked shift in taste reactivity patterns toward aversion was seen for both groups (Fig. 4). A two-way ANOVA (associative conditioning × lesion group) showed that hedonic reactions were reduced for both groups by taste aversion conditioning ($F(1,29) = 13.8$, $p < 0.01$). 6-OHDA rats did not differ from control rats in hedonic reactions on either the first (naive) day or on the test day after conditioning ($F(1,29) = 0.1$, n.s).

Conversely, the number of total aversive reactions (gapes, headshakes, face washes, forelimb flails, chin rubs, paw treads) was dramatically increased for both aphagic 6-OHDA and control groups by associative pairing with LiCl ($F(1,29) = 28.6$, $p < 0.001$; Fig. 4). Again, there was no difference between aphagic 6-HDA rats and control rats in the number of aversive reactions ($F(1,29) = 1.4$, n.s.).

These results held true for both the group of 6-OHDA rats that had > 98% depletion of neostriatal dopamine ($n = 7$), and for the subgroup that had > 99% accumbens and neostriatal depletion ($n = 3$; Fig. 4). For the > 98% neostriatal depletion group, hedonic reactions were reduced by associative conditioning ($F(1,27) = 11.2$, $p < 0.01$), whereas aversive reactions were increased ($F(1,27) = 23.9$, $p < 0.001$), and neither the hedonic nor aversive reactions of this group differed from the control group ($F(1,27) < 1.0$, n.s.). For the > 99% accumbens and neostriatal subgroup, two of the three rats reduced their hedonic reactions to zero after aversion conditioning, but the third rat emitted as many hedonic reactions as it had before, so the hedonic reduction was only marginally significant ($F(1,19) = 4.3$, $p = 0.07$). However, even this subgroup showed a robust and unanimous increase in aversive reactions to saccharin/polycose after associative conditioning ($F(1,19) = 13.7$, $p < 0.01$), equivalent to that of control rats ($F(1,19) = 0.6$, n.s.; Fig. 4).

6.3. Discussion of Experiment 2

Severe dopamine depletion did not disrupt the acquisition or expression of an associative shift from hedonic reactions to aversion. This implies that *forebrain* neural systems needed for the revaluation of rewarding stimuli remained functional. Associative taste aversions are mediated by distributed neural circuits that require the forebrain as well as the brainstem [258,318,390,426,438]. For example, Grill and Norgren [209] showed that taste-LiCl pairings fail to change behavioral taste reactivity patterns of mesencephalic decerebrate rats (which were transected above the superior colliculus). Our results indicate that forebrain evaluations of affective value still control affective taste reactivity patterns even after extensive 6-OHDA depletion of neostriatal and accumbens dopamine. Aversive reaction patterns to a LiCl-paired taste still reflect forebrain-based aversive evaluations. By implication, the normal hedonic reactions to novel polycose/saccharin prior to LiCl pairing (and to sucrose in Experiment 1) reflected a normal forebrain-based hedonic evaluation.

Our results also show that rats with extensive dopamine depletions are capable of changing their hedonic evaluation of a stimulus based on predictive relations with another event; that is, they are capable of reward learning. Associative decrements of old hedonic value and increments of new aversive value, at least, do not appear to require the integrity of ascending dopamine systems. Whether hedonic increments produced by associative pairing also persist after dopamine depletion remains an open question for the time being. But unless decreases in hedonic value are mediated by a neural system separate from that which mediates increases, it seems likely that learned hedonic increments might also be possible for these rats. And although some evidence has implicated a differential role for dopamine systems in pleasant vs. unpleasant events [301] (but see [380] and discussion below regarding dopamine mediation of aversive motivation), reward learning models have posited dopamine systems to play a similar role in learned increments and learned decrements in prediction of hedonic rewards [304,405]. Whatever role dopamine systems may play in learning about rewards, our results suggest they are not required to shift the hedonic or aversive value of rewards as a function of prior experience.

7. Experiment 3: enhancement of hedonic reaction patterns by diazepam

Experiment 2 demonstrated that dopamine depletion does not disrupt the capacity of learned negative associations to make tastes more aversive. But do 6-OHDA lesions eliminate the capacity to modulate palatability in the positive hedonic direction? Could *hedonic* reaction patterns still be enhanced? The conclusion that basic hedonic impact remains normal after dopamine depletion would be strengthened if that were true.

For normal rats hedonic reactions to taste are heightened by prior administration of benzodiazepine agonists such as diazepam, chlordiazepoxide, or midazolam [40, 43,95,97,199,328,431,465,466]. Benzodiazepine agonists also elicit feeding in normal rats [69,92,97,509]. Aphagic 6-OHDA rats would not be expected to show drug-elicited feeding. But if their deficit is primarily one of 'wanting' food rather than 'liking' food, and if their ability to modulate hedonic processes remains normal, then they ought to show enhanced hedonic reactions to a taste delivered to the mouth after treatment with a benzodiazepine agonist. Conversely, if dopamine depletion induces anhedonia, then hedonic enhancement ought to be impaired.

7.1. Methods

Seven 6-OHDA rats that had remained aphagic for 28 days after surgery, and 5 control rats, were used in this experiment. The 6-OHDA rats included the group of 6 rats that were later confirmed to have $> 98\%$ neostriatal dopamine depletion, and the subgroup of 3 rats that had $> 99\%$ depletion of both accumbens and neostriatal dopamine.

In order to minimize the sedative effects of diazepam on the day of testing, each rat received four daily pre-exposures to the drug (5 mg/kg, i.p.) prior to the day of behavioral testing. Taste reactivity tests were conducted on the fifth and sixth days.

On each test day, rats were injected with either diazepam (5 mg/kg, i.p.) or with sterile saline (0.5 ml, i.p.) in counterbalanced order across days. Oral cannulae were connected to delivery tubes, and the rats were placed in the test chamber and allowed to habituate for 10 min. An infusion of 0.3 M sucrose (1 ml) was delivered over a 1 min period, beginning 15 min after the drug injection, and taste reactivity was videorecorded for subsequent analysis, as in earlier experiments.

7.2. Results

Diazepam enhanced the hedonic reaction patterns of both control rats and aphagic 6-OHDA rats ($F(1,23) = 5.38$, $p < 0.05$; Fig. 5), and there was no difference between the two groups in hedonic enhancement ($F(1,23) = 0.5$, n.s.). Diazepam similarly enhanced hedonic reactions for the 6-OHDA group that had 98% neostriatal depletion ($F(1,21) = 6.01$; $p < 0.05$), which also did not differ from the control group ($F(1,21) = 1.13$, n.s). Even the subgroup that had 99% depletion of accumbens and neostriatal dopamine nearly tripled the number of hedonic reactions emitted to sucrose after diazepam (saline $= 4.65 + 3.2$, diazepam $= 14.3 + 2.9$; Fig. 5), although the change was not statistically significant due to the small size of the group ($F(1,5) = 6.32$, $p < 0.12$). Still, an inspection of Fig. 5 will show the reader that rats belonging to the 99% subgroup responded to the drug similarly to all other groups.

Aversive reactions were rarely emitted to sucrose even after saline, and were never altered by diazepam administration ($F(1,23) = 1.10$, n.s.).

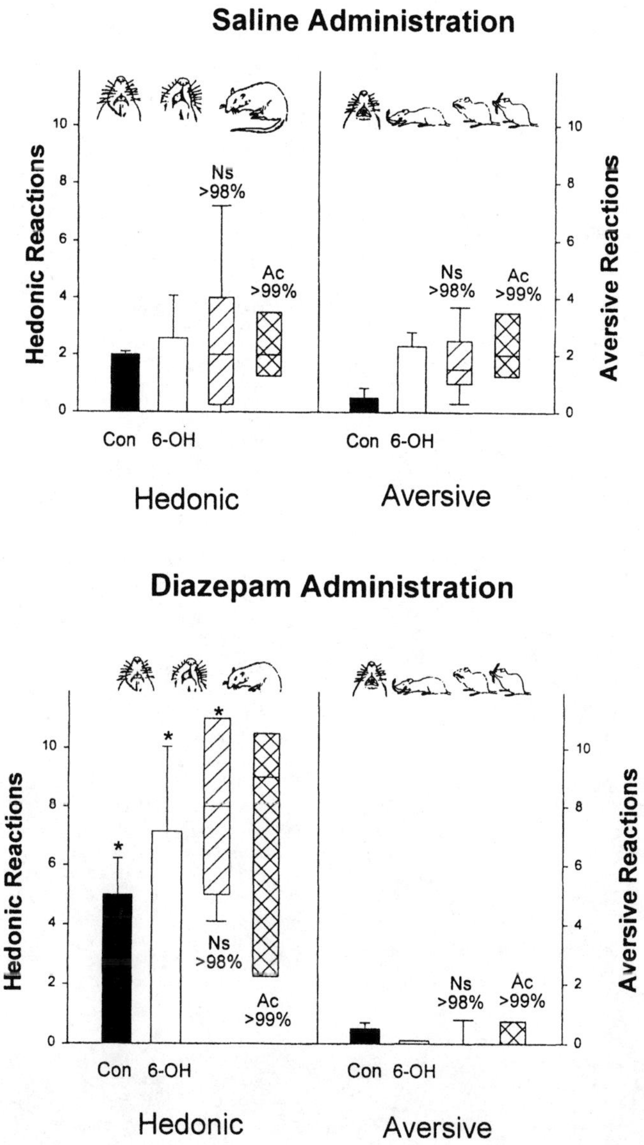

Fig. 5. Taste reactivity patterns to sucrose of 6-OHDA and control groups after diazepam (bottom) or saline (top) administration. Symbols as for Fig. 2.

7.3. Discussion of Experiment 3

The benzodiazepine agonist, diazepam, enhanced hedonic taste reactivity patterns to sucrose even in rats that had 98% to 99% depletion of dopamine. These results suggest that mesolimbic and neostriatal dopamine systems are not needed for the pharmacological enhancement of hedonic reactions. An anhedonic brain—one that was biased toward negative evaluations—might not be capable of pharmacological palatability enhancement. However, a dopamine-depleted brain still is.

8. General discussion

Are dopamine projections to the nucleus accumbens or neostriatum needed for normal hedonic evaluations, for hedonic modulation, or for learned adjustments in hedonic value? Our results indicate the answer to all three questions is 'no'.

8.1. Unconditioned hedonic reactivity.

Unconditioned affective reaction patterns to sweet and bitter tastes remained normal after 6-OHDA lesions. Dopamine depletion failed to reduce hedonic reactions to a sweet taste or to increase aversive reactions to a bitter taste. Dopamine-depleted rats remained capable of discriminating appropriately between sucrose vs. quinine, and between weak and strong concentrations of sucrose (0.3 vs. 1.0 M). These results replicate our earlier report that unconditioned affective reactions to tastes remain essentially normal after 6-OHDA lesions [45]. They extend those findings by showing that this is true even for rats that have up to 99% depletion of mesolimbic and neostriatal dopamine. This far exceeds the 85% neostriatal depletion obtained in our earlier study, and also rules out the possibility that spared dopamine in the nucleus accumbens is needed to mediate normal unconditioned hedonic/aversive reactions.

8.2. Palatability modulation.

The present results also show that dopamine projections to the neostriatum and nucleus accumbens are not necessary for the normal *modulation* of either hedonic or aversive palatability. Enhancement of *hedonic* reaction patterns to sucrose was induced pharmacologically in dopamine-depleted rats by administration of the benzodiazepine agonist, diazepam. Enhancement of *aversive* reaction patterns to an originally palatable sweet taste, and suppression of hedonic reactions, was induced in dopamine-depleted rats by associative taste aversion learning. In both cases, the magnitude of the shift in affective reaction patterns induced by these manipulations was comparable in control and dopamine-depleted rats

9. Dopamine and reward: choosing among competing explanations

Why do individuals fail to eat or drink voluntarily or show goal-directed behavior toward incentive stimuli after dopamine depletion? Competing hypotheses provide several different explanations. First, *motor deficits* produced by nigrostriatal impairment might render the animals incapable of the movements needed to eat or drink. Second, *anhedonia* caused by dopamine depletion might eliminate the hedonic impact of all food or drink reinforcers. Third, disruption of *reward learning* might make it impossible for the individual to perceive the associative relationship between food-related stimuli in the environment and the hedonic consequences of ingesting food. Fourth, disruption of *incentive salience* might abolish the incentive properties of the sight or smell of food, leaving it unattractive and incapable of eliciting approach, even if those other functions remained intact. Which of these explanations, if any, provide a plausible account of the effects of dopamine depletion on behavior directed towards food and other rewards?

9.1. Not motor deficits

The failure to eat is not likely to be explained entirely by motor deficits induced by the lesions. Although the importance of sensorimotor impairment after dopamine depletion cannot be disregarded, and needs to be better understood [216,383], it is clear that rats can still make many forelimb and mouth movements after extensive 6-OHDA lesions. For example, in the present study the action patterns elicited by tastes appeared motorically normal. Dopamine-depleted rats made normal rhythmic mouth movements, rhythmic and lateral tongue protrusions, forelimb facial strokes, etc. Forepaw and licking movements similar to those needed to eat are also preserved and sometimes even enhanced in other situations. For example, when grooming, rats with extensive 6-OHDA lesions have been found to emit the same number, as, or more, forelimb-stroke and body-lick movements than control rats [32,483] (and to further increase their emission of grooming and locomotion movements in response to a variety of drug treatments [135,288]). It is not so much that rats cannot generate the movements required for eating after 6-OHDA lesions, as that they *do not* do so.

There is no doubt that dopamine depletion impairs sensorimotor responsiveness in rats as well as in humans [46,285,287,340,379,384,386,391,392,451,485,515]. The critical question, however, is whether sensorimotor deficits alone explain the deficits in motivated behavior. Many behavioral neuroscientists have concluded that sensorimotor deficits by themselves do not suffice to explain the changes in reward effectiveness produced by dopamine manipulations [17,52,152,158,225,254,266,310,345, 347,362,401,429,505,513,518]. Thus, above and beyond sensorimotor deficits induced by dopamine depletion, the nature of the deficit in rewarded behavior needs explanation.

9.2. Not anhedonia

According to the anhedonia hypothesis dopamine depletion should reduce hedonic reactions to sucrose and/or increase aversive reaction patterns to quinine. That did not happen. Affective reaction patterns remained normal. Normal affective reaction patterns can be explained by the anhedonia hypothesis only if it is assumed that after dopamine depletion taste reactivity no longer reflects normal hedonic or aversive evaluations. In other words, the anhedonia hypothesis would be compatible with these data only if one posits that brainstem circuits were disconnected from an anhedonic forebrain by the lesion, leaving the brainstem to produce normal reflexes in the absence of affective processing by the forebrain. Do rats have an 'anhedonic-but-disconnected' forebrain after 6-OHDA lesions?

Not hedonic disconnection of the forebrain. Our observation that 6-OHDA rats retain the capacity to shift from hedonic to aversive reactions based on aversion conditioning provides strong evidence against the 'anhedonic forebrain' hypothesis. The logic of our assertion derives from the descending hierarchical control known to be exerted by forebrain neural systems over taste reactivity patterns, and the role of hierarchical control in aversion conditioning [206,207,209,211].

Studies have shown that forebrain manipulations alter the responses of neurons in the brainstem parabrachial nucleus and solitary nucleus [121,122,308,317,390], and that affective taste reactivity patterns are modulated directly by lesions and drug microinjections localized in the forebrain [106,211,335,336]. They indicate taste processing to be modulated by descending hierarchical control. This idea is supported by anatomical evidence for descending pathways from gustatory cortex and other forebrain sites to gustatory processing sites of the brainstem. Most relevant to the present study, shifts in taste reactivity patterns produced by taste aversion learning require an intact forebrain [206,209,258,426]. For example, Grill and Norgren found that decerebrate rats were not capable of changing taste reactivity patterns, even after repeated taste-LiCl pairings [206,209]. Lesions of the basolateral amygdala or gustatory cortex have also been reported to impair conditioned shifts from hedonic to aversive behavioral reactions induced by LiCl pairing [258,426]. In a vivid neuroanatomical demonstration of hierarchical control of aversion learning, Schafe et al. [390] found that the induction of c-Fos immunostaining within the nucleus of the solitary tract, a neural marker of taste aversion learning after taste-LiCl pairing, was prevented ipsilaterally by a hemitransection of connections from the forebrain. In sum, as noted by a recent review of taste aversion learning by Norgren and Grigson [318], evidence points to "the extensive projections of the PBN (parabrachial nucleus) *to the ventral forebrain* as the best candidate" for neural mediation of aversion conditioning (italics added). Associative shifts from hedonic to aversive behavioral reactions cannot be carried out by the brainstem without guidance from descending forebrain projections.

Our finding that dopamine-depleted rats switch appropriately from hedonic to aversive patterns after aversion learning rules out the possibility that the 6-OHDA lesions produce an 'anhedonic forebrain' that is somehow prevented from modulating unconditioned reactions to tastes. If the forebrain were functionally disconnected, a rat would be unable to shift its affective reaction pattern after taste-LiCl pairing. The dopamine-depleted rat is not rendered functionally decerebrate by its 6-OHDA lesion. Hierarchical controls over palatability remain intact. We conclude that the hedonic evaluation of tastes by the forebrain is not impaired by mesolimbic and neostriatal dopamine depletion.

9.2.1. Further evidence against anhedonia

9.2.1.1. Hedonic enhancement of palatability by diazepam after 6-OHDA lesions. Benzodiazepine agonists enhance palatability and induce feeding by an appetite-related process that appears to be separate from their anxiolytic and sedative effects [92,93,96,97,509] and the hypothesis of benzodiazepine hedonic enhancement has been confirmed by many taste reactivity studies [43,199,328,337,466]. Our present results indicate that the ability of diazepam to enhance taste palatability does not require accumbens or neostriatal dopamine. In one sense, this may not be surprising, because benzodiazepines seem to enhance hedonic taste palatability via actions within the brainstem [31,97,337]. On the other hand, if dopamine depletion had rendered the forebrain anhedonic, that might be expected to impair hedonic enhancement and bias affective responses toward aversion, as a variety of other forebrain lesions do [106,211,393]. But it did not.

9.2.1.2. Comparison to lesions that produce real anhedonia. The preservation of normal hedonic and aversive reaction patterns and normal palatability modulation after 6-OHDA lesions stands in stark contrast to other aphagia-producing brain lesions. Indeed, lesions that disrupt feeding typically reduce hedonic reaction patterns or enhance aversive ones. For example, hedonic reaction patterns are replaced by aversive ones after either telencephalic ablation (removal of structures rostral to thalamus), or large electrolytic lesions of the lateral hypothalamic area [164,211,306,393,446,455]). Aphagia accompanied by anhedonia (plus aversive enhancement) is also seen after excitotoxin lesions of the basal forebrain [106,138,484] that damage a small site within the ventral pallidum [34,106]. Lateral hypothalamic lesions that fail to damage the crucial ventral pallidal site produce only aphagia, and do not increase aversion or reduce hedonic reaction patterns [34,106,393,496]. Aphagia [240,529] with anhedonia can also be produced by deafferentation of the bilateral mandibular and maxillary trigeminal nerve, although the affective taste reactivity shift is more specific to hedonic affect [37]. Trigeminal deafferentation suppresses hedonic reaction patterns to sucrose and other tastes, but does not alter aversive reactions [37]. Deafferentation results in a selective anhedonia, which nonetheless *shifts* the balance between hedonic palatability and aversion, leaving foods relatively 'unliked'.

In short, most brain lesions that produce aphagia have been found to cause anhedonia, as assessed by affective taste reactivity patterns, and many aphagia-producing lesions also cause active aversion to food. Compared to other neural manipulations that produce aphagia, dopamine depletion is unusual in that it fails to alter either hedonic or aversive reactions to food. We conclude, therefore, the reason dopamine-depleted rats fail to eat is *not* because they are anhedonic.

9.3. Not reward learning?

In a prominent model of reward learning, Montague et al. (p. 1944, [304]) have argued that dopamine neurons deliver "information about prediction errors between the expected amount of reward and the actual reward". Their computational model is based on data collected primarily by Schultz and colleagues in an important series of electrophysiological studies on the relationship between the discharge rate of presumed dopamine neurons and the presentation of food rewards, and conditioned stimuli predictive of food rewards [5,277,278,300,301,371,398,399,401–403]. Accordingly, Schultz himself concurs that dopamine neurons "signal deviations from the prediction of future appetitive events" (p. 191, [400]). In a collaborative review, Schultz, Dayan, and Montague [405] concluded that "dopamine activity encodes expectations about external stimuli or reward" (p. 1594, [405]), and can signal both "changes and errors in the predictions of future salient and rewarding events" (p. 1593, [405]). Appetitive rewarding events, for Schultz, are things that "elicit approach reactions..., serve as positive reinforcers..., serve as goals of voluntary behavior...", and "have an emotional function by inducing subjective feelings of pleasure and hedonia" (p. 191, Schultz [400]), a view that seems to join both incentive 'wanting' and hedonic 'liking'. In these accounts, the activity of dopamine neurons seems to reflect reward learning in two ways. First, neuronal activation to a conditioned stimulus phasically registers an increment in the momentary strength of a prediction regarding an impending 'wanted' and 'liked' event. Second, dopamine neuronal activation to an unconditioned hedonic reward, such as the actual taste of food, encodes discrepancies between the prediction strength and the actual magnitude of 'liking' produced by the event itself [400].

Graybiel et al. have suggested a similar account for tonically active neurons (TANs) in the monkey striatum that respond to conditioned stimuli for reward [3,4,201,203]. TANs fire at 2 to 10 cycles per second, but phasically pause firing in response to certain events. For example, audible clicks or flashing lights that have been paired with a fruit juice reward gradually become able to produce phasic pauses in TAN activity on their own [3,4,201,203]. "The cells modulate their spike activity in relation to stimuli that are predictive of reward" (p. 1830, [201]). After dopamine depletion, TANs no longer modulate their firing in response to conditioned stimuli for reward [3]. Graybiel et al. conclude that TAN conditioned responses are "compatible with a 'teaching' role for reward-related nigrostriatal dopaminergic input" (p. 1830, [201]). Graybiel interprets these data, together with those of Schultz et al., to "suggest a model in which dopaminergic nigral neurons are recruited by novel rewarding stimuli, and long-term procedural memories are built up..." (p. 734, [200]). Thus, according to this account too, dopamine neurons help to entrain a type of learned *expectation* of an event that is both 'wanted' and 'liked'.

Others have similarly argued that dopamine mediates various types of reward-related *associations* between conditioned stimuli and hedonic stimuli [23,24,26,61,116,488]. For example, White (p. 181, [488]) proposed that "dopamine release in the striatal matrix acts to promote the consolidation of sensori-motor associations" whereas dopamine release in the striatal patches and nucleus accumbens primarily mediates other aspects of reward, such as 'the property to elicit approach' (p. 181, [488]) and 'responding to conditioned rewards' (p. 184, [488]). Beninger and Miller (p. 335, [26]) suggest that dopamine systems, especially D1 dopamine receptors, mediate incentive learning, "defined as the acquisition by previously neutral stimuli of the ability to elicit approach and other responses and occurs in association with the presentation of rewarding stimuli". In a related hypothesis, Di Chiara (p. 103, [116]) posited that dopamine release in accumbens and ventral striatum is crucial for "enabling the acquisition of incentive properties by stimuli (incentive learning)", specifically because of "*facilitation by dopamine of learning of the association* between the stimulus and the reinforcers" (p. 102, [116] italics added). In a more recent formulation, reminiscent of White's, Di Chiara emphasizes his belief that dopamine systems are required for the reward *association* itself: "We hypothesize that DA release in the NAc in response to a novel or relatively novel primary stimulus facilitates the association between affective and discriminative properties of stimuli" (p. 61, [117]). This 'reward association' hypothesis holds that mesolimbic dopamine is causally necessary for the formation of reward associations, and that dopamine neurotransmission is ordinarily a sufficient cause to form such associations. Di Chiara writes: "In our hypothesis, DA is not only necessary for stimulus reward and stimulus response associations (motivational learning) but phasic activation of its transmission can actually facilitate these processes" (p. 63, [117]). Thus, many authors, drawing on different lines of evidence, have emphasized that ascending dopamine systems are critical for *learning* about rewards.

9.3.1. Multiple types of reward learning?

In evaluating reward learning models of dopamine function, a question that must first be addressed is whether there is only one type of reward learning or whether there are instead multiple subtypes. If there is only one type, and if dopamine plays a critical role, then dopamine manipulations should have a very general effect on learning about rewards in many different situations. Explicit cognitive expectation (as a declarative representation), instrumental approach, conditioned hedonic reactions, and other anticipatory behavioral or physiological responses to a conditioned stimulus for reward, which are based on expectations or procedural memories: all would reflect the same learning process, and all should be influenced together by manipulations of dopamine systems.

But our results (and others [16,127,128,218,341,439]) show that reward learning cannot be a single process, and that dopamine is not necessary for all reward learning, if it is necessary for any. In our study dopamine-depleted rats learned a new Pavlovian association between a taste and its affective consequences, and used this association to transform their subsequent hedonic reaction to that taste. If reward learning takes *multiple* forms, then dopamine projections might mediate some but not others. In that case, it will be crucial for reward learning hypotheses of dopamine function to specify precisely *which* forms or aspects of reward learning depend on dopamine systems and which do not.

Which aspect of reward learning is most likely to depend on dopamine systems? Contemporary 'reward learning' models of dopamine function often emphasize the role of dopamine neurons in 'prediction of future appetitive events' and 'expectations about rewards' [400,405]. But understanding the role of dopamine systems depends on exactly what is meant by the terms 'prediction' or 'expectation'. It may be useful to distinguish between four possibilities.

First, prediction or expectation could refer to the simplest procedure that instantiates classical conditioning: a neural algorithm that underlies the formation of basic Pavlovian associations (classically-conditioned procedural memories), and generates conditioned responses based on past correlations among stimuli. However, our results suggest that dopamine projections are not needed for forming such associations or generating new responses based on newly acquired associations. [7]

Second, 'expectation of reward' might mean a process separate from associative learning, but one that is closely controlled by it as a response. For example, Pavlovian associations are translated into hedonic responses, triggering pleasant or unpleasant *affect* as a conditioned emotional response [53,358,527], including gustatory affect [42,63,113]. The ability of a conditioned stimulus to elicit *conditioned affect* is an important feature of incentive motivation theories such as those of Bindra [47–49] or Toates [460–462], and of neurobiological theories of emotion such as those of LeDoux [273] or Panksepp [322,325,347]. But again, in the present study dopamine-depleted rats were able to translate a Pavlovian association between the taste of saccharin–polycose and LiCl-induced illness into an aversive shift in the palatability of that taste. That rules out the possibility that dopamine is necessary for transformations of affect based on Pavlovian associations.

Third, 'expectation of reward' might mean activation of a psychological system that is related to hedonic impact but not identical to it. Pavlovian associations alter the *incentive motivation* properties, as well as the hedonic properties, of conditioned stimuli (see Toates [460,463], Bindra [49]). Incentive property here means the ability of the stimulus to attract approach, to elicit behavior such as feeding, to be sought after, and to elicit and maintain instrumental behavior (all of which we suggest reflects 'wanting', and hold to be separable from hedonic 'liking'). It is possible that dopamine systems play a special role in the learning of incentive properties, and in the subsequent attribution of incentive properties to conditioned stimuli ('wanting'), even if they do not contribute to learning about hedonic properties ('liking'). This possibility will be explored further below under 'Comparison of reward learning and incentive salience hypotheses'.

Fourth, 'expectation about reward' might mean exactly what it says, in the strongest sense of 'expectation'. That is, an *explicit cognitive expectation* of a specific reward. This psychological process is of course more complex than simple associative learning, and involves additional neural mechanisms [16,20,85,439]. A declarative cognitive expectation must code a future event in terms of an explicit representation of its sensory and rewarding features, and be able to draw upon that information to guide current action [123]. It is not merely a procedure for generating an anticipatory response. In humans, for example, declarative forms of expectation include imagery and symbolic or semantic representations, which can be used to make new inferences about an event that has not yet occurred.

Identifying declarative cognitive representations in animals is generally recognized to be a formidable task. But in a fascinating series of experiments, Dickinson and colleagues such as Bernard Balleine have developed methods for detecting cognitive expectations that even rats have about rewards, and separating them from simpler Pavlovian-guided processes. Although explicit cognitive representations might be expected to be more important in *primates*, the learning tasks used in most primate studies of

[7] Admittedly, our experiment induced conditioned *aversion* and a hedonic *decrement* rather than a conditioned hedonic increment. It would be of interest to obtain conditioned 'liking' in dopamine depleted rats, and some readers might suspect that associative hedonic increments would not be possible. But that is a thin reed on which to hang a hedonic learning hypothesis. Most of the reward learning hypotheses reviewed above implicate dopamine systems in hedonic decrements as well as increments. A hedonic decrement was apparent in the 6-OHDA rats' loss of hedonic reactions to saccharin–polycose. We predict that associative hedonic increments are possible too, a prediction that future experiments conceivably could test.

mesolimbic activation and reward generally have not been designed to separate associative from cognitive aspects. By contrast, Dickinson and Balleine and their colleagues have used rats as subjects in their studies of incentive learning. Yet they successfully demonstrate in these animals the existence of cognitive 'act–outcome' expectations of incentives, and show that such expectations can be experimentally teased apart from simpler Pavlovian-based aspects of reward learning [8,9,11,12,123,126–128]. Their studies indicate that animals too can form cognitive expectations of rewards, at least in certain situations (See Addendum 2 for explanation of Dickinson et al.'s analyses, and of how they dissociate 'act–outcome expectation' of reward from simpler types of reward learning).

The multiplex nature of 'reward learning' illustrated by Dickinson and Balleine and colleagues (see Addendum 2) shows that there are many different ways in which dopamine systems could contribute. Depending on which type of reward learning is meant, 'expected reward value' could have different meanings at the same time and for the same reward. The results presented here indicate that dopamine systems are not needed either for learning simple predictive associations among events that arise from their correlation, or for hedonic transformations in reward value based on those associations. But dopamine systems could conceivably be involved in the translation of hedonic value into an associatively-guided attribution of incentive salience to a conditioned stimulus, or alternatively into a cognitive representation of act–outcome value. *A critical evaluation will require 'reward learning' hypotheses of dopamine function be specific concerning the form of 'reward learning' they seek to explain* (see below for further discussion of this point).

9.4. Loss of incentive salience?

In our original report that aphagic 6-OHDA rats have normal hedonic reactions to tastes we suggested that dopamine depletion disrupts the capacity to *attribute incentive salience to neural representations* of rewards, without disrupting either their hedonic impact or their ability to enter into new associative relationships. Incentive salience, we proposed, under normal conditions must be attributed to stimuli to transform a perceived and 'liked' stimulus into one that is also 'wanted' and able to elicit voluntary action [34,45,366]. The aphagia of dopamine-depleted rats, and their lack of other motivated behavior, is compatible with this hypothesis. Even if rats still 'like' food, and retain the capacity to learn hedonic associations about it, and to make the movements needed to eat, they do not 'want' food and so do not eat it.

The incentive salience hypothesis is an extension of earlier models of incentive motivation proposed by Bolles [53] and by Bindra [48,49], and developed by Toates [460,463]. Neurobiologically, it is an extension of earlier formulations of the role of dopamine in reward by Phillips et al. [51,157,345], Wise and Bozarth [499–501,508], and by Panksepp [322–324] among others. The incentive salience hypothesis is different from previous models in that it specifies that encounters with new incentives and rewards normally activate three distinct psychological processes mediated by dissociable neural substrates [34,44,45,366]. The 3 psychological processes that compose incentive motivation and reward are posited to be: *hedonic activation* by the unconditioned stimulus, *associative learning* of the correlation between the conditioned stimulus and the unconditioned stimulus, and *attribution of incentive salience* to the conditioned stimulus or its representation on subsequent encounters (Fig. 6). Finally, the incentive salience hypothesis proposes that dopamine systems are necessary just for the third process—attribution of incentive salience.

Regarding the role of conditioned stimuli in reward, one can imagine learning about a new incentive in this way. An individual's initial contact with a hedonic reward may occur incidentally, triggering 'liking' as the individual explores its world, sampling food, etc. Such natural rewards have hedonic value presumably because of their survival value in evolutionary history [72,315]. 'Liking' or hedonic pleasure is ordinarily a necessary component of reward, leading to the acquisition of new incentives. [8] Indeed, to many, 'liking' is synonymous with reward, and the term reward is often used as a surrogate for pleasure. This is consistent with the dictionary definition of reward as 'a pleasant stimulus' (p. 2584, Shorter Oxford Dictionary) [65]. We think, however, that neural and psychological reality are more complex than the dictionary would suggest. We argue that 'liking' by itself is not true reward any more than is 'wanting' by itself: nothing need be rewarded by hedonic activation alone. Pleasure is not itself goal-directed or necessarily associated with objects or events. Pleasure by itself is simply a *triggered affective state*—there is no object of desire. It is the process of incentive salience attribution that makes a specific associated stimulus or action the *object* of desire.

[8] 'Liking' may be bypassed in reward only by special stimuli, such as electrical brain stimulation or some drug rewards, events that directly activate the neural substrate of 'wanting' or incentive salience attribution [44,366]. Such cases will look like normal reward or motivation to an external observer, who watches instrumental or goal-directed behavior, but would in a sense be mere 'sham reward', composed only of 'wanting' without 'liking'. For example, stimulation of the lateral hypothalamus makes rats 'want' food (in the sense of eliciting eating) without making them 'like' it (in the sense of enhancing hedonic reactions) [44]. Whether real reward ('wanting' plus 'liking') or sham reward (mere 'wanting' without 'liking') is evoked by an event, incentive salience will be attributed specifically to conditioned stimuli that have been associated in the past with the unconditioned activation of its neural substrate. 'Wanting' is focused on a particular target by associative learning, making it the specific object of goal-directed behavior: the object of desire.

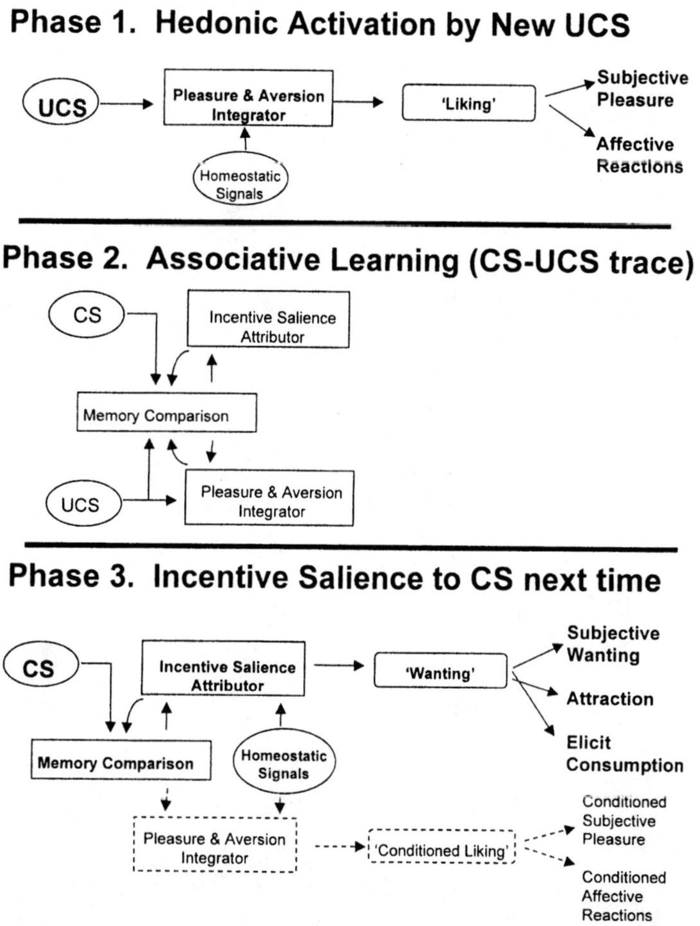

Fig. 6. Three processes in the acquisition of a new reward according to the incentive salience model. (1) The first time the unconditioned hedonic pleasure ('liking') is encountered, it acts as the normal trigger for the reward-building process, and activates the associative and incentive salience steps. But 'liking' by itself is not sufficient to motivate or direct instrumental behavior directed toward external stimuli (as the predicament of 6-OHDA rats illustrates) (2) Associative learning systems correlate the memory trace of predictive neutral events (conditioned stimuli) associated with the hedonic event. Originally the conditioned stimuli have little power to activate either 'liking' or 'wanting' systems, but associative learning links them to both. A similar process occurs during the 'reboosting' of familiar reward stimuli (3) When these conditioned stimuli are encountered on subsequent occasions, incentive salience is attributed to them by activation of dopamine-related systems, guided by associative learning. Attribution of incentive salience makes a conditioned stimulus itself the target of 'wanting', and able to act as a Bindra/Toates incentive to direct motivated behavior [49,460,463]. Separately, conditioned stimuli may also activate conditioned 'liking' (for example, as a taste paired with LiCl activates conditioned aversion). However, the burden of guiding goal-directed behavior toward Pavlovian reward stimuli falls on the incentive salience process of 'wanting'.

Associative learning, specifically Pavlovian or classical conditioning, is the second process required for a new incentive to become a 'real reward'. Associative learning identifies the correlation between hedonic activation and the predictive external event or conditioned stimulus that preceded it [355,356]. Together associative learning and hedonic/aversive activation are sufficient for the transformation of associative information into affect (i.e., a hedonic or aversive response to a conditioned stimulus), such as the conditioned taste aversion seen in dopamine-depleted rats in the present study. Without the third process of incentive salience attribution, however, associative learning and hedonic activation do not suffice for goal directed behavior, nor to make a conditioned stimulus an *attractive* event. They simply make it possible for a conditioned stimulus to activate an affective state. They cannot by themselves elicit approach, or any other instrumental action, even so simple a one as reaching out with tongue or forelimb to a goal object that is literally in front of one's face.

Incentive salience attribution is the third component of reward according to this hypothesis. It corresponds roughly to 'decision utility', as that term is used in discussions of choice theory by, for example, Kahneman et al. [243,245] and Shizgal and Conover [90,422,423]. Decision utility refers to the degree to which a goal is chosen or sought. Incentive salience is needed to transform the 'neutral' perception of a conditioned stimulus or a goal object at a distance into an attractive incentive capable of eliciting appetitive or instrumental behavior towards it. Only if this last stage of incentive salience is added does the stimulus or event become a full reward, becoming 'wanted' as well as 'liked'. Further, on each subsequent encounter with the now 'wanted' and 'liked' stimulus, its capacity to support 'wanting' is maintained or strengthened by associative reboosting of the incentive salience assigned to its representation [44,366]. Reboosting happens when a 'wanted' incentive is followed again by activation of hedonic 'liking'. If *reboosting* occurs, the reward remains 'wanted' on later occasions. In the absence of reboosting of incentive

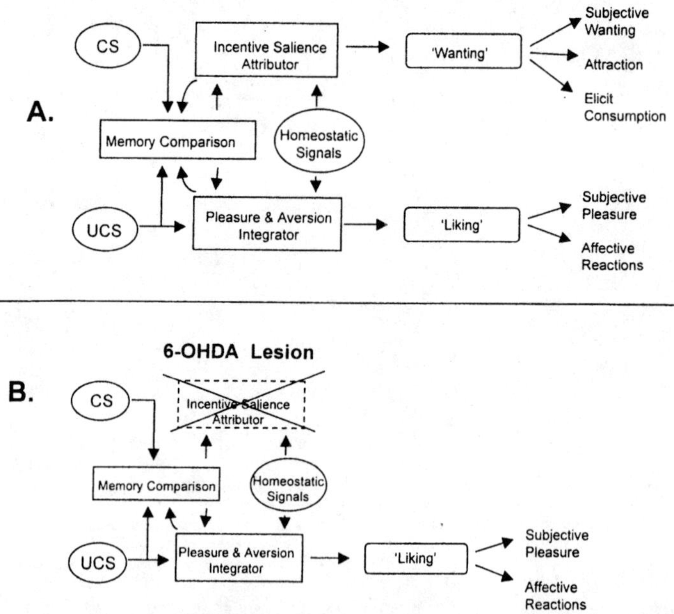

Fig. 7. Incentive salience model of incentive motivation (A; derived from Toates [460], based in part on Bindra, [49]), and of the effects of dopamine depletion on motivation and reward (B). A. 'Liking' and 'wanting' correspond to separate psychological and neural systems. Dopamine projections to the nucleus accumbens and neostriatum are needed to generate 'wanting' or incentive salience aspects of motivation, but not for hedonic 'liking' or for associative learning about rewards. Subjective pleasure and subjective wanting require further cognitive elaboration in order to produce conscious emotion from underlying 'liking' and 'wanting', but that is not depicted here. See Robinson and Berridge [366] and Berridge [34] for more discussion. B. Only incentive salience processes ('wanting') are mediated by dopamine neural systems. After 6-OHDA lesions that disrupt dopamine systems, the attribution of incentive salience is selectively abolished. Behavioral outputs of 'wanting' (appetitive, goal-directed, or instrumental action) are eliminated. Behavioral outputs of hedonic/aversive 'liking' (e.g., affective taste reactivity patterns), however, remain unimpaired. Even associative learning, which ordinarily interacts with both processes, is free to guide hedonic/aversive 'liking' after dopamine depletion (expressed in taste aversion learning in Experiment 2). But no incentive is 'wanted'. Part A modified from [366], Part B modified from [34].

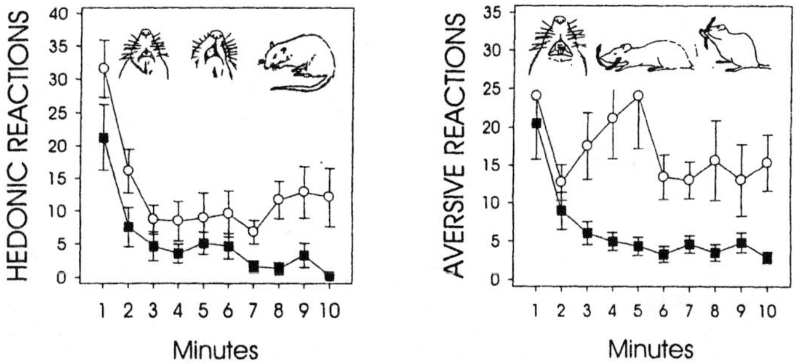

Fig. 8. Gradual sensorimotor suppression of taste reactivity by pimozide (0.5 mg/kg). Initial hedonic reactions to sucrose (left) and aversive reactions to quinine (right) are normal (pimozide = filled squares, vehicle = open circles). When the infusion continues for several minutes, a general suppression ensues for both hedonic and aversive reactions (and for other nonaffective movement patterns not shown). The suppression is equivalent regardless of hedonic/aversive or other category, and therefore does not appear to reflect a shift in palatability toward anhedonia or aversion. Modified from Peciña et al.[338].

salience, reward extinction ensues. Incentive salience is the only component of reward that we think depends upon mesolimbic and neostriatal dopamine systems.

The distinctive features of our model are that 'liking' and 'wanting' are separable psychological processes, although they typically occur together. Most important, they have separate neural substrates (Fig. 7; Fig. 8). Dopamine manipulations can directly alter 'wanting', whereas 'liking' is influenced by manipulations of other neural systems (such as GABA/benzodiazepine systems in the brainstem, ventral pallidal systems where lesions produce aversion, or opioid systems in the nucleus accumbens shell [34,40,106,337,338]). In the context of the present study incentive salience attribution is the only component of reward we posit dopamine depleted rats to lack (Fig. 7, and Berridge [34]).

10. Conditioned dopamine activity: re-examination of implications for incentive salience and reward learning hypotheses

Our hypothesis predicts that neurons which mediate incentive salience will respond to sensory stimuli that trigger 'wanting' regardless of whether they generate 'liking'. As reviewed above, both dopamine neurons themselves and their neuronal targets in the striatum respond to incentive stimuli related to food or other rewards [3–5,301,305,370,403,492]. Although anticipatory neural responses in advance of a hedonic reward are usually discussed with a *reward learning* hypothesis in mind, they are equally consistent with the *incentive salience* hypothesis. If dopamine activation is taken to reflect the attribution of incentive salience at a particular moment, then the hypothesis predicts that conditioned stimuli for hedonic events should become able to elicit activation, and that the activation will be directed by associative learning. [9]

10.1. Predictions of 'reward learning' vs. 'incentive salience' hypotheses of dopamine function

Although neuronal responses to a conditioned stimulus for a hedonic food reward are consistent with both a learning 'expectation of reward' hypothesis and the incentive salience hypothesis, the two are not identical. They may make different predictions, although the exact predictions depend, of course, on what is meant by 'reward learning'.

If a 'Bindra/Toates incentive' type of reward learning is meant, then the two hypotheses are not mutually exclusive. In this case dopamine activation could mediate specifically learning about the *incentive properties* of a classically-conditioned stimulus, as described in traditional incentive motivation theories developed by Bindra [49], Bolles [53], and Toates [460,463]. Of course, we would

[9] However, it must be granted that 'wanting' or incentive salience attribution is probably not isomorphic with the occurrence of action potentials in reward-related dopamine neurons. The firing patterns of dopamine neurons are very brief [278,301,401,405], whereas 'wanting' as a psychological process should be sustained as the goal is approached. It is plausible that the psychological process of incentive salience attribution outlasts dopamine neuronal activity in many situations. If so, the full psychological process of 'wanting' may require events later in the chain of neural causation. Dopamine neurons may well still serve to *trigger* the neuronal chain of events that instantiate incentive salience attribution. Neurons in the ventral striatum and nucleus accumbens, and their efferent targets, may mediate later events in the chain. This speculation is supported by reports that reward-related neuronal activity in the ventral striatum is more sustained than in dopamine neurons themselves, and that dopamine release in the nucleus accumbens also lasts longer [4,5,263,277,347,403,417].

argue that this does not include either acquisition of the association between the discriminative sensory properties of a stimulus and its hedonic reward properties, or the generation of a conditioned hedonic reaction when the discriminative stimulus is presented later (since we've shown these can occur without dopamine). Those would have to be mediated by non-dopaminergic systems.

The notion that there could be separate 'learning systems' for the acquisition of incentive value vs. hedonic value is not part of the original Bindra/Toates models of incentive motivation (although see Toates [463] for a formulation that incorporates the distinction). But 'liking' and 'wanting' must be separated in order to make a reward learning hypothesis of dopamine function compatible with the incentive salience model. The compatibility of specific reward learning models hinges on precisely what Montague, Schultz, Graybiel, White, Beninger, Di Chiara, et al., and other authors of reward learning hypotheses for dopamine function [3,23,26,116,117,200,304,400,401, 405,488,489] mean by 'expectation of reward'. If these reward learning hypotheses posit that dopamine mediates Pavlovian learning about *incentive value alone* (not stimulus-reward association per se, not hedonic value, not cognitive expectation of outcome), and that anticipatory neuronal responses to conditioned stimuli occur because those stimuli carry *incentive motivational* qualities, such as incentive salience, separately from mere association or from hedonic qualities, then those reward learning hypotheses are compatible with our incentive salience hypothesis. That is, predictive stimuli for reward could have associative, cognitive, hedonic, *and* incentive motivational properties, and the activation of mesolimbic dopamine systems may specifically reflect their *incentive* properties, separable from the other properties.

If, however, dopamine neurons are posited to mediate any other sense of 'expectation of reward' (see above), then either the reward learning hypothesis or the incentive salience hypothesis must be wrong. If dopamine systems mediated learning either a *conditioned hedonic response*, such as anticipatory activation of hedonic/aversive affect elicited by a conditioned stimulus, or a *cognitive expectation* of reward value in Dickinson's and Balleine's sense of instrumental incentive learning [125,128,129], then reward learning and incentive salience hypotheses would make different predictions, in at least some situations.

For instance, compare *cognitive expectancy* and *incentive salience* hypotheses. If the incentive value of a stimulus were changed *in the absence of an opportunity to learn its new reward value* (as in the experiments of Dickinson and Balleine; see Addendum 2), then an incentive salience hypothesis would expect dopamine systems to change. Without an explicit opportunity to learn the new reward value, a *cognitive expectancy* hypothesis based on Dickinson's and Balleine's concept of incentive learning would instead expect dopamine systems to follow the same expectancy value reflected in the animal's instrumental behavior. Dickinson and Balleine show that, when guided by act–outcome expectancies, the animal often behaves as if the reward will have the same value it had when it was encountered before—even under conditions when the reward won't [123,127,128]. Thus, dopamine neuron activation should remain constant under those conditions in which instrumental behavior remains constant. [10]

In contrast, the incentive salience hypothesis generally expects dopamine activation by all potent incentives. It does not matter whether the eliciting event is a conditioned stimulus that predicts a subsequent hedonic stimulus, or an unpredicted unconditioned stimulus, or the initiation of an action that is rewarding in itself (i.e., some species-specific activities [188,472]), or even perhaps merely an internal neuronal representation of the rewarding stimulus or action. And it does not matter whether a change in incentive salience has been triggered by prior associative experience or directly by a shift in physiological state (since they interact multiplicatively to control incentive value, in the Bindra/Toates sense of that term) [127,460]). This differential prediction potentially allows experimental discrimination of the incentive salience hypothesis from some forms of reward learning hypotheses of dopamine function.

Incentive reboosting and neural responses to unconditioned stimuli. The incentive salience hypothesis posits that incentive salience must be reboosted on every re-encounter with the 'wanted' stimulus and its 'liked' consequences. If this does not occur, subsequent attribution of incentive salience to the stimulus will decrease, leading to extinction of incentive value [34,45,366]. Is there direct evidence for reboosting or deboosting? Some may be

[10] A study by Balleine and Killcross [10] of instrumental performance after nucleus accumbens lesions suggests that the accumbens does *not* mediate the *cognitive representation* of act–outcome relations. They found that accumbens lesions did not impair a rat's ability to adjust its level of instrumental response based on a change in reinforcer value. They concluded that accumbens lesions "do not influence sensitivity to the instrumental contingency" (p. 191) and that the role of the accumbens is "dissociated from the control of performance mediated by the act–outcome relation" (p. 181) [10]. The lesions did impair overall rates of instrumental performance and also impaired classically-conditioned approach responses directed toward the food cup. Balleine and Killcross [10] interpreted the lesion deficit as reduced "conditioned affective arousal produced by classical conditioning" (p. 191), which seems to be more directly related to incentive salience attributions than to cognitive expectations of an outcome. Indeed, it is completely compatible with the incentive salience hypothesis, which would only assert that the 'arousal' hypothesized by Balleine and Killcross is not simply *affective* (hedonic) in nature, but reflects activation of incentive salience. It should be noted, however, that excitotoxin lesions rather than dopamine depletion were used by Balleine and Killcross, and that the test procedure was different from the extinction procedure used in the other experiments by Dickinson and Balleine described above [126–130]. Therefore a strong conclusion about dopamine's role cannot be made. Nevertheless, this study provides some evidence against the hypothesis that dopamine/accumbens systems mediate instrumental learning in the Dickinsonian sense of cognitive expectancy based on cause–outcome relations. Instead, it supports an incentive salience interpretation of accumbens function.

found in the electrophysiological studies by Schultz and colleagues.

Schultz et al. [300,405] have shown that dopamine neurons not only respond to a conditioned stimulus that predicts a hedonic reward, but *fail to respond to the unconditioned hedonic stimulus* if it has already been predicted. Dopamine neurons respond to food in the mouth if it is unexpected, but do not respond to food in the mouth that has been signaled by a predictive conditioned stimulus. At first glance, the failure to respond to a predicted event seems inconsistent with the assertion that dopamine neurons reboost incentive value on every trial. After all, the absence of neural activity seems to rule out the reboosting activity we expect.

However, the failure of dopamine neurons to fire robustly to a predicted hedonic stimulus may not reflect the complete *absence* of a response, but rather the presence of *two opposing* neuronal responses that cancel each other out [401]. This is suggested by the report by Schultz et al. that a conditioned stimulus that *fails* to be followed by the expected hedonic stimulus will elicit a decrease in firing of dopamine neurons *at the moment the hedonic stimulus usually would have been delivered* [401]. Similar firing decrements have been seen when a monkey encounters an inedible object instead of an expected food reward [371]. The demonstration of neuronal inhibition at the time an absent hedonic stimulus *should occur*, raises the possibility that such an opposing neuronal process might be generated even on trials in which the hedonic food *does occur*. In other words, on rewarded trials, excitation and inhibition might both occur and nearly cancel each other out. Consistent with this interpretation, Schultz et al. wrote, "The visual inspection of rasters and histograms (for trials on which the expected hedonic food was delivered) revealed that *depressions occurred in many neurons even in the presence of reward responses*... such that the *activating response was added on top of the depressed activity*" (p. 911, italics added [401]). In other words, the apparent lack of neuronal response to an expected hedonic event actually comprises two responses: an inhibition that corresponds to anticipation of the hedonic event, and an excitatory activation similar to that seen in naive animals.

These phenomena may provide a neuronal basis for both the 'deboosting' (i.e., extinction) of 'wanting' on nonrewarded trials (neural inhibition), and for the reboosting of incentive salience that maintains it at a constant level on trials in which the expected hedonic reward is received (neural excitation balanced together with neural inhibition). For reward extinction and deboosting, the following scenario could occur. Upon presentation of an established conditioned stimulus for reward that fails to be followed by hedonic activation, the conditioned stimulus elicits neuronal activation and is 'wanted' itself, but triggers neuronal inhibition moments later when the 'liked' hedonic unconditioned stimulus fails to materialize. If the inhibitory process is unopposed, it causes a reduction in subsequent attribution of incentive salience to the conditioned stimulus. The incentive becomes less 'wanted'.

On ordinary rewarded trials, hedonic activation does follow the conditioned stimulus. In these cases, the excitatory process *reboosts* or maintains subsequent incentive salience attributions. If the excitatory and inhibitory processes are in balance, no change occurs in the existing level of incentive salience subsequently attributed to the conditioned stimulus. 'Wanting' and instrumental performance are maintained at a constant level as long as neuronal excitation and inhibition are in balance. When the two processes are unequal, subsequent attributions of incentive salience are altered in the direction of the difference. Furthermore, not only should an *unexpected* hedonic event still activate dopamine neurons [300,301,401], but so should a *better-than-expected* hedonic reward even if *some* reward is anticipated. This would correspond to a 'positive contrast' or 'Crespi effect', in which animals over-respond to a better-than-expected reward [103,162]. Conversely, if the magnitude of the hedonic event were *less-than-expected* by the monkey an overall decrement of neuronal firing would be predicted, corresponding to a negative contrast effect [162]. Such a result would be compatible with both incentive salience and reward learning hypotheses (also see [341]).

On the other hand, the incentive salience hypothesis suggests that the balance between excitatory and inhibitory components could be altered even by manipulations that do not disturb the predictive relation between two stimuli, as long as they change their incentive value. For example, following a shift *in physiological* state a different prediction is made uniquely by the incentive salience hypothesis —and not by the 'explicit expectation of outcome' reward learning hypothesis (reward learning in Dickinson and Balleine's sense [12,127,128]). Certain physiological manipulations might shift incentive value and dopamine neuronal activity without altering either the magnitude of an unconditioned rewarding stimulus or its predictive relationship with a conditioned stimulus. This could provide a strong separation of the two hypotheses. For example, changing the physiological state of the animal to induce hunger, satiety, sodium appetite, etc., could conceivably alter the response of dopamine or striatal neurons to a conditioned stimulus for a hedonic food or salt reward, even if the stimuli themselves and their predictive relations were not changed from the animal's experience with them prior to the physiological shift.

As reviewed by Toates [460,463], the incentive value of Pavlovian conditioned stimuli (and of their hedonic unconditioned stimuli) are modulated directly by physiological states relevant to appetite, such as caloric hunger, satiety, or sodium deprivation (note: this is 'incentive value' in the Bindra/Toates and incentive salience sense of Pavlovian-acquired motivational features—not 'incentive value' in the more cognitive Dickinsonian sense [127,128] [see Addendum 2]). Such immediate shifts in the incentive value of classically-conditioned stimuli contrasts with the lack of a shift in instrumental cognitive expectancies, as reviewed by Dickinson and Balleine [127]. Thus, the incentive salience hypothesis predicts that a shift in dopamine activity should occur directly under such conditions. By contrast, a cognitive expectancy of reward hypothesis (at least, as based on the Dickinsonian concept of reward expectancy [125,127,128]) predicts that the animal would need to experience the altered hedonic value of the reward while in the altered physiological state before its instrumental behavior (and dopamine activity) would be changed. [11]

There is as yet little experimental evidence to test between incentive salience vs. reward learning predictions of dopamine function. However, in the few instances where the models diverge there is at least some suggestive evidence to support an incentive salience interpretation. For example, in a microdialysis study Fiorino, Coury, and Phillips report that an unconditional increase in the value of a sexual incentive enhanced dopamine overflow in the nucleus accumbens, even though the change in incentive value did not arise from learning, and occurred on the first experience with the new incentive [159]. Their study focused on the 'Coolidge effect' (the name based on an apocryphal remark of the late U.S. President Calvin Coolidge regarding the ability of a chicken farmer's rooster to fertilize many hens). In that phenomenon, male sexual motivation is aroused again after satiety by the presentation of a *new* female. Fiorino et al. [159] found that dopamine overflow was elicited initially by the mere presentation of a female beyond reach behind a screen, and dopamine peaked during subsequent copulation, after the screen was removed. Dopamine levels then declined over the course of successive copulation bouts with the first female, eventually returning to baseline after copulations ceased. Presentation of a second novel female behind a screen elicited a slight increase in dopamine overflow, which rose significantly during a second series of copulations (but never to the same level as with the first female) before falling again.

This pattern of results is consistent with the notion that dopamine activity reflects shifts in incentive value, even those that come about independent of learning. The second female was by definition novel, as she had never been encountered before. Therefore, her heightened motivational value, and the heightened dopamine activity she elicited, were unlikely to arise from learning (the males had not apparently ever before experienced successive copulations with multiple females in a single day, so the enhancement could not have arisen by generalization from learning). This seems to be an example, therefore, of a case where changes in dopamine activity do not reflect *predicted* reward value based on learning, but instead reflect an *unconditional modulation of incentive value*, based on a change in the unconditioned stimulus; i.e., a change in incentive salience. [12]

11. Effects of dopamine antagonists: a re-examination of anhedonia, incentive salience or anergia explanations

11.1. Comparing dopamine antagonist effects on hedonic activation

A primary conclusion of our review is that mesolimbic and neostriatal dopamine systems are not necessary for normal hedonic processes. It is reasonable to ask then, whether our conclusion can be reconciled with the wealth of evidence for *anhedonia* obtained over several decades.

[11] In order to test in practice whether dopamine firing patterns follow cognitive expectation (Dickinson's experience-dependent revaluation) vs. incentive salience predictions (Bindra/Toates direct motivational shifts) it will be important to induce *strong motivational appetites* (e.g., strong sodium depletion) when comparing predictions made by the two models. Weak physiological shifts might not be sufficient to alter neuronal response. The issue has arisen before concerning whether motivational shifts change the electrophysiological coding of gustatory reward signals in primates as in rodents, since electrophysiological studies in primate have tended to use weaker motivational shifts, for ethical and practical reasons, than comparable experiments using rodents [410,411] (for discussion see Ref. [34]). An adequate electrophysiological test would either need to induce strong motivational shifts in primates or else would have to be done using rodents as subjects and motivational procedures similar to those of Dickinson and Balleine. There is at least suggestive evidence from rodent studies to support our prediction that dopamine activation may be potentiated directly by physiological or pharmacological enhancement of incentives. Mesolimbic dopamine overflow elicited by food in rats has been suggested to be higher the hungrier they are [290,482]. The incentive salience hypothesis predicts such effects even if the experience is novel to the animal (since Pavlovian incentive value is directly enhanced by hunger state [460,463]), in contrast to predictions based on the 'cognitive expectation of incentive value' (since the expectation is based on past experience, and the work of Dickinson and Balleine [12,127,128] shows that for accurate cognitive expectation, the animal must previously experience the value of the food while hungry). Given the paucity of evidence available, the question remains open as to whether dopamine neurons will most often follow the reward learning hypothesis or the incentive salience hypothesis when their predictions diverge. But Pennartz (p. 235 [341]) draws the tentative conclusion, that "Altogether, these observations on SNpc DA neurons indicate functions in attention, orientation and the formation of behavioural responses to significant and salient stimuli, but not in reinforcement signalling per se."

[12] Furthermore, when introduced, the second female had greater incentive value than the 'spent' first female, as assessed by behavior (the male renewed copulation), but less incentive value than the first female had initially (reflected by much less vigorous copulation with the second female). This behavioral incentive value was correlated with dopamine overflow: the increase in dopamine was much less during copulation with the second female than with the first. A 'hedonic' interpretation of dopamine function is also compatible with the Coolidge effect reported by Fiorino et al. [159], since the highest dopamine levels occurred during copulation. But Fiorino et al. note that the male rats actually spent much of the 'consummatory phase' in intense appetitive pursuit of the female between intromissions, so the enhanced dopamine overflow even surrounding copulation could still reflect peak activation of a 'wanting' process during that phase [159].

Nearly all the evidence for anhedonia came, as we pointed out above, from animal studies that involved either a measure of an instrumental behavior required to obtain a reward (bar pressing, running in a runway, etc.) or a measure of choice (such as place preference or food consumption). All such studies more directly measure 'wanting' (the willingness to work for or seek an incentive) than 'liking' (the hedonic consequences of reward consumption). In all such studies the effect of any experimental manipulation (e.g., dopamine antagonist treatment) on hedonics is only *inferred* (not directly measured) by changes in 'wanting'. No such study provides, therefore, evidence of a specific role for dopamine in hedonic processes. They can be discounted because they cannot discern between a change in both 'liking' and 'wanting' vs. a change in incentive salience alone.

But two types of studies with dopamine antagonists do not fit into that category, and cannot be so easily dismissed. They are (1) animal studies of the effects of dopamine antagonists on the same affective reactions to taste studied here after 6-OHDA lesions, and (2) self-report studies in humans of the effects of dopamine antagonists on the hedonic impact of stimuli such as drugs of abuse. Are the results of such studies compatible with our conclusion?

11.2. Affective taste reactivity and dopamine antagonists: sensorimotor anergia but not anhedonia

In an early study of a dopamine antagonist's effect on hedonic and aversive reactions to taste, Treit and Berridge [465] found that haloperidol (0.5 mg/kg or 1.0 mg/kg) failed to suppress hedonic reactions of rats to a 1 min infusion of sucrose infusion, and also failed to enhance aversive reactions to quinine. Failure of a dopamine antagonist to alter affective reactions patterns is in accord with our conclusion that dopamine does not mediate hedonia. However, two taste reactivity studies conducted by Parker et al. [274,331] at about the same time suggested that a different dopamine antagonist, pimozide, did shift palatability. Leeb et al. [274] reported that pimozide suppressed hedonic reactions to sucrose if the sucrose infusion was infused over 10 min, especially in the later minutes, and especially if the trials were repeated on successive days. Conversely, Parker and Lopez [331] reported that pimozide *enhanced aversive reactions* to quinine in a similar test. The authors of those studies interpreted their results as evidence for the anhedonia hypothesis.

In order to settle the controversy, a more recent collaborative study was undertaken by Peciña et al. [339]. They concluded that both 'anhedonia' and 'increased aversion' after pimozide were illusory artifacts [339].

- First, the initial hedonic or aversive responses were generally not altered by pimozide (0.5 mg/kg) during the first minute of a sucrose or quinine infusion, supporting the conclusion that initial hedonic impact remained normal [339]. Only later responses, emitted in subsequent minutes or trials, were diminished, and that appeared to reflect a progressive sensorimotor deficit and not a shift in palatability.
- Second, a reanalysis of the data of Parker and Lopez [331] by Peciña et al. [339] showed that the apparent enhancement of aversive reactions to quinine was an artifact of the motor suppressant effects of pimozide. Pimozide reduced locomotion, and therefore, pimozide-treated rats spent more time in view of the camera, giving rise to inflated aversion scores. When the sampling error was corrected, it eliminated the enhancement of aversive reactivity originally reported by Parker and Lopez [331].
- Third, Peciña et al. [339] found that when the duration of sucrose infusions and quinine infusions were equated pimozide actually suppressed aversive reactions (rather than enhancing them) in exactly the same gradual way as it suppressed hedonic reactions. This gradual and equivalent pattern of behavioral reduction, regardless of affective category, was the principal reason for concluding that the suppression was sensorimotor in nature (similar to Salamone et al.'s concept of 'anergia' [382,383]). The sensorimotor suppression appeared only during the later minutes of a continuous oral infusion, which elicited a prolonged and vigorous response, and grew as a stimulus was repeated or sustained over several minutes or trials.

Peciña et al. [339] concluded that a progressive general sensorimotor suppression was sufficient to account for all the effects of pimozide on taste reactivity patterns. There was no reason to conclude that pimozide additionally altered hedonic or aversive palatability. In short, *pimozide does not produce anhedonic shifts in palatability*, as assessed by taste reactivity [339].

In the present study using dopamine-depleted rats we found no evidence for sensorimotor suppression. However, a 1-min infusion was used and that duration may not encroach into the temporal zone of delayed sensorimotor suppression [339]. Perhaps if a longer sustained stimulus had been used sensorimotor deficits would have been detected. Alternatively, sensorimotor suppression of taste reactivity might be more pronounced after *acute* receptor blockade than after *chronic* dopamine depletion. Whatever the case, the results of 6-OHDA lesions and dopamine antagonists are now both consistent with the conclusion that dopamine is not crucial to hedonic impact as measured by affective taste reactivity patterns.

11.3. Subjective hedonic ratings by humans and dopamine antagonists: conscious pleasure persists

What about the effects of dopamine antagonists on self-reports of subjective wanting and liking in humans? In two recent studies Brauer and de Wit report that in humans the *euphorigenic* effects of amphetamine (10 or 20 mg; euphoria assessed by subjective hedonic ratings) are not altered by co-treatment with pimozide (1, 2 or 8 mg) [58,59]. That is, pimozide did not influence subjective ratings of '*like drug*' [59]. Similarly, Ohuoha et al. [320]

reported that the ability of cocaine to produce subjective euphoria was not diminished by prior administration of either haloperidol or fluphenazine.

By contrast with unchanged ratings of 'like drug', Brauer and de Wit [59] reported that subjective ratings of '*want drug*' elicited by amphetamine were significantly suppressed by the highest dose of pimozide used. In related studies, subjective *craving* elicited by a drug or conditioned stimulus has similarly been found to be suppressed by dopamine antagonists. Modell et al. [302] primed craving in alcoholics by giving them a small drink of alcohol, and found that the elicited craving (and actual consumption) was suppressed by prior administration of haloperidol. In a study of conditioned craving, Berger et al. [28] showed videotapes of crack cocaine preparation to addicts, and found that haloperidol significantly reduced their elicited ratings of subjective craving. In the Berger et al. study, it can be noted that haloperidol also reduced ratings of the 'conditioned high' elicited by watching the video, which is inconsistent with our notion that dopamine antagonists reduce 'wanting' but not 'liking'. However, the magnitude of change in the 'high' rating was less than the effect on subjective craving. In a review of the literature on dopamine drugs and subjective *hedonic* ratings, Brauer et al. [60] note that dopamine antagonists diminished the subjective euphoric effects of amphetamine in only 2 of 10 studies they surveyed (typically at antagonist doses that were sufficiently high to produce aversive symptoms by themselves), and that dopamine antagonists were even less effective in reducing cocaine-induced euphoria. Thus, dopamine antagonists may alter human subjective ratings of wanting more reliably than they alter ratings of liking. Chronic suppression of dopamine neurotransmission, such as occurs in Parkinson's disease, may be no more effective than neuroleptic drugs in suppressing the hedonic impact of rewarding stimuli. For example, Travers et al. [464] found that Parkinson's patients rated the perceived pleasantness of sweet and salty tastes no lower than normal subjects did (and in fact gave *higher* hedonic ratings than normal to the most intense sweet solutions).

Augmentation of dopamine function may lead to converse results and to a similar conclusion regarding the role of dopamine in subjective experience. Haney et al. [219] gave pergolide (a D1/D2 dopamine receptor *agonist*) or a placebo to human addicts, and then let them perform an operant task to earn cocaine as a reward. Pre-treatment with the dopamine agonist failed to increase the addicts' subjective liking for cocaine, when rated several minutes after taking the cocaine. On the contrary, their subjective ratings of 'I like dose' or feeling 'high' or 'stimulated' were actually suppressed by pergolide [219]. By contrast, pergolide did significantly increase subjective ratings of 'I want cocaine' measured at the same time—and simultaneously increased subjective craving for other drugs too (increased ratings of 'I want alcohol' and 'I want nicotine') [219]. Heightened dopamine neurotransmission thus appears to enhance subjective wanting, but not subjective liking, for drugs such as cocaine.

Admittedly, the effects of psychoactive drugs on subjective ratings by human subjects must be interpreted cautiously. Subjective reports by humans may sometimes diverge from underlying core processes of emotion and motivation [34,41,273,307,316,494]. Subjective ratings are cognitive interpretations of the subject's own feelings, and are influenced by many cognitive factors, rather than being direct readouts of underlying 'wanting' and 'liking' processes [273,307,316,494]. Even reports that dopamine antagonists decrease subjective craving may not be able to be taken at face value, and suppression of subjective hedonic ratings also sometimes occurs. The process of incentive salience attribution is held by us to be not directly accessible to conscious introspection [34,35,41,366]. Blurring of the distinction between 'wanting' and 'liking' core processes is therefore sometimes to be expected in conscious experience and subjective reports. To conclude, more study clearly is needed, but the available evidence from studies of human subjective reports are consistent with our hypothesis that dopamine has more to do with 'wanting' rewards than with 'liking' them.

12. Phenomena that don't fit: problems for the incentive salience model?

12.1. Euphorigenic dopaminergic drugs

Probably the most convincing original evidence for the hedonia hypothesis, aside from animal studies of reward suppression by neuroleptic drugs, were demonstrations that most drugs of abuse promote activation of mesolimbic dopamine systems [266,268,505–507]. Dopamine neurotransmission is generally enhanced by rewarding drugs, and many (though not all) addictive drugs of abuse produce subjective euphoria in humans. How can it be that so many drugs that enhance dopamine neurotransmission are euphorigenic if dopamine systems do not mediate hedonia?

There are several possible answers to this question. First, all euphorigenic drugs of abuse influence multiple neurotransmitter systems, not just dopamine systems. Indeed, for many, their primary action is not on dopamine. Opiates provide an obvious example, as they produce their actions via opioid receptors, mostly located on non-dopaminergic neurons. Furthermore, unlike dopaminergic agents, opioids do alter 'liking' for food rewards, as measured by hedonic taste reactivity patterns [34,131,332, 336,338,360]. Thus, some classes of drugs may produce 'liking' (hedonia) via their direct or indirect actions on endogenous opioid or other neurotransmitter systems that mediate hedonic impact.

Even psychostimulants, such as amphetamine and cocaine, have many actions in addition to their actions on dopamine neurotransmission. For example, both drugs bind to norepinephrine and serotonin transporters, and increase the concentrations of these transmitters in dialysate, and via their actions on monoamines can influence many other transmitter systems. Serotonin systems in particular have been implicated in cocaine self-administration. For example, knockout mice lacking serotonin 1B receptors work more avidly for cocaine than wild-type controls, as indicated by higher 'breakpoints' on a progressive ratio schedule (and they also appear to be hypersensitive to the psychomotor stimulant effects of cocaine) [369,486]. Although this does not imply that serotonin, any more than dopamine, mediates the hedonic impact of cocaine, it does highlight the multiplicity of neurotransmitter systems that contribute to the rewarding effects of even psychomotor stimulant drugs. It is reasonable to hypothesize, therefore, that euphorigenic drugs produce their hedonic effects via their actions on neurotransmitter systems other than dopamine, even if their incentive properties are mediated by dopamine systems.

Furthermore, the neural circuits responsible for 'liking' and 'wanting' may be closely intertwined in the brain (albeit not identical). For example, microinjections of opioid agonists into the shell region of the nucleus accumbens enhances taste hedonics [334,338]. Thus, in the same accumbens region where dopamine plays a critical role in mediating reward 'wanting', opioid receptors have been implicated in 'liking', and there are probably direct synaptic connections between the two systems [223,246,253, 255,281,350]. Neural circuits involved in 'wanting' and 'liking' may also be found together in the ventral pallidum. The ventral pallidum receives a dopamine input from the ventral tegmental area [189,190,264], and lesions of the ventral pallidum, which produce aphagia (elimination of food 'wanting'), abolish hedonic reactions to food (elimination of 'liking'), and cause rats to respond aversively even to normally palatable food [34,106,393]. How 'wanting' and 'liking' are integrated neurobiologically remains an important challenge for future research, but some drugs that promote dopamine neurotransmission may activate both systems.

In support of our contention that dopamine is not hedonia, it is important to note that many drugs that increase dopamine neurotransmission are not euphorigenic. Rothman and Glowa [374] review evidence of multiple dissociations between the ability of drugs to enhance dopamine neurotransmission and their ability to produce euphoria. For example, there are a number of dopamine uptake blockers that are used clinically, some of which are more potent than cocaine at inhibiting [^{3}H]dopamine uptake, but many do not produce cocaine-like euphoria. One of them, mazindol, is reported to be *dysphoric* in humans. Direct dopamine receptor agonists provide another interesting example that can dissociate 'wanting' and 'liking'. Many of these agents support self-administration in animals, but the available evidence indicates people do not find them to be euphorigenic [374]. Similarly, monoamine oxidase inhibitors and L-Dopa increase extracellular dopamine but are not euphorigenic. In conclusion, the evidence reviewed by Rothman and Glowa [374] indicates that increasing dopamine neurotransmission is not a sufficient condition for producing euphoria.

Finally, in relating the effects of drugs on 'wanting' vs. 'liking' in humans it is important to keep in mind the potential for cognitive confusion regarding subjective effects. Although unlikely to explain reports of an 'orgasmic rush', a person who took a drug that made the world seem a more attractive and rewarding place, by selectively enhancing incentive salience, might find it difficult to describe those effects without invoking hedonic concepts. Also, addicts who 'want' drugs might sometimes mistakenly infer they necessarily 'like' them in order to explain to themselves their own addiction [366]. Although it may seem nonintuitive to claim that addicts could be wrong about their own feelings, there is ample evidence that people sometimes are wrong about and sometimes unaware of their own underlying emotional 'core processes' [35,141,243,244,316,494,495,528]. For a more complete discussion of addiction and drugs of abuse see Robinson and Berridge [366,367]. For discussion of how 'liking' and 'wanting' core processes contrast to subjective experience, see Berridge [35].

12.2. Paradoxical effects of dopamine antagonists

What about 'problem' phenomena from animal experiments that contradict our predictions? There are several effects of dopamine antagonists that appear to pose difficulty for an incentive salience hypothesis. First, the ability of dopamine antagonists to suppress motivated behavior is sometimes delayed. Second, under some conditions dopamine antagonists actually appear to *increase* the preference or consumption of rewards. These phenomena present a paradox in that dopamine receptor blockade, which ought to reduce incentive motivation, either apparently fails to do so or appears to do the opposite. In this section, we show how paradoxical effects can be understood in light of the incentive salience hypothesis.

12.2.1. Reinforcement extinction without motivational suppression?

Ettenberg and colleagues [82,145,148,234,235,291,292] have shown in several studies that moderate doses of pimozide, haloperidol or other dopamine antagonists can block the ability of a reward to strengthen or reinstate *future* instrumental behavior for that reward, without reducing reward-directed behavior on the trial the neuroleptic is given. This effect is similar to 'extinction mimicry', in which neuroleptics produce gradual declines in instrumental performance without altering the initial level of response when the drug is first given [175,176,179,479].

When given particular doses of pimozide or haloperidol, for example, rats may still run as fast in a runway for the reward they have received earlier as they would without neuroleptic, and a conditioned stimulus for reward still prompts locomotion [235,291]. However, subsequent running on a later drug-free day is suppressed for the reward that had been experienced earlier under the neuroleptic [291]. McFarland et al. [291] interpret the delayed effect to mean that dopamine antagonists have no effect upon the rat's motivation to run when it first receives the drug, but that neuroleptics do prevent the ability of the reward to serve as a *reinforcer*, here meaning to sustain or strengthen subsequent running. Ettenberg et al. [82,148,234,292] have also demonstrated that neuroleptics block a related reinforcement effect, namely, *reinstatement*. In reinstatement, animals are first trained on a rewarded task, and then are extinguished by the withholding of reward. They are then given a single rewarded trial—which typically reinstates future instrumental performance. Reinstatement is blocked if rats are given a neuroleptic immediately prior to the rewarded trial.

The ability of dopamine antagonists to block reinforcement and reinstatement of a subsequent response is consistent with an *anhedonia* interpretation of dopamine function [499,500,503,514]. Preventing the reward's hedonic impact should prevent reestablishment of behavior motivated to regain it, but need not impair motivation before the diminished pleasure has been experienced. Reinforcement and reinstatement suppression is also consistent with a '*reward learning*' interpretation of dopamine function [3,304,400,405]. Preventing the growth of an association between a reward and a particular stimulus or response should attenuate subsequent behavior that is guided by the association, but not necessarily other aspects of behavior. Blocking of reinforcement and reinstatement is also consistent with the *incentive salience* hypothesis if the neuroleptic prevented 'reboosting' of incentive salience (see above) [34,44,45,366]. But these results also present some unique problems for the incentive salience hypothesis. The problem for the incentive salience hypothesis is that it also predicts that *'wanting' for incentive stimuli should be impaired on the day of neuroleptic administration*, as well as on subsequent days. How can an incentive salience hypothesis reconcile the failure to observe a performance impairment on the day of neuroleptic administration with suppressed performance for the reward on a subsequent undrugged trial?

The answer may hinge in part upon the dose of neuroleptic used and in part on the conditions of testing. We posited several years ago that neuroleptics differentially impair incentive salience attributions under different conditions [34,44,366]. Neuroleptics most readily disrupt the *acquisition* of new incentive salience by conditioned stimuli and the *re-boosting* of incentive salience, both of which occur once a hedonic reward is obtained. These disruptions, we suggested, occur at *lower doses* of neuroleptic than are needed to disrupt the attribution of incentive salience to a familiar, and already 'wanted', conditioned stimulus [34,44,366]. This means that after low to moderate doses of dopamine antagonists, pre-established incentive salience may still be attributed to conditioned stimuli, but the drug may block the reboosting of incentive salience to those conditioned stimuli and the acquisition of incentive salience by new conditioned stimuli [34,44,366].

Acquisition requires an actual *increment* in incentive salience attribution. Even re-boosting that maintains the incentive value of a conditioned stimulus when hedonic reward is obtained may require an incremental process, as described earlier, to oppose the automatic de-boosting that would otherwise occur. In both acquisition and re-boosting, the occurrence of the hedonic event triggers a process that increments the incentive salience assigned to conditioned stimuli. These incremental processes may be blocked relatively easily by dopamine antagonists. By contrast, the pre-established incentive salience of a familiar 'wanted' reward is based on earlier experiences with it that occurred in the absence of a dopamine antagonist. Such pre-established attributions of incentive salience are posited by our hypothesis to be less vulnerable to neuroleptic blockade. Pre-established attributions may initially persist even if increments and re-boosting are disrupted [44,45].

If acquisition and re-boosting are preferentially blocked, then an animal may be unable to acquire a new incentive under neuroleptic blockade, but may still respond to an 'old' one. Therefore, the blocking of re-boosting for the familiar incentive may prevent reinstatement and produce 'extinction mimicry': a gradual decline in responding during or across sessions [175,176,479]. According to our hypothesis, this works as follows. First, the perception or representation of the familiar conditioned stimulus for reward triggers attribution of incentive salience based upon past associative experience with the reward and hedonic activation. The familiar conditioned stimulus is still 'wanted' since 'wanting' attributed on the basis of pre-established associations is relatively resistant to neuroleptic administration. If the individual responds and acquires the full unconditioned reward, hedonic 'liking' systems are activated just as they would be in the absence of neuroleptic. But the triggering of incentive salience systems by hedonic 'liking' is no longer sufficient to generate the re-boosting of incentive salience that would be needed to *maintain* the ability of a conditioned stimulus to elicit 'wanting' each time it is encountered [44,45]. The brain expects a 'wanted' conditioned stimulus to be followed by hedonic 'liking', just as in the past, and in a sense poses on each trial a question that has one of two answers. Does the 'wanted' reward still carry its old hedonic impact ('liking')? If hedonic activation occurs, the answer is 'yes': it triggers dopamine-related systems to reboost the incentive salience attributed to the stimulus, and the stimulus remains 'wanted' in the future. If hedonic activation fails to trigger incentive salience systems, however, the answer is 'no': then reboosting fails to occur, and 'wanting' for the conditioned stimulus is automatically devalued. [13]

Prevention of incentive salience reboosting means that the stimulus will be less 'wanted' the *next* time it is encountered: blocking reinstatement and producing 'extinction mimicry'. As Berridge and Valenstein (p. 11, [44]) put it, "reboosting appears to be especially vulnerable to neuroleptics and may be suppressed by doses that do not prevent the attribution of preestablished incentive salience". Higher doses of neuroleptics, or behavioral test procedures that more sensitively reveal modulation in appetitive motivation, would reveal motivational or 'wanting' suppression even on the day of the drug. Many studies have indeed reported an immediate motivational suppression by the dopamine antagonist drug, reducing the likelihood and strength of instrumental responding or of approach to the incentive target [17,28,50,51,157,310,382,383,429]. Extensive dopamine depletion by 6-OHDA, as in the present study, even more effectively eliminates all aspects of incentive salience attribution, leaving the individual oblivious to all incentives and rewards [287,451,452,471,531].

12.2.2. Paradoxical 'motivation increase' after dopamine antagonists?

Worse than preservation of motivation after neuroleptics, from the point of view of the incentive salience hypothesis, are *increases* in incentive motivation. In some situations, administration of a dopamine antagonist causes an animal to *increase* its self-administration of a drug or, less commonly, a food incentive.

A paradoxical enhancement of *food* intake after dopamine blockade has been reported by Salamone et al. The situation must be arranged quite carefully to achieve the effect, which actually involves a redirection of consumption from one food, which is normally preferred, toward another food, which is less preferred but more easily obtained. Rats normally ignore the nonpreferred-but-free food and work to obtain the preferred-but-hard-to-get one. After mild dopamine impairment, however, they switch to the less preferred food—and *actually increase consumption of that food relative to their normal intake of it*. For example, in a Skinner box hungry rats may choose between bar pressing to gain a preferred sweetened pellet or to eat ordinary chow that is freely available in the box. After administration of haloperidol, SCH 23990, flupenthixol, or sulpiride rats not only stop bar pressing for the preferred sweetened food, but they also *increase* their consumption of the free chow [101,382,385]. The tasty but expensive food reward loses out to bland but cheap. Similar effects are seen after localized 6-OHDA lesions of the nucleus accumbens, especially of the accumbens core [100,382,432].

Although an increase in consumption of a food, any food, might appear to be a paradoxical increase in the motivation to eat, and difficult for the incentive salience hypothesis to interpret, an increase in motivation after dopamine disruption is probably not the right explanation. Further insight into the nature of the effect is provided by additional experiments by Salamone et al. [99,382]. In these experiments rats were given a choice between two arms in a T-maze. One arm contained several food pellets, but to get to them the rats had to climb over a formidable barrier (44 cm high). The other arm contained only half the number of pellets as the first arm, but had no barrier and so was easy to reach. Normally, rats preferred to climb for the larger reward. After haloperidol or partial depletion of accumbens dopamine, however, rats switched their preference to the smaller-but-easier reward [99,382]. The failure to persist in the demanding task was not due to absolute incapacity: that was demonstrated by giving a group of rats a slightly different choice between an obstructed arm that contained the large food reward and an unobstructed arm that was *empty*. Faced with that choice, the rats continued to struggle over the obstacle to gain the food even after dopamine impairment [99,382]. The typical switch by the other groups to the less preferred reward—and their concomitant increase in consumption of the normally unchosen food—was clearly a default consequence of abandoning the difficult task in favor of any acceptable alternative. The dopamine impairment was not sufficient to eliminate all appetitive behavior and consumption. The animals were still disposed to eat some food, and the food most readily available was therefore consumed. Salamone et al. [380–383] contrast this impairment to anhedonia, and describe it instead as a form of 'anergia': a complex sensorimotor deficit manifest in motor slowing, reduced reaction to certain stimuli, and a biased response selection away from vigorous instrumental behavior toward easier alternatives (possibly related to the sensorimotor suppression of taste reactivity by neuroleptic administration described earlier [339]). Salamone et al. conclude that this impairment alters

[13] Even on the day of neuroleptic treatment, prevention of incentive salience reboosting and consequent devaluation of 'wanting' can lead to discernable consequences. Rats are reported to disengage from the food or other incentive object earlier after neuroleptic administration than they otherwise would, or similarly fail to maintain pursuit or contact as the trial goes on [175,429,430,499,512]. A possible neurological correlate consistent with this interpretation has been reported by Chang et al. [81] in an electrophysiological study of rats that bar pressed to receive cocaine infusions. Nearly 20% of neurons they recorded in the nucleus accumbens showed anticipatory responding before the cocaine was administered as the rat oriented toward the lever or began to press. Some of these neurons also responded to the cocaine itself. Pre-administration of a dopamine antagonist did not block the anticipatory neural activity correlated with incentive salience or 'wanting' triggered as the rat oriented, and the rats still pressed at the beginning of the session. The dopamine antagonist did, however, block the post-cocaine neuronal response of the same neurons [81]. That could be viewed as blocking the normal reboosting of incentive salience consequent to hedonic activation, which could cause behavioral bar pressing to extinguish.

many aspects of behavior, and that it may not be possible to parse among motivational and sensorimotor effects.

These important studies by Salamone et al. illustrate the subtle diversity of function mediated by dopamine systems. They also provide an instance in which consumption of a particular food (the normally less preferred one) is increased by a dopamine antagonist, which normally decreases food consumption. In this case the paradox of increased consumption seems easily resolved: the antagonist does not actually increase motivation to eat, it merely preserves a degree of incentive motivation (not necessarily the original level) while biasing choice away from the difficult task, probably due in part to sensorimotor effects of the drug.

Paradoxical increases in drug self-administration (e.g., cocaine or amphetamine) have also been reported to follow neuroleptic administration [112,149,267,268,522,523]. Unlike a shift in food choice, the paradoxical increase in the rate of cocaine or amphetamine self-administration reported following a dopamine antagonist cannot be explained simply by reallocation of the remaining response. In the case of drug self-administration, the *sole response* is potentiated by the dopamine antagonist. In early studies, Yokel and Wise [522,523] showed that low doses of pimozide could increase the self-administration of amphetamine by rats (followed by extinction in the case of higher doses). De Wit and Wise [112] found a similar effect of pimozide on cocaine self-administration. Increased self-administration of cocaine can be induced by low-doses of other neuroleptics such as alpha-flupenthixol too (though again, higher doses have the opposite effect of suppressing self-administration) [149]. These effects were interpreted within the anhedonia framework: reduced hedonic pleasure could prompt an individual to strive for more of the 'watered down' reward [514]. [14] The 'hedonic homeostasis' framework of Koob et al. provides essentially the same explanation as that of de Wit and Wise [112], in that it posits dopamine neurotransmission to be tied to hedonic activation [267,268]. Koob et al. (p. 514, [267]) argue that suppression of dopamine-related reward systems must blunt "in the case of cocaine,... the acute hedonic response", and that individuals must therefore work to obtain more cocaine in order to maintain their desired level of hedonic activation (i.e., hedonic homeostasis) [267,268].

This effect certainly has the appearance of an increase in incentive motivation. How can an increased rate of self-administration after treatment with a dopamine antagonist be explained by the incentive salience hypothesis, which must posit that incentive motivation, if changed at all, should be decreased by a dopamine antagonist?

First, it can safely be said that the *incentive motivation ('wanting')* to take drugs is probably never increased by neuroleptic administration. There are several reasons to believe that dopamine antagonists *reduce* the incentive value of cocaine and other drugs, even if the rate of bar pressing increases. And there are alternative explanations for the increase in response rate.

Limitations of response rate as a measure of motivation. It has been clear for nearly 4 decades that under some conditions absolute rate of response is a misleading measure of reward and motivation [473]. For example, Hodos and Valenstein [230,473] showed in 1962 that, given a choice between two levels of rewarding brain stimulation, rats typically preferred the higher intensity, even though they pressed at a faster rate for the lower intensity. Some limitations of absolute response rate as a measure of incentive value may also apply to drug reward. In a review of the usefulness of response rate measures in drug self-administration experiments, Arnold and Roberts (p. 441, [6]) concluded that "the rate of drug intake cannot directly address the issue of increased or decreased reinforcer efficacy". They note that dopamine impairments sometimes increase the rate of self-administration and sometimes reduce it, and that both effects are often taken as evidence for reduced reinforcement (i.e., reduced reward or hedonic impact): "how can both an increase and a decrease in rate of drug intake be used to draw the same conclusion? The dilemma is unmistakable: rate is an ambiguous measure of reinforcing efficacy" (p. 442, [6]).

Progressive ratio 'breakpoint designs', in which the response requirement is progressively elevated throughout a session, have been argued to provide a better measure of incentive value [6,229]. In such experiments, the first reward requires only 1 or 2 bar presses, the second reward requires more responses, the third more still, and so on. The question is, how far will an animal escalate its response to gain the reward? The results of such experiments typically indicate that motivation is *decreased*, not increased, by dopamine antagonists. For example, Depoortere et al. trained rats to bar press for cocaine on a progressive ratio schedule, and found that the D1 antagonist SCH 23390 lowered the breakpoint, so the rats quit pressing sooner [114]. This was not due to a motor deficit, Depoortere et al. [114] concluded, because rats pressed at a comparable rate under the neuroleptic as they did without it. If anything, there was a slight tendency to press more rapidly after the antagonist, again underscoring the ambiguity of absolute response rate. Similarly, Roberts et al. [364] found that preadministration of haloperidol significantly *increased* the absolute rate of cocaine self-administration, but simultaneously *lowered* the highest response ratio achieved (breakpoint). Equivalent dissociations have been reported by McGregor et al. [293,294] after microinjections of dopamine antagonists into the accumbens, and

[14] Interestingly, *decreases* in reward consumption after neuroleptics have been interpreted identically in the anhedonia framework, as reflecting reduced pleasure, on the grounds that consumption should be proportional to the hedonic intensity of the reward. For examples, see [182,429,498,499,514,517]. The contradiction points to the need for an explicit and consistent theoretical framework in which to relate behavioral changes to psychological processes.

after central 6-OHDA lesions. In all these studies there is dissociation between response rate (which typically goes up after central dopamine suppression) and breakpoint (which typically goes down). If breakpoint is a better measure of motivation than the absolute rate of self-administration, as has been suggested [6], then dopamine antagonists usually reduce the motivation for a drug reward—as the incentive salience hypothesis would suggest.

Finally, prior *sensitization* of dopamine systems has been reported by Mendrek et al. [297] to produce the *opposite* effect on progressive ratio tests, *increasing* the breakpoint for amphetamine (an effect that has been replicated by Vezina [476]). Thus, as assessed by progressive ratio schedules, manipulations that increase dopamine neurotransmission (e.g., sensitization) increase motivation for drugs, and manipulations that decrease dopamine activity (e.g., neuroleptics) decrease motivation for drugs. This is consistent with the incentive salience hypothesis that dopamine systems mediate 'wanting'. It also supports our related proposal regarding addiction, presented elsewhere, that sensitization of dopamine systems may increase 'wanting' for drugs, and produce compulsive seeking and taking of drugs (for discussion of the Incentive–Sensitization theory of addiction see Robinson and Berridge [366,367]).

12.2.3. Resolutions for the rate paradox

Still, it is important to understand why the absolute response rate of drug self-administration might increase under the influence of a neuroleptic. There are several factors that may help illuminate this phenomenon.

- First, it should be noted that neuroleptics increase response rates for cocaine or amphetamine only over a limited range of neuroleptic doses. High doses of dopamine antagonists suppress even the absolute rate of responding below baseline [149,267], which could be due to motivational deficits as well as motor deficits.
- Second, neuroleptics may diminish some of the *aversive* properties [183] (e.g., paranoia, cardiovascular responses, etc.) of cocaine or similar drugs, as well as their rewarding effects. A decrease in the aversive effects could lead an animal to increase the highest cocaine dose that it tolerates, so that it takes higher doses than normal. A rat that was still motivated at all to self-administer cocaine after a low dose of a neuroleptic might take more cocaine because its aversive impact, not its hedonic impact, was reduced.
- Third, neuroleptics themselves may sometimes have aversive effects. Dopamine antagonists, for example, can sometimes establish a conditioned place avoidance when paired associatively with a new location [78,310,361] (though not all studies find this). Dopamine antagonists by themselves also induce unpleasant symptoms in humans, manifest in subjective reports of confusion and impaired psychomotor performance [60]. To the extent that a neuroleptic has any aversive properties, cocaine and similar drugs could be an effective antidote. Animals might increase their self-administration of a drug like cocaine in part to combat the aversive effects of the neuroleptic.
- Finally, interactions among self-administered dopamine indirect agonists and low doses of neuroleptics are especially difficult to interpret. If the neuroleptic dose were low enough, the animal might soon administer sufficient indirect agonist to effectively replace any motivational impairment with dopaminergic stimulation. In that case, its neural and motivational condition early in the session (suppression of dopamine neurotransmission) would be qualitatively different from later in the same session (activation of dopamine neurotransmission). It is not clear which drug should be expected to win when the neuroleptic dose is low.

In short, increases in the rate of drug self-administration after neuroleptics are subject to a host of interpretive complications. Reward or motivation cannot be simply inferred from absolute response rate.

12.3. The 'Two Motivational Systems' hypothesis (Bechara et al.)

A different type of potential problem for the incentive salience view is posed by a novel proposal developed by Bechara et al. [17,19,310], which they call the '2 systems' hypothesis. The '2-systems' hypothesis does not propose a specific *alternative* to incentive salience ('wanting'), hedonia ('liking'), or reward learning for the *specific reward function* mediated by dopamine. Instead, it proposes a major constraint on when dopamine can mediate reward. They suggest that dopamine systems mediate reward, but only under certain conditions: *only when individuals are in a state of physiological deprivation* (e.g., caloric hunger or drug withdrawal). They suggest that an entirely separate neural system mediates the incentive value of rewards when animals are in a nondeprived state. This latter system is hypothesized to depend especially on the tegmental pedunculopontine nucleus (TPP).

Thus, Bechara et al. [22,310] suggest that there are two separate systems of reward in the brain—a dopamine-related system that is operative in the deprived state and a TPP system that is operative in the non-deprived state. The 'two systems' are held to be mutually exclusive: they contribute similarly to behavior, but at different times. At any moment only one of these neural reward systems should be active, according to their model. Activation of the dopamine reward system (deprived state) itself inhibits the TPP system (nondeprived state), they argue, and the dopamine system is activated by conditions of deprivation (for reviews, see Nader and van der Kooy, 1997 [22] and Nader et al., 1998 [310]). If the '2 systems' hypothesis of Nader et al. is true, it means that dopamine can mediate incentive salience (or hedonia or reward learning) only when individuals are in some form of a deprivation state.

Their novel suggestion is based on a series of conditioned place-preference experiments, which showed that alpha-flupentixol, a dopamine receptor antagonist, diminishes the reward value of food when rats are hungry, but not when they are sated [17,310]. Similarly, flupentixol diminishes the reward value of morphine when rats are in withdrawal, but not when they are drug-naïve [17,18,311]. By contrast, lesions of the TPP disrupt the reward value of both food and morphine only if rats are tested while sated or while drug-naïve, respectively, but not if they are hungry or in drug withdrawal [21,22].

Nader et al. make a cogent case that motivational systems are influenced by physiological depletion states and certainly show that depletion states influence the ability of neuroleptic drugs to disrupt reward. Yet there are several reasons why one might hesitate to adopt their hypothesis that reward is mediated by dopamine systems if-and-only-if an individual is in a state of physiological deprivation.

One reason is that dopamine antagonists such as pimozide, haloperidol, raclopride or SCH-23390 have been reported in many studies to suppress the reward value of food and other incentives *even in the absence of physiological depletion* [56,420,429]. Nader et al. [309,310] have attributed such apparent reward suppression during nondeprived states to the *aversive* effects of neuroleptics, rather than to putative reward-blocking effects. They argue that in tests for reward suppression it is critical that the dopamine antagonist be given only *under conditions in which it has no aversive properties* (measured by whether it supports conditioned place aversion training by itself). They suggest that in those studies where dopamine antagonists were found to suppress reward in nondeprived animals this effect was due to either the aversive consequences of antagonist treatment, or motor incapacity [22,309,310].

It must be recognized, however, that the literature on reward suppression by dopamine antagonists contains an enormous variety of test procedures, many of which contained measures intended to separate reward and motor effects. Also, many different dopamine antagonists, of various degrees of specificity for dopamine receptor subtypes, have been used to suppress reward. One might expect at least some of these drugs or test procedures to escape the confound of aversion. For example, the atypical neuroleptic drug, olanzapine, has been reported to suppress cocaine reward and food reward even at doses too low to produce a conditioned place aversion [295]. Further, it has been suggested by Shippenberg et al. [419,420] that typically only D1 receptor antagonists induce place aversions, whereas selective D2 antagonists do not. Yet D2 receptors have often been implicated in blockade of reward [13,83,88,415,429,457,458,490]. Under some conditions, even dopamine D1 antagonists may fail to produce place aversions, and may instead *inhibit* them: Acquas et al. [1] reported that, rather than produce a conditioned place aversion itself, SCH 23390 actually *blocked* the conditioned place aversion normally produced by administration of naloxone or other drugs. It seems possible, therefore, that at least *some* 'reward suppression' studies of diverse dopamine antagonists, conducted in nondeprived animals, may actually reflect the reward suppression their authors claim to have found.

Whether that is true or not, there is an additional problem for the '2 motivational systems' hypothesis. Even flupentixol, the antagonist of choice for Bechara et al., has been reported to suppress reward in the absence of a deprivation state. Van der Kooy reported, in a study with Mackey [280], that flupenthixol blocked an amphetamine conditioned place preference in naive rats. [15] There are other similar examples of reward suppression by flupenthixol in non-deprived animals. For example, Agmo et al. [2] found that flupentixol blocked the formation of a conditioned place preference normally produced in nondeprived rats by the opportunity to drink sucrose. Further, Duvauchelle et al. [139] reported that micro-injections of flupenthixol into the nucleus accumbens prevented place-preferences produced by electrical stimulation of the ventral tegmental area. It is unclear whether it is even possible for there to be a 'deprivation state' for brain stimulation reward. Yet Ettenberg et al. [147] also found that bar pressing for brain stimulation was suppressed by intra-accumbens flupenthixol and Stellar and Corbett [447] reported similar results for lateral hypothalamic stimulation after microinjection of flupenthixol into the medial fore-

[15] It should be noted that van der Kooy et al. [475] regard the amphetamine-induced place preference in nondeprived rats, or electrical brain stimulation reward, to be anomalies due to the ability of these treatments to directly activate dopamine neurotransmission, and so to bypass controls regulating physiological depletion states (personal communication). They suggest that these rewards may always be dopamine dependent because they directly activate dopamine systems. Thus, it appears that the critical variable may be not so much 'physiological deprivation state', but the ability of different rewards to directly engage dopamine-relevant motivational systems. Recent results by Laviolette and van der Kooy further suggest that it may depend even on the *direction* in which dopamine activity is directly changed: they show that reward is produced by VTA microinjections of either a GABA-A agonist (likely to inhibit dopamine neurons) or an antagonist (likely to disinhibit), but that flupentixol blocked only the agonist reward effect, and not the antagonist reward effect [272]. It is difficult to know whether the directional dependence on dopamine of VTA GABA-mediated reward reflects a 'switch' between two separate motivational systems, as its authors suggest, or is instead further evidence that no clear boundary separates the putative dopamine-dependant reward system from the dopamine-independent one. At best, the gating effect of deprivation on whether flupenthixol will block reward seems to hold for some rewards (food and opiates; GABA agonist in VTA) but not others (amphetamine, lateral hypothalamic electrical stimulation, accumbens neuropeptide Y, GABA antagonist in VTA etc.). Further, as noted above, flupentixol may block nondeprived reward value even for stimuli that do not act directly on brain dopamine systems, such as the taste of food [2]. It becomes difficult to predict, therefore, when the '2 systems' dopamine-dependence rule will apply and when it won't.

brain bundle. Related logic applies to the demonstration by Josselyn and Beninger [242] that intra-accumbens flupenthixol blocked conditioned place preferences normally produced by intra-accumbens injection of neuropeptide Y. Once again it seems difficult to posit that a deprivation state is responsible for that reward phenomenon. Finally, in non-deprived rats the intra-raphe administration of 8-OH-DPAT enhances feeding and that effect is blocked by flupenthixol [163]. The ability of flupenthixol to block the incentive motivational effects of food, drugs and electrical brain stimulation, in the absence of any physiological deprivation state, poses a serious problem for the '2 motivational systems' hypothesis. It begins to dissolve the boundary between the two motivational systems, which were posited by the hypothesis to be mutually exclusive, by showing that the dopamine system may actually mediate reward in both deprived and nondeprived states. [16]

Finally, if dopamine systems mediate reward only in deprivation states, as the '2 systems' hypothesis posits, then they *should not be activated by reward in nondeprived states*—but they apparently can be. Food rewards (the taste of saccharin or of a palatable chocolate drink, sucrose pellet, or butter cookie) can elicit dopamine overflow in the accumbens even in nondeprived rats [282,290,345,347]. Drug rewards (morphine, ethanol, nicotine, amphetamine, cocaine; given systemically or centrally) elicit dopamine overflow in accumbens the *first time they are given* [105,118,275,354,516] (when the animals are drug-naïve, and so, by definition, not in a withdrawal or deprivation state), and despite their diverse cellular mechanisms of action (only amphetamine and cocaine act directly on dopamine neurons; opiates, nicotine, ethanol must activate dopamine neurons *indirectly*). Sex elicits mesolimbic dopamine overflow in nondeprived males: a male rat who has copulated on recent days or even several times during the past hour (hardly a deprivation, no matter how 'deprived' one regards the ordinary male state), still shows elevated dopamine overflow when allowed to copulate again [159]. Sexually-receptive female rats and hamsters similarly activate mesolimbic dopamine systems when allowed to copulate under the conditions they prefer [296,299]. Maternal reward (reunion with her pups) elicits mesolimbic dopamine overflow in a mother rat after just one night away from them [220]. The list of rewards that trigger dopamine activation in 'nondeprived' rats is likely to grow. An ever growing set of deprivation states must be posited by the '2-systems' hypothesis to account for these effects (some of which appear to triggered after only hours or minutes of 'deprivation'). Otherwise it must be granted that dopamine systems are involved in many rewards (including natural rewards whose access to dopamine neurons is indirect) even in nondeprived conditions.

Our own results do not directly address this hypothesis because our 6-OHDA rats were intubated daily with food and water in order to avoid debilitation. Thus, our rats were generally not in a seriously depleted state. Nader et al. might predict that dopamine-depleted rats would show deficits only when tested in a food deprived state. However, a recent study by Qian et al. [353] examined this issue indirectly. They compared the passive consumption of an orally-infused sweet solution by aphagic 6-OHDA rats in two conditions: on a day when the rats had been artificially fed vs. after a 16-h period of caloric deprivation. There was, however, no effect of caloric deprivation on the response to food [353].

Even if dopamine mediates reward in nondeprived states, contrary to the original '2 systems' hypothesis [17,19, 310,311], there are still several ways in which deprivation states might influence the neural mediation of motivation and reward. For example, to the degree that deprivation states are unpleasant, individuals might be motivated to reduce the aversive drive-like properties of deprivation, even if incentive or hedonic reward effects of food or drugs were missing. That might be why TPP lesions do not suppress morphine's rewarding effects if animals are in withdrawal. The withdrawal state may involve different neural systems than those implicated in reward [57], and therefore, it may be possible to relieve withdrawal and thus motivate behavior after TPP lesions that impair reward systems.

It is less clear why neuroleptic suppression of dopamine systems should disrupt reward to a greater extent during deprivation states than during nondeprived states [22,310]. But one possibility is that deprivation states might activate neural systems involved in incentive motivation, including dopamine systems, to a high degree (as the value of relevant incentives increases). That might allow the impact of neuroleptics to become more visible in behavior. When the initial motivation is high, scaling effects could multiply the absolute magnitude of a neuroleptic-induced deficit, compared to when the initial state is low. A different possibility is that deprivation states might alter dopamine systems in biochemical ways that increase their vulnerability to neuroleptic blockade. For example, food restriction and weight loss have been reported to reduce levels of extracellular dopamine in the nucleus accumbens, and increase the tissue concentrations of dopamine [351]. The implication of these effects of physiological depletion for dopamine receptor blockade and reward is unclear. However, it seems safe to say that any interaction between

[16] The boundary between 'dopamine-dependent' and 'dopamine-independent' systems may be further weakened by Stefurak and van der Kooy's report that TPP lesions block the reward value of saccharin even when rats are in a deprived state [440]. The 2 systems hypothesis posits that the dopamine system *suppresses* the TPP system, and that deprivation activates the dopamine system [22,310,475]. But it appears that the TPP system may participate in reward regardless of deprivation state, just as dopamine systems do. The systems may not be mutually exclusive after all.

dopamine systems and physiological deprivation states is likely to be complex, and will not easily be reduced to a single hypothesis.

When the effect of deprivation states on dopamine systems is better understood, it may turn out that the observations that prompted the '2-systems' hypothesis will be compatible with the incentive salience distinction between 'liking' and 'wanting'. The incentive salience model and the '2 systems' model have several features in common. Both posit multiple neural systems of reward, both posit that the neural systems have functions that can be separated in behavior via experiments that manipulate dopamine systems, and both posit a modulating role for physiological deprivation states. Despite their differences regarding reward mechanisms during ordinary nondeprived states, it may yet be possible to reconcile the incentive salience hypothesis with the otherwise elegant and extraordinary hypothesis of Bechara, Nader, and van der Kooy.

13. Caveats to the 'Incentive Salience' hypothesis

13.1. Beyond reward to aversion

We would be remiss to end a discussion of the role of dopamine in reward without mention of its role in *aversive* motivational states such as fear or pain. There can be no doubt that behavior needed to actively *avoid an unpleasant outcome* is impaired as strongly by dopamine suppression as behavior directed toward a positive reward (for review, see Salamone [380]). The question is how involvement in aversive motivation bears on the role of dopamine in reward. For some investigators the involvement of dopamine in aversive motivational states raises serious doubts about whether dopamine neurons contribute to reward at all. As Gray et al. [198] put it, for example, "the most important evidence against this hypothesis (that accumbens dopamine mediates positive reinforcement or pleasure)... is that unpleasant events such as footshock increase extracellular levels of dopamine" (p. 1148, [198]).

Dopamine contributes to aversive motivational states. A variety of additional evidence supports the notion that aversive events activate dopamine systems (see below for example).

- Not only footshock but also other types of unconditioned stressors (e.g., enforced immobilization) increase dopamine overflow in accumbens and other forebrain structures [110,134,136,247,252,354,365,526]. Craig Berridge et al. [29] report neuroanatomical evidence that stress modulates dopamine neurotransmission in the caudal portion of the shell of the nucleus accumbens, via local intermingling between dopamine terminals and the norepinephrine projections from locus coeruleus that are activated in stress.
- Fear-eliciting *conditioned* stimuli, which are themselves innocuous but which have been paired with shock, also increase dopamine overflow [110,197,372,524–526]. Similarly, dopamine may be even higher during instrumental escape responding than when the unconditioned aversive stimulus is presented alone, again implicating a special involvement in aversive learning of some sort [354].
- Administration of dopamine receptor antagonist drugs suppresses behavioral performance on active avoidance learning tasks in a variety of situations [25,54,380,383].

It is possible, however, for a neural system to participate in more than one behavioral function. That dopamine systems are activated by fear-evoking stimuli, and are important for avoidance learning, says little by itself about whether they also mediate a specific aspect of reward.

In fact it is possible that dopamine systems are involved in both reward and aversively motivated behavior, and it is even possible that dopamine systems play a similar role in each. We have suggested before that a process related to incentive salience attribution might also be involved in aversively motivated behavior [35,366]. How could a positive process such as 'wanting' be involved also in aversive situations? There are several ways.

One possibility is that aversive tasks, such as active avoidance, may have a hidden appetitive component (see Gray [195]). Individuals in a fearful situation may 'want' to escape to a safe place or to perform another response that gains safety [195]. The safe place or the avoidance response may take on positive incentive properties, because they achieve a relatively positive outcome. To the degree that behavior is motivated by a desire for the more positive outcome, incentive salience, or 'wanting' for safety, could work in precisely the same way it does for conventional rewards.

'Motivational salience': Potential link between incentive and aversive states? But even in a situation in which the motivation was *entirely aversive*, a process related to incentive salience might still be at work. If so, it would no longer be appropriate to call the process *incentive* salience, but it might still be appropriate to call it *motivational* salience—with many of the same perceptual, attention-grabbing, and response-instigating properties of incentive salience. The same dopamine-based motivational salience process might be interpreted by the brain as positive incentive salience in some situations, causing events to be 'wanted', but to be perceived as *frighteningly* salient under other conditions, imbuing the attributed stimuli with a menacing motivational/perceptual tone.

What could determine whether motivational salience creates a positive incentive or an aversive fear? One way this might be achieved would be for each type of salience to be mediated by different dopamine neurons. In other words, dopaminergic labeled lines for positive vs. negative motivational salience. Separate dopamine/accumbens/amygdala subsystems could conceivably mediate 'wanting' and 'fear' as distinct processes: 'incentive salience' vs. 'aversive salience'. Consistent with the idea that dopamine systems might be segregated by motivational valence is the report by Mirenowicz and Schultz [301] that ascending dopamine neurons which are activated by a conditioned stimulus for food reward, may *not* be activated by a conditioned stimulus for an aversive air puff. Thus, dopamine neurons may be segregated by motivational valence.

An alternative possibility is that positive and negative psychological functions might be combined together into a single 'generic' motivational salience, mediated by the same dopamine neurons. In that case, the positive 'wanting' vs. negative 'frightening' valence caused by their activation would need to be gated by other mechanisms. One option is that the direction of valence could arise from the *pattern or intensity* of activation *within* the dopamine system itself. For example, low to moderate levels of activation might cause attraction, but very high levels might become frightening (as in the phenomenon of amphetamine-induced psychosis, in which the reward aspects of the drug are replaced by paranoia or frightening hallucination). A different option would be for the co-activation of non-dopaminergic neural systems to determine whether a positive valence or a negative valence would be imparted to the motivational salience of the stimulus.

The notion that dopamine systems might mediate a shared 'motivational salience' process in fear and in incentive motivation implies that dopamine activation correlates with the 'motivational attention-grabbing' properties of a particular stimulus, combining motivational and perceptual features [34,196,198,366]. That is consistent with a study on conditioned fear and latent inhibition by Young et al. [526]. Latent inhibition refers to the diminished capacity of a conditioned stimulus that is already familiar to support new learning. It is induced by presenting the conditioned stimulus (without the affective unconditioned stimulus) on occasions prior to the conditioning trial. In a microdialysis study Young, Joseph, and Gray found that following establishment of latent inhibition in a fear conditioning paradigm there was a reduction in dopamine overflow in the nucleus accumbens in response to the conditioned stimulus. This makes sense if dopamine release mediates motivational salience—in this case, a frightening motivational salience—and if the motivational salience of the conditioned stimulus was reduced by latent inhibition. That interpretation is bolstered by reports that amphetamine administration at training disrupts latent inhibition [104,197,433], an effect that appears to involve the nucleus accumbens [196]. Amphetamine, in other words, effectively re-instates the ability of the conditioned stimulus to be attributed with fearful motivational salience despite its familiarity.

For positive incentive motivation, amphetamine delivered directly into the nucleus accumbens produces comparable effects, even though the affective valence is opposite: enhancement of the ability of a conditioned stimulus to support motivated behavior. For example, Everitt and Robbins, et al. have shown in several elegant experiments that amphetamine microinjections into the accumbens potentiate the ability of a conditioned reinforcer to support incentive-oriented behavior [67,68,75,76,152–155,349,362,363]. Amphetamine microinjections increase bar pressing for conditioned reinforcers, which have previously been paired with sucrose (for hungry rats) [68,154,349], or with water (for thirsty rats) [75,76], or with a sexually-receptive female (for sexually-experienced male rats) [152,153]. Robbins and Everitt et al. offer compelling demonstrations that amphetamine microinjections even reverse, at least partly, the deficits in conditioned reinforcement that are produced by basolateral amygdala lesions [152–155,362, 363]. Kelley and Delfs further showed that microinjections of amphetamine into the anterior dorsal and ventromedial neostriatum can produce similar effects [254].

It is striking that incentive behavior for *positive* conditioned reinforcers as well as conditioning of *negative* stimuli that evoke fearful responses should be modulated together and in the same way by manipulations of dopamine activity in the accumbens or striatum. This does not negate a role for dopamine in reward. It does highlight the possibility, however, that dopamine's psychological role in reward may have common elements with its role in aversive situations—possibly involving a similar psychological 'core process' as well as a similar neural substrate [35,198,298,366,380].

13.2. Beyond the dopamine synapse

The focus of this paper has been on the motivational role of dopamine projections from the midbrain to targets in the dorsal and ventral striatum. It would be misleading, however, to simply identify incentive salience with the *activation of mesolimbic dopamine neurons, or the release of dopamine in a striatal target.* Even to the extent that dopamine neurons are the critical substrate for incentive salience, it is possible that dopamine projections to different targets mediate the incentive properties of different rewards. For example, whereas projections from the ventral tegmentum to the nucleus accumbens are clearly crucial for amphetamine reward, Gong et al. [190] have recently suggested that dopamine projections to the ventral pallidum are more important for cocaine reward. Following a similar theme, it has been reported that food may activate different neurons in the ventral striatum than cocaine even in the same monkey [55], and that cocaine and heroin may also produce neuronal patterns of activation in the nucleus accumbens that differ from each other [80]. Thus, different rewards may activate different subpopulations of dopamine/accumbens neurons.

To complicate matters more, it has been suggested that a single dopamine neuron may form different types of chemical synapses, with different morphologies, which release different neurotransmitters [453]. For example, dopamine neurons form both symmetrical synapses that are tyrosine hydroxylase-positive and asymmetrical synapses that release glutamate [221,453]. Thus, dopamine-containing neurons that project to the nucleus accumbens and neostriatum may co-release dopamine and glutamate differently at spatially-distinct sites [453]. And even the question of whether the primary action of dopamine itself is excitatory or inhibitory on post-synaptic neurons remains the subject of controversy [191]. It remains unclear what implication these issues have for the psychological functions of dopamine neurons discussed in this paper, but the interactions will surely be complex.

Further, despite our emphasis on dopamine, we caution that dopamine neurons need not be the *sole substrate* or even *chief substrate* for attributions of incentive salience to neural representations of conditioned stimuli. Other neural systems, both presynaptic and postsynaptic to dopamine neurons, may eventually prove to be even more directly related to the attribution of incentive salience than are dopamine projection systems. For example, Carlezon and Wise have suggested that the critical effect of dopamine in reward is inhibition of medium spiny neurons in the nucleus accumbens, and this may be achieved in ways other than by increasing synaptic dopamine [79]. Kelley et al. [255,256] have suggested the rewarding effects of amphetamine in the nucleus accumbens depend upon NMDA glutamate receptors there. Sarter et al. [387,388] suggest that accumbens dopamine might mediate incentive salience attribution via a GABAergic link to the basal forebrain, by triggering acetylcholine release in the neocortex.

In short, it is too simple to conclude that dopamine neurons themselves mediate incentive salience. More accurately, one can assert that the attribution of incentive salience appears to coincide with the activation of dopamine neurons, and that *incentive salience is the reward component most directly altered by manipulations of dopamine systems* (e.g., by 6-OHDA lesions, dopamine antagonist drugs, lateral hypothalamic stimulation, etc.). These manipulations reveal dissociations between 'wanting' rewards and 'liking' them, but they do not directly reveal the full nature of the psychological process or of its neurobiological substrate.

A final caveat is that it remains possible that dopamine neurons might participate in an *auxiliary* way even in reward functions we've rejected, such as associative learning or even hedonic impact. Our demonstration that dopamine-depleted rats show normal hedonics and reward learning simply means that dopamine projections are not *necessary* for normal mediation of these functions. It does not exclude the possibility that dopamine neurons normally *participate* in the neural processing of those psychological functions, as part of a neurally redundant system (providing feedback, monitoring for conveyance to other systems, etc.). Dopamine systems might participate, but we stress that these psychological functions can continue without them.

14. General conclusion

It is generally accepted that normal motivation and reward require the integrity of mesolimbic/mesostriatal dopamine systems. Some have interpreted the apparent primacy of dopamine systems to mean that these neutrons are a 'common neural currency' for pleasant rewards, mediating the *hedonic impact or pleasure of reinforcers*. Others have instead posited dopamine systems to mediate *reward learning or prediction*. But our results and those reviewed above indicate that dopamine's role in reward is not to mediate hedonic impact, nor to mediate most forms of learning about the predictive relationships between reward-relevant stimuli and their hedonic consequences. Suppression of dopamine function by massive 6-OHDA lesions does not alter the ability of rats to make hedonic evaluations, as reflected in affective taste reactivity patterns, despite obliterating the incentive value of food, water, and other rewards. Nor do 6-OHDA lesions suppress the learning of new hedonic relationships between conditioned and unconditioned stimuli, or the translating of those new reward associations into the generation of appropriate conditioned affective reactions.

We have demonstrated a dissociation between aphagia and other motivational deficits produced by 6-OHDA lesions, on one hand, and the lack of anhedonia or learning deficits on the other. We suggest this may best be explained by the hypothesis that normal reward is a multiplex process, which comprises at least three psychological components: 1) hedonic activation, 2) associative learning of the relationship between neutral events and their hedonic consequences, and 3) subsequent attribution of incentive salience to those events or their representations. Dopamine projections are not needed for either the hedonic or the associative prediction components. Instead we suggest that loss of dopamine from the nucleus accumbens and neostriatum impairs only the final component of reward, namely, the attribution of incentive salience to motivational stimuli and their representations. Lacking incentive salience attribution, dopamine-depleted rats cannot use their hedonic and associative competence to transform the perception or representation of a reward into a target incentive that is attractive and 'wanted'. Dopamine-depleted rats still 'like' rewards, and still know the rewards they 'like'. They simply fail to 'want' rewards they 'like'.

15. Addendum 1: Taste reactivity patterns as a measure of 'liking'

We do not mean to suggest that the subjective experience of pleasure is measured by the taste reactivity test. Instead, it measures a behavioral *affective reaction* [35,109,144,273]. A subjective experience need not even accompany a behavioral affective response (and almost certainly does not in some cases; for example, in the case of affective reaction patterns emitted by decerebrate animals or anencephalic human infants [211,441]). But *hedonic* and *aversive* patterns of affective reactions may still reflect a brain's underlying core evaluation of 'liking' or 'disliking' for a taste even if an evaluation is not registered by neural mechanisms of conscious awareness (for discussion of relationship between subjective pleasure and affective reactions to taste, see [34,35]).

For present purposes, our concern is whether taste reactivity patterns indeed can be used to measure the affective hedonic impact ('liking') or aversive impact ('disliking') of a stimulus. Evidence for the affective nature of hedonic/aversive taste reactivity patterns comes chiefly from the many correlations that have been found between them and the subjective ratings of taste palatability given by humans to tastes that are liked or disliked [34,206]. Human subjective reports and rat affective reactions reflect similar 'likes' and 'dislikes', and changes in their 'liking' for tastes are caused by the same manipulations.

- The sensory pleasure of sweetness to humans is enhanced by hunger and suppressed by caloric satiety [70,71,270]. Similarly, hedonic reaction patterns of rats to sweet tastes are enhanced by hunger and are suppressed by caloric satiety [33,73,74,212].
- The palatability of salt for humans is selectively enhanced by physiological sodium deficiency (salt appetite) [15,397]. Similarly, hedonic reactions of rats to NaCl are selectively increased, and aversive reactions decreased, by sodium depletion [38,178,213].
- By associative aversion conditioning procedures, taste pleasure for humans can be abolished and replaced with subjective aversion by associative pairing of a palatable food with gastrointestinal illness [377]. Similarly, hedonic reactions of rats to sweetness are abolished and replaced by aversive behavioral reactions by pairings of taste with LiCl or certain other noxious agents [30,64,209,327,329].
- Conversely, associative pairing of a palatable food with a neutral stimulus transfers the food's capacity to elicit hedonic responses to that conditioned stimulus; equivalent transfer of aversion can be obtained by pairing the stimulus with a bitter taste [42,63,113]. Similar conditioned preferences and aversions may occur for humans after associative taste pairings [377].

15.1. Insufficiency of alternative interpretations of affective taste reactivity

A reader may be tempted to reject the claim that affective patterns of taste reactivity reflect hedonic or aversive core evaluations. Instead, one might argue, taste reactivity only measures something simpler, such as a brainstem reflex, a decision whether to ingest, a consummatory phase of a behavior sequence, or a motor concomitant of swallowing or rejection. Each of these conceptual categories does apply to some aspect of reactions elicited by taste stimuli, and taste reactivity measures legitimately have been used to study each [171,205,209,210,249, 251,437]. But measurement of *hedonic vs. aversive patterns* of taste reactivity, as used here, cannot be reduced to any of those simpler categories, either alone or in combination. Since our conclusion about the role of dopamine in reward depends upon this argument regarding taste reactivity, it seems worthwhile to make clear why alternative interpretations of hedonic/aversive taste reactivity patterns are inadequate. The remark of Section 15 reviews the inadequacy of alternative interpretations, and our basis for concluding that this measure does indeed reflect core affective processes of 'liking' and 'disliking'.

15.1.1. Not mere reflex

Does taste reactivity reflect a mere brainstem reflex, or a rigid response to a sensory stimulus? No. Although the basic motor components are generated by the brainstem [211], under ordinary conditions the forebrain controls the affective pattern of response [34,206]. Evidence that the forebrain controls affective reactions comes from demonstrations that neural manipulations restricted to the forebrain produce dramatic changes in affective patterns of taste reactivity. Hedonic reaction patterns are enhanced, for example, by microinjection of an opioid agonist into the forebrain ventricles or nucleus accumbens [336,338]. Conversely, aversive reactions are enhanced by ablation lesions of the ventral pallidum and rostral structures [211], or by electrolytic or excitotoxin lesions limited to the lateral hypothalamic and ventral pallidal areas [36, 106,393,446,455]. The ability of forebrain manipulations to alter hedonic/aversive response patterns shows that forebrain neural systems control the affective pattern of response to a taste. Evidence that affective reaction patterns are not rigid S–R reflexes to a stimulus comes from demonstrations that a particular taste stimulus can elicit *opposite* affective reaction patterns if associative or physiological conditions change. Associatively conditioned aversions switch the response to sweet sucrose from hedonic to aversive [209], and conditioned preferences switch the response to a bitter taste from aversive to hedonic [42,63,530]. Similarly, changes in physiological sodium balance can switch the reaction to concentrated NaCl from aversive to hedonic, and back again with physiological state [38,42,173,178].

An alternative 'sensory reflex' interpretation of taste reactivity, offered by Nader et al. [310], attempts to account for shifts in affective reactions within a fixed (S–R) reflex framework, by positing changes in the stimulus (S). Nader et al. [310] suggest that the "taste reactivity paradigm is a better measure of the food's subjective sensory, as opposed to hedonic, properties" (p.100, [310]).

They posit taste reactivity patterns to reflect the 'discriminative properties of stimuli', or 'simply subjective sensory events' (p.101, [310]), rather than hedonic or motivational properties of the stimulus. Additionally, they suggest that conditioned *changes* in taste reactivity, such as aversion learning, are essentially a kind of conditioned *sensory illusion*. For example, an 'aversive' saccharin CS, which has been previously paired with illness, is recognized when "the first few licks will produce the normal representation of the saccharin taste" (p. 101, [310]). But its memory "will elicit conditioned aversive effects that will decrease consumption, as well as other conditioned responses such as the oro-facial behaviors that taste reactivity measures" (p. 101–102, [310]). In other words, the sweet conditioned stimulus elicits a bitter or otherwise unpleasant sensory illusion. A *conditioned hedonic enhancement* could be explained by this 'sensory reflex' interpretation as a sensory illusion of sweetness, triggered by the conditioned stimulus. Conditioned illusions cannot be invoked to explain *direct changes* in taste reactivity patterns produced either by *physiological state* (e.g., hedonic enhancement by hunger or sodium appetite) or by *pharmacological or neural manipulations* (e.g., hedonic enhancement by intracranial morphine or benzodiazepines). But presumably Nader et al. might argue that these manipulations *directly alter the 'discriminative sensory properties' of a taste*, so that the *sensation of sweetness* is enhanced by hunger, salt appetite, morphine, etc.

There are several implausibilities concerning this 'sensory reflex' interpretation as a sufficient explanation of hedonic and aversive taste reactivity patterns. First, for associative changes in affective reaction patterns, the posited sequence of 'normal representation' followed by a conditioned sensory illusion does not seem to fit the observations. Rats respond *immediately* with conditioned aversive reactions to even an isolated 50 μl squirt of the conditioned taste (about the amount ingested in a single ordinary lick) [30,209] and do not appear to require several 'normal representation' licks to recognize it [217]. More to the point, humans who have developed a conditioned taste aversion for a sweet food or drink do not report that the food subsequently has a bitter taste or otherwise changed *sensation*. Instead, the food tastes as sweet as it did before —but now they perceive it as unpleasant [376,377]. Second, regarding hunger, humans report enhanced hedonic ratings but no increase in sweetness intensity during hunger [71,270]. Unless rats experience a sensory shift during hunger or aversion learning that humans lack, these states seems more likely to alter hedonic, rather than sensory, properties of food perception. By contrast, physiological sodium depletion may indeed alter the sensory intensity coding of salty taste [91,389,418,454]. However, it is difficult for a 'sensory interpretation' to explain the dramatic shift of rats to *high* NaCl concentrations from aversive to hedonic reaction patterns on that basis (humans experience salt as *more* intense during sodium depletion [15], and a similar story is suggested for the rat in sodium depletion states by electrophysiological studies of taste sensory intensity coding in the gustatory nucleus of the solitary tract [454]), and even more difficult to explain on a 'sensory discriminative' basis why sodium deficiency also enhances hedonic reactions to a *sour or bitter taste that has been associatively paired* with salt [42]. Third, morphine and other pharmacological enhancement of hedonic taste reactivity patterns appears to similarly reflect a specific 'liking' change, since evidence indicates that opioid manipulations do *not* change the sensory discriminative properties of taste. For example, naloxone does not alter human subjective ratings of sensory sweetness intensity or of other sensory qualities of food [132], nor does it alter the ability of rats to perform a sensory discrimination task that requires them to recognize the taste of sucrose [319]. Yet opioid agonists and antagonists do alter hedonic subjective ratings in humans [132,133,520,521], and they alter hedonic/aversive taste reactivity patterns and other measures of palatability in rats [86,87,131,332,336,360]. In conclusion, evidence fails to indicate that massive shifts in taste sensory discriminative properties are caused by appetite states or conditioned food preferences/aversions, of the type sufficient to explain changes in taste reactivity patterns. It seems reasonable to conclude that taste reactivity patterns therefore do *not* reflect the *sensory discriminative* properties of a taste stimulus. Instead, hedonic and aversive reaction patterns reflect the *affective* properties of that stimulus.

15.1.2. Not mere intake

Wise has suggested that "the taste reactivity paradigm simply measures the consummatory responses of ingestion or rejection and adds little to what we can infer from other consummatory measures as to the hedonic impact of rewarding stimuli" (p. 252, [504]). Hedonic reaction patterns have often been considered as 'ingestive' [171, 205,207,209,249,406]. But on closer scrutiny, to equate taste reactivity patterns with ingestion will not stand. Although intake measures and taste reactivity patterns often change together, they can be pulled completely apart from each other and therefore must measure different processes [40]. For example, Galaverna et al. [178,412] found that the increased consumption of salt produced by physiological sodium depletion was abolished by lesions of the central nucleus of the amygdala, but this lesion had no effect on affective taste reactivity shifts. Rats failed to drink salt voluntarily from a spout after the lesion, even though they had been hormonally depleted of sodium [178]. Similarly, the rats failed to increase even their passive intake of salt solution when it was infused into their mouths [412]. Yet the same rats showed a normal increase in hedonic taste reactivity patterns to salt infusions, and reduced their aversive taste reactivity patterns [178]. In other words, after a central amygdala lesion, the rats still 'like' salt when sodium deprived, but do not seem to 'want' it. [17]

The dissociation by Galaverna et al. shows that taste reactivity patterns are separable from measures of ingestion or intake. A similar dissociation between intake and affective reaction patterns occurs naturally (even without brain damage) in the case of natural satiation at the end of a meal. After eating a certain amount, a rat refuses to ingest any more food. Its refusal is reflected both in voluntary intake tests and in passive swallowing intra-oral intake tests. However, the rejection of food caused by caloric satiation, although accompanied by reduced hedonic reactions, is *not accompanied by increased aversive reaction patterns*, even after 'super-satiation' (after the rat swallows up to 10% of its body-weight of a palatable and calorie-rich solution) [33]. Finally, in the present study, a further dissociation between affective taste reactivity patterns and intake was found: dopamine depletion reduces voluntary intake of all food and water to zero. But taste reactivity patterns remain positive to sweet tastes, negative to bitter tastes, and can be further modulated in a normal fashion by aversion learning or benzodiazepine administration. This dissociation between voluntary intake measures and taste reactivity is generally true for all neural manipulations that produce aphagia without producing aversive taste reactivity patterns [211,393].

15.1.3. Not mere consummatory behavior

Concepts of ingestion (consumption) and consummatory behavior (applied to feeding) are often combined, as in the quote from Wise above. Conceptually, however, they are not necessarily identical. 'Consummatory behavior' originally was a term introduced by the early ethologist, Craig [102], to describe the terminal phase of motivated behavior, and distinguish it from preceding phases. Is 'consummatory behavior' an adequate label to apply to taste reactivity patterns—even if consumption is not? Dopamine suppression has been suggested to disrupt appetitive but not consummatory behavior by a number of investigators [50,51,108,152,157,205,239,325,343–345]. Taste reactivity patterns have been called 'consummatory' by a number of authors (including one of us) [30,205,412]. However, there are serious difficulties with the notion that 'taste reactivity is just consummatory behavior'.

In Craig's original sense, the terms 'appetitive' and 'consummatory' refer to *temporal* phases of motivated behavior: *appetitive* behavior occurs *prior* to capture of the goal object, whereas *consummatory* behavior occurs *after* it [102]. Taken merely as a temporal label, consummatory can be applied legitimately to taste reactivity patterns, since the reactions occur after food is obtained. But as an explanatory category of brain-behavior relations (in the sense that 'consummatory behavior is mediated by neural system X'), 'consummatory' is woefully inadequate. 'Consummatory behavior' as a category includes too many different types of behavior to be changed coherently by a single brain manipulation.

Regarding eating, there are at least three types of consummatory behavior. First, consummatory ingestive behavior in Craig's original sense included the actual *licks and bites of voluntary eating* [102]. Second, the *hedonic / aversive taste reactivity patterns* studied here occur during the consummatory phase [30,205–207,210,248, 249,251,353]. Third, the act of swallowing a substance, as opposed to spitting or spilling it out of the mouth, is a form of consummatory behavior. In that sense, the consummatory label has often been used to refer to *intraoral intake*, that is, the amount passively swallowed of a solution infused into a rat's mouth via cannula by the experimenter [171,205,207,208,213,406,413]. In many cases, these various senses of 'consummatory' have been taken by their authors explicitly or implicitly to be interchangeable [30,204–207,214,249,251,406]. But it is now clear that these various types of 'consummatory behavior' are not interchangeable. They often dissociate in different directions and therefore cannot possibly be measures of the same underlying process. A few examples will suffice.

- The case of amygdala lesion-induced impairment of salt appetite discussed above provides one example of a dissociation among different 'consummatory' behaviors. Amygdala lesions disrupted the first and third senses of 'consummatory (voluntary licking of salt and intra-oral intake) but not the second sense (affective taste reactivity)' [178,412]. In the same way, caloric satiety produces rejection of food in the first sense (voluntary intake) and third sense (passive intra-oral intake) of consummatory behavior, as described above, but not in the second sense of aversive affective reaction patterns.
- Administration of bombesin and gastrin-releasing-peptide, two putative satiety peptides, has been found by Flynn and Robillard [165–170,172] to produce a similar dissociation among types of consummatory behavior. Bombesin microinjections into the 4th ventricle suppress the first sense of consummatory behavior (voluntary licking for sucrose or salt solutions) and also suppress the third sense (passive intra-oral intake [even in decerebrate rats]). However, bombesin fails to shift the second sense of consummatory behavior (hedonic or aversive taste reactivity patterns) [167,169]. Flynn concludes that these satiety peptides "inhibit intake without affecting the gustatory

[17] Electrolytic lesions of the central amygdala were used by Galaverna et al. [178,412], which destroyed both amygdala neurons and fibers of passage. Dunn and Everitt [137] have shown that taste aversion learning deficits after electrolytic amygdala lesions, once ascribed to amygdala loss, are actually due to loss of cortical fibers of passage (because they are not caused by excitotoxin amygdala lesions). It is presently unclear whether cortex or amygdala damage causes the salt appetite deficit reported by Galaverna et al. But the point remains valid that this deficit illustrates the independence of taste reactivity patterns from measures of intake or consumption, regardless of whether the dissociation is caused by destruction of amygdala neurons or of cortical fibers.

reinforcing properties of the food'' (p. 113, [169]), an interpretation similar to the 'liking' vs. 'wanting' framework we have presented.

· Even intra-oral intake (the third sense of consummatory behavior) can be detached from voluntary intake (the first sense) and from affective taste reactivity (the second sense). The intraventricular administration of neuropeptide Y is known to promote voluntary food intake, but it does not enhance the amount of a nutritive solution that rats swallow when they are fed directly by intra-oral infusion [414]. Neuropeptide Y also fails to produce strong shifts in hedonic/aversive patterns of taste reactivity to caloric solutions (R.J. Seeley, personal communication; Peciña and Berridge, personal observations).

· Disruption of dopamine neurotransmission can also dissociate the different types of consummatory behavior. After extensive 6-OHDA lesions rats fail to initiate voluntary licking or chewing even if food is placed immediately before them (loss of first sense of consummatory behavior) [471]. Dopamine antagonists can slow the rate and amount of voluntary eating for rats given food pellets [512] and suppress the duration and microstructure of bouts of voluntary licking for rats given sucrose solution [395,396,429] (effects that stand in contrast to the view that dopamine is important to appetitive but not consummatory behavior). All of these effects apply only to the voluntary chewing/licking sense of consummatory behavior (first sense), and not to the other two senses of affective reactions or passive swallowing. Dopamine antagonists do not shift consummatory behavior in the sense of hedonic/aversive patterns of taste reactivity [339,465] (although they do suppress the capacity to sustain a vigorous bout of consummatory behavior even in this sense if the eliciting stimulus is prolonged over several minutes) [339]. And consummatory behavior in the sense of intra-oral intake, or passive swallowing of an infused solution, is similarly resistant to dopamine antagonists. Tyrka and Smith [469] found that raclopride and SCH 23990, preferential D2 receptor antagonists, had no effect on the intra-oral sucrose intake of rat pups who had the solution infused directly into their mouths via an implanted cannulae. However, dopamine antagonists suppressed the free intake of sucrose if the rat pups were laid in the sucrose solution, and needed to lower their head and lap in order to ingest [468,469]. What was the difference between these two forms of consummatory behavior? Smith notes that in the free-intake test, ''pups do not make continuous contact'' with sucrose but instead ''must repeatedly initiate contact'' in order to ingest (p. 119, [429]). The need to actively re-engage an external source of sucrose, rather than respond passively to what is delivered to the mouth appears to make a crucial difference. In our view, active re-engagement with the external food requires the attribution of incentive salience to that food. The recurrence of 'wanting' is required to initiate each successive bout or lick, and is dopamine-dependent. In order to claim that consummatory behavior is not dopamine-dependent, one would have to posit that the individual fluctuates rapidly during a meal back and forth between appetitive and consummatory phases, as many times as there are bites in a meal. Although that revision is arguable, it destroys Wallace Craig's original concept of a linear progression from an appetitive to a consummatory phase of motivated behavior.

· Even the effect of dopamine manipulations on a single sense of consummatory behavior may vary, depending how it is measured. For example, Qian et al. [353] have found that the third sense of consummatory behavior (intra-oral intake) is unimpaired by 6-OHDA lesions, at least by one criterion. The aphagic rats still swallowed enough of thrice-daily infusions sufficient to maintain their body weight. However, by other criteria, the rats had a consummatory deficit even for this type of consummatory behavior. They failed to increase passive intake after food deprivation, and they generally failed to swallow as much as normal rats [353]. Such variable effects mean that it cannot be conclusively stated whether 6-OHDA rats have a consummatory behavior deficit, even in this single sense of the term. Further distinctions would need to be made in order to arrive at an answer. Clearly, consummatory behavior is not a sufficient explanatory category either to place taste reactivity in or to explain the effects of dopamine lesions. [18]

In summary, the term 'consummatory behavior' actually refers to a number of different types of behavior that follow contact with a goal. It is not a coherent single category in which to classify a response. The term can no longer be used, therefore, as an *explanation* or even as a sufficient *description* for the effects of any brain manipulation.

15.2. Conclusion: Affective reaction patterns reflect hedonic impact of 'liked' stimulus

We therefore conclude that taste reactivity patterns cannot be dismissed as an *intake* or *ingestion* measure, or as a *brainstem sensorimotor reflex*, or as a piece of homogeneous *consummatory behavior*. Although taste elicited responses partake of each of these categories, they are not reducible to any one, nor to any combination of them. These considerations can be coupled to the close relationship, summarized earlier, that rat taste reactivity patterns show to human measures of taste pleasantness or

[18] Further evidence for a role of dopamine systems in the intra-oral intake type of consummatory behavior comes from Kaplan and Södersten's [250] finding that the dopamine agonist apomorphine suppresses the consummatory intra-oral intake of an orally-infused sucrose solution by decerebrate rats. In that case, the relevant dopamine neurons must be intrinsic to the brainstem, since decerebration would eliminate the role of ascending projections to accumbens or neostriatum.

unpleasantness after many psychological and physiological manipulations. In conclusion, this compels the verdict that taste *reactivity patterns must be regarded as true affective reactions*, which connote core processes of *affective 'liking'* vs. 'disliking'.

16. Addendum 2: Measuring cognitive expectations of reward in animals (studies of incentive learning by Dickinson and Balleine)

A cognitive expectation of reward is not merely elicitation of an affective or motivational response by a conditioned stimulus. It must also, Dickinson et al. [125–127] suggest, be accompanied by the recognition by the animal that the to-be-obtained reward is *obtained by its own action*, and a *representation of the to-be-obtained reward* must be accessed to guide behavior to the goal. In other words, for an animal to have a cognitive expectation of a reward, it must *know what reward it is working for* (i.e., that it will gain a particular reward), and *understand that it is working for it* (i.e., that the reward will be the final outcome of its actions). A cognitive expectation of reward, according to Dickinson and Balleine [128] is what gives the representation of a stimulus *incentive value*. The representation of a stimulus has these properties if "instrumental behavior is mediated not only by a representation of the action-outcome relation, but also by a representation of the incentive value of the outcome, or what in common parlance would be referred to as the desire for the outcome" (p. 163, Dickinson and Balleine [128]). If dopamine systems mediated 'incentive value' in the sense of Dickinson and Balleine then dopamine must mediate learning the explicit relation between actions and specific outcomes.

It is important to stress that 'incentive learning' in Dickinson's sense implies much more than is meant by the other senses of 'expectation of reward'. It is more than a procedural associative representation of the correlation between two events. It is more than hedonic re-valuation of a conditioned stimulus based on its association with an unconditioned stimulus. It is more than the attribution of incentive salience to a stimulus that makes it motivationally attractive, or able to elicit approach. It differs from these in that it requires the expectation to be explicitly represented in a way that gives the animal prior access to features of the future reward and to the causal relations among events that predict the reward. Dickinson's use of the phrase 'incentive learning' is different from the way the term is used by other motivational theorists such as Bindra [48,49] or Toates [460–463], and is different from our use [34,366]. For Bindra or Toates, and for us, 'incentive learning' can be a simpler construct, referring merely to the process by which a Pavlovian conditioned stimulus acquires new hedonic or motivational value (i.e., it can be procedural rather than declarative, implicit rather than explicit).

In a typical experiment, Dickinson and Balleine and colleagues have assessed whether an animal has a cognitive representation of a reward by asking whether it can act appropriately when it is suddenly placed in a new motivational state. For example, if a rat had learned while hungry to perform two instrumental responses, one for sucrose solution and another for food pellets, it might be tested in a state of thirst or in a state of caloric satiety, or after one food had been associatively paired (in a different setting) with LiCl illness to induce a taste aversion. Two features of the 'new state' test are particularly important to the experiments of Dickinson and Balleine. First, the rat is tested in extinction, so that operant responses no longer earn the actual food rewards. The rat must therefore choose to work based solely on its *representation* of the rewards, since the foods themselves are not present. Second, Dickinson and Balleine take pains to arrange the experimental situation so that potential Pavlovian conditioned stimuli predict both foods equally well. This obviates control of behavior by Pavlovian-related motivational processes, which otherwise could guide behavior to one goal or the other (and which would be more related to *our* sense of incentive salience and to the Bindra/Toates sense of incentive learning).

Under these conditions, Dickinson and Balleine have shown that rats quite often fail to appropriately modify their instrumental behavior for the revalued food. If a rat had worked vigorously for a food when it was trained, it often continues to work hard in the test—even if the food would now have reduced hedonic value (e.g., because now the food would evoke a conditioned aversion). If a rat had not worked vigorously before, because the food did not have great value during training, it still does not work harder during the test, even though the food would now have enhanced hedonic value (e.g., because now the rat is hungrier). If the two foods now have different values, rats often seem not to recognize that difference, and work similarly for both (although see Rescorla [357] for instances in which the specific inference transfers successfully to behavior; these, however, may be at least partly accounted for by noncognitive factors [12,127]). In such cases, Dickinson's and Balleine's rats, at any rate, appear to behave based on the 'predicted reward value' of the food. That is, the rats behave as if the food's value is *equivalent to the value it last had when it was previously experienced.* The rat's 'expectation of reward' apparently is that the reward will be the same as before—even though it won't. In these situations a rat can be said to have a 'cognitive expectation of reward' in one sense, but it is an incorrect one. The rat has not yet fully learned about the new value of the food (its cognitive representation is not updated), and its behavior is not guided by an accurate representation of the food at that moment. In the strict Dickinsonian sense, therefore, its behavior does not reflect the incentive value of the reward: it lacks incentive learning.

There are two ways Dickinson et al. have found in which a rat can be provided with information sufficient to correct its mistake, allowing it to change its instrumental behavior appropriate to the new incentive value of the food or water.

The primary way is to let a rat experience the changed hedonic value of the reward while it is in the changed state. [19] This would ordinarily happen naturally if the test were not conducted under extinction conditions. If it was not tested in extinction the rat would simply sample both rewards, and quickly experience which was better in the new state, and modify its behavior accordingly. But the same outcome is obtained, Dickinson and Balleine show, by simply allowing a rat to taste the revalued reward elsewhere (while the rat is in the state to be tested later), and thus to experience its new hedonic value prior to the instrumental extinction test. Armed with that information, a rat will later employ the now-known value of the food in the cognitive representation it has of the food's value, and of the food's causal relationship to the two different actions. It then modifies its instrumental response in the extinction test appropriate to the re-valued food. Other instrumental responses, used to obtain another reward that was not re-valued, are not altered. For Dickinson, Balleine and colleagues this selective and intelligent change in behavior demonstrates true 'incentive learning'. It demonstrates that a rat knows what it is working for, and how to get it. Anything else falls short. Future studies of dopamine systems regarding the learning and prediction of reward stimuli will need to incorporate this distinction in order to parse among the multiple possible meanings of 'reward learning'.

[19] The second way is to provide during extinction testing a simple *Pavlovian conditioned stimulus* that had previously been paired with the re-valued food specifically. For example, Dickinson and Dawson [130] presented a conditioned stimulus for a sucrose solution to thirsty rats while they performed two responses in extinction. The two responses had previously delivered sucrose solution or food pellets when they had been hungry. Presentation of the conditioned stimulus for sucrose solution caused the rats to work harder on both responses: it energized their motivation. A conditioned stimulus for dry food pellets, by contrast, did not energize performance. This is especially relevant to the Bindra/Toates account of incentive motivation theory, by which the sucrose conditioned stimulus evoked the same hedonic and incentive processes that the watery sucrose solution would have evoked if it had been present. In a sense, it called to mind the properties of sucrose solution more vividly, and the rats responded to the conditioned stimulus as they would have to the sucrose itself. This kind of effect is both *associative* in a Pavlovian sense and *motivational*, in the sense that the stimulus has hedonic and incentive impact. It is essentially what is meant by 'incentive learning' in theories of motivation such as Bindra's [47–49] and Toates' [460,463]. It is also what we have meant by 'learned incentive salience' [44,45,366]. But the classically-conditioned motivational process is not *cognitive*, and Dickinson and Dawson [130] conclude that it does not convey information about the *differential relation between sucrose solution and the two responses*. For this reason, the energized rats could—in a sense—be said not to know what they were working for.

17. Note added in proof

An important review was published after this article went to press: W. Schultz, Predictive reward signals of dopamine neurons. J. Neurophysiol. 80 (1998) 1–27. In it, Schultz provides an excellent overview and adds substantial detail to the 'reward learning' hypothesis of dopamine function. However, the theory remains similar in its essential points to that outlined in earlier reviews by Schultz and colleagues, and so we stand by our comments regarding the 'dopamine reward learning' hypothesis.

Acknowledgements

Without implying acquiescence to the ideas presented here, we thank Drs. J. Wayne Aldridge, Steven Cooper, Howard (Casey) Cromwell, Anthony Dickinson, Susana Peciña, Per Södersten, Roland Suri, and Frederick Toates for helpful comments on earlier versions of this manuscript. We also thank Drs. Antoine Bechara, Karim Nader, and Derek van der Kooy for stimulating discussion of their reward hypothesis, and Gaetano Di Chiara for supplying an advance copy of a manuscript. Finally, we thank Dr. Diane Camp for assistance with the dopamine assay, and Darlene Tansil for assistance with the taste reactivity experiments.

References

[1] E. Acquas, E. Carboni, P. Leone, G. Dichiara, SCH 23390 blocks drug-conditioned place-preference and place- aversion—anhedonia (lack of reward) or apathy (lack of motivation) after dopamine-receptor blockade, Psychopharmacology 99 (1989) 151–155.

[2] A. Agmo, A. Galvan, B. Talamantes, Reward and reinforcement produced by drinking sucrose: two processes that may depend on different neurotransmitters, Pharmacol. Biochem. Behav. 52 (1995) 403–414.

[3] T. Aosaki, A.M. Graybiel, M. Kimura, Effect of the nigrostriatal dopamine system on acquired neural responses in the striatum of behaving monkeys, Science 265 (1994) 412–415.

[4] T. Aosaki, M. Kimura, A.M. Graybiel, Temporal and spatial characteristics of tonically active neurons of the primate's striatum, J. Neurophysiol. 73 (1995) 1234–1252.

[5] P. Apicella, T. Ljungberg, E. Scarnati, W. Schultz, Responses to reward in monkey dorsal and ventral striatum, Exp. Brain Res. 85 (1991) 491–500.

[6] J.M. Arnold, D.C. Roberts, A critique of fixed and progressive ratio schedules used to examine the neural substrates of drug reinforcement, Pharmacol. Biochem. Behav. 57 (1997) 441–447.

[7] C.S. Bailey, S. Hsiao, J.E. King, Hedonic reactivity to sucrose in rats: modification by pimozide, Physiol. Behav. 38 (1986) 447–452.

[8] B. Balleine, J. Ball, A. Dickinson, Benzodiazepine-induced outcome revaluation and the motivational control of instrumental action in rats, Behav. Neurosci. 108 (1994) 573–589.

[9] B. Balleine, A. Dickinson, Instrumental performance following reinforcer devaluation depends upon incentive learning, Q. J. Exp. Psychol. [B] 45B (1991) 285–301.

[10] B. Balleine, S. Killcross, Effects of ibotenic acid lesions of the nucleus accumbens on instrumental action, Behav. Brain Res. 65 (1994) 181–193.

[11] B.W. Balleine, A. Dickinson, The role of incentive learning in instrumental outcome revaluation by sensory-specific satiety, Anim. Learn and Behav. 26 (1998) 46–59.

[12] B.W. Balleine, A. Dickinson, Goal-directed instrumental action: contingency and incentive learning and their cortical substrates, Neuropharmacol. (in press).

[13] M.T. Bardo, Neuropharmacological mechanisms of drug reward: Beyond dopamine in the nucleus accumbens, Crit. Rev. Neurobiol. 12 (1998) 37–67.

[14] V. Bassareo, G. Di Chiara, Differential influence of associative and nonassociative learning mechanisms on the responsiveness of prefrontal and accumbal dopamine transmission to food stimuli in rats fed ad libitum, J. Neurosci. 17 (1997) 851–861.

[15] G.K. Beauchamp, M. Bertino, D. Burke, K. Engelman, Experimental sodium depletion and salt taste in normal human volunteers, Am. J. of Clinical Nutrition 51 (1990) 881–889.

[16] A. Bechara, H. Damasio, D. Tranel, A.R. Damasio, Deciding advantageously before knowing the advantageous strategy, Science 275 (1997) 1293–1295.

[17] A. Bechara, F. Harrington, K. Nader, D. van der Kooy, Neurobiology of motivation: double dissociation of two motivational mechanisms mediating opiate reward in drug-naive versus drug-dependent animals, Behav. Neurosci. 106 (1992) 798–807.

[18] A. Bechara, K. Nader, D. van der Kooy, Neurobiology of withdrawal motivation: evidence for two separate aversive effects produced in morphine-naive versus morphine-dependent rats by both naloxone and spontaneous withdrawal, Behav. Neurosci. 109 (1995) 91–105.

[19] A. Bechara, K. Nader, D. Van der Kooy, A two-separate-motivational-systems hypothesis of opioid addiction, Pharmacol. Biochem. Behav. 59 (1998) 1–17.

[20] A. Bechara, D. Tranel, H. Damasio, R. Adolphs, C. Rockland, A.R. Damasio, Double dissociation of conditioning and declarative knowledge relative to the amygdala and hippocampus in humans, Science 269 (1995) 1115–1118.

[21] A. Bechara, D. van der Kooy, The tegmental pedunculopontine nucleus: a brain-stem output of the limbic system critical for the conditioned place preferences produced by morphine and amphetamine, J. Neurosci. 9 (1989) 3400–3409.

[22] A. Bechara, D. van der Kooy, A single brain stem substrate mediates the motivational effects of both opiates and food in nondeprived rats but not in deprived rats, Behav. Neurosci. 106 (1992) 351–363.

[23] R.J. Beninger, The role of dopamine in locomotor activity and learning, Brain Res. 287 (1983) 173–196.

[24] R.J. Beninger, C.M. D'Amico, R. Ranaldi, Microinjections of flupenthixol into the caudate putamen of rats produce intrasession declines in food-rewarded operant responding, Pharmacol. Biochem. Behav. 45 (1993) 343–350.

[25] R.J. Beninger, S.T. Mason, A.G. Phillips, H.C. Fibiger, The use of conditioned suppression to evaluate the nature of neuroleptic-induced avoidance deficits, J. Pharmacol. Exp. Ther. 213 (1980) 623–627.

[26] R.J. Beninger, R. Miller, Dopamine D-1 like receptors and reward-related incentive learning, Neurosci. and Biobehav. Rev. 22 (1998) 335–345.

[27] J. Benjamin, L. Li, C. Patterson, B.D. Greenberg, D.L. Murphy, D.H. Hamer, Population and familial association between the D4 dopamine receptor gene and measures of novelty seeking, Nature Genet. 12 (1996) 81–84.

[28] S.P. Berger, S. Hall, J.D. Mickalian, M.S. Reid, C.A. Crawford, K. Delucchi, K. Carr, S. Hall, Haloperidol antagonism of cue-elicited cocaine craving, Lancet 347 (1996) 504–508.

[29] C.W. Berridge, T.L. Stratford, S.L. Foote, A.E. Kelley, Distribution of dopamine beta-hydroxylase-like immunoreactive fibers within the shell subregion of the nucleus accumbens, Synapse 27 (1997) 230–241.

[30] K. Berridge, H.J. Grill, R. Norgren, Relation of consummatory responses and preabsorptive insulin release to palatability and learned taste aversions, J. Comp. Physiol. Psychol. 95 (1981) 363–382.

[31] K.C. Berridge, Brainstem systems mediate the enhancement of palatability by chlordiazepoxide, Brain Res. 447 (1988) 262–268.

[32] K.C. Berridge, Substantia nigra 6-OHDA lesions mimic striatopallidal disruption of syntactic grooming chains: a neural systems analysis of sequence control, Psychobiology 17 (1989) 377–385.

[33] K.C. Berridge, Modulation of taste affect by hunger, caloric satiety, and sensory-specific satiety in the rat, Appetite 16 (1991) 103–120.

[34] K.C. Berridge, Food reward: brain substrates of wanting and liking, Neurosci. Biobehav. Rev. 20 (1996) 1–25.

[35] K.C. Berridge, Pleasure, pain, desire, and dread: Hidden core processes of emotion, in: D. Kahneman, E. Diener, N. Schwarz, (Eds.), Foundations of Hedonic Psychology: Scientific Understanding of Enjoyment and Suffering, Russell Sage Foundation, New York, in press.

[36] K.C. Berridge, H.C. Cromwell, Motivational-sensorimotor interaction controls aphagia and exaggerated treading after striatopallidal lesions, Behav. Neurosci. 104 (1990) 778–795.

[37] K.C. Berridge, J.C. Fentress, Trigeminal-taste interaction in palatability processing, Science 228 (1985) 747–750.

[38] K.C. Berridge, F.W. Flynn, J. Schulkin, H.J. Grill, Sodium depletion enhances salt palatability in rats, Behav. Neurosci. 98 (1984) 652–660.

[39] K.C. Berridge, H.J. Grill, Isohedonic tastes support a two-dimensional hypothesis of palatability, Appetite 5 (1984) 221–231.

[40] K.C. Berridge, S. Peciña, Benzodiazepines, appetite, and taste palatability, Neurosci. Biobehav. Rev. 19 (1995) 121–131.

[41] K.C. Berridge, T.E. Robinson, The mind of an addicted brain: sensitization of wanting versus liking, Cur. Dir. Psychol. Sci. 4 (1995) 71–76.

[42] K.C. Berridge, J. Schulkin, Palatability shift of a salt-associated incentive during sodium depletion, Q. J. Exp. Psychol. [B] 41 (1989) 121–138.

[43] K.C. Berridge, D. Treit, Chlordiazepoxide directly enhances positive ingestive reactions in rats, Pharmacol. Biochem. Behav. 24 (1986) 217–221.

[44] K.C. Berridge, E.S. Valenstein, What psychological process mediates feeding evoked by electrical stimulation of the lateral hypothalamus?, Behav. Neurosci. 105 (1991) 3–14.

[45] K.C. Berridge, I.L. Venier, T.E. Robinson, Taste reactivity analysis of 6-hydroxydopamine-induced aphagia: implications for arousal and anhedonia hypotheses of dopamine function, Behav. Neurosci. 103 (1989) 36–45.

[46] K.P. Bhatia, C.D. Marsden, The behavioural and motor consequences of focal lesions of the basal ganglia in man, Brain 117 (1994) 859–876.

[47] D. Bindra, A unified interpretation of emotion and motivation, Ann New York Acad. Sci. 159 (1969) 1071–1083.

[48] D. Bindra, A motivational view of learning, performance, and behavior modification, Psychol. Rev. 81 (1974) 199–213.

[49] D. Bindra, How adaptive behavior is produced: a perceptual-motivation alternative to response reinforcement, Behav. Brain Sci. 1 (1978) 41–91.

[50] J.R. Blackburn, J.G. Pfaus, A.G. Phillips, Dopamine functions in appetitive and defensive behaviours, Prog. Neurobiol. 39 (1992) 247–279.

[51] J.R. Blackburn, A.G. Phillips, H.C. Fibiger, Dopamine and preparatory behavior: I Effects of pimozide, Behav. Neurosci. 101 (1987) 352–360.

[52] J.R. Blackburn, A.G. Phillips, A. Jakubovic, H.C. Fibiger, Dopamine and preparatory behavior: II A neurochemical analysis, Behav. Neurosci. 103 (1989) 15–23.
[53] R.C. Bolles, Reinforcement, expectancy, and learning, Psychol. Rev. 79 (1972) 394–409.
[54] T.B. Borowski, L. Kokkinidis, Contribution of ventral tegmental area dopamine neurons to expression of conditional fear: effects of electrical stimulation, excitotoxin lesions, and quinpirole infusion on potentiated startle in rats, Behav. Neurosci. 110 (1996) 1349–1364.
[55] E.M. Bowman, T.G. Aigner, B.J. Richmond, Neural signals in the monkey ventral striatum related to motivation for juice and cocaine rewards, J. Neurophysiol. 75 (1996) 1061–1073.
[56] M.A. Bozarth, R.A. Wise, Heroin reward is dependent on a dopaminergic substrate, Life Sci. 29 (1981) 1881–1886.
[57] M.A. Bozarth, R.A. Wise, Anatomically distinct opiate receptor fields mediate reward and physical dependence, Science 224 (1984) 516–517.
[58] L.H. Brauer, H. de Wit, Subjective responses to D-amphetamine alone and after pimozide pretreatment in normal, healthy volunteers, Biol. Psychiatry 39 (1996) 26–32.
[59] L.H. Brauer, H. De Wit, High dose pimozide does not block amphetamine-induced euphoria in normal volunteers, Pharmacol. Biochem. Behav. 56 (1997) 265–272.
[60] L.H. Brauer, A.J. Goudie, H. de Wit, Dopamine ligands and the stimulus effects of amphetamine: animal models versus human laboratory data, Psychopharmacology 130 (1997) 2–13.
[61] T.S. Braver, J.D. Cohen, An integrated computational model of dopamine function in reinforcement learning and working memory, Journal of Cognitive Neuroscience (1998) 82-82.
[62] H.C. Breiter, R.L. Gollub, R.M. Weisskoff, D.N. Kennedy, N. Makris, J.D. Berke, J.M. Goodman, H.L. Kantor, D.R. Gastfriend, J.P. Riorden, R.T. Mathew, B.R. Rosen, S.E. Hyman, Acute effects of cocaine on human brain activity and emotion, Neuron 19 (1997) 591–611.
[63] P.A. Breslin, T.L. Davidson, H.J. Grill, Conditioned reversal of reactions to normally avoided tastes, Physiol. Behav. 47 (1990) 535–538.
[64] P.A. Breslin, A.C. Spector, H.J. Grill, A quantitative comparison of taste reactivity behaviors to sucrose before and after lithium chloride pairings: a unidimensional account of palatability, Behav. Neurosci. 106 (1992) 820–836.
[65] L. Brown, The New Shorter Oxford English Dictionary on Historical Principles, Clarendon Press: Oxford Univ. Press, Oxford and New York, 1993.
[66] V.J. Brown, P.J. Brasted, E.M. Bowman, The effect of systemic D-amphetamine on motor versus motivational processes in the rat, Psychopharmacology 128 (1996) 171–180.
[67] L.H. Burns, B.J. Everitt, A.E. Kelley, T.W. Robbins, Glutamate-dopamine interactions in the ventral striatum: role in locomotor activity and responding with conditioned reinforcement, Psychopharmacology 115 (1994) 516–528.
[68] L.H. Burns, T.W. Robbins, B.J. Everitt, Differential effects of excitotoxic lesions of the basolateral amygdala, ventral subiculum and medial prefrontal cortex on responding with conditioned reinforcement and locomotor activity potentiated by intra-accumbens infusions of D-amphetamine, Behav. Brain Res. 55 (1993) 167–183.
[69] M.J. Burton, S.J. Cooper, A. Posadas-Andrews, Interactions between chlordiazepoxide and food deprivation determining choice in food-preference test [proceedings], Br. J. Pharmacol. 68 (1980) 157P–158P.
[70] M. Cabanac, Physiological role of pleasure, Science 173 (1971) 1103–1107.
[71] M. Cabanac, Sensory pleasure, Q. Rev. Biol. 54 (1979) 1–29.
[72] M. Cabanac, On the origin of consciousness, a postulate and its corollary, Neurosci. and Biobehav. Rev. 20 (1996) 33–40.
[73] M. Cabanac, L. Lafrance, Postingestive alliesthesia: the rat tells the same story, Physiol. Behav. 47 (1990) 539–543.
[74] M. Cabanac, L. Lafrance, Facial consummatory responses in rats support the ponderostat hypothesis, Physiol. Behav. 50 (1991) 179–183.
[75] M. Cador, T.W. Robbins, B.J. Everitt, Involvement of the amygdala in stimulus-reward associations: interaction with the ventral striatum, Neuroscience 30 (1989) 77–86.
[76] M. Cador, T.W. Robbins, B.J. Everitt, H. Simon, M. Le Moal, L. Stinus, Limbic-striatal interactions in reward-related processes: Modulation by the dopaminergic system, in: P. Willner, J. Scheel-Kruger (Eds.), The Mesolimbic Dopamine System: From Motivation to Action, Wiley, New York, 1991, pp. 225–250.
[77] S.B. Caine, G.F. Koob, L.H. Parsons, B.J. Everitt, J.C. Schwartz, P. Sokoloff, D3 receptor test in vitro predicts decreased cocaine self-administration in rats, Neuroreport 8 (1997) 2373–2377.
[78] D.J. Calcagnetti, M.D. Schechter, Conditioned place aversion following the central administration of a novel dopamine release inhibitor CGS 10746B, Pharmacol. Biochem. Behav. 40 (1991) 255–259.
[79] W.A. Carlezon Jr., R.A. Wise, Rewarding actions of phencyclidine and related drugs in nucleus accumbens shell and frontal cortex, J. Neurosci. 16 (1996) 3112–3122.
[80] J.Y. Chang, P.H. Janak, D.J. Woodward, Comparison of mesocorticolimbic neuronal responses during cocaine and heroin self-administration in freely moving rats, J. Neurosci. 18 (1998) 3098–3115.
[81] J.Y. Chang, S.F. Sawyer, R.S. Lee, D.J. Woodward, Electrophysiological and pharmacological evidence for the role of the nucleus accumbens in cocaine self-administration in freely moving rats, J. Neurosci. 14 (1994) 1224–1244.
[82] A.L. Chausmer, A. Ettenberg, A role for D2, but not D1, dopamine receptors in the response-reinstating effects of food reinforcement, Pharmacol. Biochem. Behav. 57 (1997) 681–685.
[83] A.L. Chausmer, C.M. Reals, A. Ettenberg, Comparison of the effects of D1 and D2 dopamine receptor antagonist on the response-reinstating properties of food reinforcement, Soc. Neurosci. 21 (1995) 1674, Abstract.
[84] D. Clark, L.A. Chiodo, Electrophysiological and pharmacological characterization of identified nigrostriatal and mesoaccumbens dopamine neurons in the rat, Synapse 2 (1988) 474–485.
[85] R.E. Clark, L.R. Squire, Classical conditioning and brain systems: The role of awareness, Science 280 (1998) 77–81.
[86] S.N. Clarke, L.A. Parker, Morphine-induced modification of quinine palatability: effects of multiple morphine-quinine trials, Pharmacol. Biochem. Behav. 51 (1995) 505–508.
[87] J. Cleary, D.T. Weldon, E. Hare, C. Billington, A.S. Levine, Naloxone effects on sucrose-motivated behavior, Psychopharmacology 126 (1996) 110–114.
[88] P.G. Clifton, I.N. Rusk, S.J. Cooper, Effects of dopamine D1 and dopamine D2 antagonists on the free feeding and drinking patterns of rats, Behav. Neurosci. 105 (1995) 272–281.
[89] J.D. Cohen, D. Servan-Schreiber, A theory of dopamine function and its role in cognitive deficits in schizophrenia, Schizophrenia Bulletin 19 (1993) 85–104.
[90] K.L. Conover, P. Shizgal, Competition and summation between rewarding effects of sucrose and lateral hypothalamic stimulation in the rat, Behav. Neurosci. 108 (1994) 537–548.
[91] R.J. Contreras, M. Frank, Sodium deprivation alters neural responses to gustatory stimuli, J. General Physiology 73 (1979) 569–594.
[92] S.J. Cooper, Benzodiazepines as appetite-enhancing compounds, Appetite 1 (1980) 7–19.
[93] S.J. Cooper, L.B. Estall, Behavioural pharmacology of food, water and salt intake in relation to drug actions at benzodiazepine receptors, Neurosci. Biobehav. Rev. 9 (1985) 5–19.
[94] S.J. Cooper, J. Francis, D.J. Barber, Selective dopamine D-1

receptor agonists, SK and F 38393 and CY 208-243 reduce sucrose sham-feeding in the rat, Neuropharmacology 32 (1993) 101–102.
[95] S.J. Cooper, S. Higgs, The benzodiazepine agonist midazolam microinjected into the rat parabrachial nucleus produces hyperphagia, Soc. Neurosci. Abst. 20 (1994) 1285.
[96] S.J. Cooper, S. Higgs, Neuropharmacology of appetite and taste preferences, in: C.R. Legg, D.A. Booth, (Eds.), Appetite: Neural and Behavioural Bases, Oxford Univ. Press, New York, 1994, pp. 212–242.
[97] S.J. Cooper, S. Higgs, P.G. Clifton, Behavioral and neural mechanisms for benzodiazepine-induced hyperphagia, Appetite 24 (1995) 78–79.
[98] S.J. Cooper, A. Jackson, R. Morgan, R. Carter, Evidence for opiate receptor involvement in the consumption of a high palatability diet in nondeprived rats, Neuropeptides 5 (1985) 345–348.
[99] M.S. Cousins, A. Atherton, L. Turner, J.D. Salamone, Nucleus accumbens dopamine depletions alter relative response allocation in a T-maze cost/benefit task, Behav. Brain Res. 74 (1996) 189–197.
[100] M.S. Cousins, J.D. Salamone, Nucleus accumbens dopamine depletions in rats affect relative response allocation in a novel cost/benefit procedure, Pharmacol. Biochem. Behav. 49 (1994) 85–91.
[101] M.S. Cousins, W. Wei, J.D. Salamone, Pharmacological characterization of performance on a concurrent lever pressing/feeding choice procedure: effects of dopamine antagonist, cholinomimetic, sedative and stimulant drugs, Psychopharmacology 116 (1994) 529–537.
[102] W. Craig, Appetites and aversions as constituents of instincts, Biological Bulletin of Woods Hole 34 (1918) 91–107.
[103] L.P. Crespi, Quantitative variation of incentive and performance in the white rat, Am. J. Psychol. 55 (1942) 467–517.
[104] A. Crider, P.R. Solomon, M.A. McMahon, Disruption of selective attention in the rat following chronic D-amphetamine administration: relationship to schizophrenic attention disorder, Biol. Psychiatry. 17 (1982) 351–361.
[105] D. Crippens, T.E. Robinson, Withdrawal from morphine or amphetamine: Different effects on dopamine in the ventral–medial striatum studied with microdialysis, Brain Res. 650 (1994) 56–62.
[106] H.C. Cromwell, K.C. Berridge, Where does damage lead to enhanced food aversion: the ventral pallidum/substantia innominata or lateral hypothalamus?, Brain Res. 624 (1993) 1–10, [published erratum appears in Brain Res 1994 Apr 11;642(1-2):355].
[107] C.A. Dackis, M.S. Gold, New concepts in cocaine addiction: the dopamine depletion hypothesis, Neurosci. Biobehav. Rev. 9 (1985) 469–477.
[108] G. Damsma, J.G. Pfaus, D. Wenkstern, A.G. Phillips, H.C. Fibiger, Sexual behavior increases dopamine transmission in the nucleus accumbens and striatum of male rats: comparison with novelty and locomotion, Behav. Neurosci. 106 (1992) 181–191.
[109] C. Darwin, P. Ekman, The Expression of the Emotions in Man and Animals, Harper Collins—Oxford Univ. Press, Oxford, 1998 (originally published 1872).
[110] M. Davis, J.M. Hitchcock, M.B. Bowers, C.W. Berridge, K.R. Melia, R.H. Roth, Stress-induced activation of prefrontal cortex dopamine turnover: blockade by lesions of the amygdala, Brain Res. 664 (1994) 207–210.
[111] M. de Ryck, P. Teitelbaum, The postures of catecholamine-depletion catalepsy: their possible adaptive value in thermoregulation, Physiol. Behav. 21 (1978) 817–820.
[112] H. De Wit, R.A. Wise, Blockade of cocaine reinforcement in rats with the dopamine receptor blocker pimozide, but not with the noradrenergic blockers phentolamine or phenoxybenzamine, Can. J. Psychol. 31 (1977) 195–203.
[113] A.R. Delamater, V.M. LoLordo, K.C. Berridge, Control of fluid palatability by exteroceptive Pavlovian signals, J. Exp. Psychol. [Anim. Behav.] 12 (1986) 143–152.
[114] R.Y. Depoortere, D.H. Li, J.D. Lane, M.W. Emmett-Oglesby, Parameters of self-administration of cocaine in rats under a progressive-ratio schedule, Pharmacol. Biochem. Behav. 45 (1993) 539–548.
[115] R.A. Depue, Collins P.F., Neurobiology of the structure of personality: dopamine, facilitation, and extraversion, Behav. Brain Sci. (in press).
[116] G. Di Chiara, The role of dopamine in drug abuse viewed from the perspective of its role in motivation, Drug Alcohol Depend. 38 (1995) 95–137.
[117] G. Di Chiara, A motivational learning hypothesis of the role of mesolimbic dopamine in compulsive drug use, J. Psychopharmacol. 12 (1998) 54–67.
[118] G. Di Chiara, A. Imperato, Drugs abused by humans preferentially increase synaptic dopamine concentrations in the mesolimbic system of freely moving rats, Proc. Natl. Acad. Sci. U.S.A. 85 (1988) 5274–5278.
[119] G. Di Chiara, G. Tanda, Blunting of reactivity of dopamine transmission to palatable food: a biochemical marker of anhedonia in the CMS model?, Psychopharmacology 134 (1997) 351–353, discussion 371-377.
[120] P. Di Ciano, C.D. Blaha, A.G. Phillips, Conditioned changes in dopamine oxidation currents in the nucleus accumbens of rats by stimuli paired with self-administration or yoked-administration of d-amphetamine, Euro. J. Neurosci. 10 (1998) 1121–1127.
[121] P.M. Di Lorenzo, S. Monroe, Corticofugal input to taste-responsive units in the parabrachial pons, Brain Res. Bull. 29 (1992) 925–930.
[122] P.M. Di Lorenzo, S. Monroe, Corticofugal influence on taste responses in the nucleus of the solitary tract in the rat, J. Neurophysiol. 74 (1995) 258–272.
[123] A. Dickinson, Intentionality in animal conditioning, in: L. Weiskrantz (Ed.), Thought Without Language: A Fyssen Foundation Symposium., Clarendon Press/Oxford Univ. Press, Oxford, England, 1988, pp. 305–325.
[124] A. Dickinson, Expectancy theory in animal conditioning, in: R.R.M. Stephen, B. Klein (Eds.), Contemporary Learning Theories: Pavlovian Conditioning and the Status of Traditional Learning Theory., Lawrence Erlbaum Associates, Hillsdale, NJ, USA, 1989, pp. 279–308.
[125] A. Dickinson, Instrumental conditioning, in: N.J. Mackintosh (Ed.), Animal Learning and Cognition, Academic Press, New York, 1994, pp. 45–79.
[126] A. Dickinson, B. Balleine, Motivational control of instrumental performance following a shift from thirst to hunger, Q. J. Exp. Psychol. [B] 42 (1990) 413–431.
[127] A. Dickinson, B. Balleine, Motivational control of goal-directed action, Anim. Learn. and Behav. 22 (1994) 1–18.
[128] A. Dickinson, B. Balleine, Motivational control of instrumental action, Cur. Dir. Psychol. Sci. 4 (1995) 162–167.
[129] A. Dickinson, J. Campos, Z.I. Varga, B. Balleine, Bidirectional instrumental conditioning, Q. J. Exp. Psychol. [B] 49 (1996) 289–306.
[130] A. Dickinson, G.R. Dawson, Pavlovian processes in the motivational control of instrumental performance, Q. J. Exp. Psychol. [B] B (1987) 201–213.
[131] T.G. Doyle, K.C. Berridge, B.A. Gosnell, Morphine enhances hedonic taste palatability in rats, Pharmacol. Biochem. Behav. 46 (1993) 745–749.
[132] A. Drewnowski, D.D. Krahn, M.A. Demitrack, K. Nairn, B.A. Gosnell, Taste responses and preferences for sweet high-fat foods: evidence for opioid involvement, Physiol. Behav. 51 (1992) 371–379.
[133] A. Drewnowski, D.D. Krahn, M.A. Demitrack, K. Nairn, B.A. Gosnell, Naloxone, an opiate blocker, reduces the consumption of sweet high-fat foods in obese and lean female binge eaters, Am. J. Clin. Nutr. 61 (1995) 1206–1212.
[134] A.J. Dunn, Stress-related activation of cerebral dopaminergic systems, Ann. New York Acad. Sci. 537 (1988) 188–205.

[135] A.J. Dunn, J.E. Alpert, S.D. Iversen, Dopamine denervation of frontal cortex or nucleus accumbens does not affect ACTH-induced grooming behaviour, Behav. Brain Res. 12 (1984) 307–315.

[136] A.J. Dunn, C.W. Berridge, Physiological and behavioral-responses to corticotropin-releasing factor administration—Is CRF a mediator of anxiety or stress responses, Brain Res. Rev. 15 (1990) 71–100.

[137] L.T. Dunn, B.J. Everitt, Double dissociations of the effects of amygdala and insular cortex lesions on conditioned taste aversion, passive avoidance, and neophobia in the rat using the excitotoxin ibotenic acid, Behav. Neurosci. 102 (1988) 3–23.

[138] S.B. Dunnett, I.Q. Whishaw, G.H. Jones, S.T. Bunch, Behavioural, biochemical and histochemical effects of different neurotoxic amino acids injected into nucleus basalis magnocellularis of rats, Neuroscience 20 (1987) 653–669.

[139] C.L. Duvauchelle, M. Levitin, L.A. MacConell, L.K. Lee, A. Ettenberg, Opposite effects of prefrontal cortex and nucleus accumbens infusions of flupenthixol on stimulant-induced locomotion and brain stimulation reward, Brain Res. 576 (1992) 104–110.

[140] P. Ekman, An argument for basic emotions, Cognition and Emotion 6 (1992) 169–200.

[141] P.C. Ellsworth, Levels of thought and levels of emotion, in: P. Ekman, R.J. Davidson (Eds.), The Nature of Emotion: Fundamental Questions, Oxford Univ. Press, New York, 1994, pp. 192–196.

[142] Epictetus, E. Carter, All the works of Epictetus, which are now extant; consisting of his Discourses, preserved by Arrian, in four books, the Enchiridion, and fragments, J. and F. Rivington, London, 1768.

[143] Epictetus, T.W. Higginson, The works of Epictetus. Consisting of his Discourses, in four books, the Enchiridion, and Fragments, Little Brown, Boston, 1897.

[144] A.N. Epstein, Instinct and motivation as explanations for complex behavior, in: D.W. Pfaff (Ed.), The Physiology of Motivation, Springer-Verlag, New York, 1982, pp. 25–58.

[145] A. Ettenberg, Dopamine, neuroleptics and reinforced behavior, Neurosci. and Biobehav. Rev. 13 (1989) 105–111.

[146] A. Ettenberg, C.H. Camp, Haloperidol induces a partial reinforcement extinction effect in rats: implications for a dopamine involvement in food reward, Pharmacol. Biochem. Behav. 15 (1986) 813–821.

[147] A. Ettenberg, G.F. Koob, F.E. Bloom, Response artifact in the measurement of neuroleptic-induced anhedonia, Science 213 (1981) 357–359.

[148] A. Ettenberg, L.A. MacConell, T.D. Geist, Effects of haloperidol in a response-reinstatement model of heroin relapse, Psychopharmacology 124 (1996) 205–210.

[149] A. Ettenberg, H.O. Pettit, F.E. Bloom, G.F. Koob, Heroin and cocaine intravenous self-administration in rats: mediation by separate neural systems, Psychopharmacology 78 (1982) 204–209.

[150] K.R. Evans, F.J. Vaccarino, Intra-nucleus accumbens amphetamine: dose-dependent effects on food intake, Pharmacol. Biochem. Behav. 25 (1986) 1149–1151.

[151] K.R. Evans, F.J. Vaccarino, Amphetamine- and morphine-induced feeding: evidence for involvement of reward mechanisms, Neurosci. Biobehav. Rev. 14 (1990) 9–22.

[152] B.J. Everitt, Sexual motivation: a neural and behavioural analysis of the mechanisms underlying appetitive and copulatory responses of male rats, Neurosci. Biobehav. Rev. 14 (1990) 217–232.

[153] B.J. Everitt, M. Cador, T.W. Robbins, Interactions between the amygdala and ventral striatum in stimulus-reward associations: studies using a second-order schedule of sexual reinforcement, Neuroscience 30 (1989) 63–75.

[154] B.J. Everitt, K.A. Morris, O.B. A, T.W. Robbins, The basolateral amygdala-ventral striatal system and conditioned place preference: further evidence of limbic-striatal interactions underlying reward-related processes, Neuroscience 42 (1991) 1–18.

[155] B.J. Everitt, T.W. Robbins, Amygdala-ventral striatal interactions and reward-related processes, in: J.P. Aggleton (Ed.), The Amygdala: Neurobiological Aspects of Emotion, Memory, and Mental Dysfunction, Wiley, New York, 1992, pp. 401–429.

[156] M.B. Feigin, A. Sclafani, S.R. Sunday, Species differences in polysaccharide and sugar taste preferences, Neurosci. Biobehav. Rev. 11 (1987) 231–240.

[157] H.C. Fibiger, A.G. Phillips, Reward, motivation, cognition: Psychobiology of mesotelencephalic systems, Handbook of Physiology—The Nervous System, 4 (1986) 647–675.

[158] H.C. Fibiger, A.G. Phillips, E.E. Brown, The neurobiology of cocaine-induced reinforcement, Ciba Found. Symp. 166 (1992) 96–111, discussion 111-24.

[159] D.F. Fiorino, A. Coury, A.G. Phillips, Dynamic changes in nucleus accumbens dopamine efflux during the Coolidge effect in male rats, J. Neurosci. 17 (1997) 4849–4855.

[160] L.L. Firestone, F. Gyulai, M. Mintun, L.J. Adler, K. Urso, P.M. Winter, Human brain activity response to fentanyl imaged by positron emission tomography, Anesth. Analg. 82 (1996) 1247–1251.

[161] M.W. Fischman, Relationship between self-reported drug effects and their reinforcing effects: studies with stimulant drugs, NIDA Res. Monogr. 92 (1989) 211–230.

[162] C.F. Flaherty, Incentive Relativity, Cambridge Univ. Press, New York, 1996.

[163] P.J. Fletcher, Dopamine receptor blockade in nucleus accumbens or caudate nucleus differentially affects feeding induced by 8-OH-DPAT injected into dorsal or median raphe, Brain Res. 552 (1991) 181–189.

[164] S.J. Fluharty, H.J. Grill, Taste reactivity of lateral hypothalamic lesioned rats: effects of deprivation and tube feeding, Neurosci. Abstr. 7 (1981) 29.

[165] F.W. Flynn, Fourth ventricle bombesin injection suppresses ingestive behaviors in rats, Am. J. Physiol. 256 (1989) R590–R596.

[166] F.W. Flynn, Effects of fourth ventricle bombesin injection on meal-related parameters and grooming behavior, Peptides 12 (1991) 761–765.

[167] F.W. Flynn, Caudal brain stem systems mediate effects of bombesin-like peptides on intake in rats, Am. J. Physiol. 262 (1992) R37–R44.

[168] F.W. Flynn, Fourth ventricular injection of selective bombesin receptor antagonists facilitates feeding in rats, Am. J. Physiol. 264 (1993) R218–R221.

[169] F.W. Flynn, Applications of taste reactivity to the study of the neural-hormonal controls of ingestive behavior, Neurosci. Biobehav. Rev. 19 (1995) 109–120.

[170] F.W. Flynn, Mammalian bombesin-like peptides suppress sham drinking of salt by sodium-deficient rats, Peptides 17 (1996) 951–956.

[171] F.W. Flynn, H.J. Grill, Intraoral intake and taste reactivity responses elicited by sucrose and sodium chloride in chronic decerebrate rats, Behav. Neurosci. 102 (1988) 934–941.

[172] F.W. Flynn, L. Robillard, Inhibition of ingestive behavior following fourth ventricle bombesin injection in chronic decerebrate rats, Behav. Neurosci. 106 (1992) 1011–1014.

[173] F.W. Flynn, J. Schulkin, M. Havens, Sex differences in salt preference and taste reactivity in rats, Brain Res. Bull. 32 (1993) 91–95.

[174] G. Fouriezos, P. Hansson, R.A. Wise, Neuroleptic-induced attenuation of brain stimulation reward in rats, J. Comp. Physiol. Psychol. 92 (1978) 661–671.

[175] G. Fouriezos, R.A. Wise, Pimozide-induced extinction of intracranial self-stimulation: response patterns rule out motor or performance deficits, Brain Res. 103 (1976) 377–380.

[176] K.B.J. Franklin, S.N. McCoy, Pimozide-induced extinction in rats: stimulus control of responding rules out motor deficits, Pharmacol. Biochem. Behav. 11 (1979) 71–75.

[177] N.H. Frijda, A. Tcherkassof, Facial expressions as modes of action readiness, in: J.A. Russell, J.M. Fernández-Dols (Eds.), The Psy-

chology of Facial Expression, Cambridge Univ. Press, Cambridge, 1997, pp. 78–102.
[178] O.G. Galaverna, R.J. Seeley, K.C. Berridge, H.J. Grill, A.N. Epstein, J. Schulkin, Lesions of the central nucleus of the amygdala. I: Effects on taste reactivity, taste aversion learning and sodium appetite, Behav. Brain Res. 59 (1993) 11–17.
[179] C.R. Gallistel, M. Boytim, Y. Gomita, L. Klebanoff, Does pimozide block the reinforcing effect of brain stimulation?, Pharmacol. Biochem. Behav. 17 (1982) 769–781.
[180] E.L. Gardner, Brain reward mechanisms, in: J.H. Lowinson, P. Ruiz, R.B. Millman, J.G. Langrod (Eds.), Substance Abuse: A Comprehensive Textbook, Williams and Wilkin, Baltimore, 1997, pp. 51–85.
[181] E.L. Gardner, J.H. Lowinson, Drug craving and positive–negative hedonic brain substrates activated by addicting drugs, Sem. Neurosci. 5 (1993) 359–368.
[182] N. Geary, G.P. Smith, Pimozide decreases the positive reinforcing effect of sham fed sucrose in the rat, Pharmacol. Biochem. Behav. 22 (1985) 787–790.
[183] T.D. Geist, A. Ettenberg, Concurrent positive and negative goalbox events produce runway behaviors comparable to those of cocaine-reinforced rats, Pharmacol. Biochem. Behav. 57 (1997) 145–150.
[184] A.N. Gilbert, A.J. Fridlund, J. Sabini, Hedonic and social determinants of facial displays to odors., Chem. Senses 12 (1987) 355–363.
[185] D.B. Gilbert, S.J. Cooper, 7-OH-DPAT injected into the accumbens reduces locomotion and sucrose ingestion: D3 autoreceptor-mediated effects?, Pharmacol. Biochem. Behav. 52 (1995) 275–280.
[186] S.Q. Giraudo, M.K. Grace, C.C. Welch, C.J. Billington, A.S. Levine, Naloxone's anorectic effect is dependent upon the relative palatability of food, Pharmacol. Biochem. Behav. 46 (1993) 917–921.
[187] B.K. Giza, T.R. Scott, A. Sclafani, R.F. Antonucci, Polysaccharides as taste stimuli: their effect in the nucleus tractus solitarius of the rat, Brain Res. 555 (1991) 1–9.
[188] S.E. Glickman, B.B. Schiff, A biological theory of reinforcement, Psychol. Rev. 74 (1967) 81–109.
[189] W. Gong, D. Neill, J.B. Justice Jr., Conditioned place preference and locomotor activation produced by injection of psychostimulants into ventral pallidum, Brain Res. 707 (1996) 64–74.
[190] W. Gong, D. Neill, J.B. Justice Jr., 6-Hydroxydopamine lesion of ventral pallidum blocks acquisition of place preference conditioning to cocaine, Brain Res. 754 (1997) 103–112.
[191] F. Gonon, Prolonged and extrasynaptic excitatory action of dopamine mediated by D1 receptors in the rat striatum in vivo, J. Neurosci. 17 (1997) 5972–5978.
[192] A.A. Grace, Phasic versus tonic dopamine release and the modulation of dopamine system responsivity: a hypothesis for the etiology of schizophrenia, Neuroscience 41 (1991) 1–24.
[193] A.A. Grace, B.S. Bunney, The control of firing pattern in nigral dopamine neurons: burst firing, J. Neurosci. 4 (1984) .
[194] A. Gratton, R.A. Wise, Drug- and behavior-associated changes in dopamine-related electrochemical signals during intravenous cocaine self-administration in rats, J. Neurosci. 14 (1994) 4130–4146.
[195] J.A. Gray, Elements of a Two-Process Theory of Learning, Academic Press, New York, 1975.
[196] J.A. Gray, Dopamine release in the nucleus accumbens: the perspective from aberrations of consciousness in schizophrenia, Neuropsychologia 33 (1995) 1143–1153.
[197] J.A. Gray, P.M. Moran, G. Grigoryan, S.L. Peters, A.M. Young, M.H. Joseph, Latent inhibition: the nucleus accumbens connection revisited, Behav. Brain Res. 88 (1997) 27–34.
[198] J.A. Gray, A.M. Young, M.H. Joseph, Dopamine's role [letter], Science 278 (1997) 1548–1549.
[199] R.W. Gray, S.J. Cooper, Benzodiazepines and palatability: taste reactivity in normal ingestion, Physiol. Behav. 58 (1995) 853–859.
[200] A.M. Graybiel, Building action repertoires: memory and learning functions of the basal ganglia, Cur. Opin. Neurobiol. 5 (1995) 733–741.
[201] A.M. Graybiel, T. Aosaki, A.W. Flaherty, M. Kimura, The basal ganglia and adaptive motor control, Science 265 (1994) 1826–1831.
[202] A.M. Graybiel, E.C. Hirsch, Y. Agid, The nigrostriatal system in Parkinson's disease, Adv. Neurol. 53 (1990) 17–29.
[203] A.M. Graybiel, M. Kimura, Adaptive neural networks in the basal ganglia, in: J.C. Houk, J.L. Davis, D.G. Beiser (Eds.), Models of Information Processing in the Basal Ganglia, MIT, Cambridge, 1995, pp. 103–116.
[204] P.S. Grigson, J.M. Kaplan, M.F. Roitman, R. Norgren, H.J. Grill, Reward comparison in chronic decerebrate rats, Am. J. Physiol. 273 (1997) R479–R486.
[205] H.J. Grill, Production and regulation of ingestive consummatory behavior in the chronic decerebrate rat, Brain Res. Bull. 5 (1980) 79–87.
[206] H.J. Grill, K.C. Berridge, Taste reactivity as a measure of the neural control of palatability, in: J.M. Sprague, A.N. Epstein (Eds.), Progress in Psychobiology and Physiological Psychology, Vol. 11, Academic Press, Orlando, 1985, pp. 1–61.
[207] H.J. Grill, J.M. Kaplan, Caudal brainstem participates in the distributed neural control of feeding, in: E.M. Stricker (Ed.), Neurobiology of Food and Fluid Intake, Vol. 10, Plenum, New York, 1990, pp. 125–149.
[208] H.J. Grill, R.R. Miselis, Lack of ingestive compensation to osmotic stimuli in chronic decerebrate rats, Am. J. Physiol. 240 (1981) R81–R86.
[209] H.J. Grill, R. Norgren, Chronically decerebrate rats demonstrate satiation but not bait shyness, Science 201 (1978) 267–269.
[210] H.J. Grill, R. Norgren, The taste reactivity test: I. Mimetic responses to gustatory stimuli in neurologically normal rats, Brain Res. 143 (1978) 263–279.
[211] H.J. Grill, R. Norgren, The taste reactivity test: II. Mimetic responses to gustatory stimuli in chronic thalamic and chronic decerebrate rats, Brain Res. 143 (1978) 281–297.
[212] H.J. Grill, M.F. Roitman, J.M. Kaplan, A new taste reactivity analysis of the integration of taste and physiological state information, Am. J. Physiol. 271 (1996) R677–R687.
[213] H.J. Grill, J. Schulkin, F.W. Flynn, Sodium homeostasis in chronic decerebrate rats, Behav. Neurosci. 100 (1986) 536–543.
[214] H.J. Grill, A.C. Spector, G.J. Schwartz, J.M. Kaplan, F.W. Flynn, Evaluating taste effects on ingestive behavior, in: F.M. Toates, N.R. Rowland (Eds.), Feeding and Drinking, Vol. 1, Elsevier, Amsterdam, 1987, pp. 151–188.
[215] A. Hajnal, G.P. Mark, P.V. Rada, L. Lenard, B.G. Hoebel, Norepinephrine microinjections in the hypothalamic paraventricular nucleus increase extracellular dopamine and decrease acetylcholine in the nucleus accumbens: Relevance to feeding reinforcement, J. Neurochem. 68 (1997) 667–674.
[216] S. Hall, T. Schallert, Striatal dopamine and the interface between orienting and ingestive functions, Physiol. Behav. 44 (1988) 469–471.
[217] B.P. Halpern, D.N. Tapper, Taste stimuli: quality coding time, Science 171 (1971) 1256–1258.
[218] S.B. Hamann, L. Cahill, L.R. Squire, Emotional perception and memory in amnesia, Neuropsychology 11 (1997) 104–113.
[219] M. Haney, R.W. Foltin, M.W. Fischman, Effects of pergolide on intravenous cocaine self-administration in men and women, Psychopharmacology 137 (1998) 15–24.
[220] S. Hansen, A.H. Bergvall, S. Nyiredi, Interaction with pups enhances dopamine release in the ventral striatum of maternal rats—a microdialysis study, Pharmacol. Biochem. Behav. 45 (1993) 673–676.
[221] T. Hattori, Conceptual history of the nigrostriatal dopamine system, Neurosci. Res. 16 (1993) 239–262.
[222] T.G. Heffner, J.A. Hartman, L.S. Seider, A rapid method for the

regional dissection of the rat brain, Pharmacol. Biochem. Behav. 13 (1980) 453–456.

[223] L. Heimer, D.S. Zahm, L. Churchill, P.W. Kalivas, C. Wohltmann, Specificity in the projection patterns of accumbal core and shell in the rat, Neuroscience 41 (1991) 89–125.

[224] S.E. Hemby, C. Co, T.R. Koves, J.E. Smith, S.I. Dworkin, Differences in extracellular dopamine concentrations in the nucleus accumbens during response-dependent and response-independent cocaine administration in the rat, Psychopharmacology 133 (1997) 7–16.

[225] L. Hernandez, B.G. Hoebel, Food reward and cocaine increase extracellular dopamine in the nucleus accumbens as measured by microdialysis, Life Sci. 42 (1988) 1705–1712.

[226] S. Higgs, S.J. Cooper, Midazolam-induced rapid changes in licking behaviour: evidence for involvement of endogenous opioid peptides, Psychopharmacology 131 (1997) 278–286.

[227] K.G. Hill, S.W. Kiefer, Naltrexone treatment increases the aversiveness of alcohol for outbred rats, Alcohol Clin. Exp. Res. 21 (1997) 637–641.

[228] P.K. Hitchcott, C.M. Bonardi, G.D. Phillips, Enhanced stimulus-reward learning by intra-amygdala administration of a D3 dopamine receptor agonist, Psychopharmacology 133 (1997) 240–248.

[229] W. Hodos, Progressive ratio as a measure of reward strength, Science 134 (1961) 943–944.

[230] W.H. Hodos, E.S. Valenstein, An evaluation of response rate as a measure of rewarding intracranial stimulation, J. Comp. Physiol. Psychol. 55 (1962) 80–84.

[231] B.G. Hoebel, Brain-stimulation reward in relation to behavior, in: A. Waquier, E.T. Rolls (Eds.), Brain-Stimulation Reward, Elsevier, New York, 1976, pp. 335–372.

[232] B.G. Hoebel, Neuroscience and motivation: pathways and peptides that define motivational systems, in: R.C. Atkinson, R.J. Herrnstein, G. Lindzey, R.D. Luce (Ed.), Stevens' Handbook of Experimental Psychology, Vol. 1, Wiley, New York, 1988, pp. 547–626.

[233] B.G. Hoebel, G.P. Mark, H.L. West, Conditioned release of neurotransmitters as measured by microdialysis, Clin. Neuropharmacol. 15 (Suppl 1) (1992) 704A–705A, Pt A.

[234] J.C. Horvitz, A. Ettenberg, Haloperidol blocks the response-reinstating effects of food reward: a methodology for separating neuroleptic effects on reinforcement and motor processes, Pharmacol. Biochem. Behav. 31 (1988) .

[235] J.C. Horvitz, A. Ettenberg, Conditioned incentive properties of a food-paired conditioned stimulus remain intact during dopamine receptor blockade, Behav. Neurosci. 105 (1991) 536–541.

[236] S. Hsiao, G.P. Smith, Raclopride reduces sucrose preference in rats, Pharmacol. Biochem. Behav. 50 (1995) 121–125.

[237] C.L. Hull, Essentials of Behavior, Yale Univ. Press, New Haven, 1951.

[238] C.L. Hull, A. Amsel, M.E. Rashotte, Mechanisms of Adaptive Behavior: Clark L. Hull's Theoretical Papers, with Commentary, Columbia Univ. Press, New York, 1984.

[239] S. Ikemoto, J. Panksepp, Dissociations between appetitive and consummatory responses by pharmacological manipulations of reward-relevant brain regions, Behav. Neurosci. 110 (1996) 331–345.

[240] M.F. Jacquin, H.P. Zeigler, Trigeminal orosensation and ingestive behavior in the rat, Behav. Neurosci. 97 (1983) 62–97.

[241] W. James, What is an emotion, Mind 9 (1884) 188–205.

[242] S.A. Josselyn, R.J. Beninger, Neuropeptide Y: intraaccumbens injections produce a place preference that is blocked by *cis*-flupenthixol, Pharmacol. Biochem. Behav. 46 (1993) 543–552.

[243] D. Kahneman, Assessments of individual well-being: a bottom-up approach, in: D. Kahneman, E. Diener, N. Schwartz (Eds.), Foundations of Hedonic Psychology: Scientific Perspectives on Enjoyment and Suffering, Russel Sage Foundation, New York, in press.

[244] D. Kahneman, B.L. Fredrickson, C.A. Schreiber, D.A. Redelmeier, When more pain is preferred to less: adding a better end, Psychological Science 4 (1993) 401–405.

[245] D. Kahneman, P.P. Wakker, R. Sarin, Back to Bentham? Explorations of experienced utility, Q. J. Econ. 112 (1997) 375–405.

[246] P.W. Kalivas, Interactions between dopamine and excitatory amino acids in behavioral sensitization to psychostimulants, Drug and Alcohol Dependence 37 (1995) 95–100.

[247] P.W. Kalivas, P. Duffy, Selective activation of dopamine transmission in the shell of the nucleus accumbens by stress, Brain Res. 675 (1995) 325–328.

[248] J.M. Kaplan, I. Bednar, P. Södersten, Simultaneous display of sexual and ingestive behaviour by rats, J. Neuroendocrin. 4 (1993) 381–392.

[249] J.M. Kaplan, M.F. Roitman, H.J. Grill, Ingestive taste reactivity as licking behavior, Neurosci. Biobehav. Rev. 19 (1995) 89–98.

[250] J.M. Kaplan, P. Södersten, Apomorphine suppresses ingestive behaviour in chronic decerebrate rats, Neuroreport 5 (1994) 1839–1840.

[251] J.M. Kaplan, A.C. Spector, H.J. Grill, Ingestion rate as an independent variable in the behavioral analysis of satiation, Am. J. Physiol. 258 (1990) R662–R671.

[252] A. Katoh, T. Nabeshima, A. Kuno, M. Wada, R. Ukai, T. Kameyama, Changes in striatal dopamine release in stress-induced conditioned suppression of motility in rats, Behav. Brain Res. 77 (1996) 219–221.

[253] A.E. Kelley, E.P. Bless, C.J. Swanson, Investigation of the effects of opiate antagonists infused into the nucleus accumbens on feeding and sucrose drinking in rats, J. Pharmacol. Exp. Ther. 278 (1996) 1499–1507.

[254] A.E. Kelley, J.M. Delfs, Dopamine and conditioned reinforcement: I. Differential effects of amphetamine microinjections into striatal subregions, Psychopharmacology 103 (1991) 187–196.

[255] A.E. Kelley, S.L. Smith-Roe, M.R. Holahan, Response-reinforcement learning is dependent on *N*-methyl-D-aspartate receptor activation in the nucleus accumbens core, Proc. Natl. Acad. Sci. U.S.A. 94 (1997) 12174–12179.

[256] A.E. Kelley, L.C. Throne, NMDA receptors mediate the behavioral effects of amphetamine infused into the nucleus accumbens, Brain Res. Bull. 29 (1992) 247–254.

[257] T.H. Kelly, R.W. Foltin, L. King, M.W. Fischman, Behavioral response to diazepam in a residential laboratory, Biol. Psychiatry 31 (1992) 808–822.

[258] S.W. Kiefer, M.R. Orr, Taste avoidance, but not aversion, learning in rats lacking gustatory cortex, Behav. Neurosci. 106 (1992) 140–146.

[259] E.A. Kiyatkin, Functional significance of mesolimbic dopamine, Neurosci. Biobehav. Rev. 19 (1995) 573–598.

[260] E.A. Kiyatkin, A. Gratton, Electrochemical monitoring of extracellular dopamine in nucleus accumbens of rats lever-pressing for food, Brain Res. 652 (1994) 225–234.

[261] E.A. Kiyatkin, G.V. Rebec, Activity of presumed dopamine neurons in the ventral tegmental area during heroin self-administration, Neuroreport 8 (1997) 2581–2585.

[262] E.A. Kiyatkin, E.A. Stein, Conditioned changes in nucleus accumbens dopamine signal established by intravenous cocaine in rats, Neurosci. Lett. 211 (1996) 73–76.

[263] E.A. Kiyatkin, R.A. Wise, A. Gratton, Drug- and behavior-associated changes in dopamine-related electrochemical signals during intravenous heroin self-administration in rats, Synapse 14 (1993) 60–72.

[264] M.A. Klitenick, A.Y. Deutch, L. Churchill, P.W. Kalivas, Topography and functional role of dopaminergic projections from the ventral mesencephalic tegmentum to the ventral pallidum, Neuroscience 50 (1992) 371–386.

[265] M.J. Koepp, R.N. Gunn, A.D. Lawrence, V.J. Cunningham, A.

Dagher, T. Jones, D.J. Brooks, C.J. Bench, P.M. Grasby, Evidence for striatal dopamine release during a video game, Nature 393 (1998) 266–268.

[266] G.F. Koob, Neural mechanisms of drug reinforcement, Ann. New York Acad. Sci. 654 (1992) 171–191.

[267] G.F. Koob, S.B. Caine, L. Parsons, A. Markou, F. Weiss, Opponent process model and psychostimulant addiction, Pharmacol. Biochem. Behav. 57 (1997) 513–521.

[268] G.F. Koob, M. Le Moal, Drug abuse: hedonic homeostatic dysregulation, Science 278 (1997) 52–58.

[269] A.E. Kosobud, G.C. Harris, J.K. Chapin, Behavioral associations of neuronal activity in the ventral tegmental area of the rat, J. Neurosci. 14 (1994) 7117–7129.

[270] B. Laeng, K.C. Berridge, C.M. Butter, Pleasantness of a sweet taste during hunger and satiety: effects of gender and 'sweet tooth', Appetite 21 (1993) 247–254.

[271] R.J. Lamb, K.L. Preston, C.W. Schindler, R.A. Meisch, F. Davis, J.L. Katz, J.E. Henningfield, S.R. Goldberg, The reinforcing and subjective effects of morphine in post-addicts: a dose-response study, J. Pharmacol. Exp. Ther. 259 (1991) 1165–1173.

[272] S. Laviolette, D. van der Kooy, GABA-A receptor signalling in the ventral tegmental area dissociates separate dopamine-dependent and dopamine-independent motivational systems, Neurosci. Abstr, 24 (in press).

[273] J. LeDoux, The Emotional Brain: The Mysterious Underpinnings of Emotional Life, Simon and Schuster, New York, 1996.

[274] K. Leeb, L. Parker, R. Eikelboom, Effects of pimozide on the hedonic properties of sucrose: analysis by the taste reactivity test, Pharmacol. Biochem. Behav. 39 (1991) 895–901.

[275] P. Leone, D. Pocock, R.A. Wise, Morphine–dopamine interaction —ventral tegmental morphine increases nucleus-accumbens dopamine release, Pharmacol. Biochem. Behav. 39 (1991) 469–472.

[276] A.S. Levine, D.T. Weldon, M. Grace, J.P. Cleary, C.J. Billington, Naloxone blocks that portion of feeding driven by sweet taste in food-restricted rats, Am. J. Physiol. 268 (1995) R248–R252.

[277] T. Ljungberg, P. Apicella, W. Schultz, Responses of monkey midbrain dopamine neurons during delayed alternation performance, Brain Res. 567 (1991) 337–341.

[278] T. Ljungberg, P. Apicella, W. Schultz, Responses of monkey dopamine neurons during learning of behavioral reactions, J. Neurophysiol. 67 (1992) 145–163.

[279] Y. Lu, J.L. Peters, A.C. Michael, Direct comparison of the response of voltammetry and microdialysis to electrically evoked release of striatal dopamine, J. Neurochem. 70 (1998) 584–593.

[280] W.B. Mackey, D. van der Kooy, Neuroleptics block the positive reinforcing effects of amphetamine but not of morphine as measured by place conditioning, Pharmacol. Biochem. Behav. 22 (1985) 101–105.

[281] C.S. Maldonado-Irizarry, C.J. Swanson, A.E. Kelley, Glutamate receptors in the nucleus accumbens shell control feeding behavior via the lateral hypothalamus, J. Neurosci. 15 (1995) 6779–6788.

[282] G.P. Mark, D.S. Blander, B.G. Hoebel, A conditioned stimulus decreases extracellular dopamine in the nucleus accumbens after the development of a learned taste aversion, Brain Res. 551 (1991) 308–310.

[283] G.P. Mark, S.E. Smith, P.V. Rada, B.G. Hoebel, An appetitively conditioned taste elicits a preferential increase in mesolimbic dopamine release, Pharmacol. Biochem. Behav. 48 (1994) 651–660.

[284] A. Markou, G.F. Koob, Postcocaine anhedonia. An animal model of cocaine withdrawal, Neuropsychopharmacology 4 (1991) 17–26.

[285] C.D. Marsden, Which motor disorder in Parkinson's disease indicates the true motor function of the basal ganglia? in: D. Evered, M. O'Conner (Eds.), Functions of the Basal Ganglia, Pitman, London, 1984, pp. 225–237.

[286] C.D. Marsden, Dopamine and basal ganglia disorders in humans, Semin. Neurosci. 4 (1992) 171–178.

[287] J.F. Marshall, J.S. Richardson, P. Teitelbaum, Nigrostriatal bundle damage and the lateral hypothalamic syndrome, J. Comp. Physiol. Psychol. 87 (1974) 808–830.

[288] J.F. Marshall, B.H. Turner, P. Teitelbaum, Compulsive, abnormal walking caused by anticholinergics in akinetic, 6-hydroxydopamine-treated rats, Science 199 (1978) 1461–1463.

[289] P. Martel, M. Fantino, Influence of the amount of food ingested on mesolimbic dopaminergic system activity: a microdialysis study, Pharmacol. Biochem. Behav. 55 (1996) 297–302.

[290] P. Martel, M. Fantino, Mesolimbic dopaminergic system activity as a function of food reward: a microdialysis study, Pharmacol. Biochem. Behav. 53 (1996) 221–226.

[291] K. McFarland, A. Ettenberg, Haloperidol differentially affects reinforcement and motivational processes in rats running an alley for intravenous heroin, Psychopharmacology 122 (1995) 346–350.

[292] K. McFarland, A. Ettenberg, Reinstatement of drug-seeking behavior produced by heroin-predictive environmental stimuli, Psychopharmacology 131 (1997) 86–92.

[293] A. McGregor, G. Baker, D.C. Roberts, Effect of 6-hydroxydopamine lesions of the amygdala on intravenous cocaine self-administration under a progressive ratio schedule of reinforcement, Brain Res. 646 (1994) 273–278.

[294] A. McGregor, D.C. Roberts, Dopaminergic antagonism within the nucleus accumbens or the amygdala produces differential effects on intravenous cocaine self-administration under fixed and progressive ratio schedules of reinforcement, Brain Res. 624 (1993) 245–252.

[295] W.M. Meil, M.D. Schechter, Olanzapine attenuates the reinforcing effects of cocaine, Eur. J. Pharmacol. 340 (1997) 17–26.

[296] R.L. Meisel, D.M. Camp, T.E. Robinson, A microdialysis study of ventral striatal dopamine during sexual behavior in female Syrian hamsters, Behav. Brain Res. 55 (1993) 151–157.

[297] A. Mendrek, C.D. Blaha, A.G. Phillips, Pre-exposure of rats to amphetamine sensitizes self-administration of this drug under a progressive ratio schedule, Psychopharmacology 135 (1998) 416–422.

[298] Z. Merali, J. McIntosh, P. Kent, D. Michaud, H. Anisman, Aversive and appetitive events evoke the release of corticotropin-releasing hormone and bombesin-like peptides at the central nucleus of the amygdala, J. Neurosci. 18 (1998) 4758–4766.

[299] P.G. Mermelstein, J.B. Becker, Increased extracellular dopamine in the nucleus accumbens and striatum of the female rat during paced copulatory behavior, Behav. Neurosci. 109 (1995) 354–365.

[300] J. Mirenowicz, W. Schultz, Importance of unpredictability for reward responses in primate dopamine neurons, J. Neurophysiol. 72 (1994) 1024–1027.

[301] J. Mirenowicz, W. Schultz, Preferential activation of midbrain dopamine neurons by appetitive rather than aversive stimuli, Nature 379 (1996) 449–451.

[302] J.G. Modell, J.M. Mountz, F.B. Glaser, J.Y. Lee, Effect of haloperidol on measures of craving and impaired control in alcoholic subjects, Alcohol Clin. Exp. Res. 17 (1993) 234–240.

[303] G.J. Mogenson, C.R. Yang, The contribution of basal forebrain to limbic-motor integration and the mediation of motivation to action, Adv. Exp. Med. Biol. 295 (1991) 267–290.

[304] P.R. Montague, P. Dayan, T.J. Sejnowski, A framework for mesencephalic dopamine systems based on predictive Hebbian learning, J. Neurosci. 16 (1996) 1936–1947.

[305] F. Mora, G.J. Mogenson, E.T. Rolls, Activity of neurons in the region of the substantia nigra during feeding in the monkey, Brain Res. 133 (1977) 267–276.

[306] P.J. Morgane, Alterations in feeding and drinking behavior of rats with lesions of the globus pallidi, Am. J. Physiol. 201 (1961) 420–428.

[307] S.T. Murphy, R.B. Zajonc, Affect, cognition, and awareness: affective priming with optimal and suboptimal stimulus exposures, J. Pers. Soc. Psychol. 64 (1993) 723–739.

[308] E. Murzi, L. Hernandez, T. Baptista, Lateral hypothalamic sites eliciting eating affect medullary taste neurons in rats, Physiol. Behav. 36 (1986) 829–834.
[309] K. Nader, A. Bechara, D.C. Roberts, D. van der Kooy, Neuroleptics block high- but not low-dose heroin place preferences: further evidence for a two-system model of motivation, Behav. Neurosci. 108 (1994) 1128–1138.
[310] K. Nader, A. Bechara, D. van der Kooy, Neurobiological constraints on behavioral models of motivation, An. Rev. Psychol. 48 (1997) 85–114.
[311] K. Nader, D. van der Kooy, Deprivation state switches the neurobiological substrates mediating opiate reward in the ventral tegmental area, J. Neurosci. 17 (1997) 383–390.
[312] S. Nakajima, R.L. Patterson, The involvement of dopamine D2 receptors, but not D3 or D4 receptors, in the rewarding effect of brain stimulation in the rat, Brain Res. 760 (1997) 74–79.
[313] K. Nakamura, R. Norgren, Taste response of neurons in the nucleus of the solitary tract of awake rats: an extended stimulus array, J. Neurophysiol. 70 (1993) 879–891.
[314] M.J. Nash, Addicted: Why do people get hooked? Mounting evidence points to a powerful brain chemical called dopamine, Time, 1997, pp. 68–76.
[315] R.M. Nesse, K.C. Berridge, Psychoactive drug use in evolutionary perspective, Science 278 (1997) 63–66.
[316] R.W. Nisbett, T.D. Wilson, Telling more than we can know: verbal reports on mental processes, Psychol. Rev. 84 (1978) 231–259.
[317] R. Norgren, Gustatory system, in: G. Paxinos (Ed.) The Rat Nervous System, Academic Press, San Diego, 1995, pp. 751–771.
[318] R. Norgren, P.S. Grigson, The role of the central gustatory system in learned taste aversions, in: T. Onon, B.L. McNaughton, S. Molotchnikoff, E.T. Rolls, H. Nishijo (Eds.), Perception, Memory, and Emotion: Frontiers in Neuroscience. Eds., Pergamon, Oxford, UK, 1996, pp. 479–497.
[319] E. O'Hare, J. Cleary, P.J. Bartz, D.T. Weldon, C.J. Billington, A.S. Levine, Naloxone administration following operant training of sucrose/water discrimination in the rat, Psychopharmacology 129 (1997) 289–294.
[320] D.C. Ohuoha, J.A. Maxwell, L.E. Thomson 3rd, J.L. Cadet, R.B. Rothman, Effect of dopamine receptor antagonists on cocaine subjective effects: a naturalistic case study, J. Subst. Abuse Treat. 14 (1997) 249–258.
[321] P.G. Overton, D. Clark, Burst firing in midbrain dopaminergic neurons, Brain Res. Rev. 25 (1997) 312–334.
[322] J. Panksepp, The anatomy of emotions, in: R. Plutchik, H. Kellerman (Eds.), Emotion: Theory, Research, and Experience., Vol. 3: Biological Foundation of Emotions, Academic Press, New York, 1986, pp. 91–124.
[323] J. Panksepp, The neurochemistry of behavior, An. Rev. Psychol. 37 (1986) 77–107.
[324] J. Panksepp, Brain emotional circuits and psychopathologies, in: J.P. Manfred Clynes (Ed.), Emotions and Psychopathology., Plenum, New York, NY, US, 1988, pp. 37–76.
[325] J. Panksepp, Affective Neuroscience: the Foundations of Human and Animal Emotions, Oxford Univ. Press, Oxford, U.K., 1998.
[326] L. Parker, K. Leeb, Amphetamine-induced modification of quinine palatability: Analysis by the taste reactivity test, Pharmacol. Biochem. Behav. 47 (1994) 413–420.
[327] L.A. Parker, Behavioral conditioned responses across multiple conditioning/testing trials elicited by lithium- and amphetamine-paired flavors, Behav. Neural. Biol. 41 (1984) 190–199.
[328] L.A. Parker, Chlordiazepoxide enhances the palatability of lithium-, amphetamine-, and saline-paired saccharin solution, Pharmacol. Biochem. Behav. 50 (1995) 345–349.
[329] L.A. Parker, Rewarding drugs produce taste avoidance, but not taste aversion, Neurosci. Biobehav. Rev. 19 (1995) 143–151.
[330] L.A. Parker, T. Carvell, Orofacial and somatic responses elicited by lithium-, nicotine- and amphetamine-paired sucrose solution, Pharmacol. Biochem. Behav. 24 (1986) 883–887.
[331] L.A. Parker, N. Lopez Jr., Pimozide enhances the aversiveness of quinine solution, Pharmacol. Biochem. Behav. 36 (1990) 653–659.
[332] L.A. Parker, S. Maier, M. Rennie, J. Crebolder, Morphine- and naltrexone-induced modification of palatability: analysis by the taste reactivity test, Behav. Neurosci. 106 (1992) 999–1010.
[333] I.P. Pavlov, Conditioned reflexes; an Investigation of the Physiological Activity of the Cerebral Cortex, Oxford Univ. Press: Humphrey Milford, [London], 1927.
[334] S. Pecina, K. Berridge, Opioid feeding site objectively mapped within shell of nucleus accumbens, Neurosci. Abstr. 23 (1997) 529.
[335] S. Peciña, K.C. Berridge, Comparison of systemic and intracranial administration of morphine: effects on hedonic taste reactivity (in rats), Neurosci. Abstr. 19 (1993) 1820.
[336] S. Peciña, K.C. Berridge, Central enhancement of taste pleasure by intraventricular morphine, Neurobiology 3 (1995) 269–280.
[337] S. Peciña, K.C. Berridge, Brainstem mediates benzodiazepine enhancement of taste palatability: comparison of diazepam microinjections into fourth versus lateral ventricles, Brain Res. 727 (1996) 22–30.
[338] S. Peciña, K.C. Berridge, Morphine microinjections enhance feeding and palatability in the shell but not core of nucleus accumbens, Neurosci. Abstr. 22 (1996) 1408.
[339] S. Peciña, K.C. Berridge, L.A. Parker, Pimozide does not shift palatability: separation of anhedonia from sensorimotor effects, Pharmacol. Biochem. Behav. 58 (1997) 801–811.
[340] S.M. Pellis, V.C. Pellis, R.M. Chesire, N. Rowland, P. Teitelbaum, Somnolence, akinesia, and sensory activation of motivated behavior in the lateral hypothalamic syndrome, Proc. Natl. Acad. Sci. U.S.A. 72 (1975) 2819–2823.
[341] C.M. Pennartz, The ascending neuromodulatory systems in learning by reinforcement: comparing computational conjectures with experimental findings, Brain Res. Rev. 21 (1996) 219–245.
[342] J.L. Peters, A.C. Michael, Modeling voltammetry and microdialysis of striatal extracellular dopamine: The impact of dopamine uptake on extraction and recovery ratios, J. Neurochem. 70 (1998) 594–603.
[343] J.G. Pfaus, Homologies of animal and human sexual behaviors, Horm. Behav. 30 (1996) 187–200.
[344] J.G. Pfaus, G. Damsma, D. Wenkstern, H.C. Fibiger, Sexual activity increases dopamine transmission in the nucleus accumbens and striatum of female rats, Brain Res. 693 (1995) 21–30.
[345] A.G. Phillips, J.G. Pfaus, C.D Blaha, Dopamine and motivated behavior: insights provided by in vivo analyses, in: P. Willner, J. Scheel-Kruger, (Ed.), The Mesolimbic Dopamine System: From Motivation to Action, Wiley, Chichester, 1991, pp. 199–224.
[346] A.G. Phillips, L.J. Atkinson, J.R. Blackburn, C.D. Blaha, Increased extracellular dopamine in the nucleus accumbens of the rat elicited by a conditional stimulus for food: an electrochemical study, Can. J. Physiol. Pharmacol. 71 (1993) 387–393.
[347] A.G. Phillips, C.D. Blaha, J.G. Pfaus, J.R. Blackburn, Neurobiological correlates of positive emotional states: Dopamine, anticipation, and reward, in: K.T. Strongman (Ed.), International Review of Studies on Emotion, Vol. 2, Wiley, New York, 1992, pp. 31–50.
[348] A.G. Phillips, R.S. Nikaido, Disruption of brain stimulation-induced feeding by dopamine receptor blockade, Nature 258 (1975) 750–751.
[349] G.D. Phillips, T.W. Robbins, B.J. Everitt, Mesoaccumbens dopamine-opiate interactions in the control over behaviour by a conditioned reinforcer, Psychopharmacology 114 (1994) 345–359.
[350] R.C. Pierce, P.W. Kalivas, A circuitry model of the expression of behavioral sensitization to amphetamine-like psychostimulants, Brain Res. Rev. 25 (1997) 192–216.
[351] E.N. Pothos, I. Creese, B.G. Hoebel, Restricted eating with weight loss selectively decreases extracellular dopamine in the nucleus

accumbens and alters dopamine response to amphetamine, morphine, and food intake, J. Neurosci. 15 (1995) 6640–6650.

[352] M.T. Price, H.C. Fibiger, Discriminated escape learning and response to electric shock after 6-hydroxydopamine lesions of the nigro-neostriatal dopaminergic projection, Pharmacol. Biochem. Behav. 3 (1975) 285–290.

[353] M. Qian, A.E. Johnson, P. Södersten, CCK-8 inhibits ingestive behaviour in rats with lateral hypothalamic 6-OHDA lesions, Neuroreport (in press).

[354] P.V. Rada, P.M.G., G.H.B., Dopamine release in the nucleus accumbens by hypothalamic stimulation-escape behavior, Brain Res. 782 (1998) 228–234.

[355] R.A. Rescorla, Behavioral studies of Pavlovian conditioning, Ann. Rev. Neurosci. 11 (1988) 329–352.

[356] R.A. Rescorla, Pavlovian conditioning. It's not what you think it is, Am. Psychol. 43 (1988) 151–160.

[357] R.A. Rescorla, Control of instrumental performance by Pavlovian and instrumental stimuli, J. Exp. Psychol. Anim. Behav. Process 20 (1994) 44–50.

[358] R.A. Rescorla, R.L. Solomon, Two-process learning theory: Relationships between Pavlovian conditioning and instrumental learning, Psychol. Rev. 74 (1967) 151–182.

[359] N.R. Richardson, A. Gratton, Behavior-relevant changes in nucleus accumbens dopamine transmission elicited by food reinforcement: an electrochemical study in rat, J. Neurosci. 16 (1996) 8160–8169.

[360] H.J. Rideout, L.A. Parker, Morphine enhancement of sucrose palatability: analysis by the taste reactivity test, Pharmacol. Biochem. Behav. 53 (1996) 731–734.

[361] F.O. Risinger, S.D. Dickinson, C.L. Cunningham, Haloperidol reduces ethanol-induced motor activity stimulation but not conditioned place preference, Psychopharmacology 107 (1992) 453–456.

[362] T.W. Robbins, M. Cador, J.R. Taylor, B.J. Everitt, Limbic-striatal interactions in reward-related processes, Neurosci. Biobehav. Rev. 13 (1989) 155–162.

[363] T.W. Robbins, B.J. Everitt, Neurobehavioural mechanisms of reward and motivation, Curr. Opin. Neurobiol. 6 (1996) 228–236.

[364] D.C. Roberts, E.A. Loh, G. Vickers, Self-administration of cocaine on a progressive ratio schedule in rats: dose–response relationship and effect of haloperidol pretreatment, Psychopharmacology 97 (1989) 535–538.

[365] T.E. Robinson, A.L. Angus, J.B. Becker, Sensitization to stress: the enduring effects of prior stress on amphetamine-induced rotational behavior, Life Sci. 37 (1985) 1039–1042.

[366] T.E. Robinson, K.C. Berridge, The neural basis of drug craving: an incentive-sensitization theory of addiction, Brain Res. Rev. 18 (1993) 247–291.

[367] T.E. Robinson, K.C. Berridge, The psychology and neurobiology of addiction: an incentive sensitization view, Addiction, in press (1998).

[368] T.E. Robinson, D.M. Camp, The effects of 4 days of continuous striatal microdialysis on indexes of dopamine and serotonin neurotransmission in rats, J. Neurosci. Meth. 40 (1991) 211–222.

[369] B.A. Rocha, K. Scearce-Levie, J.J. Lucas, N. Hiroi, N. Castanon, J.C. Crabbe, E.J. Nestler, R. Hen, Increased vulnerability to cocaine in mice lacking the serotonin-1B receptor, Nature 393 (1998) 175–178.

[370] E.T. Rolls, The neurophysiology of feeding, Proc. Nutr. Soc. 40 (1981) 361–362.

[371] R. Romo, W. Schultz, Dopamine neurons of the monkey midbrain: contingencies of responses to active touch during self-initiated arm movements, J. Neurophysiol. 63 (1990) 592–606.

[372] J.B. Rosen, J. Schulkin, From normal fear to pathological anxiety, Psychol. Rev. 105 (1998) 325–350.

[373] Z.L. Rossetti, Y. Hmaidan, G.L. Gessa, Marked inhibition of mesolimbic dopamine release: a common feature of ethanol, morphine, cocaine and amphetamine abstinence in rats, Eur. J. Pharmacol. 221 (1992) 227–234.

[374] R.B. Rothman, J.R. Glowa, A review of the effects of dopaminergic agents on humans, animals, and drug-seeking behavior, and its implications for medication development—focus on GBR-12909, Molecular Neurobiology 11 (1995) 1–19.

[375] N. Rowland, D.M. Marques, A.E. Fisher, Comparison of the effects of brain dopamine-depleting lesions upon oral behaviors elicited by tail pinch and electrical brain stimulation, Physiol. Behav. 24 (1980) 273–281.

[376] P. Rozin, A. Fallon, The acquisition of likes and dislikes for foods., What is America Eating?: Proceedings of a Symposium. (National Research Council), National Academy Press, Washington, DC, US, 1986, pp. 58–71.

[377] P.N. Rozin, J. Schulkin, Food selection, in: E.M. Stricker (Ed.), Neurobiology of Food and Fluid Intake, Vol. 10, Plenum, New York, 1990, pp. 297–328.

[378] J.D. Salamone, Behavioral pharmacology of dopamine systems: a new synthesis, in: P. Willner, J. Scheel-Kruger (Eds.), The Mesolimbic dopamine system: from motivation to action, Wiley, New York, 1991, pp. 599–611.

[379] J.D. Salamone, Complex motor and sensorimotor functions of striatal and accumbens dopamine: involvement in instrumental behavior processes, Psychopharmacology 107 (1992) 160–174.

[380] J.D. Salamone, The involvement of nucleus accumbens dopamine in appetitive and aversive motivation, Behav. Brain Res. 61 (1994) 117–133.

[381] J.D. Salamone, The behavioral neurochemistry of motivation: methodological and conceptual issues in studies of the dynamic activity of nucleus accumbens dopamine, J. Neurosci. Meth. 64 (1996) 137–149.

[382] J.D. Salamone, M.S. Cousins, S. Bucher, Anhedonia or anergia? Effects of haloperidol and nucleus accumbens dopamine depletion on instrumental response selection in a T-maze cost/benefit procedure, Behav. Brain. Res. 65 (1994) 221–229.

[383] J.D. Salamone, M.S. Cousins, B.J. Snyder, Behavioral functions of nucleus accumbens dopamine: empirical and conceptual problems with the anhedonia hypothesis, Neurosci. Biobehav. Rev. 21 (1997) 341–359.

[384] J.D. Salamone, K. Mahan, S. Rogers, Ventrolateral striatal dopamine depletions impair feeding and food handling in rats, Pharmacol. Biochem. Behav. 44 (1993) 605–610.

[385] J.D. Salamone, R.E. Steinpreis, L.D. McCullough, P. Smith, D. Grebel, K. Mahan, Haloperidol and nucleus accumbens dopamine depletion suppress lever pressing for food but increase free food consumption in a novel food choice procedure, Psychopharmacology 104 (1991) 515–521.

[386] J.D. Salamone, M.J. Zigmond, E.M. Stricker, Characterization of the impaired feeding behavior in rats given haloperidol or dopamine-depleting brain lesions, Neuroscience 39 (1990) 17–24.

[387] M. Sarter, G.G. Berntson, J.T. Cacioppo, Brain imaging and cognitive neuroscience. Toward strong inference in attributing function to structure, Am. Psychol. 51 (1996) 13–21.

[388] M. Sarter, J.P. Bruno, Dopamine role [letter], Science 278 (1997) 1549–1550.

[389] G. Scalera, P.S. Grigson, R. Norgren, Gustatory functions, sodium appetite, and conditioned taste aversion survive excitotoxic lesions of the thalamic taste area, Behav. Neurosci. 111 (1997) 633–645.

[390] G.E. Schafe, R.J. Seeley, I.L. Bernstein, Forebrain contribution to the induction of a cellular correlate of conditioned taste aversion in the nucleus of the solitary tract, J. Neurosci. 15 (1995) 6789–6796.

[391] T. Schallert, S. Hall, 'Disengage' sensorimotor deficit following apparent recovery from unilateral dopamine depletion, Behav. Brain Res. 30 (1988) 15–24.

[392] T. Schallert, M. Upchurch, N. Lobaugh, S.B. Farrar, W.W. Spirduso, P. Gilliam, D. Vaughn, R.E. Wilcox, Tactile extinction: distinguishing between sensorimotor and motor asymmetries in rats with unilateral nigrostriatal damage, Pharmacol. Biochem. Behav. 16 (1982) 455–462.

[393] T. Schallert, I.Q. Whishaw, Two types of aphagia and two types of sensorimotor impairment after lateral hypothalamic lesions: observations in normal weight, dieted, and fattened rats, J. Comp. Physiol. Psychol. 92 (1978) 720–741.
[394] T. Schallert, I.Q. Whishaw, V.D. Ramirez, P. Teitelbaum, Neurotransmitters and the regulation of food intake, Prog. Brain Res. 42 (1975) 235–249.
[395] L.H. Schneider, J.D. Davis, C.A. Watson, G.P. Smith, Similar effect of raclopride and reduced sucrose concentration on the microstructure of sucrose sham feeding, Eur. J. Pharmacol. 186 (1990) 61–70.
[396] L.H. Schneider, C.A. Watson, J.D. Davis, J. Gibbs, G.P. Smith, Microstructural analysis of the inhibition of sucrose sham feeding by SCH 23390, Appetite 12 (1989) 122–124.
[397] J. Schulkin, Sodium Hunger: the Search for a Salty Taste, Cambridge Univ. Press, New York, 1991.
[398] W. Schultz, Responses of midbrain dopamine neurons to behavioral trigger stimuli in the monkey, J. Neurophysiol. 56 (1986) 1439–1461.
[399] W. Schultz, Activity of dopamine neurons in the behaving primate, Sem. Neurosci. 4 (1992) 129–138.
[400] W. Schultz, Dopamine neurons and their role in reward mechanisms, Cur. Opin. Neurobio. 7 (1997) 191–197.
[401] W. Schultz, P. Apicella, T. Ljungberg, Responses of monkey dopamine neurons to reward and conditioned stimuli during successive steps of learning a delayed response task, J. Neurosci. 13 (1993) 900–913.
[402] W. Schultz, P. Apicella, T. Ljungberg, R. Romo, Activity of monkey striatal and dopamine neurons during the performance of delayed response tasks, in: G. Percheron, J.S. McKenzie, J. Feger (Eds.), The Basal Ganglia IV, Plenum, New York, 1995, pp. 305–316.
[403] W. Schultz, P. Apicella, T. Ljungberg, R. Romo, E. Scarnati, Reward-related activity in the monkey striatum and substantia nigra, Prog. Brain Res. 99 (1993) 227–235.
[404] W. Schultz, P. Apicella, E. Scarnati, T. Ljungberg, Neuronal activity in monkey ventral striatum related to the expectation of reward, J. Neurosci. 12 (1992) 4595–4610.
[405] W. Schultz, P. Dayan, P.R. Montague, A neural substrate of prediction and reward, Science 275 (1997) 1593–1599.
[406] G.J. Schwartz, H.J. Grill, Relationships between taste reactivity and intake in the neurologically intact rat, Chem. Senses 9 (1984) 249–272.
[407] M. Schwartz, P. Teitelbaum, Nigrostriatal bundle damage and the lateral hypothalamic syndrome, J. Comp. Physiol. Psychol. 87 (1974) 808–830.
[408] A. Sclafani, L.T. Einberg, J.W. Nissenbaum, Influence of saccharin on Polycose, sucrose, and glucose intake and preference in rats, Neurosci. Biobehav. Rev. 11 (1987) 223–229.
[409] A. Sclafani, J.W. Nissenbaum, M. Vigorito, Starch preference in rats, Neurosci. Biobehav. Rev. 11 (1987) 253–262.
[410] T.R. Scott, The effect of physiological need on taste, in: E.D. Capaldi, T.L. Powley (Eds.), Taste, Experience, and Feeding, American Psychological Association, Washington, DC, 1990, pp. 45–61.
[411] T.R. Scott, S. Yaxley, Z.J. Sienkiewicz, E.T. Rolls, Gustatory responses in the nucleus tractus solitarius of the alert cynomolgus monkey, J. Neurophysiol. 55 (1986) 182–200.
[412] R.J. Seeley, O. Galaverna, J. Schulkin, A.N. Epstein, H.J. Grill, Lesions of the central nucleus of the amygdala: II. Effects on intraoral NaCl intake, Behav. Brain Res. 59 (1993) 19–25.
[413] R.J. Seeley, J.M. Kaplan, H.J. Grill, Effects of interrupting an intraoral meal on meal size and meal duration in rats, Appetite 20 (1993) 13–20.
[414] R.J. Seeley, C.J. Payne, S.C. Woods, Neuropeptide Y fails to increase intraoral intake in rats, Am. J. Physiol. 268 (1995) R423–R427.
[415] D.W. Self, W.J. Barnhart, D.A. Lehman, E.J. Nestler, Opposite modulation of cocaine-seeking behavior by D1- and D2-like dopamine receptor agonists, Science 271 (1996) 1289–1586.
[416] D. Servan-Schreiber, R.M. Bruno, C.S. Carter, J.D. Cohen, Dopamine and the mechanisms of cognition: Part I. A neural network model predicting dopamine effects on selective attention, Biological Psychiatry 43 (1998) 713–722.
[417] M. Shidara, T.G. Aigner, B.J.R., Neuronal signals in the monkey ventral striatum related to progress through a predictable series of trials, J. Neurosci. 16 (1998) 2613–2625.
[418] T. Shimura, M. Komori, T. Yamamoto, Acute sodium deficiency reduces gustatory responsiveness to NaCl in the parabrachial nucleus of rats, Neurosci. Lett. 236 (1997) 33–36.
[419] T.S. Shippenberg, R. Bals-Kubik, A. Huber, A. Herz, Neuroanatomical substrates mediating the aversive effects of D-1 dopamine receptor antagonists, Psychopharmacology 103 (1991) 209–214.
[420] T.S. Shippenberg, A. Herz, Motivational effects of opioids: influence of D-1 versus D-2 receptor antagonists, Eur. J. Pharmacol. 151 (1988) 233–242.
[421] P. Shizgal, Neural basis of utility estimation, Cur. Opin. Neurobio. 7 (1997) 198–208.
[422] P. Shizgal, On the neural computation of utility: implications from studies of brain stimulation reward, in: D. Kahneman, E. Deiner, N. Schwartz (Eds.), Foundations of Hedonic Psychology: Scientific Perspectives on Enjoyment and Suffering, Russel Sage Foundation, New York, in press.
[423] P. Shizgal, K. Conover, On the neural computation of utility, Cur. Dir. Psychol. Sci. 5 (1996) 37–43.
[424] T.L. Sills, J.P. Baird, F.J. Vaccarino, Individual differences in the feeding effects of amphetamine: role of nucleus accumbens dopamine and circadian factors, Psychopharmacology 112 (1993) 211–218.
[425] K.J. Simansky, K.A. Bourbonais, G.P. Smith, Food-related stimuli increase the ratio of 3,4-dihydroxyphenylacetic acid to dopamine in the hypothalamus, Pharmacol. Biochem. Behav. 23 (1985) 253–258.
[426] L.C. Simbayi, R.A. Boakes, M.J. Burton, Effects of basolateral amygdala lesions on taste aversions produced by lactose and lithium chloride in the rat, Behav. Neurosci. 100 (1986) 455–465.
[427] B.F. Skinner, The Behavior of Organisms: An Experimental Analysis, D. Appleton-Century Company incorporated, New York, London, 1938.
[428] B.F. Skinner, Cumulative Record: A Selection of Papers, 3rd edn., Appleton-Century-Crofts, New York, 1972.
[429] G.P. Smith, Dopamine and food reward, in: A.M. Morrison, S.J. Fluharty (Eds.), Progress in Psychobiology and Physiological Psychology, Vol. 15, Academic Press, New York, 1995, pp. 83–144.
[430] G.P. Smith, L.H. Schneider, Relationships between mesolimbic dopamine function and eating behavior, Ann. New York Acad. Sci. 537 (1988) 254–261.
[431] A.H.V. Söderpalm, S. Hansen, Benzodiazepines enhance the consumption and palatability of alcohol in the rat, Psychopharmacology 137 (1998) 215–222.
[432] J.D. Sokolowski, J.D. Salamone, The role of accumbens dopamine in lever pressing and response allocation: Effects of 6-OHDA injected into core and dorsomedial shell, Pharmacol. Biochem. Behav. 59 (1998) 557–566.
[433] P.R. Solomon, A. Crider, J.W. Winkelman, A. Turi, R.M. Kamer, L.J. Kaplan, Disrupted latent inhibition in the rat with chronic amphetamine or haloperidol-induced supersensitivity: relationship to schizophrenic attention disorder, Biol. Psychiatry 16 (1981) 519–537.
[434] R.L. Solomon, Addiction: An opponent-process theory of acquired motivation: The affective dynamics of addiction, in: M.E.P.S. Jack, D. Maser (Eds.), Psychopathology: Experimental Models, W. H. Freeman, Publishers, San Francisco, CA, US, 1977, pp. 66–103.

[435] R.L. Solomon, J.D. Corbit, An opponent-process theory of motivation: I Temporal dynamics of affect, Psychol. Rev. 81 (1974) 119–145.
[436] R. Soussignan, B. Schall, Children's facial responsiveness to odors: Influences of hedonic valence of odor, gender, age, and social presence, Developmental Psychology 32 (1996) 367–379.
[437] A.C. Spector, P. Breslin, H.J. Grill, Taste reactivity as a dependent measure of the rapid formation of conditioned taste aversion: a tool for the neural analysis of taste-visceral associations, Behav. Neurosci. 102 (1988) 942–952.
[438] A.C. Spector, R. Norgren, H.J. Grill, Parabrachial gustatory lesions impair taste aversion learning in rats, Behav. Neurosci. 106 (1992) 147–161.
[439] L.R. Squire, S.M. Zola, Structure and function of declarative and nondeclarative memory systems, Proc. Natl. Acad. Sci. U.S.A. 93 (1996) 13515–13522.
[440] T.L. Stefurak, D. van der Kooy, Tegmental pedunculopontine lesions in rats decrease saccharin's rewarding effects but not its memory-improving effect, Behav. Neurosci. 108 (1994) 972–980.
[441] J.E. Steiner, The gustofacial response: observation on normal and anencephalic newborn infants, Symp. Oral Sens. Percept. 4 (1973) 254–278.
[442] J.E. Steiner, Human facial expressions in response to taste and smell stimulation, Adv. Child Dev. Behav. 13 (1979) 257–295.
[443] J.E. Steiner, D. Glaser, Differential behavioral responses to taste stimuli in non-human primates, J. Human Evol. 13 (1984) 709–723.
[444] J.E. Steiner, D. Glaser, Taste-induced facial expressions in apes and humans, Human Evol. 10 (1995) 97–105.
[445] J.E. Steiner, D. Glaser, M.E. Hawilo, K.C. Berridge, Evolutionary continuum of facial expression: human newborn versus nonhuman primate reaction to sensory pleasure, Manuscript in preparation. (1998).
[446] J.R. Stellar, F.H. Brooks, L.E. Mills, Approach and withdrawal analysis of the effects of hypothalamic stimulation and lesions in rats, J. Comp. Physiol. Psychol. 93 (1979) 446–466.
[447] J.R. Stellar, D. Corbett, Regional neuroleptic microinjections indicate a role for nucleus accumbens in lateral hypothalamic self-stimulation reward, Brain Res. 477 (1989) 126–143.
[448] J.R. Stellar, E. Stellar, The Neurobiology of Motivation and Reward, Springer-Verlag, New York, 1985.
[449] J. Stewart, Normal hedonic reactions to sucrose by 6-OHDA rats may reflect 'functional decerebration'. Communicated at Society for Neuroscience meeting, New Orleans, 1991.
[450] R.E. Strecker, G.F. Steinfels, B.L. Jacobs, Dopaminergic unit activity in freely moving cats: lack of relationship to feeding, satiety, and glucose injections, Brain Res. 260 (1983) 317–321.
[451] E.M. Stricker, M.J. Zigmond, Brain catecholamines and the lateral hypothalamic syndrome, in: D. Novin, W. Wyrwicka, G. Bray (Eds.), Hunger: Basic Mechanisms and Clinical Implications, Raven Press, New York, 1976, pp. 19–32.
[452] E.M. Stricker, M.J. Zigmond, Brain monoamines, homeostasis, and adaptive behavior., Handbook of Physiology: Intrinsic Regulatory Systems of the Brain, Vol. 4, American Physiological Society, Bethesda, MD, 1986, pp. 677–696.
[453] D. Sulzer, M.P. Joyce, L. Lin, D. Geldwert, S.N. Haber, T. Hattori, S. Rayport, Dopamine neurons make glutamatergic synapses in vitro, J. Neurosci. 18 (1998) 4588–4602.
[454] R. Tamura, R. Norgren, Repeated sodium depletion affects gustatory neural responses in the nucleus of the solitary tract of rats, Am. J. Physiol. 273 (1997) R1381–R1391.
[455] P. Teitelbaum, A.N. Epstein, The lateral hypothalamic syndrome: recovery of feeding and drinking after lateral hypothalamic lesions, Psychol. Rev. 69 (1962) 74–90.
[456] P. Teitelbaum, D.L. Wolgin, Abnormal gait sequence in locomotion after atropine treatment of catecholamine-deficient akinetic rats, Proc. Natl. Acad. Sci. U.S.A. 84 (1987) 8750–8753.
[457] P. Terry, Dopamine receptor subtypes and ingestive behavior, in: S.J. Cooper, P.G. Clifton (Eds.), Drug Receptor Subtypes and Ingestive Behavior, Academic Press, San Diego, 1995.
[458] P. Terry, D.B. Gilbert, S.J. Cooper, Dopamine receptor subtype agonists and feeding behavior, Obesity Res. 3 (1995) 515S–523S.
[459] E.L. Thorndike, Animal Intelligence: An Experimental Study of the Associative Processes in Animals, Macmillan, New York, 1898.
[460] F. Toates, Motivational Systems, Cambridge Univ. Press, Cambridge, 1986.
[461] F. Toates, The interaction of cognitive and stimulus-response processes in the control of behaviour, Neurosci. Biobehav. Rev. 22 (1998) 59–83.
[462] F.M. Toates, The control of ingestive behaviour by internal and external stimuli—a theoretical review, Appetite 2 (1981) 35–50.
[463] F.M. Toates, Comparing motivational systems—an incentive motivation perspective, in: C.R. Legg, D.A. Booth (Eds.), Appetite: Neural and Behavioural Bases, Oxford Univ. Press, New York, 1994, pp. 305–327.
[464] J.B. Travers, L.R. Akey, S.C. Chen, S. Rosen et al., Taste preferences in Parkinson's disease patients, Chem. Senses 18 (1993) 47–55.
[465] D. Treit, K.C. Berridge, A comparison of benzodiazepine, serotonin, and dopamine agents in the taste-reactivity paradigm, Pharmacol. Biochem. Behav. 37 (1990) 451–456.
[466] D. Treit, K.C. Berridge, C.E. Schultz, The direct enhancement of positive palatability by chlordiazepoxide is antagonized by Ro 15-1788 and CGS 8216, Pharmacol. Biochem. Behav. 26 (1987) 709–714.
[467] M.E. Trulson, D.W. Preussler, Dopamine-containing ventral tegmental area neurons in freely moving cats: activity during the sleep–waking cycle and effects of stress, Exp. Neurol. 83 (1984) 367–377.
[468] A. Tyrka, C. Gayle, G.P. Smith, Raclopride decreases sucrose intake of rat pups in independent ingestion tests, Pharmacol. Biochem. Behav. 43 (1992) 863–869.
[469] A. Tyrka, G.P. Smith, Potency of SCH 23390 for decreasing sucrose intake in rat pups depends on mode of ingestion, Pharmacol. Biochem. Behav. 39 (1991) 955–961.
[470] U. Ungerstedt, Is interruption of the nigro-striatal dopamine system producing the 'lateral hypothalamus syndrome'?, Acta Physiol. Scand. 80 (1970) 35A–36A.
[471] U. Ungerstedt, Adipsia and aphagia after 6-hydroxydopamine induced degeneration of the nigro-striatal dopamine system, Acta Physiol. Scand. Suppl. 367 (1971) 95–122.
[472] F.J. Vaccarino, B.B. Schiff, S.E. Glickman, Biological view of reinforcement, in: S.B. Klein, R.R. Mowrer (Eds.), Contemporary Learning Theories: Instrumental Conditioning Theory and the Impact of Biological Constraints on Learning, Lawrence Erlbaum Associates, Hillsdale, NJ, 1989, pp. 111–142.
[473] E.S. Valenstein, Problems of measurement and interpretation with reinforcing brain stimulation, Psychol. Rev. 71 (1964) 415–437.
[474] E.S. Valenstein, The interpretation of behavior evoked by brain stimulation, in: A. Wauquier, E.T. Rolls (Eds.), Brain-Stimulation Reward, Elsevier, New York, 1976, pp. 557–575.
[475] D. van der Kooy, K. Nader, A. Bechara, Role of dopamine in reward. Personal communication (email discussion), 1998.
[476] P. Vezina, Sensitization by prior drug exposure increases break point for self-administration of drug reward by rats, Personal Communication, 1998.
[477] N.D. Volkow, G.J. Wang, J.S. Fowler, J. Logan, S.J. Gatley, R. Hitzemann, A.D. Chen, S.L. Dewey, N. Pappas, Decreased striatal dopaminergic responsiveness in detoxified cocaine-dependent subjects, Nature 386 (1997) 830–833.
[478] C.T. Wang, R.L. Huang, M.Y. Tai, Y.F. Tsai, M.T. Peng, Dopamine release in the nucleus accumbens during sexual behavior in prenatally stressed adult male rats, Neurosci. Lett. 200 (1995) 29–32.

[479] E.M. Wasserman, Y. Gomita, C.R. Gallistel, Pimozide blocks reinforcement but not priming from MFB stimulation in the rat, Pharmacol. Biochem. Behav. 17 (1982) 783–787.

[480] F. Weiss, A. Markou, M.T. Lorang, G.F. Koob, Basal extracellular dopamine levels in the nucleus accumbens are decreased during cocaine withdrawal after unlimited-access self-administration, Brain Res. 593 (1992) 314–318.

[481] C.C. Welch, E.M. Kim, M.K. Grace, C.J. Billington, A.S. Levine, Palatability-induced hyperphagia increases hypothalamic Dynorphin peptide and mRNA levels, Brain Res. 721 (1996) 126–131.

[482] B.H. Westerink, A. Teisman, J.B. de Vries, Increase in dopamine release from the nucleus accumbens in response to feeding: a model to study interactions between drugs and naturally activated dopaminergic neurons in the rat brain, Naunyn-Schmiedeberg's Arch. Pharmacol. 349 (1994) 230–235.

[483] I.Q. Whishaw, S.B. Dunnett, Dopamine depletion, stimulation or blockade in the rat disrupts spatial navigation and locomotion dependent upon beacon or distal cues, Behav. Brain Res. 18 (1985) 11–29.

[484] I.Q. Whishaw, W.T. O'Connor, S.B. Dunnett, Disruption of central cholinergic systems in the rat by basal forebrain lesions or atropine: effects on feeding, sensorimotor behaviour, locomotor activity and spatial navigation, Behav. Brain Res. 17 (1985) 103–115.

[485] I.Q. Whishaw, W.T. O'Connor, S.B. Dunnett, The contributions of motor cortex, nigrostriatal dopamine and caudate-putamen to skilled forelimb use in the rat, Brain 109 (1986) 805–843.

[486] F.J. White, Cocaine and the serotonin saga, Nature 393 (1998) 118–119.

[487] N.M. White, Control of sensorimotor function by dopaminergic nigrostriatal neurons: influence on eating and drinking, Neurosci. Biobehav. Rev. 10 (1986) 15–36.

[488] N.M. White, Reward or reinforcement: what's the difference?, Neurosci. Biobehav. Rev. 13 (1989) 181–186.

[489] N.M. White, Addictive drugs as reinforcers: multiple partial actions on memory systems, Addiction 91 (1996) 921–949, discussion 951-965.

[490] N.M. White, M.G. Packard, N. Hiroi, Place conditioning with dopamine D1 and D2 agonists injected peripherally or into nucleus accumbens, Psychopharmacology 103 (1991) 271–276.

[491] I. Wickelgren, Getting the brain's attention [news], Science 278 (1997) 35–37.

[492] G.V. Williams, E.T. Rolls, C.M. Leonard, C. Stern, Neuronal responses in the ventral striatum of the behaving macaque, Behav. Brain Res. 55 (1993) 243–252.

[493] C. Wilson, G.G. Nomikos, M. Collu, H.C. Fibiger, Dopaminergic correlates of motivated behavior: importance of drive, J. Neurosci. 15 (1995) 5169–5178.

[494] T.D. Wilson, J.W. Schooler, Thinking too much: introspection can reduce the quality of preferences and decisions, J. Pers. Soc. Psychol. 60 (1991) 181–192.

[495] P. Winkielman, R.B. Zajonc, N. Schwarz, Subliminal affective priming resists attributional interventions, Cognition and Emotion 11 (1997) 433–465.

[496] P. Winn, The lateral hypothalamus and motivated behavior: an old syndrome reassessed and a new perspective gained, Cur. Dir. Psychol. Sci. 4 (1995) 182–187.

[497] R.A. Wise, The dopamine synapse and the notion of 'pleasure centers' in the brain, Trends Neurosci. 3 (1980) 91–95.

[498] R.A. Wise, Common neural basis for brain stimulation reward, drug reward, and food reward, in: B.G. Hoebel, D. Novin (Eds.), The Neural Basis of Feeding and Reward, Haer Institute for Electrophysiological Research, Brunswick, Maine, 1982, pp. 445–454.

[499] R.A. Wise, Neuroleptics and operant behavior: the anhedonia hypothesis, Behav. Brain Sci. 5 (1982) 39–87.

[500] R.A. Wise, The anhedonia hypothesis: Mark III, Behav. Brain Sci. 8 (1985) 178–186.

[501] R.A. Wise, Sensorimotor modulation and the variable action pattern (VAP): Toward a noncircular definition of drive and motivation, Psychobiology 15 (1987) 7–20.

[502] R.A. Wise, The brain and reward, in: J.M. Liebman, S.J. Cooper (Eds.), The Neuropharmacological Basis of Reward, Clarendon Press, Oxford, U.K., 1989, pp. 377–424.

[503] R.A. Wise, Neuroleptic-induced anhedonia: Recent studies, in: C.A. Tamminga, C.S. Schulz (Eds.), Schizophrenia Research. Advances in Neuropsychiatry and Psychopharmacology, Vol. 1., Raven Press, Publishers, New York, NY, US, 1991, pp. 323–331.

[504] R.A. Wise, A brief history of the anhedonia hypothesis, in: C.R. Legg, D. Booth (Eds.), Appetite: Neural and Behavioural Bases, Oxford Univ. Press, New York, 1994, pp. 243–263.

[505] R.A. Wise, Addictive drugs and brain stimulation reward, An. Rev. Neurosci. 19 (1996) 140–319.

[506] R.A. Wise, Neurobiology of addiction, Cur. Opin. Neurobio. 6 (1996) 243–251.

[507] R.A. Wise, M.A. Bozarth, Brain mechanisms of drug reward and euphoria, Psychiat. Med. 3 (1985) 445–460.

[508] R.A. Wise, M.A. Bozarth, A psychomotor stimulant theory of addiction, Psychol. Rev. 94 (1987) 469–492.

[509] R.A. Wise, V. Dawson, Diazepam-induced eating and lever pressing for food in sated rats, J. Comp Physiol. Psychol. 86 (1974) 930–941.

[510] R.A. Wise, P. Leone, R. Rivest, K. Leeb, Elevations of nucleus accumbens dopamine and DOPAC levels during intravenous heroin self-administration, Synapse 21 (1995) 140–148.

[511] R.A. Wise, P. Newton, K. Leeb, B. Burnette, D. Pocock, J.B. Justice Jr., Fluctuations in nucleus accumbens dopamine concentration during intravenous cocaine self-administration in rats, Psychopharmacology 120 (1995) 10–20.

[512] R.A. Wise, L. Raptis, Effects of naloxone and pimozide on initiation and maintenance measures of free feeding, Brain Res. 368 (1986) 62–68.

[513] R.A. Wise, P.-P. Rompre, Brain dopamine and reward, An. Rev. Psychol. 40 (1989) 191–225.

[514] R.A. Wise, J. Spindler, H. deWit, G.J. Gerberg, Neuroleptic-induced 'anhedonia' in rats: pimozide blocks reward quality of food, Science 201 (1978) 262–264.

[515] D.L. Wolgin, J. Cytawa, P. Teitelbaum, Sensory neglect produced by lateral hypothalamic damage, Science 174 (1971) 523–525.

[516] P.L. Wood, T.S. Rao, Morphine stimulation of mesolimbic and mesocortical but not nigrostriatal dopamine release in the rat as reflected by changes in 3-methoxytyramine levels, Neuropharmacology 30 (1991) 399–401.

[517] S. Xenakis, A. Sclafani, The effects of pimozide on the consumption of a palatable saccharin-glucose solution in the rat, Pharmacol. Biochem. Behav. 15 (1981) 435–442.

[518] S. Xenakis, A. Sclafani, The dopaminergic mediation of a sweet reward in normal and VMH hyperphagic rats, Pharmacol. Biochem. Behav. 16 (1982) 293–302.

[519] J.S. Yeomans, A. Mathur, M. Tampakeras, Rewarding brain stimulation: role of tegmental cholinergic neurons that activate dopamine neurons, Behav. Neurosci. 107 (1993) 1077–1087.

[520] M.R. Yeomans, R.W. Gray, Effects of naltrexone on food intake and changes in subjective appetite during eating: evidence for opioid involvement in the appetizer effect, Physiol. Behav. 62 (1997) 15–21.

[521] M.R. Yeomans, P. Wright, H.A. Macleod, J.A. Critchley, Effects of nalmefene on feeding in humans. Dissociation of hunger and palatability, Psychopharmacology 100 (1990) 426–432.

[522] R.A. Yokel, R.A. Wise, Increased lever pressing for amphetamine after pimozide in rats: implications for a dopamine theory of reward, Science 187 (1975) 547–549.

[523] R.A. Yokel, R.A. Wise, Attenuation of intravenous amphetamine reinforcement by central dopamine blockade in rats, Psychopharmacology 48 (1976) 311–318.

[524] M. Yoshioka, M. Matsumoto, H. Togashi, H. Saito, Effect of conditioned fear stress on dopamine release in the rat prefrontal cortex, Neurosci. Lett. 209 (1996) 201–203.

[525] A.M. Young, R.G. Ahier, R.L. Upton, M.H. Joseph, J.A. Gray, Increased extracellular dopamine in the nucleus accumbens of the rat during associative learning of neutral stimuli, Neuroscience 83 (1998) 1175–1183.

[526] A.M. Young, M.H. Joseph, J.A. Gray, Latent inhibition of conditioned dopamine release in rat nucleus accumbens, Neuroscience 54 (1993) 5–9.

[527] P.T. Young, The role of affective processes in learning and motivation, Psychol. Rev. 66 (1959) 1104–1125.

[528] R.B. Zajonc, Feeling and thinking: preferences need no inferences, Am. Psychol. 35 (1980) 151–175.

[529] H.P. Zeigler, M.F. Jacquin, M.G. Miller, Trigeminal sensorimotor mechanisms and ingestive behavior, Neurosci. Biobehav. Rev. 8 (1984) 415–423.

[530] D.A. Zellner, K.C. Berridge, H.J. Grill, J.W. Ternes, Rats learn to like the taste of morphine, Behav. Neurosci. 99 (1985) 290–300.

[531] M.J. Zigmond, E.M. Stricker, Deficits in feeding behavior after intraventricular injection of 6-hydroxydopamine in rats, Science 177 (1972) 1211–1214.

Neuron, Vol. 19, 591–611, September, 1997, Copyright ©1997 by Cell Press

Acute Effects of Cocaine on Human Brain Activity and Emotion

Hans C. Breiter,[1,2,9] Randy L. Gollub,[2]
Robert M. Weisskoff,[1] David N. Kennedy,[1,3]
Nikos Makris,[3] Joshua D. Berke,[5] Julie M. Goodman,[1,2]
Howard L. Kantor,[1,6] David R. Gastfriend,[2,4]
Jonn P. Riorden,[2,4] R. Thomas Mathew,[2,4,7]
Bruce R. Rosen,[1] and Steven E. Hyman[2,8]
[1]Nuclear Magnetic Resonance Center
Department of Radiology
[2]Department of Psychiatry
[3]Center for Morphometric Analysis
Department of Neurology
Massachusetts General Hospital and Harvard Medical School
Boston, Massachusetts 02129
[4]Addictions Services
Department of Psychiatry
Massachusetts General Hospital and Harvard Medical School
Boston, Massachusetts 02114
[5]Program in Neuroscience
Harvard University
Boston, Massachusetts 02115
[6]Department of Cardiology
Massachusetts General Hospital and Harvard Medical School
Boston, Massachusetts 02114

Summary

We investigated brain circuitry mediating cocaine-induced euphoria and craving using functional MRI (fMRI). During double-blind cocaine (0.6 mg/kg) and saline infusions in cocaine-dependent subjects, the entire brain was imaged for 5 min before and 13 min after infusion while subjects rated scales for rush, high, low, and craving. Cocaine induced focal signal increases in nucleus accumbens/subcallosal cortex (NAc/SCC), caudate, putamen, basal forebrain, thalamus, insula, hippocampus, parahippocampal gyrus, cingulate, lateral prefrontal and temporal cortices, parietal cortex, striate/extrastriate cortices, ventral tegmentum, and pons and produced signal decreases in amygdala, temporal pole, and medial frontal cortex. Saline produced few positive or negative activations, which were localized to lateral prefrontal cortex and temporo-occipital cortex. Subjects who underwent repeat studies showed good replication of the regional fMRI activation pattern following cocaine and saline infusions, with activations on saline retest that might reflect expectancy. Brain regions that exhibited early and short duration signal maxima showed a higher correlation with rush ratings. These included the ventral tegmentum, pons, basal forebrain, caudate, cingulate, and most regions of lateral prefrontal cortex. In contrast, regions that demonstrated early but sustained signal maxima were more correlated with craving than with rush ratings; such regions included the NAc/SCC, right parahippocampal gyrus, and some regions of lateral prefrontal cortex. Sustained negative signal change was noted in the amygdala, which correlated with craving ratings. Our data demonstrate the ability of fMRI to map dynamic patterns of brain activation following cocaine infusion in cocaine-dependent subjects and provide evidence of dynamically changing brain networks associated with cocaine-induced euphoria and cocaine-induced craving.

[7]Present address: Tri-County Center for Substance Abuse Treatment, Wilmington, North Carolina, 28402.
[8]Present address: Office of the Director, National Institute of Mental Health, Bethesda, Maryland, 20892.
[9]To whom correspondence should be addressed.

Introduction

Cocaine is one of the most reinforcing drugs known, both in humans and in animals (Johanson and Fischman, 1989). With repetitive use, cocaine may produce a profound state of addiction in humans characterized by compulsive drug use and inability to control use despite significant adverse consequences (Gawin, 1991; American Psychiatric Association, 1994). Progress toward understanding the neural substrates of addiction to cocaine has been substantial in recent years but has been focused on animal models that permit invasive studies. Noninvasive functional neuroimaging approaches, such as functional magnetic resonance imaging (fMRI), now allow studies of neural circuit function to be extended to the human. This has the advantage of being able to correlate subjective information about emotional and cognitive responses with observed patterns of brain activation.

Based on extensive investigations of rodent and primate models, the mesoaccumbens dopamine pathway, extending from the ventral tegmentum of the midbrain (VT) to the nucleus accumbens, appears to be the critical shared substrate of the reinforcing effects of cocaine (Louilot et al., 1989; Williams, 1989; Apicella et al., 1991; Schultz et al., 1992) and other addictive drugs (reviewed in Koob, 1996). Using nondrug stimuli, the nucleus accumbens has also been shown to play a critical role in learning associated with reinforcement (Mirenowicz and Schultz, 1996). Reinforcement in animals depends on the increase in synaptic dopamine levels in the mesoaccumbens circuit produced by cocaine-like drugs via blockade of the dopamine reuptake transporter (DAT) (DeWit and Wise, 1977; Ritz et al., 1987). In both animals and humans, the acutely reinforcing effects of psychostimulant drugs can produce a pattern of repeated self-administration. Human users may initially self-administer cocaine to gain pleasure, to conform to peer behavior, or to relieve stress and other dysphoric feelings. An accelerated pattern of drug use in vulnerable individuals may produce increasing levels of dependence and, eventually, addiction (Hyman, 1996).

While the mesoaccumbens dopamine pathway has been most closely implicated in the acutely rewarding actions of cocaine, other circuits have also been implicated in reward processes, including the basal forebrain, which receives major afferents from the nucleus accumbens and itself receives dopaminergic input (Heimer et al., 1997). Brain stimulation reward (BSR) experiments have directly implicated the basal forebrain in reinforcement (Rompre and Shizgal, 1986; Shizgal et al., 1989; Arvanitogiannis et al, 1996). The nucleus accumbens is also strongly linked to the amygdala (Ito et al., 1974; Yim and Mogenson, 1982; Russchen et al., 1985; Amaral, et al., 1992), a linkage thought to be important for the formation of stimulus–reward associations (Jones and Mishkin, 1972; Spiegler and Mishkin, 1981; Gaffan and Harrison, 1987; Gaffan et al., 1988). Recently, PET scanning has demonstrated amygdala activation during cocaine craving in abstinent cocaine-abusing subjects relative to normal controls (Childress et al., 1996, Soc. Neurosci., abstract; Grant et al., 1996; Schweitzer et al., 1996, Soc. Neurosci., abstract). Thus, according to current neurobiological models, the nucleus accumbens, amygdala, basal forebrain, and VT are central components of circuitry mediating brain processes underlying reward and memory of that reward.

A number of human studies using cocaine infusions (Fowler et al., 1989; London et al., 1990; Pearlson et al., 1993; Volkow et al., 1997a) and withdrawing subjects (Volkow et al., 1990, 1991, 1992, 1993, 1997b) have implicated the striatum in human cocaine use, withdrawal, and craving. Given the spatial resolution of the techniques utilized, they may not have fully distinguished the dorsal and ventral striatum, in particular the nucleus accumbens. None of these studies reported specific sampling of other regions implicated with reward processes, such as the VT, basal forebrain, or amygdala. Only three of these studies approached the 1–2 min temporal resolution needed to resolve components of cocaine-induced euphoria (Fowler et al., 1989; Pearlson et al., 1993; Volkow et al., 1997a).

To investigate activity in reward circuitry in humans during cocaine infusions and to associate this activity with subjective reports for both cocaine-induced euphoria and postcocaine craving, we used fMRI (Bandettini et al., 1992; Kwong et al., 1992; Ogawa et al., 1992) in conjunction with physiological monitoring and online evaluation of computerized behavioral rating scales. FMRI with a 1.5 T instrument has higher resolution than previous PET and SPECT studies of cocaine effects, permitting investigation of regions with relatively small volume, such as the nucleus accumbens and the amygdala. For these experiments, cocaine-dependent volunteers underwent an unblinded cocaine infusion the night before the fMRI experiment for clinical screening and for training with behavioral assessments on scales of rush, high, low, and craving. During the subsequent double-blind cocaine (0.6 mg/kg) and saline infusions, subjects rated these four scales every 15 s during multiple fMRI acquisitions (Figure 1). Pilot results from this study have previously been presented (Breiter et al., 1996c; Gollub et al., 1996), and data regarding global versus regional cocaine effects is presented elsewhere (Gollub et al., submitted).

Based upon animal data (Koob and Bloom, 1988; Brown et al., 1992; Stein and Fuller, 1992, 1993), we set out to study whether putative brain reward circuitry such as the nucleus accumbens and VT along with other known sites of cocaine binding such as the caudate nucleus would exhibit blood oxygen level–dependent (BOLD) signal changes (Ogawa et al., 1992) for cocaine and not for saline. We were also interested in studying other regions associated with reward and reward-based memory (e.g., basal forebrain and amygdala) and paralimbic structures reported activated in animal studies of acute cocaine administration (Brown et al., 1992; Stein and Fuller, 1992, 1993; Graham and Porrino, 1995; Hammer et al., 1995; Lyons et al., 1996). We predicted that fMRI activation in the nucleus accumbens would be correlated with behavioral reports of cocaine-induced subjective rush and high in dependent subjects. The results in this report will be focused on subcortical limbic structures and paralimbic cortex, though all regions found activated will be discussed in the text and included as a supplemental table available on the Internet.

Results

Clinical and Physiological Data

Seventeen subjects were infused with cocaine while being scanned with fMRI. Scans affected by uncorrectable gross movement were rejected as uninterpretable. Of these 17 subjects, ten had interpretable fMRI data for the cocaine infusions, and ten had interpretable data for the saline infusions after motion correction (seven studies with usable matched infusions).

Following the cocaine infusion (0.6 mg/kg over 30 s), there was an increase in heart rate (HR) within the first minute, while the increase in mean blood pressure (MBP) was slower. Similarly, the drop in end-tidal carbon dioxide ($ETCO_2$) was also slower. Cocaine ($N = 17$) caused the HR to increase rapidly from a preinfusion value of 60 ± 7 beats per minute (bpm) to 79 ± 16 bpm at 2 min postinfusion ($p < 0.0001$), to 82 ± 12 bpm at 5 min postinfusion ($p < 1 \times 10^{-6}$), to 93 ± 14 bpm at 10 min postinfusion ($p < 1 \times 10^{-8}$). Normal sinus rhythm was observed in all subjects throughout the study (Gollub et al., 1996).

MBP rose slightly from 96 ± 12 torr before the infusion to 101 ± 12 torr at 2 min postinfusion ($p < 0.11$, NS), then up to 111 ± 15 torr at 5 min ($p < 0.002$) before starting to slowly decline. The $ETCO_2$ dropped slowly from a baseline of 39 ± 4 mm Hg to 36 ± 4 mm Hg by 10 min ($p < 0.02$). In all subjects scanned, these three measures had returned to baseline by 2 hr, the interinfusion interval (Gollub et al., 1996). Physiologic responses to the 0.6 mg/kg cocaine infusion are in close accord with previously published studies in experienced cocaine abusers (Fischman and Schuster, 1982; Fischman et al., 1985; Foltin and Fischman, 1991).

Plasma samples taken before the first infusion demonstrated absence of residual cocaine at the time of the first infusion in all of the subjects studied. Peak plasma cocaine levels (C_{max}) following the cocaine infusion ranged from 197 to 893 mcg/l with a mean of 388.7 ± 233.0 ($N = 7$ subjects with complete data). The time to peak cocaine plasma concentration varied from 3 to 15 min for subjects in the initial series of experiments (mean $\pm$ SD: 7.6 ± 4.2 min) and the four subjects with interpretable retest experiments (mean $\pm$ SD: 6.0 ± 2.9 min).

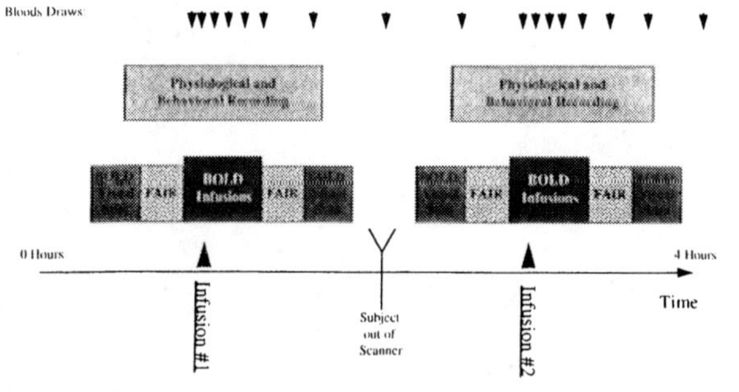

Figure 1. Experiment Design

Over a 5 hr period, subjects participated in ten experimental scans. The experimental runs were grouped, five apiece, around each of the double-blind infusions. Details of each acquisition are presented in Experimental Procedures. Physiological recording along with behavioral ratings were initiated prior to the first FAIR scan and continued through the second FAIR scan of each infusion block. After the first infusion, the second double-blind infusion could not be initiated until the 120 min blood sample had been collected. In between the sets of functional scans for each infusion, clinical scans were acquired for neuroradiolgical assessment. These scans included sagital T1 images, axial proton density and T2 images, and 3-D time-of-flight angiogram.

Scores for the Profile of Mood States (POMS) inventory, assessed before, between, and after the two infusions, showed no change in five of the six POMS measures (i.e., tension, depression, vigor, fatigue, confusion) over the total scan time. Vigor increased in the second infusion for both cocaine and saline infusions. Spielberger scores assessed before, between, and after both infusions indicated no significant change in anxiety levels across scans. These observations would be consistent with the interpretation that subjects did not experience increased discomfort or anxiety in the scanner environment over the course of the experiment.

Behavioral Measures

All ten subjects with interpretable cocaine fMRI data reported clear cocaine effects (see Figure 2). Both peak rush (max score = 3; mean $\pm$ SD = 2.2 $\pm$ 1.1) and peak high (2.1 $\pm$ 0.8) occurred, in the average data, 3 min postinfusion. Peak low (primarily reports of dysphoria and paranoia: 0.9 $\pm$ 0.8) occurred 11 min postinfusion, while peak craving (1.3 $\pm$ 0.9) occurred 12 min postinfusion. No subject reported effects from the saline infusion on any of the four measures. Ratings obtained for rush, high, low, and craving measures at the 0.6 mg/kg blinded cocaine dosage, given in the fMRI scanner, were higher compared to those obtained at the unblinded 0.2 mg/kg dosage administered in the Massachusetts General Hospital (MGH) Mallinckrodt General Clinical Research Center (GCRC) (rush: 1.2 $\pm$ 1.1; high: 1.7 $\pm$ 1.2; low: 0.8 $\pm$ 0.8; craving: 1.0 $\pm$ 1.3). For the four subjects with interpretable test–retest cocaine data, behavioral measures were unchanged on average for the two conditions (retest results, rush: 1.8 $\pm$ 1.0; high: 2.3 $\pm$ 0.5; low: 1.0 $\pm$ 0.8; craving: 1.0 $\pm$ 1.2).

Cocaine Infusion

Foci of Signal Change

Cocaine caused regional signal increases (Kolmogorov-Smirnov, $p < 7.1 \times 10^{-6}$) (see Tables 1–4 for multiple limbic and paralimbic regions, supplemental Table 6 http://www.neuron.org/cgi/content/full/19/3/591/T6, and Figures 3a and 3b) in discrete foci in the nucleus accumbens/subcallosal cortex (NAc/SCC), caudate nucleus,

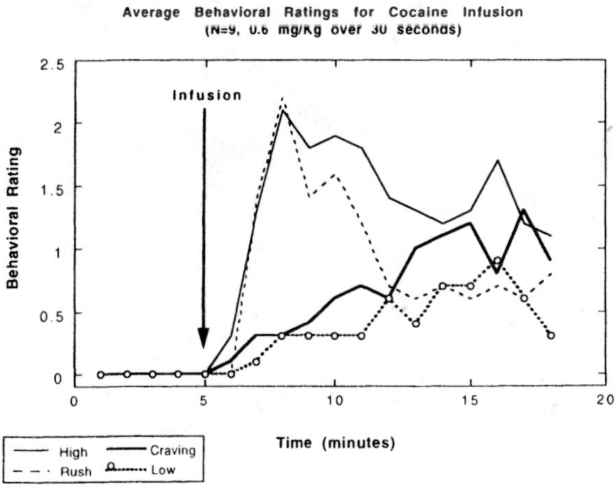

Figure 2. Graph of Average Behavioral Measures

The rush, high, low, and craving ratings were averaged within category for the nine of ten subjects who had interpretable cocaine fMRI data after motion correction and behavioral ratings time-locked to the scanner.

Table 1. Characterization of Cocaine Effects on FMRI Signal in Subcortical Gray Structures

Anatomic Region		Tal Coordinates R/L	Tal Coordinates A/P	Tal Coordinates S/I	P Value (KS Statistic)	% Signal Change (Pre versus Post Drug)	Proportion Individuals ($p < 0.001$)	Multiple Correlation Analysis: Rush	Multiple Correlation Analysis: Craving
NAc/SCC	R	6	7	−9	7×10^{-6}	1.5	9/10	ϕ	+
	L	−6	13	0	4×10^{-6}	1.5	8/10	ϕ	+
Caudate	R	13	−3	22	5×10^{-7}	0.8	8/10	+	−
	L	−9	−3	19	3×10^{-7}	1.0	7/10	+	ϕ
Putamen	R	28	7	−3	4×10^{-8}	1.4	8/10	+	−
	L	−28	7	−3	NS (5×10^{-5})	0.5	5/10	ϕ	ϕ
BF/GP	R	22*	1*	−6*	NS	ϕ	6/10	ϕ	+
	L	−19	0	−3	6×10^{-9}	1.8	7/10	+	−
Thalamus									
aThal	R	3	−18	13	6×10^{-8}	0.4	8/10	ϕ	ϕ
	L	ϕ	ϕ	ϕ	NS	ϕ	7/10	ϕ	ϕ
pThal	R	6	−25	16	9×10^{-7}	1.4	8/10	+	ϕ
	L	−6*	−31*	9*	NS	ϕ	8/10	+	ϕ
LGN	R	19	−25	0	NS (8×10^{-5})	0.8	8/10	+	ϕ
	L	−19	−25	−3	2×10^{-7}	0.5	7/10	+	ϕ

Table 2. Characterization of Cocaine Effects on FMRI Signal in Temporal Lobe

Anatomic Region		Tal Coordinates R/L	Tal Coordinates A/P	Tal Coordinates S/I	P Value (KS Statistic)	% Signal Change (Pre versus Post Drug)	Proportion Individuals ($p < 0.001$)	Multiple Correlation Analysis: Rush	Multiple Correlation Analysis: Craving
Hippocampus									
aHip	R	28*	−18*	−9*	NS	ϕ	9/10	ϕ	−
	L	−28*	−17*	−16*	NS	ϕ	10/10	ϕ	±∇
pHip	R	34	−28	−13	2×10^{-8}	1.8	9/10	+	+
	L	−22	−37	0	NS (1×10^{-5})	0.9	10/10	+	ϕ
Insula									
aINS	R	34	13	6	3×10^{-8}	0.9	10/10	+	ϕ
	L	−28	19	−6	5×10^{-6}	0.5	8/10	+	ϕ
pINS	R	41	−15	0	2×10^{-9}	1.1	8/10	+	ϕ
	L	−41	−12	−3	3×10^{-11}	1.0	7/10	+	+
Amygdala	R	22	−6	−13	NS (-7×10^{-5})	−1.2	4/10 (+), 5/10 (−)	ϕ	−
	L	−25	−9	−19	-1×10^{-6}	−0.3	3/10 (+), 5/10 (−)	ϕ	−

Table 3. Characterization of Cocaine Effects on FMRI Signal in Medial Paralimbic Cortices

Anatomic Region		Tal Coordinates R/L	Tal Coordinates A/P	Tal Coordinates S/I	P Value (KS Statistic)	% Signal Change (Pre versus Post Drug)	Proportion Individuals ($p < 0.001$)	Multiple Correlation Analysis: Rush	Multiple Correlation Analysis: Craving
Cingulate G.									
aCG (BA 24/32)	R	9	13	34	1×10^{-8}	0.9	9/10	+	ϕ
(BA 32)	R	3	26	28	3×10^{-7}	0.8		+	ϕ
(BA 24)	B	0	−3	31	3×10^{-8}	1.0	9/10	+	+
pCG (BA 31)	R	3	−31	38	3×10^{-6}	0.5	8/10	+	ϕ
(BA 31)	L	−9	−28	41	NS (1×10^{-5})	0.5	5/10	+	+
Parahippocampal G.									
(BA 28)	R	22	−21	−22	6×10^{-6}	2.7	9/10	+	++
(BA 28)	L	−19	−28	−9	2×10^{-8}	0.5	9/10	+	+
(BA 35)	R	16*	−40*	−6*	NS	ϕ	ϕ	+	ϕ
(BA 19)	L	−30*	−50*	2*	NS	ϕ	ϕ	+	+

Table 4. Characterization of Cocaine Effects on FMRI Signal in Brainstem

Anatomic Region		Tal Coordinates R/L	Tal Coordinates A/P	Tal Coordinates S/I	P Value (KS Statistic)	% Signal Change (Pre versus Post Drug)	Proportion Individuals ($p < 0.001$)	Multiple Correlation Analysis: Rush	Multiple Correlation Analysis: Craving
VT (SN)	R	9	−15	−13	4×10^{-6}	1.1	6/10	+	ϕ
	L	−16	−21	−6	3×10^{-9}	1.5	6/10	+	ϕ

putamen, basal forebrain, thalamus, insula, hippocampus, parahippocampal region, cingulate, lateral frontal cortices, lateral temporal cortex, parietal cortex, striate and extrastriate cortices, along with regional decreases in signal in amygdala (see Tables 1–4 and Figure 3b), temporal pole, and medial frontal cortex (see supplemental Table 7 http://www.neuron.org/cgi/content/full/19/3/591/T7). Negative activation in the temporal pole and medial frontal cortex lay in close proximity to regions of susceptibility artifact. Positive signal change was also noted in the vicinity of the VT and the pons.

Across most positive and negative activations with cocaine, plots of signal intensity versus time showed early signal maxima with rapid (starting within 1 min of the signal maxima) decrease toward baseline. Some activations, however, demonstrated early signal maxima that were sustained at a plateau level for time periods ranging from 5 min to the end of the scanning interval. These differences in time course appeared to correlate with different behavioral states.

Large activations in a few individuals may result in statistically significant activations in the averaged group data. To determine the extent to which the averaged data reflects common activations, statistical maps were analyzed for 16 subcortical regions (see Figure 4 for examples of anatomic definitions and Tables 1–4 for results) in the ten subjects used for the average map. The data is presented as the ratio of the number of subjects who showed activation in that structure at a less stringent p value threshold ($p < 0.001$); this type of analysis has previously been reported (Breiter et al., 1996b). The individual data analysis strongly supports the average results in the NAc/SCC, thalamus, hippocampus, insula, cingulate gyrus, and parahippocampal gyrus with eight or nine of ten subjects contributing to the group activation. Other regions including caudate, putamen, basal forebrain, and VT also reflected majority activation with six to eight subjects showing activation. One exception was noted: the amygdala demonstrated response heterogeneity across individuals. This heterogeneity suggests caution in the interpretation of the negative amygdala activation in the average map.

Correlation Maps

Multiple correlation analysis was used to determine whether activations observed for the baseline versus postinfusion comparison were associated with specific behavioral states. We calculated a correlation value (R) for each behavioral measure to describe the strength of similarity between the signal time course of each brain voxel to that behavioral measure. We used a multiple correlation technique with the rush and the craving ratings, because these measures were the most temporally distinct from each other (see Figure 2). Namely, rush ratings had early and transient maxima, while craving ratings had a longer latency to reaching maximum following infusion. The resulting correlation data are shown in Tables 1–4 and in Figure 5.

Regions that correlated with rush had early and transient signal maxima. Strong correlations were noted for the left basal forebrain and bilateral VT. In addition, many other regions of brain activation on our KS maps due to cocaine were positively correlated with rush ratings, including sections of the right cingulate gyrus, bilateral insula, bilateral thalamus, bilateral caudate nucleus, bilateral pontine brainstem, and the majority of activations in the prefrontal cortex.

Regions that showed significant correlation with craving had early signal maxima (or minima for the negative activations) followed by sustained signal change. The sustained signal change (see Figures 3a and 3b) in these regions produced the strong correlation with craving. Thus, while regions hypothesized to be involved in brain reward (NAc/SCC) and reinforcement-based memory (amygdala) showed signal changes (positive and negative changes, respectively) early, at the time of subjective rush and high, both regions showed persistent signal changes that correlated significantly with subjective reports of craving and not rush. Another region that showed a positive correlation with craving was a region of the right parahippocampal gyrus.

Finally, other regions demonstrated significant correlation with both rush and craving ratings, identified in Tables 1–4 by a plus sign in the columns for both ratings. Of these regions, those that overlapped with activations

Tables 1–4 summarize activation due to cocaine infusion. Anatomic Region identifies the structure on the basis of subcortical location, lobe, gyrus (if medial paralimbic cortex), or placement in the brainstem. See Experimental Procedures for details regarding anatomic definitions and localization. BA indicates the probable Brodmann area, for cortical areas, of activation in the group average data as determined from the atlas of Talairach and Tournoux (1988). Activation laterality is denoted by R and L; when bilateral, a B is used. Tal Coordinates denotes the Talairach coordinates using the atlas of Talairach and Tournoux (1988) of the voxel with the maximum p value for the KS maps of pre- versus postinfusion time points and overlapping correlation regions (except where denoted by an asterisk, in which case the coordinates denote the location of the voxel with maximum p value for the correlational analysis when no significant activation was present in the KS maps of the group average data). Coordinates are expressed in mm from the anterior commissure: R/L, right (+)/left (−); A/P, anterior (+)/posterior (−); S/I, superior (+)/inferior (−). P value indicates the maximum p value for each activated cluster of voxels on the unsmoothed Kolmogorov-Smirnov statistical map. Regions are listed as significant if $p < 7.1 \times 10^{-6}$ (see Experimental Procedures). When NS (nonsignificant) is followed by a p value in parentheses, this indicates a region of activation that did not meet our significance threshold, yet due to symmetric placement with respect to another activation in the opposite hemisphere was included. Percent signal change was determined for each activation by taking all voxels around the max vox with $p < 10^{-5}$ and comparing the first 38 fMRI time points with the subsequent 98 time points. Proportion Individuals lists the number of subjects to the total number of subjects (N = 10) who showed activation ($p < 10^{-3}$ for each voxel) in each anatomically defined region of interest; these regions of interest may include one or more activations from the group average statistical analysis. Correlation Analysis lists the results of a multiple correlational analysis of the fMRI time data to the behavioral measures of rush and craving. A plus sign indicates a positive correlation, a minus sign indicates a negative correlation, and a ϕ indicates no correlation to the measure. To be tabulated, a correlation region had to have five voxels with $R > 0.70$ for each voxel (see Experimental Procedures). The symbol ± indicates two nearby correlation regions of opposite sign in the same anatomic region. In Table 3, note that two plus signs are placed in the craving column for one activation; in this case, one correlation region was correlated to similar degree with both rush and craving measures, while the other correlation region was uniquely correlated to craving alone.

a

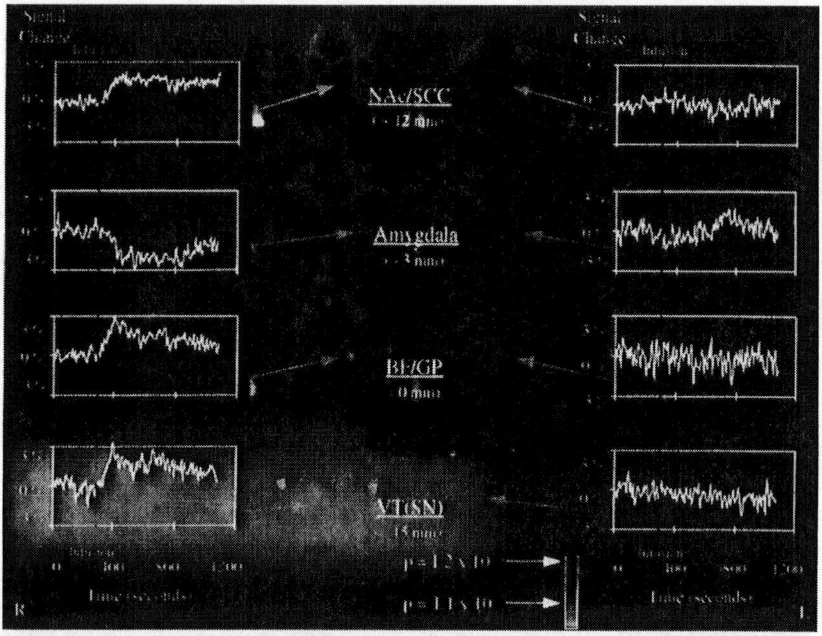
Signal
Change
NAc/SCC
Amygdala
BF/GP
VT(SN)
Time (seconds)
R
L

b

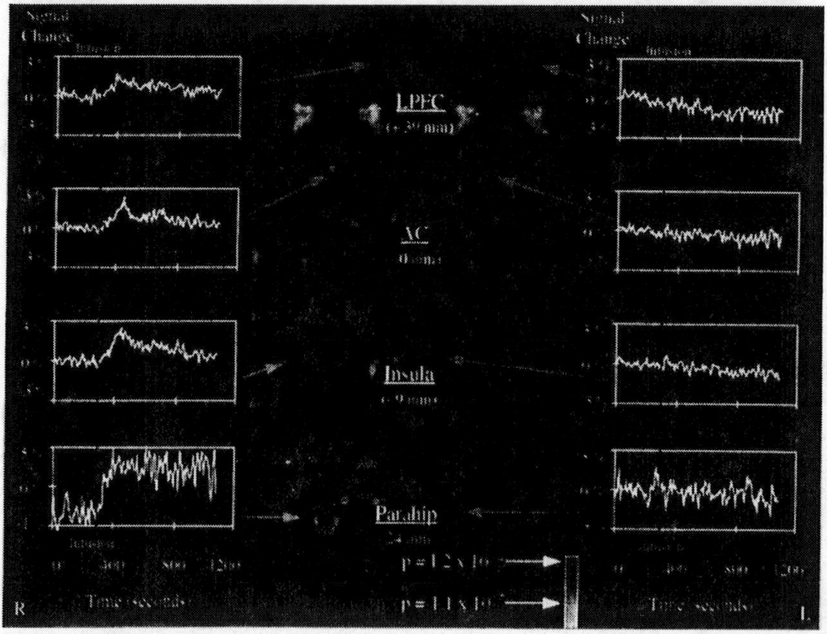
Signal
Change
LPFC
AC
Insula
Parahip
R
L

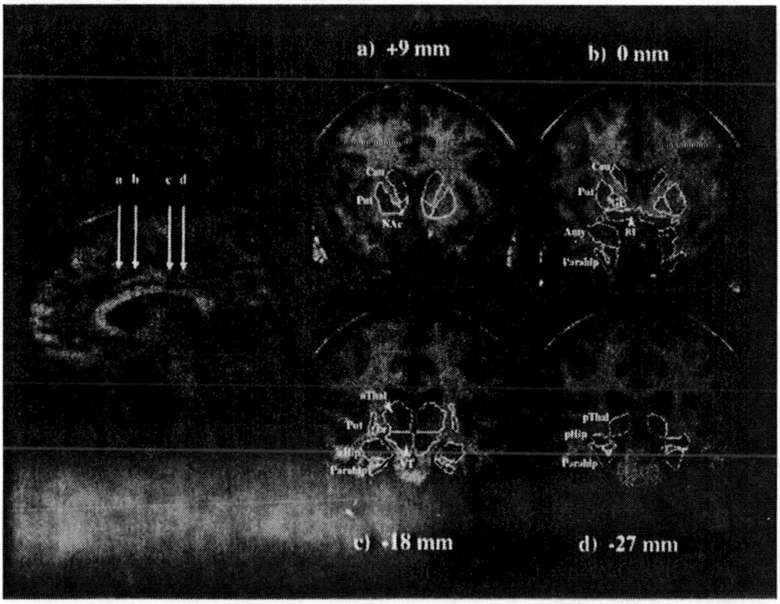

Figure 4. Selected Anatomic Definitions Used for Average and Individual Activation Localization

Structural T1 images from one individual are shown in the same orientation as the Talairach coronal position. Regions of interest for localization of statistical map activations are indicated in white on top of these gray scale structural images. Coronal slice planes are given with respect to the anterior commissure. The abbreviations and definitions used in this image are defined in the Expermental Procedures section on anatomic localization of activations. It has to be pointed out that the nucleus accumbens (NAc in the figure) can be distinguished on this individual's image from the subcallosal cortex that is adjacent and medial to it. This distinction between nucleus accumbens and subcallosal cortex is not possible on averaged images and is not always possible on individual images. Therefore, we refer to a nucleus accumbens/ subcallosal cortex region of interest for both our averaged data and our individual data.

seen in the comparison of preinfusion versus postinfusion time points include sections of the left parahippocampal gyrus, left cingulate gyrus, left insula, and right hippocampus.

Test–Retest Comparisons

Seven subjects had retest infusions at times ranging from 3.5 to 4 months after the first experiment. Of these seven, four subjects had interpretable cocaine infusion data after motion correction for test–retest comparison. These four subjects received their double-blind cocaine and saline infusions in the same order for the retest experiments as for the test experiments. To keep expectancies as similar as possible between test and retest conditions, subjects had been informed on several occasions that the identity of the first retest infusion did not imply the identity of the second retest infusion and that the MGH pharmacy maintained a double-blind experimental design for subjects and researchers during all retest infusions. Regions of positive signal change that were similar between average maps of the test and retest cocaine infusions are listed in Table 5. Note that activations that overlapped did not necessarily have statistical maxima in the exact same anatomic region. However, their statistical maxima were within 1.5 cm of each other or the two activation clusters had overlapping voxels at a high statistical threshold. Twenty-six of

Figure 3. Regional Brain Activation with Cocaine and Saline

(a) Images of subcortical brain regions showing significant fMRI signal changes after cocaine, but not after saline, infusions. On the left are Kolmogorov-Smirnov (KS) statistical maps at four coronal levels of pre- versus postinfusion time points for the average fMRI data from ten subjects who received cocaine. These KS statistical maps are overlaid in pseudocolor on corresponding gray scale average structural maps. Activations with positive signal change include the NAc/SCC, BF/GP, and VT, while activations with negative signal change include the amygdala. The signal intensity versus time graph for the activations (for all voxels with $p < 10^{-6}$ within the named region) is placed next to each image. On the right are identical slice planes overlaid with the KS statistical map for the saline infusion; the saline signal intensity versus time graphs for the same anatomic regions active during cocaine are placed next to the saline images to demonstrate the absence of comparable change.

(b) Images of other paralimbic and heteromodal cortex activations after cocaine and after saline infusions. Regions shown include the lateral prefrontal cortex (LPFC), anterior cingulate, insula, and parahippocampal gyrus. Image and graph layout follow the conventions described in (a).

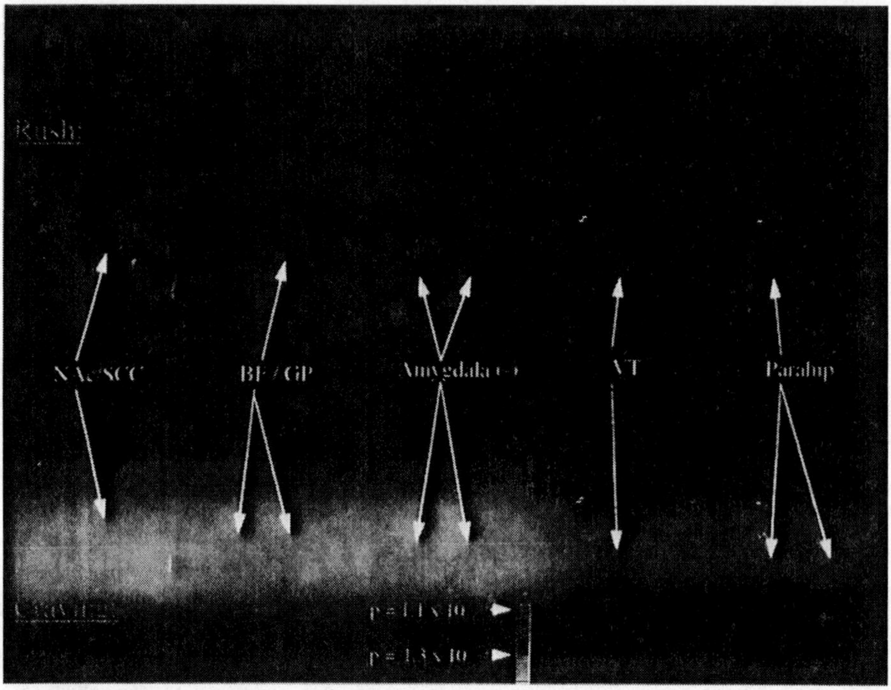

Figure 5. Multiple Correlation Images

Correlation images associated with rush and with craving are displayed as coronal images, respectively, in the top row and the bottom row. Each correlation map is presented as a pseudocolor p value map superimposed on a gray scale structural image. Coronal images represent slices from +15 mm, 0 mm, −3 mm, −18 mm, and −24 mm with respect to the anterior commissure. Regions highlighted in this figure were more strongly correlated with one behavioral measure than another and include the NAc/SCC, BF/GP, Amygdala, VT, and parahippocampal gyrus.

thirty-two postcocaine activations in the test sample were matched by similar activations in the retest experiments, including subcortical regions originally hypothesized to be activated, namely the NAc/SCC (see Figure 6), basal forebrain, and caudate. For regions such as the NAc/SCC, the percent signal change for voxels meeting the threshold of $p < 10^{-5}$ in the test condition (left = 3.8%, right = 2.4%) was marginally higher than the percent signal change for the retest condition (left = 2.3%, right = 2.1%), though more voxels met the $p < 10^{-5}$ threshold on retest.

Other areas of activation that matched between test and retest conditions included parahippocampal regions, thalamic, insular, and cingulate regions. For the average map of four subjects in the test condition, there were fewer activations overall (N = 32) than for the average map with ten subjects (N = 92 activations with positive signal change). This raises the possibility that the smaller cohort had insufficient power to identify smaller magnitude signal changes, thus the test cohort's activation profile may be a subset of the larger group's activation profile. In support of this possibility is the observation that of the 56 regions observed with the cocaine retest experiment, 28 regions were not matched by previous test activations, but 22 of these directly matched activations seen with the total cohort of ten subjects. Other factors that might contribute to the heterogeneity include the current level of cocaine usage or altered anxiety or positive expectancy related to the prior experience with our experimental procedures.

Saline Infusion

Foci of Signal Change

In the ten subjects with interpretable data, saline infusions produced no positive signal change in limbic or paralimbic regions. One focus of negative signal change was noted in the left temporal pole, which approximated a similar activation for the cocaine infusion. For areas outside of limbic and paralimbic regions, positive signal changes were noted in the inferior frontal gyrus, inferior/middle temporal gyri, and extrastriate region (see supplemental Table 8 http://www.neuron.org/cgi/content/full/19/3/591/T8) and negative signal changes in lateral frontal cortex, superior temporal gyri, and extrastriate cortex (see supplemental Table 9 http://www.neuron.org/cgi/content/full/19/3/591/T9). All five positive activations with saline matched the location of activations

Table 5. Test–Retest Cocaine Infusions: Regions of Similarity for Foci of Positive Signal Change

Test					Retest					
Anatomy (Region/BA)	Tal Coordinate R/L	A/P	S/I	Vox #	Anatomy (Region/BA)	Tal Coordinate R/L	A/P	S/I	Vox #	Proximity (<1.5 cm)
Subcortical Gray Structures										
Caudate/NAc	25	−27	18	8	Caudate	18	−12	21	77	−
Caudate/NAc	9	15	−3	81	GO a11	3	15	−6	160	+
BF/GP	−21	0	−6	10	BF/GP	−15	3	0	23	+
Thalamus/pThal	6	−27	12	62	Caudate	18	−12	21	77	−
					Cingulate a23	3	−27	28	43	−
Temporal Lobe										
Lateral and Intrasylvian Surfaces										
GTm a21	43	−6	−15	28	GTm a21	46	−18	−9	26	+[a]
Insula	37	−15	−3	38						+
Insula	−40	−15	−6	129	Insula	−40	−9	0	63	+
					GTm a21	−46	−24	−3	57	+
Insula	−40	6	0	45	Insula	−40	−9	0	63	+
Insula	−34	12	18	12	Insula	−37	18	6	66	+[a]
Medial Paralimbic Cortices										
Cingulate a24	0	−3	40	8	Cingulate a24	3	9	34	83	+
Cingulate a23/31	21	−27	34	13	Cingulate a23	12	−18	34	18	+
					Cingulate a23	3	−27	28	43	−
Parahip a35	18	−36	−12	89	GF a37	46	−51	−21	152	−
					GF a20/36	34	−33	−15	26	+[a]
Parahip a28/36	−21	−24	−21	83	Thalamus/pThal	−18	−15	3	17	−
					Parahip a35/36	−28	−27	−15	150	+

Table 5 shows which activations were similar between test and retest conditions for the cocaine infusions. Specific anatomic regions are described using the nomenclature discussed in Experimental Procedures with the exception of the following terms: GTm (gyrus temporalis medius), GF (gyrus fusiformis), GO (gyrus orbitales). BA indicates the probable Brodman area, for cortical areas, of activation. Under Tal Coordinate are the Talairach coordinates (Talairach and Tournoux, 1988) of the voxel with the maximum p value as determined from the KS maps (Breiter et al., 1996b). Coordinates are expressed in mm from the anterior commissure: R/L, right (+)/left (−); A/P, anterior (+)/posterior (−); S/I, superior (+)/inferior (−). The number of voxels around the max vox that meet the p value threshold of $p < 10^{-5}$ are listed under Vox #. Proximity lists whether the voxels with the maximum p values for each activation are within 1.5 cm of each other; thus a plus sign is placed in the last column if they are <1.5 cm apart, or a minum sign is placed if they are more than 1.5 cm apart.

[a] Indicates there is no overlap, but the max vox of the two activations are within 1.5 cm of each other.

seen in the cocaine maps; only one negative saline signal change, in the superior temporal gyrus, matched the location of an activation with negative signal change following cocaine infusion.

Test–Retest Comparisons

As with the cocaine test–retest comparisons, four of seven subjects had interpretable saline infusion data for test–retest comparison after motion correction. For the saline test–retest comparison with four individuals, no limbic or paralimbic regions were activated. For regions outside of limbic and paralimbic regions, six of the test activations were also similar to those seen with retest. Of these six activations, four of the six approximated activations seen with the average saline map of ten individuals, suggesting that the subgroup of four represent a good approximation of the group of ten.

The saline retest data evidenced multiple new activations not seen during the first saline test. The majority of these (10/16) were in the striate, extrastriate, and ventral temporal cortex implicated in ventral stream information processing for vision (Tootell et al., 1995). Eleven of the sixteen activations were similar to activations seen with the initial cocaine infusion for the total cohort and the retest cocaine infusions in the subgroup of four individuals (Table 5). Most striking was the appearance of activations in the bilateral NAc/SCC (Talairach coordinates: R/L −9, A/P 18, S/I 3; R/L 9, A/P 15, S/I −3) and the right insula (Talairach coordinates: R/L 40, A/P −15, S/I 0). The saline retest NAc/SCC (Figure 7) and insula activations closely approximated the same activations seen for the initial cocaine infusion in the total cohort (see Tables 1–4) and the cocaine NAc/SCC activation that correlated more with maximum ratings of craving than with rush (Tables 1–4). Moreover, these NAc/SCC and insula activations were similar to the same activations in the cocaine condition that showed good cocaine test–retest reproducibility (Table 5). Compared to the bilateral NAc/SCC activations seen with cocaine test–retest infusions, the bilateral NAc/SCC activations seen with saline retest infusion demonstrated a lower percent signal change (left = 0.4%, right = 1.5%) for all voxels meeting the threshold of $p < 10^{-5}$. On the basis of location of activation maxima, 11 of the 16 new activations seen with saline retest infusion in the NAc/SCC, the frontal cortex, and the temporal cortex were seen with either the cocaine test or retest infusions.

Discussion

Following an infusion of cocaine under double-blind conditions, cocaine-dependent subjects demonstrated significant increases in HR and MBP and decreases in $ETCO_2$. Cocaine plasma concentration reached maximum at ~7 min after infusion. Subjects reported early

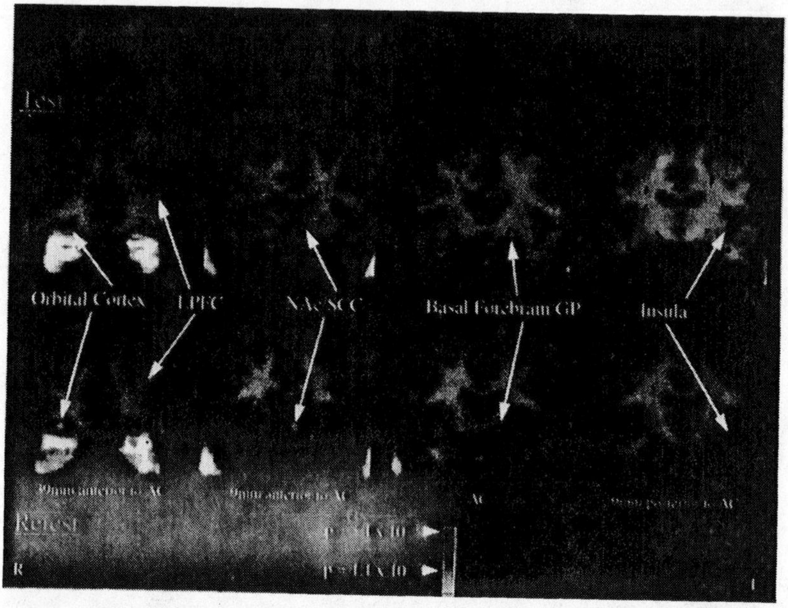

Figure 6. Test–Retest Cocaine Experiments

The Kolmogorov-Smirnov (KS) statistical maps (unsmoothed) for the average fMRI data in Talairach space from four subjects who had test–retest cocaine infusions are displayed in pseudocolor on top of gray scale structural images from these same subjects. Coronal slices are identified by their relationship in mm to the anterior commissure (AC).

maxima ~3 min after infusion for behavioral ratings of rush and high and later maxima for behavioral ratings of craving and low. Thus, maximal subjective euphoria was reported during the distribution phase of cocaine plasma kinetics, before maximal intravascular cocaine levels had been attained.

Brain regions that showed focal increases in BOLD signal at the time of onset of subjective measures of euphoria included putative brain reward circuitry (NAc/SCC, basal forebrain, and VT), caudate, putamen, thalamus, medial temporal and paralimbic regions (hippocampus, parahippocampal gyrus, cingulate cortex, and insula), brainstem (pons), and neocortical regions such as the lateral prefrontal cortex, lateral temporal cortex, parietal cortex, and occipital cortex. Decreases in fMRI signal were also noted in the amygdala, temporal pole, and medial frontal cortex, although the latter regions were in close proximity to areas of susceptibility artifact (see below). In comparison to cocaine, saline produced few regions of fMRI signal increase, limited to lateral prefrontal and temporo-occipital cortex. Small regions of signal decrease were also noted in the lateral prefrontal cortex and temporal cortex. All of the four positive temporal lobe activations seen during the saline infusion, along with the negative temporal pole activation, were also seen in the cocaine condition.

Multiple correlational analysis of averaged behavioral ratings with averaged cocaine fMRI data indicated differences in the temporal pattern of activation, which can be associated with rush and with craving ratings (Figure 8). Brain activation correlated with rush ratings was noted in a subset of regions associated in animal experiments with brain reward such as the VT, left basal forebrain, midbrain and pontine brainstem, bilateral caudate nucleus, and right cingulate gyrus. All of these regions are directly connected with the VT or the nucleus accumbens. Other brain activations in regions not previously implicated in animal models of drug self-administration or BSR, which showed a similar pattern of early transient signal maxima, included regions of prefrontal, parietal, temporal, and occipital cortex. Brain activation correlated with craving measures was noted in the NAc/SCC and right parahippocampus. A negative correlation with craving was also noted in the amygdala (a region with negative fMRI signal change on the average maps).

Limitations

In this study, subjects exhibited head movement following both cocaine and placebo infusions despite use of a bite bar. Complete movement correction was possible for some subjects with maximal displacements up to ~3 mm, although in some subjects, complex movements of similar magnitude produced unacceptable residual motion artifacts. As with our previous experience with a psychiatric population (Breiter et al., 1996b), a significant proportion of studies (6/17 cocaine infusions and 4/15 saline infusions) had to be discarded due to uncorrectable movement.

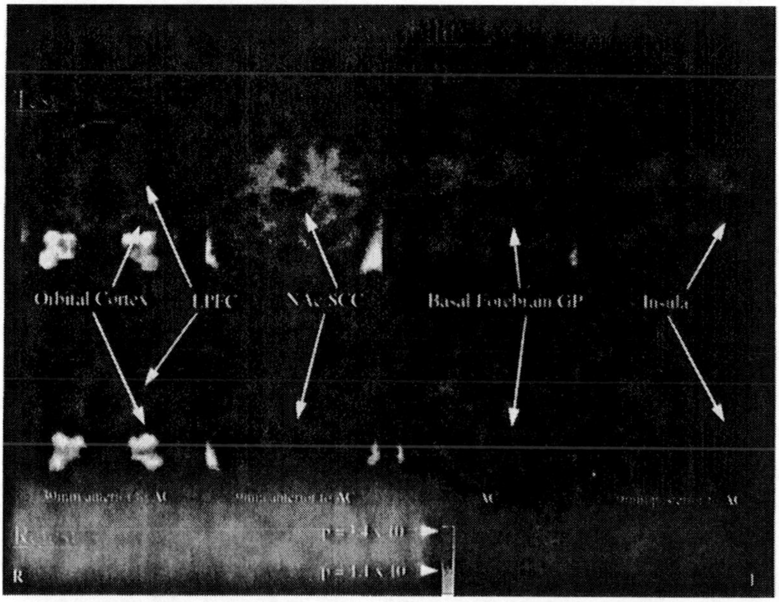

Figure 7. Test–Retest Saline Experiments

The Kolmogorov-Smirnov (KS) statistical maps (unsmoothed) are displayed as described in Figure 6, but for the four subjects who had test–retest saline infusions. Note the NAc/SCC activaton in the cocaine test (Figure 6) but not the saline test condition (this figure). By the retest, NAc/SCC activation could also be observed in response to the saline condition. Despite this generalization of response, NAc/SCC activation still represented a larger percent signal change for both the test and retest cocaine conditions.

Motion correction must also be considered in the context of its contribution to altered spatial resolution. Our voxel size during imaging was $3.125 \times 3.125 \times 8$ mm, which would appear adequate to resolve some subnuclei of larger subcortical structures. But, the combination of (1) motion correction, (2) transformation into Talairach space, and (3) averaging alter our effective spatial resolution to approximately 1 cm^3. Activations from averaged data in our study, thus, cannot be attributed with certainty to specific subnuclei of larger gray matter structures. Indeed, any anatomic localization with averaged data sets and superimposition of different structural and functional data acquisitions must be considered in probabilistic terms. This is the case even for individual statistical maps superimposed on structural images, albeit to a lesser degree, since images are superimposed from different acquisitions with the potential for movement between them, as well as different spatial warping and signal-to-noise characteristics. These issues are apparent with the test–retest data, where some activations that overlap do not necessarily have statistical maxima in the identical anatomic spot. This could be due to limitations imposed by our effective spatial resolution or noise of physiological origin in our underlying fMRI measurements.

Some regions, such as the NAc/SCC, basal forebrain, hypothalamus, and amygdala, are near areas with a high potential for magnetic susceptibility artifact, primarily seen on echo-planar images as signal dropout. Given unpredictable effects on T2*-weighted signal change from regions with high susceptibility, especially with concurrent motion, we checked and confirmed that activations seen with the cocaine and saline infusions did not overlap regions of susceptibility artifact on the functional images. For this reason, regions such as the medial frontal cortex and temporal pole, which showed large negative signal changes that were proximal to areas of susceptibility artifact, cannot be considered reliable activations.

Two issues regarding experimental design need to be mentioned. This study incorporated double-blind conditions and subject instructions designed to equalize cocaine expectancy for each infusion, in both test and retest conditions. Despite these precautions, since subjects knew they would only receive a single infusion per scan and could feel the infusion volume as it was administered, the blind only lasted a few minutes past the infusion, after which all subjects knew whether they had received cocaine or saline. This was clearly reflected, for both test and retest conditions, in the absolutely uniform zero ratings for rush and high following saline.

Secondly, in the design of the overall study, multiple attempts were made to distinguish BOLD fMRI signal

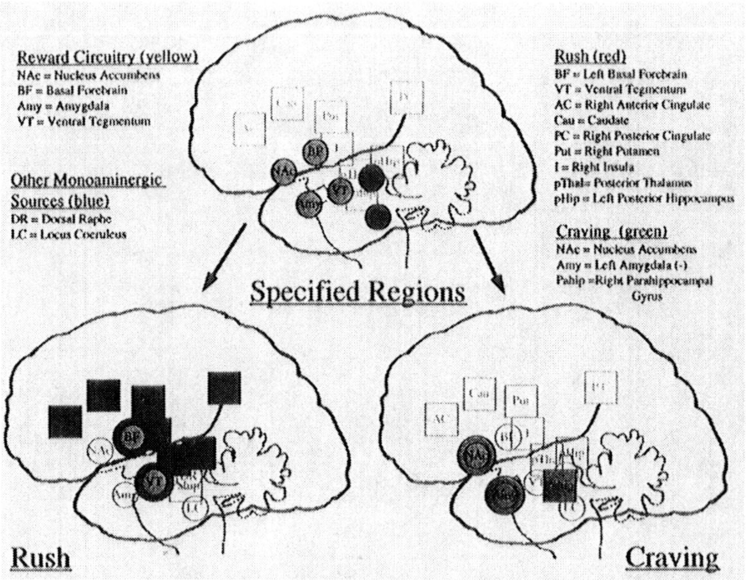

Figure 8. Summary Schematic of Limbic and Paralimbic Brain Regions that Correlate with Euphoria (in Red) Versus Those Regions that Correlate with Craving (in Green)

Above these summary schematics is a schematic of the brain regions (in yellow) we predicted to be active after the infusion of cocaine. Two other brainstem monoaminergic regions, potentially encompassed in a pontine activation seen in our baseline versus postinfusion comparison, are also illustrated in blue. This pontine activation did correlate with behavioral ratings for rush.

changes due to region specific activation from changes due to systemic physiological or direct vascular effects of cocaine. Each infusion scan (see Figure 1) was bracketed by control experiments to determine whether regionally specific primary visual cortex activation was altered by the cocaine or placebo infusion, and how much change there was in global cerebral blood flow (Gollub et al., submitted). The results of these control experiments clearly support our interpretation of focal regional activation following cocaine infusion. Focal primary visual cortical activation was quantitatively unchanged following cocaine or saline. Moreover, although the flow-sensitive scan revealed an approximate 14% decrease in flow-related signal in cortical gray matter, no such change was measured during BOLD scanning. Even with these reassurances, though, a strong caveat should be added to the results of local gray matter changes related to cocaine; namely, that they were observed in the presence of significant cardiovascular and respiratory effects from cocaine.

Finally, a general issue regarding the linkage of fMRI signal to underlying neuronal activity must be mentioned. At this time, the relationship of BOLD signal to pre- and postsynaptic mechanisms of neurotransmission is unknown. Thus, it is conceivable that increased fMRI signal in the NAc/SCC, for example, could be due to increased activity of inhibitory (GABAergic) nerve terminals, which produce a decrease in neuronal cell body activity in the NAc/SCC rather than excitatory input to or output from the NAc/SCC, which would be associated with a regional increase in neuronal cell body activity. The linkage of fMRI signal to underlying neuronal activity remains an area of continuing research, which is needed to connect more directly the results of this neuroimaging study and others to the body of basic substance abuse research using animals.

Regions with Short Duration Signal Change and Relation to Euphoria

Two of the behavioral ratings used in this experiment, rush and high, described separable features of the subjective experience of euphoria or pleasure. Such subjective measures can only be obtained with human subjects. With animal experiments, behavioral scientists have been limited to investigation of the effects of "rewarding" stimuli on observable behavior (White et al., 1987) based on repeated approach behaviors or response repetitions. It can be hypothesized that acutely rewarding behavioral stimuli (i.e., cocaine) administered to a conscious (human) subject produce not only behavioral effects (reinforcement) and lead to encoding of emotional memories but also produce subjective pleasure that can be reported.

Behavioral research with animal models has shown that increased dopamine transmission in the nucleus accumbens is associated with behavioral responses to rewards. However, the exact relationship of mesoaccumbens dopamine function to the action of a reward as an incentive or as a reinforcement has been an area of controversy (Richardson and Gratton, 1996). The implicit assumption in relating dopamine transmission in the nucleus accumbens to cocaine use is that dopamine transmission is a central correlate of the reinforcing actions of rewards (Wise et al., 1978; Wise, 1982; Koob, 1992). Thus, in humans, we postulated that an acute change in fMRI activation in the nucleus accumbens area (NAc/SCC) would be correlated with behavioral measures of euphoria. The pattern of fMRI signal change could not be predicted, since dopamine produces complex modulatory effects on postsynaptic neurons and because the relationship of the BOLD signal to pre- and postsynaptic mechanisms of neurotransmission is unknown. What we found was that fMRI activation in the VT (the source of dopamine for the nucleus accumbens), basal forebrain, pontine brainstem, caudate, insula, cingulate gyrus, and prefrontal cortex were correlated with behavioral measures of euphoria.

Computational models of the output of VT neurons suggest that they code for a deviation between the experienced reward and the previous predictions for reward. VT neurons would accordingly report ongoing prediction errors for reward and deliver a signal to forebrain targets to alter ongoing processing of reward predictions and the direction of reward-maximizing actions (Schultz et al., 1997). Thus, in the naive state, VT neuronal firing is increased in nonhuman primates early in the acquisition of lever pressing behavior (Schultz, 1986; Nishino et al., 1987; Romo and Schultz, 1990; Schultz and Romo, 1990; Ljungberg et al., 1992; Schultz et al., 1993). However, after several lever press trials in the same experiments, simulating a more chronic state of drug use, VT neurons demonstrate electrophysiological decreases in response. In our fMRI study, subjects were chronic users but were naive to cocaine use in the fMRI environment. They showed a pattern of early but transient signal change in VT, which is analogous to the response of primates naive to cocaine. Perhaps the novelty of cocaine administration in the fMRI setting may have contributed to the observed VT activation. This formulation regarding learning effects could be confirmed by serial retest studies with larger cohorts than our current study.

Regions to which VT input might be important in mediating the subjective concomitants of reward and that demonstrated activation with early signal maxima and short duration and thus correlation with rush ratings include the cingulate gyrus and the basal forebrain. The cingulate gyrus has been associated both with euphoric experiences in humans induced by procaine (Ketter et al., 1996) but also, in direct contrast, with the emotional intensity of aversive events (Talbot et al., 1991; Sikes and Vogt, 1992; Coghill et al., 1994; Casey et al., 1996; Craig et al., 1996). The basal forebrain has also been implicated in affective function, in that it has been directly implicated in the results from BSR experiments. Since BSR was first observed by Olds and Milner (1954), evidence has accumulated that regions such as VT, lateral hypothalamus (Murray and Shizgal, 1991, 1996), and basal forebrain (Rompre and Shizgal, 1986; Shizgal et al., 1989; Arvanitogiannis et al., 1996) contain the neuron somata that generate this effect. It is important to note that the basal forebrain constitutes one of the primary outputs of both the nucleus accumbens and the amygdala (Heimer et al., 1997).

In our study, extensive brainstem activation distinct from the VT was also observed, including activation in the vicinity of regions for other monoaminergic systems such as the serotonergic system (primarily the dorsal raphe) and the noradrenergic system (the locus coeruleus). This other brainstem activation also demonstrated early signal maxima with rapid return to basal levels that correlated with rush ratings. FMRI BOLD scans in the brainstem are confounded by cardiac-induced motion. Thus, replication of our brainstem observations using a recently developed technique of cardiac gating with a subsequent T1 correction algorithm (Guimares et al., 1996) will be important.

Regions of Sustained Signal Change and Possible Relation to Cocaine-Induced Craving

In this study, no brain region showed statistically significant signal intensity changes that directly paralleled the change in behavioral ratings for cocaine-induced craving or dysphoria (i.e., with slow onset of signal change and peak effects after approximately 10 min). To a first approximation, the ramp function of the craving ratings is the same as the average motion displacement detected by the AIR algorithm. Since our baseline drift correction removed signal changes that would be correlated with this motion, the absence of brain regions with time course changes specific for cocaine-induced craving is a matter to be interpreted with caution.

Some brain regions did however show sustained activation that led to a higher degree of correlation with the craving ratings. Our observation, for instance, of sustained signal change in the NAc/SCC is the explanation for its stronger association with craving than with rush ratings. In general, the differences at high thresholds between the rush and craving correlation maps reflect a distinction between behavioral ratings with early peaks and shorter duration (i.e., rush) and ratings with prolonged time courses (i.e., craving; see signal time courses in Figures 3a and 3b). It is significant that subtraction of fMRI time courses with early maxima and short duration from those with prolonged time courses would produce a time course closely resembling that of the craving ratings. This suggests a possible model for craving in humans. Craving may not be mediated by one or two distinct brain regions; rather, postcocaine craving may reflect a change over time in the pattern of brain activation from cocaine. Many brain regions are active at the time that subjects report euphoria. Over time, though, only a few brain regions remain activated; this change in the pattern of brain regions activated may be causally related to the subjective experience of craving.

The observation of sustained activation in the NAc/SCC, which occurred over the time interval that subjects experienced cocaine-induced rush and then craving, links the NAc/SCC with both reinforcement and with incentive functions. This contrasts with the simple view that dopamine transmission in the nucleus accumbens area (NAc/SCC) is the central correlate of reward and therefore subjective euphoria. Although some studies have reported an association between feeding or consummatory behavior and elevated dopamine levels in the nucleus accumbens (Heffner et al., 1980; Hernandez and Hoebel, 1988; Radhakishun et al., 1988; Yoshida et al., 1992), other studies suggest that the increases in nucleus accumbens dopamine transmission do not result from consummatory behavior (Blackburn et al., 1986, 1989, 1992; Chance et al., 1987; Weatherford et al., 1991; McCullough and Salamone, 1992; Elbaz et al., 1993, Soc. Neurosci., abstract; McCullough et al., 1993; Phillips et al., 1993; Salamone et al., 1994) and that mesoaccumbens dopamine neurons respond to incentive rather than to reinforcing components of rewards (Kiyatkin and Gratton, 1994; Richardson and Gratton, 1996). Our fMRI data, showing a correlation between cocaine-induced craving and sustained activation in the NAc/SCC, supports a complex role for the NAc/SCC in the human, with a potential role in incentive as well as reinforcement.

Other brain regions with sustained signal change after early signal maxima included several lateral prefrontal regions and one section of the parahippocampal gyrus (see Figure 3b), though other parahippocampal activations did not display this behavior (see Tables 1–4). The parahippocampal gyrus has efferents to the nucleus accumbens and amygdala, is a primary input source for the hippocampus, and has been implicated not only in explicit memory (Squire and Knowlton, 1995) but also in the association of context to emotionally relevant stimuli during fear conditioning (LeDoux, 1993). The common sustained activation of the NAc/SCC and parahippocampal gyrus, along with relatively discrete sections of lateral prefrontal cortex, points to a distributed network of brain regions involved with the cocaine-induced craving.

Sustained negative signal change in the left amygdala was also observed. This left amygdala signal change needs to be discussed with the caveat that inspection of individual maps showed some heterogeneity of activation, in that three subjects evidenced positive signal change and only five subjects displayed negative signal change. Such heterogeneity in amygdala activation resembles electrophysiologic findings in rodents, in that acute intravenous cocaine produces mixed suppression and excitation in amygdalar neurons (Cunningham, 1995). In contrast, microiontophoretic application of cocaine in the amygdala uniformly produces suppression of spontaneous neuronal discharges (Cunningham, 1995), indicating that functional connectivity is important for mediating amygdala response to cocaine.

Our left amygdala data appear to contrast with other reports of positive correlation between amygdala activation and cue-elicited craving (Childress et al., 1996, Soc. Neurosci., abstract; Grant et al., 1996; Schweitzer et al., 1996, Soc. Neurosci., abstract). The amygdala has been implicated in the orientation to and remembering of affectively salient stimuli for social interaction (Leonard et al., 1985; Rolls, 1992; Breiter et al., 1996d). Interpretation of our current negative amygdala activation in the context of this other work can only be speculative. It is possible that cocaine-induced craving represents a distinct process from that of cue-conditioned craving (Everitt, 1997). Given the potential for expectancy effects in the current double-blind infusion experiment, order effects in each of the cue-conditioned craving experiments (Childress et al., 1996, Soc. Neurosci., abstract; Grant et al., 1996; Schweitzer et al., 1996, Soc. Neurosci., abstract), and differences in neuroanatomical resolution between our fMRI work and the PET studies of other investigators (Childress et al., 1996, Soc. Neurosci., abstract; Grant et al., 1996; Schweitzer et al., 1996, Soc. Neurosci., abstract), further work will be needed to assert that differences exist between craving during acute cocaine withdrawal and craving elicited by cues.

Signal Changes During Saline and Possible Relation to Expectancy and Craving

The lateral prefrontal and temporo-occipital activations observed with saline infusion were similar to activations after cocaine infusion and might represent a common effect from expectation or a chance similarity given the number of regions activated during the cocaine condition. It is unlikely they represent chance, since they were mostly replicated in saline retest experiments. The saline activations might be considered in the context of the results from a recent PET study of cue-induced cocaine craving in cocaine addicts (Grant et al., 1996), if one considers the saline infusion as a potential cue. In the study of Grant and colleagues (1996), increased glucose metabolism was reported in the lateral prefrontal and temporo-occipital cortices. It is interesting to note the similarity of regional activation between studies, even though our subjects rated craving at zero throughout the saline infusion.

The issue of cocaine expectancy also arises with regard to new activations observed with the saline retest experiments. Orbital cortex activation was noted bilaterally on saline retest; this region has been implicated in the suppression of expectancies in animals (Morgan et al., 1993; Morgan and LeDoux, 1995). Bilateral NAc/SCC activation was also observed with saline retest. Given theorized involvement of the nucleus accumbens with the processing of predictions of reward (Schultz et al., 1997) and observations of altered conditioned responses in animals after only one cocaine dose (Weiss et al., 1989), it is possible the NAc/SCC activation on saline retest may represent one-trial learning. Further work will be needed to evaluate the time course of change in regions such as the NAc/SCC to determine if these represent learning effects (Schultz et al., 1997).

Conclusions

During double-blind infusion experiments in cocaine-dependent subjects, we observed dramatic effects from cocaine in physiology, behavioral report, and fMRI brain activation that were not found following saline. A significant feature of this study was the continuous sampling of brain blood oxygenation changes to intravenous cocaine over 18 min, which was exploited for multiple correlational analysis with the behavioral data. Several brain regions showed short duration of activation that was well correlated with the reinforcement-related rating of rush, while other regions showed sustained activation, demonstrating some of the features associated with the incentive-related measure of craving. In particular, the VT and basal forebrain correlated more strongly with rush measures, while the NAc/SCC and amygdala correlated more strongly with craving measures, even though these latter two regions had early signal maxima as seen with the rush measures. Early but sustained activation in the NAc/SCC implies that it is activated during both rush and craving experiences, which contrasts with the general view of circuitry mediating reinforcement (Wise et al., 1978; Wise, 1982; Koob, 1992) and suggests the NAc/SCC is also involved with incentive functions.

In contrast to cocaine effects, saline produced activations in prefrontal cortex and lateral temporo-occipital cortex, most of which were also found active with cocaine, and resembled findings from other investigators during cue-induced craving in abstinent cocaine-dependent subjects (Childress et al., 1996, Soc. Neurosci., abstract; Grant et al., 1996; Schweitzer et al., 1996, Soc. Neurosci., abstract). The observation of NAc/SCC activation on saline retest infusion raises the possibility that generalization of expectancy across the two infusion conditions may occur within one trial; this hypothesis needs confirmation.

Our cocaine results provide evidence in the human for a functional integration of circuits involved with reinforcement and circuits involved with drug craving (see Figure 8). The known anatomic interconnections between limbic and paralimbic regions with short duration versus sustained alteration in BOLD signal converge on a core set of brain regions: the NAc/SCC, basal forebrain, amygdala, and VT. From animal research, there is evidence that the VT is necessary for reward prediction (summarized in Schultz et al., 1997), the amygdala for orienting to and remembering affectively significant stimuli (Everitt et al., 1991; LeDoux, 1992; Hatfield et al., 1996) and attentional modulation of perceptional function (Leonard et al., 1985; Rolls, 1992), the nucleus accumbens for determination and modulation of motoric responses toward perceptual stimuli and internal homeostatic needs (Le Moal et al., 1977; Kelley and Stinus, 1985; Fibiger and Phillips, 1986; White, 1986; Blackburn et al., 1989), and the basal forebrain for attention to internal state and attribution of primary reward (Shizgal et al., 1989; Arvanitogiannis et al., 1996). Future research will be important for determining whether or not these regions function in this manner in humans and how these functions produce incentive and reward.

Experimental Procedures

Subjects

Of the 17 subjects who completed the experimental protocol, 13 were men and four were women (mean age = 34.5 ± 4.6 years; education = 12.2 ± 1.6 years; weight = 79.6 ± 17.8 kg; Addiction Severity Index [McLellan et al., 1980] Composite Score [0 to 1.00] on the drug dimension = 0.18 ± 0.13 and on the alcohol dimension = 0.27 ± 0.25; Hamilton Anxiety Scale [0 to 54] 2.94 ± 2.08; Hamilton Depression Scale [0 to 52] 7.53 ± 5.66). All subjects were right-handed. Except for cocaine addiction, they were medically and neurologically normal by physical exam, review of systems, blood work including electrolytes, liver function tests, cell blood count, and toxicology. No subject had a history of head trauma with loss of consciousness or had any family history of sudden cardiac death or cardiac disease. All subjects tested negative for human immunodeficiency virus (HIV). Women were not pregnant by βHCG testing and were scanned at the midfollicular phase of their menstrual cycle. All subjects fulfilled criteria for cocaine dependence, with or without comorbid alcohol or marihuana abuse, by Mini-Structured Clinical Interview for DSM-IV (SCID) (American Psychiatric Association, 1994). Our subjects were selected to be heavy, long-term cocaine users (mean = 7.8 ± 6.0 years; days of cocaine use in 30 days prior to experiment = 16.2 ± 8.2 days). Current monetary expenditure for cocaine was $397.0 ± 318.0 over the week prior to the experiment. No subjects were seeking or receiving treatment for substance abuse at the time of the study. To be accepted into the imaging protocol, during screening, subjects had to have one positive urinalysis to confirm recent cocaine use, but had to be abstinent from cocaine and alcohol for at least 18 hr before the infusion. Approximately 18 hr before each imaging session, subjects underwent a screening IV test dose of 0.2 mg/kg in the MGH Mallinckrodt GCRC under the supervision of a cardiologist and psychiatrist to ascertain cardiac and neurological tolerance of the experimental procedures. They were subsequently monitored in the GCRC until the time of scanning. All subjects gave informed consent to participate in these procedures following the rules of the Subcommittee on Human Studies at MGH. Subjects were reimbursed for participation in this protocol on the basis of days in the hospital and could earn a bonus for completion of all scans. Reimbursement was with noncash vouchers (e.g., nontransferrable food coupons).

Experimental Design

Subjects were admitted to the MGH GCRC for the screening procedures; those meeting all criteria were boarded overnight on the unit in preparation for imaging the following day. The following morning, the subject had bilateral intravenous catheters placed (right forearm for cocaine or saline infusion, left forearm for serial venous blood sampling for quantitative cocaine levels). Scanning was performed between 11 AM and 3 PM, during which the subject was in the scanner for two periods of time, each lasting from 45 to 90 min. During each scanning period, one infusion was given, either cocaine (0.6 mg/kg, maximum dose 40 mg) or saline (both in a volume of 10 ml given over 30 s IV) in a randomized, double-blind order. Five different scans were performed during each period. The infusion itself was made 5 min into an 18-minute-long BOLD scan. The BOLD infusion scan was bracketed by flow-sensitive alternating inversion recovery (FAIR) and visual stimulation BOLD scans (the data from these scans were used to delineate the global versus regional signal changes from cocaine and are reported in a separate manuscript [Gollub et al., submitted]). The time interval between functional scans within a period was kept to a minimum. The entire sequence of five functional scans was completed within 45–60 min. The subject was removed from the scanner for a 15–30 min rest and then was returned to magnet and the sequence was repeated for the second infusion. A minimum of 2 hr had to pass between each double-blind infusion.

Subject Instructions

For the preexperiment test infusion with 0.2 mg/kg cocaine on the night before scanning, subjects were informed they would receive a small dose of intravenous cocaine in the presence of a cardiologist and a psychiatrist to screen for medical side effects from intravenous cocaine and to train them in making behavioral ratings of their experience.

For experiments performed in the magnet, subjects were informed they would receive two infusions to which both they and the experimenters were blind. Infusions could either be saline or 0.6 mg/kg of cocaine in saline; the experience of one infusion did not imply what would be the identity of the other. Subjects were further asked to continue behavioral ratings throughout the FAIR and BOLD infusion scans (~40 min in total) and to remain as motionless as possible to minimize fMRI movement artifacts. All subjects understood they could terminate the experiment at any time without explanation.

Plasma/Urine Monitoring

Sequential 4 ml venous blood samples were collected immediately before and at 1, 3, 5, 10, 15, 30, 60, 90, and 120 min following each infusion. The 120 min sample for the first infusion was also the preinfusion sample for the second infusion.

Physiological Monitoring

Physiologic monitoring was conducted using an InVivo OmniTrak 3100 patient monitoring system (Orlando, FL) modified to permit on-line computer acquisition of physiologic measurements. Each subject was fitted with chest leads to record the electrocardiogram (ECG) and to measure heart rate (HR), a nasal cannula to measure respiratory rate and $ETCO_2$, and a blood pressure cuff to measure noninvasively systemic MBP. The temporal resolution of the system for sampling blood pressure was once every 2 min. The InVivo system sampled and displayed updated values for each of the other parameters once per second except for the ECG trace, which was digitized at a rate of 100 Hz.

The measured physiologic parameters were ported to a Macintosh Power PC 7100 running a custom National Instruments LabView data acquisition program. This program allowed the simultaneous acquisition of (1) the digitized analog ECG trace signal acquired using a National Instruments MIO16L board, (2) the GE scanner J8 trigger pulse that indicated when the gradient coils of the magnet were firing, and (3) serial port read of ASCII characters reporting physiologic measures from the InVivo system.

Precautions taken to ensure safe conduct of the study included use of ACLS trained personnel, frequent running of mock codes with clocked performance of tasks and strict definition of individual tasks, and presence of a cardiologist at the time of all infusions whose sole responsibility was to monitor subject safety. Before and after completion of both infusions, subjects underwent a 12-lead ECG to determine the absence of any interval change from the experiments and to clear them for discharge home. Because of magnetohydrodynamic effects on the ECG tracing, a baseline rhythm strip was obtained prior to each drug infusion and all subsequent tracings were compared to that one.

Behavioral Monitoring

For both infusions, analog scales for behavioral response were projected via the LabView program and a back projection television system (Sharp Liquid Crystal, RU2000) outside the Faraday shield of the scanner. These projected stimuli were then focused via a biconvex lens (Buhl Optical) inside the Faraday shield onto a rear projection screen that was viewed through an overhead mirror in the magnet bore. For both infusions, subjects viewed images prior to actual experimentation so that images could be focused and centered in each subject's visual field.

During FAIR and BOLD infusion scans, behavioral measures of rush, high, low, and craving were obtained in a continuous sequence each minute. Thus, over each 15 s epoch, one rating scale would be projected for the subject's response. Given four scales, it took 1 min to cycle through the complete set of scales. Timing of scan initiation, infusion onset and offset, and scan completion were linked with ongoing behavioral reports to allow subsequent correlational analysis between behavioral ratings and fMRI acquisitions. Behavioral responses were acquired with a four-button button press that had been adapted to the magnet environment by construction with nonmagnetic components and filtering of its output at the Faraday shield.

To obtain meaningful behavioral ratings during scanning, subjects were trained beforehand. The day before scanning, subjects were interviewed in depth by one of two board-certified psychiatrists to describe fully their experience of cocaine intake. These descriptions were then categorized by the psychiatrist and subject into four components: the rush, high, low, and craving that were to be rated on an integer scale of 0 (none) to 3 (maximum). The individualized conventions for description of subjective responses were then tested, during the unblinded preinfusion with 0.2 mg/kg cocaine, on a portable computer with a program simulating that used in the MRI.

Of the four behavioral measures, only craving was defined operationally in terms of the action the individual wanted to engage in (to get more cocaine). The other three behavioral measures, rush, high, and low, were defined in terms of subjective feelings that were not necessarily associated with a behavioral output or associated with the planning and implementation of physical activity. Thus, by definition, only craving was defined as a motivational state. In general, rush experiences involved physical sensations of elevated heart rate and sweating, along with internal feelings variously characterized as "speeding" sensations and sensations of "being out of control". In contrast, the high experience was generally associated with feelings of self-confidence, well-being, and sociability. The low experience encompassed all negative subjective feelings potentially associated with cocaine use, such as anxiety, paranoia, dysphoria, or anhedonia; the majority of subjects in this study discussed the low in terms of dysphoric effect distinct from a diminishment in the high experience.

Imaging

Scanning was performed with a quadrature head coil and a 1.5 T MR scanner (General Electric) modified for echo-planar imaging (Advanced NMR). Imaging involved the following protocol. First, a sagittal localizer scan (conventional T1-weighted spoiled gradient refocused gradient echo [SPGR] sequence; through-plane resolution = 2.8 mm; 60 slices) was performed to orient, for subsequent scans, 15 contiguous axial slices covering the whole brain. This scan was also used as the structural scan for Talairach transformation. Next, an automated shimming technique was used to optimize B_0 homogeneity (Reese et al., 1995). This was followed by an SPGR T1-weighted flow-compensated scan (resolution = 1.6 mm × 1.6 mm × 8 mm), which was primarily obtained to aid Talairach transformation during data analysis (see Breiter et al., 1996b). The fourth scan was a T1-weighted echo-planar inversion recovery sequence (TI = 1200 ms, in-plane resolution = 1.57 mm) for high resolution structural images to be used in preliminary statistical maps but not with Talairach transformed or averaged maps. Finally, BOLD imaging was performed using an asymmetric spin echo $T2^*$-weighted sequence (TR = 8000, TE = 50, 180° refocusing pulse offset by −25 ms; FOV = 40 × 20 cm; in-plane resolution = 3.125 mm; through-plane resolution = 8 mm; 15 contiguous axial slices covering the whole brain) to measure "activation" (local changes in blood flow and oxygenation) (Bandettini et al., 1992; Kwong et al., 1992; Ogawa et al., 1992). Images were acquired interleaved for 136 time points for each infusion.

Data Analysis

Plasma/Urine Levels

Cocaine quantitative assays were performed by the MGH Clinical Chemistry Laboratory using a liquid chromatography with photodiode array detection method they developed (Puopolo et al., 1992), with minor modifications (flow rate increased from 2.0 to 2.6 ml/min and LCPCN column length increased from 150 to 250 mm). Intra-assay imprecision at 100, 20, and 10 mg/l for cocaine is 5.1%, 5.7%, and 6.6%, respectively.

Physiological Data

The data analysis and graphing program IGOR (WaveMetrics, Inc.) was used to analyze the data. Data were first analyzed by a two-way ANOVA with drug treatment (saline, cocaine) and time of measurement as factors. When significant F values were obtained for one of the physiologic measures, individual time points were compared by posthoc t tests to determine if (and at what times) the change from baseline was significant. The Bonferroni correction for multiple comparisons was used; the criteria for significance at the 0.05 level was $p < 0.007$.

Behavioral Data

The integer output for each behavioral rating was segregated by category of rush, high, low, and craving. For the group data in Figure 2, the 18 measures for each behavioral category obtained during the 18 min BOLD infusion scan were averaged for the nine subjects with both interpretable behavioral data and fMRI data. This averaged data was then utilized in the correlational analysis of the cocaine fMRI data.

BOLD Data for Initial fMRI Experiments and for Test/Retest Experiments

Motion Correction. To reduce head motion, each subject was positioned using a bite bar, and echo-planar data was motion corrected using an algorithm (Jiang et al., 1995) adapted from Woods et al.

(1992) and described elsewhere (Breiter et al., 1996b). Motion correction of the BOLD saline infusion data revealed an average maximal displacement of 1.8 ± 2.3 mm, resulting in a mean correction per time point of 0.6 ± 0.5 mm. For the cocaine infusion data, there was an average maximal displacement of 1.1 ± 0.7 mm, resulting in a mean correction per time point of 0.6 ± 0.4 mm. After motion correction, time series data were inspected to assure that no data set evidenced residual motion in the form of cortical rim or ventricular artifacts >1 voxel. There was no statistically significant difference in maximal displacement between paired groups of saline versus cocaine infusions ($p < 0.4$).

TALAIRACH TRANSFORMATION. Each individual's set of infusion-related functional images, along with the associated conventional structural scans, were transformed into Talairach space (Talairach and Tournoux, 1988; Breiter et al., 1996b, 1996d) and resliced in the coronal orientation over 57 slices with isotropic voxel dimensions (x, y, z = 3.125 mm). Because of possible movement between acquisitions of structural and functional scans, functional data were further fit to the structural scan by translation of exterior contours. For the cocaine and saline infusions, two subjects evidenced movement between structural and functional scans of >2 voxels in magnitude, and, therefore, were discarded from further analysis.

NORMALIZATION, AVERAGING, AND CONCATENATION. For cocaine and saline infusions, Talairach-transformed functional data were intensity scaled (i.e., normalized relative to a standard preinfusion epoch) so that all mean baseline raw magnetic resonance signals were equal. Talairach-transformed structural and functional data were then averaged by run across the ten subjects with interpretable cocaine infusion data and the ten subjects with interpretable saline infusion data; similar averaging of Talairach-transformed structural and functional data was performed for the four subjects used in the test/retest analysis (Breiter et al., 1995, Proc. Soc. Magn. Reson./Euro. Soc. Magn. Reson. Med. Biol., abstract; Breiter et al., 1995, Proc. Soc. Neurosci., abstract; Brieter et al., 1996b, 1996d).

VOXEL-BY-VOXEL STATISTICAL MAPPING. Unsmoothed Kolmogorov-Smirnov (KS) statistical images were constructed (Breiter et al., 1996b, 1996d) from these averaged data sets comparing baseline (N = 38 time points) and postinfusion (N = 98 time points) epochs. Drift correction (i.e., removal of a first-order linear function) was incorporated in the statistical calculation but not for the signal intensity time courses shown. Subsequently, clusters of activation were determined on data that were smoothed by a 0.7 pixel gaussian filter (~ Hamming filter in the spatial domain). To guide the determination of activation clusters, smoothed data sets were subjected to a cluster-growing algorithm (Jiang et al., 1996, Neuroimage, abstract; Bush et al., 1996, Neuroimage, abstract) and activation clusters listed that met a corrected p value threshold. The cluster-growing algorithm was set to select activations with maximum p values below $p < 10^{-5}$ and to separate activations with pixels of $p < 10^{-4}$ between them. All activation clusters were then evaluated on the unsmoothed data to ascertain that they met cluster constraints, did not overlap areas of susceptibility, had time courses consistent with the experimental paradigm, and could be anatomically localized (see below for details). The correction for multiple comparisons of this data, in order to maintain an overall $\alpha < 0.05$, was the Bonferroni correction for all gray matter voxels sampled in the brain, or $p < 7.1 \times 10^{-6}$ (Breiter et al., 1996d). To be tabulated, activations had to meet cluster constraints on the unsmoothed KS statistical maps as follows: for subcortical gray matter, three contiguous voxels with one voxel at $p < 7.1 \times 10^{-6}$ and two voxels at $p < 10^{-5}$; and for cortical activations, five contiguous voxels with one voxel at $p < 7.1 \times 10^{-6}$ and four voxels at $p < 10^{-5}$. The effect of such cluster constraints on statistical significance have been discussed previously by our group (Breiter et al., 1996b).

The time course of signal change was evaluated for each putative activation identified on statistical maps of averaged data by the cluster-growing algorithm. These signal intensity versus time curves were assessed to ascertain that activation did not precede infusion onset. All activations had to meet this constraint, along with anatomical constraints that the Talairach coordinate of their maximum voxel (i.e., the voxel with the lowest p value) was in the brain as assessed by the Talairach atlas (Talairach and Tournoux, 1988) and that the activation, when thresholded at $p < 10^{-5}$, did not extend outside the brain when superimposed over the Talairach-transformed structural images.

NEUROANATOMICAL ANALYSIS. We used a combined approach to anatomic localization of functional data. The group average data (GAD) were mapped using an approach focused on Talairach coordinates. In addition, the individual data (ID) were mapped using a region of interest-based approach, focused on the limbic and paralimbic areas.

Anatomic Localization of GAD. Statistical maps of group averaged data were superimposed over high resolution conventional T1-weighted images that had been transformed into the Talairach domain and averaged. Primary anatomic localization of activation foci was performed by inspection of these coronally resliced T1-weighted scans and via the Talairach coordinates of the maximum voxel from each activation cluster (see section on determination of activation clusters). Subcortical localization of activations followed the region of interest conventions described below and demonstrated in Figure 4. All activations were checked against the functional image data to ascertain that they did not overlap areas of susceptibility artifact. Such overlap was determined by whether or not a voxel's signal intensity during the baseline was less than the average voxel in its slice by 50% of the difference between the average voxel signal intensity in the slice and the average voxel signal intensity outside of the slice.

Anatomic Localization of ID. To assess the degree to which subcortical activations seen in the group represent common activations across the population, as opposed to the effect of strong activations in a few subjects, each individual's Talairach-transformed T1 high resolution scan was inspected and regions of interest (ROIs) defined. Visual inspection of the superimposed KS statistical maps, thresholded at a liberal statistical threshold (KS, $p < 0.001$), was then performed to determine if activation was present in each of the anatomic structures discussed below. These results were tabulated as a ratio of individuals showing lateralized activation in that structure to the total number of subjects evaluated (N = 10). As our predictions involved only subcortical structures, our individual analysis also focused on noncortical regions, with the exception of medial paralimbic and intrasylvian cortices.

The methods used for definition of the subcortical ROIs followed the conventions of the MGH Center for Morphometric Analysis. These ROIs were defined by use of specific anatomic landmarks identified by direct visualization of each individual Talairach-transformed T1 anatomic scan. These coronal scans had voxel dimensions of x, y, z = 3.125 mm, a matrix of 49 × 37 × 57, and were viewed on the computer monitor with a size of 38 mm × 31 mm (see Figure 4). Key landmarks necessary for anatomic localization included the anterior commissure (AC), posterior commissure (PC), lateral geniculate nucleus (LGN), mammillary body (MB), substantia nigra (SN), anterior and posterior extents of amygdala, anterior and posterior extents of hippocampus, posterior extent of pulvinar, collateral sulcus, and splenium of corpus callosum.

Sixteen ROIs were defined to encompass the following structures: the caudate nucleus (Cau), the nucleus accumbens and subcallosal cortex (NAc/SCC), the putamen (Put), the pallidum (GP), the amygdala (Amy), the anterior and posterior insula (aINS and pINS), the anterior and posterior hippocampus (aHip and pHip), the parahippocampal gyrus (Parahip), the precommissural and postcommissural cingulate gyrus (aCG and pCG), the basal forebrain (BF), the precommissural and postcommissural thalamus (aThal and pThal), the lateral geniculate nucleus (LGN), and the ventral tegmentum (VT: including SN and surrounding region). Definitions for each of these ROIs were as follows: Cau extents reached from the anterior tip of its head to the part of its body corresponding at the coronal level of the LGN. NAc/SCC was identified at the inferior junction between the head of Cau and the Put. It was delimited superiorly by a line connecting the inferior corner of the lateral ventricle and the inferiormost point of the internal capsule abutting NAc/SCC and laterally by a vertical line passing from the latter point. Put, GP, VT, LGN, and Amy were directly visualized, and the posterior extent of Amy was at the identical coronal plane as the anterior tip of aHip. The posterior extent of the aHip was the coronal plane in front of the PC; the PC plane was the anterior border of pHip. The posterior border of the pHip was identified by direct visualization. Parahip was limited superiorly by the hippocampus or the amygdala and inferiorly by the collateral sulcus. By convention, we did not consider Parahip activation behind the posterior end of the hippocampus.

The insula was directly identified on the coronal plane throughout its anteroposterior extent; its anterior portion (aINS) continued to the coronal plane before the AC while its posterior extent (pINS) included the coronal plane with the AC. The precommissural cingulate (aCG) extended from the paracingulate sulcus anteriorly to the coronal plane anterior to the posterior commissure. Its superior border was determined by the paracingulate sulcus through the coronal slice containing the AC and, behind this plane, the cingulate sulcus. Its inferior border was defined by the paracingulate sulcus (curving portion) anteriorly and the callosal sulcus posteriorly. The postcommissural cingulate (pCG) extended from the coronal plane of the PC anteriorly to the subparietal sulcus posteriorly. Its superior border was defined by the cingulate sulcus and the subparietal sulcus, whereas its inferior border was the anterior portion of the calcarine sulcus (Damasio, 1995; Caviness et al., 1996). BsFor region extended anteroposteriorly from the NAc level to the SN coronal section and medially to the hypothalamus (which extended anteroposteriorly from AC to include posteriorly the MB, having a vertical line at the level of the optic tract or the lateralmost extent of the optic chiasm of the internal capsule as its lateral border and the interhemispheric midline as its medial border). The thalamus was divided anteroposteriorly in two sectors. The aThal extended from the anterior tip of the thalamus to the coronal plane anterior to the posterior commissure, and pThal extended posterior to the PC, including the PC coronal section. The thalamic ROIs were defined inferiorly by the hypothalamic fissure.

Correlational Analysis of BOLD Data from the FMRI Experiments

A multiple correlational analysis was performed between group-averaged behavioral data ($N = 9$), and group-averaged fMRI data ($N = 10$). In one subject, the behavioral data was not time locked to the scanner due to computer malfunction, thus these data were not used in the group average of behavioral data. The multiple correlation technique involved cross-correlation of the group average behavioral ratings for rush and craving with the group average fMRI data to generate correlation coefficient (R value) maps and transformation of the R value maps via the Fischer transform into p value maps. To be tabulated, an activation had to have five contiguous voxels with $R > 0.70$ for each voxel. For 136 time points, an $R > 0.70$ corresponds to a $p < 10^{-20}$. Because we averaged ten subjects, this $R > 0.70$ corresponds to an $R > 0.22$ in the individual. The resultant maps illustrated the brain regions whose signal change resembled the time course of rating change for each category of subjective rating.

Comparison of BOLD Data from Test Experiments with Retest Experiments

For the subgroups of subjects that had interpretable repeat cocaine infusion scan data ($N = 4$) and those with interpretable repeat saline infusion scan data ($N = 4$), data analysis involving Talairach transformation, signal normalization, averaging, and statistical mapping followed the procedures described above. Also, as above, activations were determined using the same cluster-growing algorithm; activations were interrogated regarding proximity to susceptibility, relationship to experimental paradigm, and anatomy in similar manner. Activations were tabulated with the number of unsmoothed voxels in each activation cluster that met the criteria of $p < 10^{-6}$. Similarity of activation between test and retest conditions was determined by the proximity of the maximum voxels (i.e., with reference to p value threshold) for each activation and by overlap between the set of voxels in each cluster that met the threshold of $p < 10^{-6}$ (note: the Bonferroni threshold for multiple comparisons is $p < 7.1 \times 10^{-6}$). To be considered "similar" activations, they had to have their maximum voxels within 1.5 cm of each other or have at least one overlapping voxel at the strict $p < 10^{-6}$ threshold.

Acknowledgments

This work was supported by grants to H. C. B., R. L. G., and B. R. R. from the National Institute of Drug Abuse (grants #00265, #00275, and #09467) and to B. R. R. from the Heart, Lung, and Blood Institute of the NIH (grant #39810), Bethesda, Maryland. This work was also supported by a Young Investigator Award to H. C. B. from the National Alliance for Research on Schizophrenia and Depression (NARSAD).

We thank Terry Campbell and Mary Foley for technical assistance, Drs. Peter Fox, Nora Volkow, Anna-Rose Childress, Ron Hammer, and Steve Grant for critical review of the pilot data for this study, Drs. Joseph Coyle and Barry Kosofsky for critical comments on the manuscript, the clinical staff of the MGH GCRC for their clinical and technical assistance, Dr. Verne Caviness for consultation regarding anatomic localization of activation foci, Dr. Alex Guimares for technical assistance initiating these experiments, along with Monica Strauss, Elizabeth Huffman, Etienne Benson and William Kennedy for assistance with data analysis and manuscript preparation.

Received August 22, 1997; revised September 8, 1997.

References

Amaral, D.G., Price, J.L., Pitkanen, A., and Carmichael, S.T. (1992). Anatomical organization of the primate amygdala complex. In The Amygdala, J.P. Aggleton, ed. (New York: John Wiley-Liss), pp. 1–66.

American Psychiatric Association. (1994). DSM-IV: Diagnostic and Statistical Manual of Mental Disorders, 3rd Ed. Rev. (Washington, DC: American Psychiatric Association).

Apicella, P., Ljungberg, T., Scarnati, E., and Schultz, W. (1991). Responses to reward in monkey dorsal and ventral striatum. Exp. Brain Res. *85*, 491–500.

Arvanitogiannis, A., Waraczynski, M., and Shizgal, P. (1996). Effects of excitotoxic lesions of the basal forebrain on MFB self-stimulation. Physiol. Behav. *59*, 795–806.

Bandettini, P.A., Wong, E.C., Hinks, R.S., Tikofsky, R.S., and Hyde, J.S. (1992). Time course EPI of human brain function during task activation. Magn. Reson. Med. *25*, 390–397.

Blackburn, J., Phillips, A., Jakubovic, A., and Fibiger, H. (1986). Increased dopamine metabolism in the nucleus accumbens and striatum following consumption of a nutritive meal but not a palatable non-nutritive saccharine solution. Pharmacol. Biochem. Behav. *25*, 1095–1100.

Blackburn, J., Phillips, A., Jakubovic, A., and Fibiger, H. (1989). Dopamine and preparatory behavior: II. a neurochemical analysis. Behav. Neurosci. *103*, 15–23.

Blackburn, J., Pfaus, J., and Phillips, A. (1992). Dopamine functions in appetitive and defensive behaviors. Prog. Neurobiol. *3*, 247–279.

Breiter, H.C., Berke, J.D., Kennedy, W.A., Rosen, B.R., and Hyman, S.E. (1996a). Activation of striatum and amygdala during reward conditioning: an fMRI study. NeuroImage *3*, S220.

Breiter, H.C., Rauch, S.L., Kwong, K.K., Baker, J.R., Weisskoff, R.M., Kennedy, D.N., Kendrick, A.D., Davis, T.L., Jiang, A., Cohen, M.S., et al. (1996b). Functional magnetic resonance imaging of symptom provocation in obsessive-compulsive disorder. Arch. Gen. Psychiatry *53*, 595–606.

Breiter, H.C., Gollub, R., Weisskoff, R., Kennedy, W., Kantor, H., Gastfriend, D., Berke, J., Riorden, J., Matthew, T., Makris, N., et al. (1996c). Activation of human brain reward circuitry by cocaine observed using fMRI. Proc. Soc. Neurosci. *3*, 1933.

Breiter, H.C., Etcoff, N.L., Whalen, P.J., Kennedy, W.A., Rauch, S.L., Buckner, R.L., Strauss, M.M., Hyman, S.E., and Rose, B.R. (1996d). Response and habituation of the human amygdala during visual processing of facial expression. Neuron *17*, 875–887.

Brown, E.E., Robertson, G.S., and Fibiger, H.C. (1992). Evidence for conditional neuronal activation following exposure to a cocaine-paired environment: role of forebrain limbic structures. J. Neurosci. *12*, 4112–4121.

Casey, K.L., Minoshima, S., Morrow, T.J., and Koeppe, R.A. (1996). Comparison of human cerebral activation pattern during cutaneous warmth, heat pain, and deep cold pain. J. Neurophysiol. *76*, 571–581.

Caviness, V.S., Meyer, J., Makris, N., and Kennedy, D.N. (1996). MRI-based topographic parcellation of human neocortex: an anatomically specified method with estimate of reliability. J. Cog. Neurosci. *8*, 566–587.

Chance, W.T., Foli-Nelson, T., Nelson, J.L., and Fischer, J.E. (1987). Neurotransmitter alterations associated with feeding and satiety. Brain Res. *416*, 228–234.

Coghill, R.C., Talbot, J.D., Evans, A.C., Meyer, E., Gjedde, A., Bushnell, M.C., and Duncan, G.H. (1994). Distributed processing of pain and vibration by the human brain. J. Neurosci. *14*, 4095–4108.

Craig, A.D., Reiman, E.M., Evans, A., and Bushnell, M.C. (1996). Functional imaging of an illusion of pain. Nature *384*, 259–260.

Cunningham, K.H. (1995). Modulation of serotonin function by acute and chronic cocaine: neurophysiological analyses. In The Neurobiology of Cocaine, R.P. Hammer, ed. (Boca Raton, FL: CRC Press), pp. 121–143.

Damasio, H. (1995). Human Brain Anatomy in Computerized Images. (Oxford: Oxford University Press).

DeWit, H., and Wise, R.A. (1977). Blockade of cocaine reinforcement in rats with the dopamine receptor blocker pimozide, but not with the noradrenergic blockers phentolamine or phenoxybenzamine. Can. J. Psychol. *31*, 195–203.

Everitt, B.J. (1997). Craving cocaine cues: cognitive neuroscience meets drug addiction research. Trends Cogn. Sci. *1*, 1–2.

Everitt, B.J., Morris, K.A., O'Brien, A., and Robbins, T.W. (1991). The basolateral amygdala-ventral striatal system and conditioned place preference: further evidence of limbic-striatal interactions underlying reward-related processes. J. Neurosci. *42*, 1–18.

Fibiger, H., and Phillips, A. (1986). Reward, motivation, cognition: psychobiology of neotelencephalic dopamine systems. In Handbook of Physiology: The Nervous System, Vol. 4, V.B. Mountcastle, F.E. Bloom, and S.R. Geiger, eds. (Bethesda, MD: American Physiological Society), pp. 647–675.

Fischman, M.W., and Schuster, C.R. (1982). Cocaine self-administration in humans. Fed. Proceed. *41*, 241–246.

Fischman, M.W., Schuster, C.R., Javaid, J., Hatano, Y., and Davis, J. (1985). Acute tolerance development to the cardiovascular and subjective effects of cocaine. J. Pharm. Exper. Ther. *235*, 677–682.

Foltin, R.W., and Fischman, M.W. (1991). Smoked and intravenous cocaine in humans: acute tolerance, cardiovascular and subjective effects. J. Pharm. Exper. Ther. *257*, 247–261.

Fowler, J.S., Volkow, N.D., Wolf, A.P., et al. (1989). Mapping cocaine binding sites in human and baboon brain in vivo. Synapse *4*, 371–377.

Gaffan, D., and Harrison, S. (1987). Amygdalectomy and disconnection in visual learning for auditory secondary reinforcement by monkeys. J. Neurosci. *7*, 2285–2292.

Gaffan, D., and Harrison, S. (1988). Disconnection of the amygdala from visual association cortex impairs visual reward-association learning in monkeys. J. Neurosci. *8*, 3144–3150.

Gawin, F.H. (1991). Cocaine addiction: psychology and neurophysiology. Science *251*, 1580–1586.

Gollub, R., Breiter, H., Weisskoff, R., Kennedy, W., Kantor, H., Gastfriend, D., Berke, J., Riordon, J., Matthew, T., Makris, N., et al. (1996). Global responses to cocaine during fMRI do not obscure regional activation. Proc. Soc. Neurosci. *3*, 1933.

Graham, J.H., and Porrino, L.J. (1995). Neuroanatomical basis of cocaine self-administration. In The Neurobiology of Cocaine, R.P. Hammer, ed. (New York: CRC Press, Inc.), pp. 3–14.

Grant, S., London, E., Newlin, D., Villemagne, V., Liu, X., Contoreggi, C., Phillips, R., and Margolin, A. (1996). Activation of memory circuits during cue-elicited cocaine craving. Proc. Natl. Acad. Sci. USA *93*, 12040–12045.

Guimares, A.R., Melcher, J.R., Talavage, T.M., Baker, J.R., Rosen, B.R., and Weisskoff, R.M. (1996). Detection of inferior colliculus activity during auditory stimulation using cardiac gated functional MRI with T1 correction. NeuroImage *3*, S9.

Hammer, R.P., Young, B.B., and Thomas, W.L. (1995). Regional metabolic manifestations of cocaine sensitization, tolerance, and withdrawal. In The Neurobiology of Cocaine, R.P. Hammer, ed. (New York: CRC Press, Inc.), pp. 15–29.

Hatfield, T., Han, J.-S., Conley, M., Gallagher, M., and Holland, P. (1996). Neurotoxic lesions of basolateral, but not central, amygdala interfere with pavlovian second-order conditioning and reinforcer devaluation effects. J. Neurosci. *16*, 5256–5265.

Heffner, T., Hartman, J., and Seidan, L. (1980). Feeding increases dopamine metabolism in the rat brain. Science *208*, 1168–1170.

Heimer, L., Harlan, R.E., Alheid, G.F., Garcia, M.M., and DeOlmos, J. (1997). Substantia innominata: a notion which impedes clinical-anatomical correlations in neuropsychiatric disorders. Neuroscience *76*, 957–1006.

Hernandez, L., and Hoebel, B. (1988). Food reward and cocaine increase extracellular dopamine in the nucleus accumbens as measured by microdialysis. Life Sci. *42*, 1705–1712.

Hyman, S.E. (1996). Addiction to cocaine and amphetamine. Neuron *16*, 901–904.

Ito, N., Ishida, H., Miyakawa, F., Naito, H. (1974). Microelectrode study of projections from the amygdaloid complex to the nucleus accumbens in the cat. Brain Res. *67*, 338–341.

Jiang, A., Kennedy, D.N., Baker, J.R., Weisskoff, R.M., Tootell, R.B.H., Woods, R.P., Benson, R.R., Kwong, K.K., Brady, T.J., Rosen, B.R., and Belliveau, J.W. (1995). Motion detection and correction in functional MR imaging. Hum. Brain Mapp. *3*, 1–12.

Johanson, C.E., and Fischman, M.W. (1989). The pharmacology of cocaine related to its abuse. Pharmacol. Rev. *41*, 3–52.

Jones, B., and Mishkin, M. (1972). Limbic lesion and the problem of stimulus-reinforcement association. Expl. Neurol. *36*, 362–377.

Kelley, A., and Stinus, L. (1985). Disappearance of hoarding behavior after 6-hydroxydopamine lesions of the mesolimbic dopamine neurons and its reinstatement with L-dopa. Behav. Neurosci. *99*, 531–545.

Ketter, T., Andreason, P., George, M., Lee, C., Gill, D., Parekh, P., Willis, M., Herscovitch, P., and Post, R. (1996). Anterior paralimbic mediation of procaine-induced emotional and psychosensory experiences. Arch. Gen. Psychiatry *53*, 59–69.

Kiyatkin, E., and Gratton, A. (1994). Electrochemical monitoring of extracellular dopamine in nucleus accumbens of rats lever-pressing for food. Brain Res. *652*, 225–234.

Koob, G.F. (1992). Neurobiological mechanisms of cocaine and opiate dependence. In Addictive States, C.P. O'Brien and J.H. Jaffe, eds. (New York: Raven Press), pp. 171–191.

Koob, G.F. (1996). Drug addiction: the yin and yang of hedonic homeostasis. Neuron *16*, 893–896.

Koob, G.F., and Bloom, F.E. (1988). Cellular and molecular mechanisms of drug dependence. Science *242*, 715–723.

Kwong, K.K., Belliveau, J.W., Chesler, D.A., Goldberg, I.E., Weiskoff, R.M., Poncelet, B.P., Kennedy, D.N., Hoppel, B.E., Cohen, M.S., Turner, R., et al. (1992). Dynamic magnetic resonance imaging of human brain activity during primary sensory stimulation. Proc. Natl. Acad. Sci. USA *89*, 5675–5679.

LeDoux, J.E. (1992). Emotion and the amygdala. In The Amygdala: Neurobiological Aspects of Emotion, Memory, and Mental Dysfunction, J.P. Aggleton, ed. (New York: John Wiley-Liss), pp. 339–351.

LeDoux, J.E. (1993). Emotional memory: in search of systems and synapses. Ann. N Y Acad. Sci. *702*, 149–157.

Le Moal, M., Stinus, L., Simon, H., Tassin, J., Thierry, A., Blanc, G., Glowinski, J., and Cardo, B. (1977). Behavioral effects of a lesion in the ventral mesencephalic tegmentum: evidence for involvement of A10 dopaminergic neurons. In Advances in Biochemical Psychopharmacology, Vol. 16, E. Costa and G.L. Gessa, eds. (New York: Raven Press), pp. 237–245.

Leonard, C.M., Rolls, E.T., Wilson, F.A.W., and Baylis, G.C. (1985). Neurons in the amygdala of the monkey with responses selective for faces. Behav. Brain Res. *15*, 159–176.

Ljungberg, T., Apicella, P., and Schultz, W. (1992). Responses of monkey dopamine neurons during learning of behavioral reactions. J. Neurophysiol. *67*, 145–163.

London, E.D., Cascella, N.G., Wong, D.F., Phillips, R.L., Dannals, R.F., Links, J.M., Herning, R., Grayson, R., Jaffe, J.H., and Wagner, H.N. (1990). Cocaine-induced reduction of glucose utilization in human brain. Arch. Gen. Psychiatry *47*, 567–574.

Louilot, A., Taghzouti, K., Simon, H., and Le Moal, M. (1989). Limbic system, basal ganglia and dopaminergic neurons. Brain Behav. Evol. *33*, 157–161.

Lyons, D., Friedman, D.P., Nader, M.A., and Porrino, L.J. (1996). Cocaine alters cerebral metabolism within the ventral striatum and limbic cortex of monkeys. J. Neurosci. *16*, 1230–1236.

McCullough, L., and Salamone, J. (1992). Involvement of nucleus accumbens dopamine in the motor activity induced by periodic food presentation: a microdialysis and behavioral study. Brain Res. *592*, 29–36.

McCullough, L., Cousins, M., and Salamone, J. (1993). The role of nucleus accumbens dopamine in responding on a continuous reinforcement operant schedule: a neurochemical and behavioral study. Pharmacol. Biochem. Behav. *46*, 581–586.

McLellan, A.T., Luborsky, L., and Woody, G.E. (1980). An improved diagnostic evaluation instrument for substance abuse patients: the addiction severity index. J. Nerv. Ment. Disord. *168*, 26–33.

Mirenowicz, J., and Schultz, W. (1996). Preferential activation of midbrain dopamine neurons by appetitive rather than aversive stimuli. Nature *379*, 449–451.

Morgan, M.A., and LeDoux, J.E. (1995). Differential contribution of dorsal and ventral medial prefrontal cortex to the acquisition and extinction of conditioned fear in rats. Behav. Neurosci. *109*, 681–688.

Morgan, M.A., Romanski, L.M.., and LeDoux, J.E. (1993). Extinction of emotional learning: contribution of medial prefrontal cortex. Neurosci. Lett. *163*, 109–113.

Murray, B., and Shizgal, P. (1991). Anterolateral lesions of the medial forebrain bundle increases the frequency threshold for self-stimulation of the lateral hypothalamus and ventral tegmental area in the rat. Psychobiology *19*, 135–146.

Murray, B., and Shizgal, P. (1996). Attenuation of medial forebrain bundle reward by anterior lateral hypothalamic lesions. Behav. Brain Res. *75*, 33–47.

Nishino, H., Ono, T., Muramoto, K., Fukuda, M., and Sasaki, K. (1987). Neuronal activity in the ventral tegmental area during motivated bar press feeding in the monkey. Brain Res. *413*, 302–313.

Ogawa, S., Tank, D.W., Menon, R., Ellermann, J.M., Kim, S.G., Merkle, H., and Ugurbil, K. (1992). Intrinsic signal changes accompanying sensory stimulation: functional brain mapping using MRI. Proc. Natl. Acad. Sci. USA *89*, 5951–5955.

Olds, J., and Milner, P.M. (1954). Positive reinforcement produced by electrical stimulation of septal area and other regions of rat brain. J. Comp. Physiol. Psychol. *47*, 419–427.

Pearlson, G.D., Jeffery, P.J., Harris, G.J., Ross, C.A., Fischman, M.W., and Camargo, E.E. (1993). Correlation of acute cocaine-induced changes in local cerebral blood flow with subjective effects. Am. J. Psych. *150*, 495–497.

Phillips, A., Atkinson, L., Blackburn, J., and Blaha, C. (1993). Increased extracellular dopamine in the nucleus accumbens of the rat elicited by a conditional stimulus for food: an electrochemical study. Can. J. Physiol. Pharmacol. *71*, 387–393.

Puopolo, P.R., Chamberlin, P., and Flood, J.G. (1992). Detection and confirmation of cocaine and cocaethylene in serum emergency toxicology specimens. Clin. Chem. *38*, 1838–1842.

Radhakishun, F., van Ree, J., and Westerink, B. (1988). Scheduled eating increases dopamine release in the nucleus accumbens of food-deprived rats as assessed with on-line brain dialysis. Neurosci. Lett. *85*, 351–356.

Reese, T.G., Davis, T.L., and Weisskoff, R.M. (1995). Automated shimming at 1.5T using echo planar image frequency maps. J. Magn. Reson. Imaging *5*, 739–745.

Richardson, N., and Gratton, A. (1996). Behavior-relevant changes in nucleus accumbens dopamine transmission elicited by food reinforcement: an electrochemical study in rat. J. Neurosci. *16*, 8160–8169.

Ritz, M.C., Lamb, R.J., Goldberg, S.R., and Kuhar, M.J. (1987). Cocaine receptors on dopamine transporters are related to self-administration of cocaine. Science *237*, 1219–1223.

Rolls, E.T. (1992). Neurophysiology and function of the primate amygdala. In The Amygdala: Neurobiological Aspects of Emotion, Memory, and Mental Dysfunction, J.P. Aggleton, ed. (New York: John Wiley-Liss), pp. 143–165.

Romo, R., and Schultz, W. (1990). Dopamine neurons in the monkey midbrain: contingencies of responses to acute touch during self-initiated arm movements. J. Neurophysiol. *63*, 592–606.

Rompre, P.-P., and Shizgal, P. (1986). Electrophysiological characteristics of neurons in forebrain regions implicated in self-stimulation of the medial forebrain bundle in the rat. Brain Res. *364*, 338–349.

Russchen, F.T., Bakst, I., Amaral, D.G., and Price, J.L. (1985). The amygdalostiatal projections in the monkey. An anterograde tracing study. Brain Res. *329*, 241–257.

Salamone, J., Cousins, M., McCullough, L., Carriero, D., and Berkowitz, R. (1994). Nucleus accumbens dopamine release increases during instrumental lever pressing for food but not free food consumption. Pharmacol. Biochem. Behav. *49*, 25–31.

Schultz, W. (1986). Responses of midbrain dopamine neurons to behavioral trigger stimuli in the monkey. J. Neurophysiol. *56*, 1439–1461.

Schultz, W., and Romo, R. (1990). Dopamine neurons of the monkey midbrain: contingencies of responses to stimuli eliciting immediate behavioral reactions. J. Neurophysiol. *63*, 607–624.

Schultz, W., Apicella, P., Scarnati, E., and Ljungberg, T. (1992). Neuronal activity in monkey ventral striatum related to the expectation of reward. J. Neurosci. *12*, 4595–4610.

Schultz, W., Apicella, P., and Ljungberg, T. (1993). Responses of monkey dopamine neurons to reward and conditioned stimuli during successive steps of learning a delayed response task. J. Neurosci. *13*, 900–913.

Schultz, W., Dayan, P., and Montague, P.R. (1997). A neural substrate of prediction and reward. Science *275*, 1593–1599.

Shizgal, P., Schindler, D., and Rompre, P.-P. (1989). Forebrain neurons driven by rewarding stimulation of the medial forebrain bundle in the rat: comparison of psychophysical and electrophysiological estimates of refractory periods. Brain Res. *499*, 234–248.

Sikes, R.W., and Vogt, B.A. (1992). Nociceptive neurons in area 24 of rabbit cingulate cortex. J. Neurophysiol. *68*, 1720–1732.

Spiegler, B.J., and Mishkin, M. (1981). Evidence for the sequential participation of inferior temporal cortex and amygdala in the acquisition of stimulus-reward associations. Behav. Brain Res. *3*, 303–317.

Squire, L.R., and Knowlton, B.J. (1995). In The Cognitive Neurosciences, M.S. Gazzaniga, ed. (Cambridge, MA: MIT Press), pp. 825–837.

Stein, E.A., and Fuller, S.A. (1992). Selective effects of cocaine on regional cerebral blood flow in the rat. J. Pharmacol. Exp. Ther. *262*, 327–334.

Stein, E.A., and Fuller, S.A. (1993). Cocaine's time action profile on regional cerebral blood flow in the rat. Brain Res. *626*, 117–126.

Talairach, J., and Tournoux, P. (1988). C0-planar Stereotaxic Atlas of the Human Brain (New York: Thieme Medical Publishers).

Talbot, J.D., Marrett, S., Evans, A.C., Meyer, E., Bushell, M.C., and Duncan, G.H. (1991). Multiple representations of pain in human cerebral cortex. Science *251*, 1355–1358.

Tootell, R.B.H., Reppas, J.B., Kwong, K.K., Malach, R., Born, R.T., Brady, T.J., Rosen, B.R., and Belliveau, J.W. (1995). Functional analysis of human MT and related visual cortical areas using magnetic resonance imaging. J. Neurosci. *15*, 3215–3230.

Volkow, N.D., Fowler, J.S., Wolf, A.P., Schlyer, D., Chyng-Yann, S., Alpert, R., Dewey, S., Logan, J., Bendriem, B., Christman, D., et al. (1990). Effects of chronic cocaine abuse on postsynaptic dopamine receptors. Am. J. Psychiatry *147*, 719–724.

Volkow, N.D., Fowler, J.S., and Wolf, A.P. (1991). Changes in brain glucose metabolism in cocaine dependence and withdrawal. Am. J. Psychiatry *148*, 621–626.

Volkow, N.D., Hitzemann, R., and Wang, G.-J. (1992). Long-term frontal brain metabolic changes in cocaine abusers. Synapse *11*, 184–190.

Volkow, N.D., Fowler, J.S., and Wang, G.-J. (1993). Decreased dopamine D2 receptor availability is associated with reduced frontal metabolism in cocaine abusers. Synapse *14*, 169–177.

Volkow, N.D., Wang, G.-J., Fischman, M.W., Foltin, R.W., Fowler, J.S., Abumrad, N.N., Vitkun, S., Logan, J., Gatley, S.J., Pappas, N., et al. (1997a). Relationship between subjective effects of cocaine and dopamine transporter occupancy. Nature *386*, 827–830.

Volkow, N.D., Wang, G.-J., Fowler, J.S., Logan, J., Gatley, S.J., Hitzemann, R., Chen, A.D., Dewey, S.L., and Pappas, N. (1997b). Decreased striatal dopaminergic responsiveness in detoxified cocaine-dependent subjects. Nature *386*, 830–833.

Weatherford, S., Greenberg, D., Melville, L., Jerome, C., Gibbs, J., and Smith, G. (1991). Failure to detect increases in brain dopamine metabolism in rats sham feeding sucrose and corn oil. Pharmacol. Biochem. Behav. *39*, 1025–1028.

Weiss, S.R.B., Post, R.M., Pert, A., Woodward, R., and Murman, D. (1989). Context-dependent cocaine sensitization: differential effect of haloperidol on development versus expression. Pharmacol. Biochem. Behav. *34*, 655.

White, N. (1986). Control of sensorimotor function by dopaminergic nigrostriatal neurons: influence on eating and drinking. Neurosci. Biobehav. Rev. *10*, 15–36.

White, N.M., Messier, C., and Carr, G.D. (1987). Operationalizing and measuring the organizing influence of drugs on behavior. In Methods of Assessing the Reinforcing Properties of Abused Drugs, M.A. Bozarth, ed. (New York: Springer-Verlag), pp. 591–617.

Williams, G.V. (1989). Neuronal activity in the primate caudate nucleus and ventral striatum reflects the association between stimuli determining behavior. In Neural Mechanisms in Disorders of Movement, A.R. Crossman and M.A. Sambrook, eds. (London: John Libbey), pp. 63–73.

Wise, R.A. (1982). Neuroleptics and operant behavior: the anhedonia hypothesis. Behav. Brain Sci. *5*, 39–87.

Wise, R., Spinder, J., DeWit, H., and Gerber, G. (1978). Neuroleptic-induced "anhedonia" in rats: pimozide blocks the reward quality of food. Science *201*, 262–264.

Woods, R.P., Cherry, S.R., and Mazziotta, J.C. (1992). Rapid automated algorithm for aligning and reslicing PET images. J. Comput. Assist. Tomogr. *16*, 620–633.

Yim, C.Y., and Mogenson, G.J. (1982). Response of nucleus accumbens neurons to amygdala stimulation and its modification by dopamine. Brain Res. *239*, 401–415.

Yoshida, M., Yokoo, H., Mizoguchi, K., Kawahara, H., Tsuda, A., Nishikawa, T., and Tanaka, M. (1992). Eating and drinking cause increased dopamine release in the nucleus accumbens and ventral tegmental area in the rat: measurement by in vivo microdialysis. Neurosci. Lett. *139*, 73–76.

ORIGINAL ARTICLE

Illicit Psychoactive Substance Use, Heavy Use, Abuse, and Dependence in a US Population-Based Sample of Male Twins

Kenneth S. Kendler, MD; Laura M. Karkowski, PhD; Michael C. Neale, PhD; Carol A. Prescott, PhD

Background: In order to develop informed approaches to prevention and treatment of illicit psychoactive substance use, abuse, and dependence, we need to understand the sources of individual differences in risk.

Methods: In personal interviews with 1198 male-male twin pairs (708 monozygotic and 490 dizygotic) ascertained from a population-based registry, we assessed lifetime use, heavy use, and abuse of and dependence on cannabis, sedatives, stimulants, cocaine, opiates, and hallucinogens. Twin resemblance was assessed by probandwise concordance, odds ratio, tetrachoric correlations, and biometrical model fitting.

Results: Twin resemblance for substance use, heavy use, abuse, and dependence was substantial, and consistently greater in monozygotic than in dizygotic twins. For any drug use and for cannabis and hallucinogen use, model fitting suggested that twin resemblance was due to both genetic and familial-environmental factors. Twin resemblance for sedative, stimulant, cocaine, and opiate use, however, was caused solely by genetic factors. With 2 exceptions (cocaine abuse and stimulant dependence), twin resemblance for heavy use, abuse, and dependence resulted from only genetic factors, with heritability of liability usually ranging from 60% to 80%. No consistent evidence was found for violations of the equal environment assumption.

Conclusions: In accord with prior results in studies of women, the family environment plays a role in twin resemblance for some forms of substance use in men. However, twin resemblance for heavy use, abuse, and dependence in men is largely caused by genetic factors, and heritability estimates are high.

Arch Gen Psychiatry. 2000;57:261-269

ILLICIT PSYCHOACTIVE substance use, abuse, and dependence are major public health problems. To develop informed approaches to prevention and treatment, we need to understand the sources of individual differences in risk. Substantial evidence suggests that the liability to psychoactive substance use disorder (PSUD) aggregates in families.[1-6] Both twin[7-10] and adoption[11-13] studies suggest that part of this familial aggregation is due to genetic factors.

In the first phase of a comprehensive study of PSUD in a US population-based twin population, we examined cannabis, cocaine, hallucinogen, opiate, sedative, and stimulant use, abuse, and dependence in personally interviewed members of more than 800 female-female twin pairs.[14-16] In a separate and recently completed study, we have interviewed personally, with the same assessment instrument, both members of 1193 male-male (MM) pairs ascertained from the same twin registry. In this article, therefore, we examine the results for the use, heavy use, and abuse of and dependence on these categories of psychoactive substances in these MM pairs.

From the Departments of Psychiatry (Drs Kendler, Karkowski, Neale, and Prescott) and Human Genetics (Drs Kendler and Neale), Medical College of Virginia, and the Virginia Institute for Psychiatric and Behavioral Genetics (Drs Kendler, Karkowski, Neale, and Prescott), Virginia Commonwealth University, Richmond.

RESULTS

POTENTIAL BIASES

Noncooperation of the cotwin predicted an increased risk for psychoactive substance use, heavy use, abuse, and dependence in the twin in 10 of 36 analyses. For MZ twins, it predicted sedative use; sedative, stimulant, and opiate heavy use; cocaine abuse; and cocaine and opiate dependence. For DZ twins, it predicted sedative use and marijuana and sedative dependence. Although the findings were replicated across zygosity groups only once (for sedative use), these many significant findings—all in the same direction—were unlikely to occur by chance ($P = .005$).[24]

Controlling for zygosity, the similarity of childhood and adult environments

SUBJECTS AND METHODS

SUBJECTS

This report is based on data collected in the second wave of interviews in a new study of adult twins from the Virginia Twin Registry (now part of the Mid-Atlantic Twin Registry). The Virginia registry was formed by a systematic search of all Virginia birth certificates since 1918. Subjects from multiple births are matched by names and birth dates from state records to obtain addresses and telephone numbers. Twins were eligible for participation in this study if one or both twins were successfully matched, were members of a multiple birth that included at least 1 male, were white, and were born between 1940 and 1974. Of 9417 individuals eligible for the first wave, 6814 (72.4%) had completed interviews, 1163 (12.4%) refused, 33 (0.4%) had incomplete interviews, 388 (4.1%) did not agree within the study time limit, 862 (9.1%) could not be located, and 157 (1.7%) were deceased or too ill to be interviewed. At least 1 year after the completion of the first-wave interview (performed by telephone in most instances), we contacted the twins again and attempted to schedule a second-wave interview. The number of subjects eligible for wave-2 interviews included the 6814 with complete wave-1 interviews as well as 3 subjects interviewed at wave 2 who were eligible at wave 1 but from whom completed wave-1 interviews were not obtained. Whenever possible, this interview was completed face-to-face (79.4% of sample). Of the 6817 individuals eligible for the wave-2 interview, 5629 (82.6%) were successfully interviewed while 852 (12.5%) refused, 22 (0.3%) had incomplete interviews, 237 (3.5%) did not agree within the study time limit, 51 (0.7%) could not be located, and 26 (0.4%) were deceased or too ill to be interviewed. To assess the test-retest reliability of our assessments, 131 members of MM twins were reinterviewed 4.4 ± 1.1 months (mean ± SEM) after their initial interview.

The current report is based on 1198 MM pairs with complete data on PSUD from the wave-2 interview. There were 1184 male-male twins, with 12 pairs from 4 all-male triplet births and 1 pair each from a male-male-female triplet birth and a male-male-female-female quadruplet birth. In addition, this sample includes 534 subjects whose cotwins did not complete a wave 2 interview, of whom 247 came from monozygotic (MZ) and 287 from dizygotic (DZ) pairs.

At the time of second-wave interview (1994-1998), subjects were 20 to 58 years old (mean [SD], 36.8 [9.1]), and had a mean of 13.4 years of education (SD, 2.6). Interviewers had a master's degree in a mental health–related field or a bachelor's degree in this area plus 2 years of clinical experience. They received 40 hours of classroom training plus regular individual and group review sessions. Two senior staff reviewed each interview for completeness and consistency. Members of a twin pair were interviewed by different interviewers who were blind to clinical information about the cotwin.

ZYGOSITY DIAGNOSIS

We began assessing zygosity by genotyping 227 twin pairs with 8 or more highly polymorphic DNA markers. Using these pairs, we developed a Fisher discriminant function with PROC DISCRIM in SAS[17] using height, weight, 6 standard zygosity questions, and the twins' history of any blood tests. Using this discriminant function, we could confidently assign zygosity to all of the remaining sample (operationalized as an estimated probability of monozygosity of ≤10% or ≥90%) except for 97 pairs. Of these, we had usable DNA from both members of 65 pairs, from which we obtained zygosities. All available information on the remaining 32 cases, including photographs, was reviewed by 2 of us (K.S.K. and C.A.P.), who assigned final zygosities. Assignment of zygosity for twins without an interviewed cotwin was done using the discriminant function analysis. These analyses were based on 708 complete MZ pairs and 490 complete DZ pairs.

MEASURES

Lifetime use, heavy use, abuse, and dependence were assessed separately for 7 categories of substances using an adaptation of the Structured Clinical Interview for *DSM-III-R*.[18] With illustrative specific forms, these categories were cannabis (marijuana and hashish); sedatives (quaalude, Seconal, and Valium); stimulants (speed, ecstasy, and Ritalin); cocaine (intranasal, freebase, and crack); opiates (heroin, Demerol [meperidine hydrochloride], morphine); hallucinogens (lysergic acid diethylamide, mescaline, and phencyclidine); and "other," including inhalants (glue and nitrous oxide), over-the-counter medications (diet and sleeping pills), and miscellaneous (steroids and poppers). For those substances that could be legally obtained, we told respondents that we were interested solely in nonmedical use, defined as use (1) without a physician's prescription; (2) in greater amounts than prescribed; (3) more often than prescribed; or (4) for any other reason than that a physician said they should be taken. Heavy

significantly predicted twin resemblance 7 out of 56 times: (1) For childhood environment, it predicted stimulant and hallucinogen use, cannabis, and any heavy use. (2) For adult environment, it predicted cocaine heavy use, hallucinogen abuse, and sedative dependence. Although there was no replication across substances or levels of use or misuse, this number of significant findings would occur by chance approximately 2% of the time,[24] and all the significant effects were in the predicted direction.

For most drug use categories, rates were higher in DZ than MZ twins. Although these differences were usually modest, they reached significance for cannabis use and abuse; sedative abuse; opiate heavy use; hallucinogen use; and any use, heavy use, and abuse.

TEST-RETEST RELIABILITY

Drug use was assessed with excellent reliability ($\kappa > 0.70$ and $r > 0.90$ for all), as was heavy use except with sedatives (**Table 1**). The test-retest reliabilities for drug abuse and dependence (where available) were in the fair to good range (most κ values between 0.50 and 0.70 and most r values > 0.80).

use was defined as ever using the substance more than 10 times per month.

Drug abuse and dependence were diagnosed using *DSM-IV* criteria,[19] except that we ignored criterion B for substance abuse, which rules out abuse in the presence of dependence. Thus, we diagnosed abuse and dependence nonhierarchically. Use and misuse of the *other* category were too rare to usefully analyze separately, but the *other* category was added to the category of *any* PSUD.

STATISTICAL ANALYSIS

We assess twin resemblance in 3 ways. First, proband concordance is the proportion of affected individuals among cotwins of affected twins. This statistic ignores information from pairs in which both twins are unaffected. Second, the odds ratio (OR) reflects the risk of being affected (or using a substance) among cotwins of affected twins compared with the risk of being affected among cotwins of unaffected twins.

Third, we use a liability-threshold model to estimate the genetic and environmental contributions to twin resemblance for substance use, abuse, and dependence. For categorical characteristics, such as lifetime use or dependence, the estimates reflect resemblance in twins pairs for their liability to develop the disorder.[20] Liability is assumed to be continuous and normally distributed in the population, with individuals who exceed a theoretical threshold expressing the disorder.

Individual differences in liability are assumed to arise from 3 sources: additive genetic (A), from genes with allelic effects that combine additively; common environment (C), which includes all sources shared by members of a twin pair, including family environment, social class, schools; and specific environment (E), which includes all remaining environmental factors not shared within a twin pair plus measurement error. Monozygotic twins within a pair resemble one another because they share all of their A and C components, while DZ pairs share (on average) half of their A and all of their C components. It is possible to include nonadditive genetic effects, such as dominance or epistasis, but these have not been implicated in prior studies of PSUD and their inclusion did not improve the fit of our models, so we did not consider them further.

Our model also assumes independence and additivity of the 3 components and the equality of shared environmental effects. The equal environment assumption requires that MZ and DZ pairs be equally similar in the etiologically relevant aspects of their shared environments. To test this assumption, we assessed twin similarity for environmental exposure in childhood using standard questions.[21] Similarity of their adult environment is assessed by measures of current frequency of contact. We examine whether, when controlling for zygosity, pairs with greater environmental similarity are more similar for substance use, heavy use, abuse, or dependence.

Since drug use, abuse, and dependence are correlated in twin pairs, twin studies provide a method for detecting cooperation bias. If, for example, drug use predicts noncooperation, then drug use in one twin should predict a decreased probability that the cotwin would be successfully interviewed.

Traditional twin modeling examines only pairs concordant for assessment. However, information about diagnostic thresholds is contained in twins whose cotwin was not interviewed. Using a recently developed option in the software package Mx,[22] we fitted models including single twins by the method of maximum likelihood. During optimization, trial values of the parameters were used to generate an overall predicted covariance matrix and an overall matrix of thresholds. For any particular observation, the overall matrix was filtered to create a submatrix matching those observations that were present. Likewise, the corresponding subset of the matrix of thresholds is created. These matrices are then used to compute the log-likelihood of the observation in question. The log-likelihoods of all cases were summed to obtain the log-likelihood of the sample, which was maximized using numerical optimization software.

Maximum likelihood analysis of raw ordinal data does not directly provide an overall test of goodness of fit of the model. However, it is possible to perform such a test by comparing the fit of the model being used with the sum of the fits of models (MZ and DZ fitted separately) in which every correlation and every threshold are estimated as free parameters. Twice the difference in log-likelihood between this saturated model and the model being tested yields a statistic that is (under certain regularity conditions) asymptotically distributed as χ^2 values with degrees of freedom equal to the difference in the number of parameters in the 2 models. Tests between alternative models may be carried out the same way.

Alternative models are evaluated by comparing the difference in their χ^2 values relative to the difference in their degrees of freedom, according to the principle of parsimony—models with fewer parameters are preferable if they do not provide significantly worse fit. We operationalize parsimony by using the Akaike information criterion (AIC) statistic,[23] calculated as $\chi^2 - 2\,df$, where df indicates degrees of freedom.

PREVALENCES AND PATTERNS OF TWIN RESEMBLANCE

Table 2 presents, for MZ and DZ twins, the prevalence, probandwise concordance, OR, and difference in ORs between zygosities for the use, heavy use, and abuse of and dependence on any illicit substance and for the 6 specific classes of illicit substances. The following results are noteworthy: (1) Prevalences of the various drug use categories differ widely. Rates for cannabis are consistently the highest and opiates among the lowest. (2) Across the various substances, abuse is usually more frequently reported than heavy use, while dependence is substantially rarer. (3) In MZ twins, ORs were significantly greater than 1 for all categories of use; all categories of heavy use and abuse except opiates; and all categories of dependence except sedatives, opiates, and hallucinogens. For DZ twins, ORs significantly exceeded unity for all forms of use except opiates; for cannabis, stimulant, and cocaine heavy use; for cannabis and cocaine abuse; and for cocaine dependence. (4) In MZ twins, higher ORs were consistently seen for heavy use and abuse than for use. This trend was less clear in DZ twins. (5) Odds ratios were estimable in both MZ and DZ twins in 20 sub-

Table 1. Test-Retest Reliability of Psychoactive Substance Use, Heavy Use, Abuse, and Dependence (n = 131)*

Substance	Use κ	Use r	Heavy Use κ	Heavy Use r	Abuse κ	Abuse r	Dependence κ	Dependence r
Cannabis	+0.91	0.99	+0.84	0.98	+0.67	0.89	+0.60	0.89
Sedatives	+0.79	0.97	+0.39	0.79	+0.51	0.82	...	...
Stimulants	+0.72	0.92	+0.72	0.95	+0.60	0.92	+0.66	0.94
Cocaine	+0.93	0.99	+0.72	0.95	+0.68	0.92	+0.47	0.80
Opiates	+0.74	0.96	+0.66	0.94	+0.49	0.86	...	...
Hallucinogens	+0.88	0.99	...	...	+0.59	0.91	...	...
Any	+0.89	0.99	+0.74	0.93	+0.65	0.89	+0.63	0.92

Ellipses indicate that fewer than 4 individuals met the criteria on either occasion of measurement.

stance category combinations. The OR was greater in MZ twins in all 20 categories and this difference was significant in 18. The 2 categories in which MZ resemblance did not significantly exceed DZ resemblance were cannabis use and cocaine abuse.

TETRACHORIC CORRELATIONS

As with the ORs, the tetrachoric correlations were consistently higher in MZ than in DZ twins (**Table 3**). With 2 exceptions (sedative heavy use and stimulant dependence), tetrachoric correlations in MZ twins exceeded 0.55, indicating a high degree of twin resemblance. Tetrachoric correlations in DZ twins were more variable, ranging from nearly 0 for opiate use and sedative abuse to greater than 0.40 for stimulant use, marijuana heavy use, and cocaine heavy use and abuse.

MODEL-FITTING RESULTS

Use

For model fitting, we will describe the results in each category for cannabis, as it is the most commonly used substance and provides, therefore, the greatest statistical power. We comment more briefly on results for other substances. For use, the full or ACE model fit moderately well for cannabis (χ^2_3 = 7.40, P = .06). Compared with this model, we could reject, by the χ^2 difference test, the AE (χ^2_1 = 7.43, P = .006); CE (χ^2_1 = 5.41, P = .02); and E-only models (χ^2_2 = 218.67, P<.001). The best-fit ACE model, which produced the lowest AIC value, suggested that one third of the variance in liability to cannabis use was due to additive genetic factors, one third to family environment, and one third to unique environment.

Similar results were found for any substance use and hallucinogen use. For both these categories, the AE and CE models could be rejected at or nearly at the .05 level and the E-only model could be rejected at the .0001 level. From the best-fit ACE model, family environment was seen to account for approximately 35% of the variance in liability, while genetic factors were considerably more important for hallucinogens than for any drug use.

For sedative, stimulant, cocaine, and opiate use, however, the best-fit model was the simple AE model, with the heritability of liability to use being estimated in the range of 50% to 70%. Against the ACE model, the CE models could be rejected at the .05 level and the E-only models at the .0001 level for all these substances. It is noteworthy that in models containing both A and C, the positive correlation of these parameter estimates produces quite large confidence intervals (CIs). That is, when there is evidence of an effect of both genes and family environment for a dichotomous trait like substance use, even with relatively large sample sizes, parameter estimates for these 2 factors are known with little precision. In AE models, by contrast, the CIs are narrower.

Heavy Use

The results for heavy use of cannabis differed substantially from those for use. The full model fit well (χ^2_3 = 5.81, P = .12). Against the ACE model, the AE model could not be rejected (χ^2_1 = 1.26, P = .26), but both the CE (χ^2_1 = 18.79, P<.001) and E-only (χ^2_2 = 203.87, P<.001) models could be strongly rejected. The best-fit model was AE, with an estimated heritability of liability to cannabis heavy use of 84%. The absence of twin pairs concordant for opiate heavy use, abuse, or dependence made model fitting impossible. For heavy use of all other substances and any substance, the AE model provided the best fit, with estimated heritabilities that ranged from 45% for sedatives to 83% for any substance. The CE model could be rejected against the ACE model at the .05 level only for stimulant and any substance. The E-only model could be rejected for stimulants, cocaine, and any substance. The low prevalence of sedative and hallucinogen heavy use resulted in heritability estimates with wide CIs.

Abuse

Results for cannabis abuse resembled those seen for heavy use. While the AE model gave the same fit as the ACE model, the CE (χ^2_1 = 20.22, P<.001) and E-only (χ^2_2 = 158.64, P<.001) models could be rejected with high levels of statistical confidence. The heritability estimated from the best-fit AE model was high (76%), with a relatively narrow CI. Qualitatively similar results were obtained with abuse of any substance, as well as abuse of sedatives, stimulants, and hallucinogens. For all of the categories, both the CE and E-only models could be rejected against the ACE model by the χ^2 difference test. The rarer the rates of abuse, the broader were the CIs around the parameter estimates of the best-fit models.

Table 2. Prevalence, Probandwise Concordance, and Odds Ratios for Illicit Psychoactive Substance Use, Heavy Use, Abuse, and Dependence in Monozygotic (MZ) and Dizygotic (DZ) Twins*

Substance	Prevalence ± SE		Probandwise Concordance ± SE		Odds Ratio (95% CI)		Difference in Odds Ratios	
	MZ	DZ	MZ	DZ	MZ	DZ	χ^2 (df = 1)	P
Use								
Cannabis	50.4 ± 1.3	55.9 ± 1.8	0.73 ± 0.01	0.71 ± 0.02	7.5† (5.4-10.5)	4.2† (2.9-6.2)	0.95	.33
Sedatives	10.1 ± 0.8	11.5 ± 1.0	0.44 ± 0.03	0.25 ± 0.03	11.7† (6.7-20.6)	3.1† (1.6-6.3)	8.57	.003
Stimulants	17.7 ± 1.0	19.8 ± 1.3	0.52 ± 0.03	0.40 ± 0.03	9.5† (6.1-14.9)	3.9† (2.4-6.4)	7.00	.008
Cocaine	16.0 ± 1.0	18.2 ± 1.2	0.52 ± 0.03	0.36 ± 0.03	11.0† (6.9-17.5)	3.4† (2.0-5.7)	11.22	.001
Opiates	5.9 ± 0.6	6.0 ± 0.8	0.29 ± 0.04	0.07 ± 0.02	8.9† (4.1-19.2)	1.2 (0.3-5.1)	6.78	.009
Hallucinogens	12.9 ± 0.9	16.4 ± 1.2	0.62 ± 0.03	0.45 ± 0.03	26.7† (15.5-46.0)	6.7† (3.9-11.5)	12.82	<.001
Any	52.6 ± 1.3	59.0 ± 1.6	0.74 ± 0.01	0.73 ± 0.02	6.8† (4.9-9.4)	4.2† (2.8-6.1)	3.55	.06
Heavy Use								
Cannabis	14.5 ± 0.9	17.2 ± 1.2	0.63 ± 0.03	0.41 ± 0.03	26.2† (15.5-44.2)	5.2† (3.0-8.7)	18.87	<.001
Sedatives	1.1 ± 0.3	2.0 ± 0.5	0.13‡ ± 0.06	0.00‡	15.4† (1.6-145.5)	...	2.60	.11
Stimulants	4.0 ± 0.5	5.6 ± 0.7	0.36 ± 0.05	0.15 ± 0.04	20.7† (8.3-51.2)	3.2§ (1.0-10.0)	6.96	.008
Cocaine	3.0 ± 0.5	3.7 ± 0.6	0.42 ± 0.06	0.22 ± 0.05	40.4† (14.4-113.9)	9.4† (2.7-32.0)	3.32	.07
Opiates	0.8 ± 0.2	2.0 ± 0.5	0.00‡	0.00‡	...	...	...	...
Hallucinogens	0.8 ± 0.2	1.5 ± 0.4	0.18‖ ± 0.09	0.00‡	38.8¶ (3.5-428.1)	...	3.22	.07
Any	16.3 ± 1.0	19.8 ± 1.3	0.63 ± 0.03	0.43 ± 0.04	22.5† (13.7-36.8)	4.7† (2.9-7.7)	19.76	<.001
Abuse								
Cannabis	16.6 ± 1.0	20.1 ± 1.3	0.58 ± 0.03	0.38 ± 0.03	15.0† (9.4-24.0)	3.2† (2.0-5.3)	20.23	<.001
Sedatives	2.3 ± 0.5	4.3 ± 0.7	0.24 ± 0.06	0.05 ± 0.02	18.1† (5.1-64.3)	1.2 (0.2-9.0)	7.01	.008
Stimulants	7.1 ± 0.7	8.7 ± 0.9	0.40 ± 0.04	0.16 ± 0.03	14.8† (7.4-29.3)	2.3 (1.0-5.6)	11.49	.001
Cocaine	4.6 ± 0.6	5.7 ± 0.7	0.31 ± 0.04	0.25 ± 0.04	13.4† (5.7-31.9)	7.1† (2.7-18.5)	0.96	.33
Opiates	1.5 ± 0.3	2.3 ± 0.5	0.00	0.00	...	...	...	...
Hallucinogens	3.3 ± 0.5	3.5 ± 0.6	0.34 ± 0.05	0.00	24.3† (8.8-67.0)	...	9.37	.002
Any	19.8 ± 1.1	23.6 ± 1.4	0.61 ± 0.02	0.42 ± 0.03	14.5† (9.3-22.5)	3.2† (2.1-5.1)	22.02	<.001
Dependence								
Cannabis	4.1 ± 0.5	4.4 ± 0.7	0.28 ± 0.04	0.09 ± 0.03	12.4† (4.9-31.4)	2.4 (0.5-11.1)	3.56	.06
Sedatives	0.4 ± 0.2	0.8 ± 0.3	0.33‖ ± 0.15	0.00‖	...	...	3.38	.07
Stimulants	2.1 ± 0.4	2.1 ± 0.5	0.13 ± 0.04	0.10‡ ± 0.05	8.5¶ (1.7-42.0)	5.6 (0.6-49.1)	0.09	.76
Cocaine	2.8 ± 0.4	3.1 ± 0.6	0.41 ± 0.06	0.13 ± 0.04	41.0† (14.0-120.2)	5.6§ (1.1-27.5)	4.56	.03
Opiates	0.4 ± 0.2	1.0 ± 0.3	0.00‖	0.00‖	...	...	...	...
Hallucinogens	0.5 ± 0.2	1.0 ± 0.3	0.29‖ ± 0.13	0.00‖	...	...	4.27	.04
Any	6.9 ± 0.7	8.6 ± 0.9	0.41 ± 0.04	0.24 ± 0.04	15.5† (7.8-30.8)	4.2† (1.9-9.4)	6.10	.01

*Ellipses indicate that the value was not calcuated. CI indicates confidence interval.
†$P<.001$.
‡$n\leq 20$.
§$P<.05$.
‖$n\leq 10$.
¶$P<.01$.

However, cocaine abuse was an exception to this pattern. Here, the tetrachoric correlation was only modestly greater in MZ than DZ twins (+0.61 vs +0.49). The full-model estimates of a^2, c^2, and e^2 were 32%, 32%, and 37%, respectively. The E-only model could be confidently rejected against the ACE model (χ^2_2 = 39.12, $P<.001$), but neither the AE nor the CE model could be rejected (χ^2_1 = 1.51, P = .22; and χ^2_1 = 0.94, P = .33; respectively). Although the CE model produced the best fit by AIC, the fact that the fits of the AE and CE models were within 0.57 χ^2 units of each other suggested that we had little power to determine the contribution of genetic vs environmental factors to the familial resemblance for cocaine abuse.

Dependence

The findings for cannabis dependence resembled those obtained for cannabis heavy use and abuse. Against the ACE model, the E-only model could be confidently rejected (χ^2_1 = 21.47, $P<.001$) and the CE model could be rejected at marginal levels of significance (χ^2_1 = 3.42, P = .06). By AIC, the AE model produced the best fit, with an estimated heritability of 58%. Because of its greater rarity, the CIs on heritability estimates for cannabis dependence are considerably larger than those seen for cannabis abuse.

For both any cocaine use and cocaine dependence, the pattern of results was similar and the CE models could be rejected at the .05 level against the ACE models (χ^2_1 = 6.68, P = .01; and χ^2_1 = 4.90, P = .03; respectively). Estimates of heritability were high (71% and 79%, respectively). Results were less certain for sedative, stimulant, and hallucinogen dependence. For all 3 substances, the E-only model could be rejected (χ^2_2 = 7.73, P = .02; χ^2_2 = 5.98, P = .05; and χ^2_2 = 6.34, P = .04; respectively), supporting the evidence of aggregation of risk within twin pairs. For both sedative and hallucinogen

Table 3. Tetrachoric Correlations, Model Fitting, and Parameter Estimates of Best-Fit Model for Illicit Psychoactive Substance Use, Heavy Use, Abuse, and Dependence in Monozygotic (MZ) and Dizygotic (DZ) Twins*

Substance	Tetrachoric Correlations		Model Fit in χ^2 Units				Parameter Estimates for Full and Best-Fit Models (95% CI)			
	MZ	DZ	ACE†	AE‡	CE‡	E§	F, B	a^2	c^2	e^2
Use										
Cannabis	0.67	0.51	7.4‖	14.8	12.8	226.1	F, B	0.33 (0.05-0.60)	0.34 (0.10-0.58)	0.33 (0.26-0.40)
Sedatives	0.67	0.34	3.4	3.4‖	12.8	80.3	F	0.68 (0.25-0.77)	0.00 (0.00-0.38)	0.32 (0.24-0.45)
							B	0.68 (0.55-0.78)		0.32 (0.22-0.45)
Stimulants	0.67	0.45	4.9	6.5‖	11.9	133.9	F	0.47 (0.12-0.75)	0.21 (0.00-0.50)	0.33 (0.24-0.43)
							B	0.69 (0.60-0.77)		0.31 (0.23-0.40)
Cocaine	0.69	0.40	3.3	3.6‖	14.5	127.3	F	0.61 (0.25-0.77)	0.09 (0.00-0.40)	0.30 (0.22-0.40)
							B	0.70 (0.61-0.78)		0.30 (0.22-0.39)
Opiates	0.55	0.03	3.5	3.5‖	8.9	26.1	F	0.52 (0.11-0.69)	0.00 (0.00-0.33)	0.48 (0.32-0.69)
							B	0.52 (0.31-0.68)		0.48 (0.32-0.69)
Hallucinogens	0.82	0.58	5.4‖	9.3	18.1	205.8	F, B	0.53 (0.23-0.85)	0.30 (0.00-0.57)	0.17 (0.11-0.17)
Any	0.64	0.51	6.9‖	15.1	10.6	199.3	F, B	0.27 (0.00-0.55)	0.38 (0.12-0.46)	0.36 (0.29-0.44)
Heavy Use										
Cannabis	0.83	0.51	5.8	7.1‖	24.6	209.7	F	0.66 (0.35-0.89)	0.18 (0.00-0.46)	0.17 (0.11-0.24)
							B	0.84 (0.77-0.89)		0.17 (0.11-0.23)
Sedatives	0.49	0.00	2.8	2.8‖	5.3	5.3	F	0.45 (0.00-0.82)	0.00 (0.00-0.40)	0.55 (0.18-0.98)
							B	0.45 (0.00-0.82)		0.55 (0.18-0.98)
Stimulants	0.69	0.28	1.7	1.7‖	8.3	38.4	F	0.70 (0.20-0.84)	0.00 (0.00-0.42)	0.30 (0.16-0.49)
							B	0.70 (0.51-0.84)		0.30 (0.16-0.49)
Cocaine	0.78	0.51	0.3	0.8‖	3.5	48.1	F	0.55 (0.00-0.90)	0.23 (0.00-0.74)	0.22 (0.10-0.41)
							B	0.80 (0.62-0.90)		0.20 (0.10-0.38)
Hallucinogens	0.63	0.00	4.0	4.0‖	5.7	8.1	F	0.62 (0.00-0.91)	0.00 (0.00-0.65)	0.38 (0.09-0.98)
							B	0.62 (0.02-0.91)		0.38 (0.09-0.98)
Any	0.81	0.50	4.9	6.1‖	24.6	215.3	F	0.65 (0.36-0.88)	0.17 (0.14-0.44)	0.18 (0.12-0.25)
							B	0.83 (0.76-0.88)		0.17 (0.12-0.24)
Abuse										
Cannabis	0.75	0.39	5.4	5.4‖	25.6	164.0	F	0.76 (0.42-0.82)	0.01 (0.00-0.31)	0.23 (0.17-0.33)
							B	0.76 (0.68-0.83)		0.24 (0.17-0.32)
Sedatives	0.61	0.03	10.8	10.8‖	15.3	23.0	F	0.59 (0.06-0.81)	0.00 (0.00-0.37)	0.41 (0.20-0.73)
							B	0.59 (0.27-0.80)		0.41 (0.20-0.73)
Stimulants	0.68	0.22	5.0	5.0‖	15.1	57.6	F	0.66 (0.30-0.77)	0.00 (0.00-0.29)	0.34 (0.22-0.50)
							B	0.66 (0.50-0.78)		0.34 (0.22-0.50)
Cocaine	0.61	0.49	2.6	4.1	3.5‖	41.7	F	0.32 (0.00-0.78)	0.32 (0.00-0.68)	0.37 (0.37-0.37)
							B		0.57 (0.40-0.70)	0.43 (0.30-0.60)
Hallucinogens	0.70	0.00	8.0	8.0‖	14.9	32.3	F	0.65 (0.24-0.82)	0.00 (0.00-0.34)	0.35 (0.19-0.58)
							B	0.65 (0.41-0.82)		0.35 (0.18-0.59)
Any	0.76	0.40	4.6	4.6‖	26.6	186.6	F	0.74 (0.42-0.83)	0.03 (0.02-0.31)	0.23 (0.17-0.31)
							B	0.77 (0.69-0.83)		0.23 (0.17-0.31)
Dependence										
Cannabis	0.59	0.20	4.0	4.0‖	7.4	25.5	F	0.58 (0.00-0.75)	0.00 (0.00-0.02)	0.42 (0.42-0.65)
							B	0.58 (0.35-0.75)		0.42 (0.26-0.66)
Sedatives	0.83	0.00	4.5	4.5‖	7.3	12.2	F	0.87 (0.00-0.99)	0.00 (0.00-0.80)	0.13 (0.01-0.68)
							B	0.87 (0.32-0.99)		0.13 (0.01-0.67)
Stimulants	0.43	0.34	1.9	2.1	2.0‖	7.9	F	0.22 (0.00-0.72)	0.21 (0.00-0.62)	0.57 (0.28-0.92)
							B		0.39 (0.08-0.64)	0.61 (0.36-0.92)
Cocaine	0.77	0.37	1.1	1.1‖	6.0	39.8	F	0.79 (0.09-0.90)	0.00 (0.00-0.62)	0.21 (0.17-0.28)
							B	0.79 (0.59-0.90)		0.21 (0.10-0.42)
Hallucinogens	0.80	0.00	4.1	4.1‖	6.5	10.4	F	0.79 (0.00-0.90)	0.00 (0.00-0.73)	0.21 (0.03-0.80)
							B	0.79 (0.20-0.97)		0.21 (0.04-0.80)
Any	0.69	0.39	4.1	4.2‖	10.8	68.2	F	0.65 (0.16-0.81)	0.05 (0.00-0.48)	0.29 (0.18-0.44)
							B	0.71 (0.57-0.82)		0.29 (0.18-0.43)

**A indicates additive genes; C, common or familial environment; E, individual specific environment; CI, confidence interval; F, full model; and B, best-fit model by Akaike information criteria. Results could not be estimated for opiate heavy use, abuse, or dependence because of the absence of concordant pairs.*

†*Using 3* df.

‡*Using 4* df.

§*Using 5* df.

‖*Best-fit model using Akaike information criteria.*

dependence, c^2 was estimated at 0 in the ACE model, but the deterioration in fit from the ACE to CE models was modest (χ^2_1 = 2.76, P = .10; and χ^2_1 = 2.36, P = .12; respectively). For stimulant dependence, the full model produced estimates of a^2, c^2, and e^2 of 0.22, 0.21, and 0.57, respectively. The CE model produced the best fit by AIC, but the fact that the fits of the ACE, AE, and CE models were within 0.18 χ^2 units of one another indicated that we have little power to determine the source of familial resemblance for stimulant dependence.

COMMENT

The goal of this article was to determine the sources of individual differences in risk for the use, heavy use, and abuse of and dependence on illicit psychoactive substances in men from a US population-based twin sample.

How representative of US men were the twins assessed in this study? In 1996, during the data-collection phase of this study, the National Household Survey on Drug Abuse assessed lifetime psychoactive substance use in more than 18 000 individuals.[25] Using the age categories for non-Hispanic white males in their report (reweighted to approximate the age distribution of our sample), the predicted lifetime rates for the 3 categories of drug use in which our data were most comparable were cannabis, 41.2%; cocaine, 14.7%; and hallucinogens, 13.5%. Weighted estimates for lifetime use and dependence in US males are also available from the National Comorbidity Survey, conducted from 1990 through 1992. They reported lifetime use (dependence) rates for categories similar to 5 of our 6 categories: cannabis, 51.7% (6.2%); sedatives, 14.0% (1.0%); stimulants, 18.4% (1.8%); cocaine, 19.5% (3.5%); and hallucinogens, 14.1% (0.7%). The rates found in our twin sample (Table 2) were nearly all within the range found in these 2 comparable epidemiologic studies. Consistent with other studies, which showed that twins do not differ from the general population in rates of psychopathologic conditions,[26-28] these results suggest that our sample is likely to be broadly representative of US men.

Two large-scale general population twin studies of psychoactive substance use and misuse are particularly comparable with this study: the male Vietnam Era Twin Registry[8] and female-female twin pairs previously studied from the Virginia Twin Registry.[14-16] Results from the Vietnam Era Twin Registry were reported for a category closest to our definition of abuse.[8] Uniformly, across substance categories, the Vietnam era sample produced lower levels of heritability and more evidence for family environment than found in our sample. For the comparable categories of any substance, cannabis, and hallucinogen abuse, the heritability values reported from the Vietnam era study were below the lower 95% CIs of our estimates. While these differences could be caused by many factors, the 2 cohorts differed substantially in mode of ascertainment (birth certificates vs both members inducted into the armed services). Furthermore, the Vietnam era sample may have had a unique historical experience of drug exposure.

Our results were more similar to those found in adult female-female twin pairs from the Virginia Twin Registry.[14-16] For example, in women, the best-fit models for cannabis use and abuse produced estimates of a^2, c^2, and e^2 of 0.40, 0.35, and 0.25 and 0.72, 0.0, and 0.28, respectively, close to the estimates for men (Table 3). Some differences were noteworthy. In women, we found strong evidence that family environment affected risk for cocaine and stimulant use.[15,16] In men, by contrast, the evidence, while present for both cocaine and stimulant use (ie, DZ correlations greater than half the MZ correlations), was slight and the AE model fit best for both substances.

Our findings are also relatively similar to those recently reported from a treated sample of US twins. Like us, van den Bree et al[9] found, in men, more evidence for familial-environmental effects on use than on abuse/dependence; heritability estimates for abuse and/or dependence were mostly in the range of 0.60 to 0.80. As in our study, a recent investigation of adolescent Virginia twins reports that family environment substantially influences the risk for use of marijuana or any illicit substance.[29]

The results of this study should be interpreted in the light of 6 potential methodologic limitations. First, although our sample size was large, the numbers of twins with certain forms of heavy use, abuse, and especially dependence were small. As reflected by the large CIs of our model-fitting results, this sample was insufficient to determine, with high precision, the magnitude of the genetic and environmental effects for a number of subtypes of PSUD.

Second, as this sample was restricted to whites, it is not possible to extrapolate these results to other ethnic groups. Third, while our sample was derived from a population-based twin registry and our prevalences were in the range of those reported elsewhere, results suggested that for several categories of drug use and misuse, the final study sample was unlikely to be completely representative of the original twin population. This is consistent with prior evidence that individuals with substance abuse are somewhat less likely to cooperate in general population surveys.[30,31] The impact of differential cooperation on the results from twin studies is complex and not entirely predictable,[32,33] but underestimation of heritability is probably more likely than overestimation.[32] Furthermore, our analyses using Mx software[22] included twins whose cotwins were not interviewed, which eliminates some of the bias. Essentially, we used information on potential differences in the prevalence of PSUD in those twins with vs without a cotwin participating to obtain a better estimate of the prevalence of PSUD in the population. The method is a binary data maximum likelihood application of the "missing at random" principle expounded by Little and Rubin.[34]

Fourth, we found higher rates of substance use and misuse in DZ vs MZ twins. This pattern of findings could result from "true" differences (eg, higher average cotwin social support in MZ vs DZ twins) and/or methodologic factors (higher MZ correlations for noncooperativity leading to more effective screening of MZ vs DZ pairs[32]). From whatever cause, the differences were modest and unlikely to substantially influence the results obtained.

Fifth, we assessed PSUD in this sample with a single structured interview. In this design, unreliability is confounded with individual-specific environment[35] and produces a downward bias in estimates of heritability. We can roughly assess the magnitude of this problem by examining the tetrachoric correlations from our test-retest reliability study (Table 1). These suggest that with the possible exceptions of sedative heavy use and abuse and cocaine dependence, the magnitude of diagnostic error was insufficient to produce large downward biases in our parameter estimates. However, some of the estimates reported here for individual-specific environment undoubtedly reflect diagnostic unreliability.

Finally, the human twin study is a quasiexperimental method that cannot approach the methodologic rigor possible in controlled genetic experiments.[35] With a phenotype such as illicit substance use and misuse, which is strongly correlated with a range of social factors,[36,37] it is a particular concern that excess environmental resemblance of MZ vs DZ twins might upwardly bias heritability estimates.[35] We found modest evidence for such an effect using standard measures of the correlated childhood and adult environments. To further evaluate this possible bias, we fitted structural equation models designed to detect and correct for the effects of the equal environment assumption[38] to the 7 conditions in which we found evidence for its violation. For sedative dependence, too few affected twins were available to permit stable model estimation. For the remaining 6 conditions, the proportion of variance in liability in the full model accounted for by the correlated environment averaged 7%. However, in all but one of these models, this correlated environmental factor could be set to 0 with an improvement in the model AIC. The one exception was frequency of adult contact and heavy cocaine use, for which, with the inclusion of a parameter reflecting equal environment assumption violations, the heritability of liability declined from 80% to 60%. It is unlikely that the overall results of this investigation were substantially biased by violations of the equal environment assumption.

These results reinforce a growing body of family,[1-6] twin,[7-10,14-16,39,40] and adoption studies[11-13] that suggest that the risk for psychoactive substance use and misuse is substantially influenced by genetic factors. Our results also support the hypothesis that family environment is important at the stage of substance initiation. The magnitude of genetic influences on PSUD is striking and exceeds that seen in our sample for common psychiatric disorders, such as major depression,[41,42] panic disorder,[43] and phobias.[44]

The demonstration of genetic variance in risk is only the beginning rather than the conclusion of a research program. Of the many questions that can now be asked, 4 are noteworthy. (1) What are the pathways from genes to substance misuse and to what extent do they involve personality, psychopathologic processes, variations in metabolism, target receptors, and/or postreceptor mechanisms? (2) What is the relationship between the genetic and environmental factors that influence initiation vs subsequent misuse?[45] (3) How specific are genetic risks for the use and misuse of individual psychoactive substances?[10] (4) What are the chromosomal locations of susceptibility genes for PSUD?[46]

Accepted for publication December 1, 1999.

This work was supported by grants MH/DA-49492 and DA-11287 from the National Institutes of Health and by Research Scientist Award MH-01277 from National Institute of Mental Health (Dr Kendler), Bethesda, Md. The Virginia Twin Registry, established by W. Nance, MD, PhD, and maintained by L. Corey, PhD, is supported by grants HD-26746 and NS-31564 from the National Institutes of Health.

Reprints: Kenneth S. Kendler, MD, Department of Psychiatry, Medical College of Virginia, Virginia Commonwealth University, Box 980126, Richmond, VA 23298-0126.

REFERENCES

1. Croughan JL. The contributions of family studies to understanding drug abuse. In: Robins LN, ed. *Studying Drug Abuse.* New Brunswick, NJ: Rutgers University Press; 1985:240-264.
2. Mirin SM, Weiss RD, Sollogub A, Michael J. Psychopathology in families of drug abusers. In: Mirin SM, ed. *Substance Abuse and Psychopathology.* Washington, DC: American Psychiatric Association Press; 1984:79-106.
3. Rounsaville BJ, Kosten TR, Weissman MM, Prusoff R, Pauls D, Anton SF, Merikangas K. Psychiatric disorders in relatives of probands with opiate addiction. *Arch Gen Psychiatry.* 1991;48:33-42.
4. Dinwiddie SH, Reich T. Genetic and family studies in psychiatric illness and alcohol and drug dependence. *J Addict Dis.* 1993;12:17-27.
5. Merikangas K, Stolar M, Stevens DE, Goulet J, Preisig MA, Fenton B, Zhang H, O'Malley SS, Rounsaville BJ. Familial transmission of substance use disorders. *Arch Gen Psychiatry.* 1998;55:973-979.
6. Bierut LJ, Dinwiddie SH, Begleiter H, Crowe RR, Hesselbrock V, Nurnberger JI Jr, Porjesz B, Schuckit MA, Reich T. Familial transmission of substance dependence: alcohol, marijuana, cocaine, and habitual smoking: a report from the Collaborative Study on the Genetics of Alcoholism. *Arch Gen Psychiatry.* 1998;55: 982-988.
7. Grove WM, Eckert ED, Heston L, Bouchard TJ Jr, Segal N, Lykken DT. Heritability of substance abuse and antisocial behavior: a study of monozygotic twins reared apart. *Biol Psychiatry.* 1990;27:1293-1304.
8. Tsuang MT, Lyons MJ, Eisen SA, Goldberg J, True W, Meyer JM, Eaves LJ. Genetic influences on abuse of illicit drugs: a study of 3,297 twin pairs. *Am J Med Genet.* 1996;67:473-477.
9. van den Bree MB, Johnson EO, Neale MC, Pickens RW. Genetic and environmental influences on drug use and abuse/dependence in male and female twins. *Drug Alcohol Depend.* 1998;52:231-241.
10. Tsuang MT, Lyons MJ, Meyer JM, Doyle T, Eisen SA, Goldberg J, True W, Lin N, Toomey R, Eaves L. Co-occurence of abuse of different drugs in men: the role of drug-specific and shared vulnerabilities. *Arch Gen Psychiatry.* 1998;55:967-972.
11. Cadoret RJ, Troughton E, O'Gorman TW, Heywood E. An adoption study of genetic and environmental factors in drug abuse. *Arch Gen Psychiatry.* 1986;43: 1131-1136.
12. Cadoret RJ, Yates WR, Troughton E, Woodworth G, Stewart MA. Adoption study demonstrating two genetic pathways to drug abuse. *Arch Gen Psychiatry.* 1995; 52:42-52.
13. Cadoret RJ, Yates WR, Troughton E, Woodworth G, Stewart MA. An adoption study of drug abuse/dependency in females. *Compr Psychiatry.* 1996;37:88-94.
14. Kendler KS, Prescott CA. Cannabis use, abuse and dependence in a population-based sample of female twins. *Am J Psychiatry.* 1998;155:1016-1022.
15. Kendler KS, Prescott CA. Cocaine use, abuse and dependence in a population-based sample of female twins. *Br J Psychiatry.* 1998;173:345-350.
16. Kendler KS, Karkowski LM, Prescott CA. Hallucinogen, opiate, sedative and stimulant use and abuse in a population-based sample of female twins. *Acta Psychiatr Scand.* 1999;99:368-376.
17. SAS Institute. *SAS/STAT User's Guide, Version 6, Fourth Edition.* Vols 1 and 2. Cary, NC: SAS Institute Inc; 1990.
18. Spitzer RL, Williams JB, Gibbon J. *Structured Clinical Interview for DSM-III-R-Patient Version.* New York: New York State Psychiatric Institute; 1987.
19. American Psychiatric Association. *Diagnostic and Statistical Manual of Mental Disorders, Fourth Edition.* Washington, DC: American Psychiatric Association; 1994.

20. Falconer DS. The inheritance of liability to certain diseases, estimated from the incidence among relatives. *Ann Hum Genet.* 1965;29:51-76.
21. Loehlin JC, Nichols RC. *Heredity, Environment and Personality: A Study of 850 Sets of Twins.* Austin: University of Texas Press; 1976.
22. Neale MC. *Statistical Modelling With Mx.* Richmond: Dept of Psychiatry, Medical College of Virginia, Virginia Commonwealth University; 1991.
23. Akaike H. Factor analysis and AIC. *Psychometrika.* 1987;52:317-332.
24. Feild HS, Armenakis AA. On use of multiple tests of significance in psychological research. *Psychol Rep.* 1974;35:427-431.
25. *SAMHSA: National Household Survey on Drug Abuse Main Findings 1996.* Rockville, Md: National Clearinghouse for Alcohol and Drug Information; 1998.
26. Kendler KS, Martin NG, Heath AC, Eaves LJ. Self-report psychiatric symptoms in twins and their nontwin relatives: are twins different? *Am J Med Genet.* 1995; 60:588-591.
27. Rutter M, Redshaw J. Annotation: growing up as a twin: twin-singleton differences in psychological development. *J Child Psychol Psychiatry.* 1991;32:885-895.
28. Kendler KS, Pedersen NL, Farahmand BY, Persson PG. The treated incidence of psychotic and affective illness in twins compared to population expectation: a study in the Swedish Twin and Psychiatric Registries. *Psychol Med.* 1996;26: 1135-1144.
29. Maes HH, Woodard CE, Murrelle L, Meyer JM, Silberg JL, Hewitt JK, Rutter M, Simonoff E, Pickles A, Carbonneau R, Neale MC, Eaves LJ. Tobacco, alcohol and drug use in eight-to-sixteen-year-old twins: the Virginia Twin Study of Adolescent Behavioral Development. *J Stud Alcohol.* 1999;60:293-305.
30. Allgulander C. Psychoactive drug use in a general population sample, Sweden: correlates with perceived health, psychiatric diagnoses, and mortality in an automated record-linkage study. *Am J Public Health.* 1989;79:1006-1010.
31. Kessler RC, Little RJ, Groves RM. Advances in strategies for minimizing and adjusting for survey nonresponse. *Epidemiol Rev.* 1995;17:192-204.
32. Kendler KS, Holm NV. Differential enrollment in twin registries: its effect on prevalence and concordance rates and estimates of genetic parameters. *Acta Genet Med Gemellol (Roma).* 1985;34:125-140.
33. Neale MC, Eaves LJ. Estimating and controlling for the effects of volunteer bias with pairs of relatives. *Behav Genet.* 1993;23:271-277.
34. Little RJ, Rubin DB. *Statistical Analysis With Missing Data.* New York, NY: John Wiley & Sons; 1987.
35. Kendler KS. Twin studies of psychiatric illness: current status and future directions. *Arch Gen Psychiatry.* 1993;50:905-915.
36. Hawkins JD, Catalano RF, Miller JY. Risk and protective factors for alcohol and other drug problems in adolescence and early adulthood: implications for substance abuse prevention. *Psychol Bull.* 1992;112:64-105.
37. Webster RA, Hunter M, Keats JA. Peer and parental influences on adolescents' substance use: a path analysis. *Int J Addict.* 1994;29:647-657.
38. Hettema JM, Neale MC, Kendler KS. Physical similarity and the equal-environment assumption in twin studies of psychiatric disorders. *Behav Genet.* 1995;25:327-335.
39. Gynther LM, Carey G, Gottesman II, Vogler GP. A twin study of non-alcohol substance abuse. *Psychiatry Res.* 1995;56:213-220.
40. Jang KL, Livesley WJ, Vernon PA. Alcohol and drug problems: a multivariate behavioural genetic analysis of co-morbidity. *Addiction.* 1995;90:1213 1221.
41. Kendler KS, Neale MC, Kessler RC, Heath AC, Eaves LJ. A population-based twin study of major depression in women: the impact of varying definitions of illness. *Arch Gen Psychiatry.* 1992;49:257-266.
42. Kendler KS, Prescott CA. A population-based twin study of lifetime major depression in men and women. *Arch Gen Psychiatry.* 1999;56:39-44.
43. Kendler KS, Neale MC, Kessler RC, Heath AC, Eaves LJ. Panic disorder in women: a population-based twin study. *Psychol Med.* 1993;23:397-406.
44. Kendler KS, Neale MC, Kessler RC, Heath AC, Eaves LJ. The genetic epidemiology of phobias in women: the interrelationship of agoraphobia, social phobia, situational phobia, and simple phobia. *Arch Gen Psychiatry.* 1992;49:273-281.
45. Kendler KS, Neale MC, Sullivan PF, Corey LA, Gardner CO, Prescott CA. A population-based twin study in women of smoking initiation and nicotine dependence. *Psychol Med.* 1999; 29:299-308.
46. Straub RE, Sullivan PF, Ma Y, Myakishev MV, Harris-Kerr C, Wormley B, Kadambi B, Sadek H, Silverman MA, Webb BT, Neale MC, Bulik CM, Joyce PR, Kendler KS. Susceptibility genes for nicotine dependence: a genome scan and follow-up in an independent sample suggest that regions on chromosomes 2, 4, 10, 16, 17 and 18 merit further study. *Mol Psychiatry.* 1999;4:129-144.

Predictive Reward Signal of Dopamine Neurons

WOLFRAM SCHULTZ
Institute of Physiology and Program in Neuroscience, University of Fribourg, CH-1700 Fribourg, Switzerland

Schultz, Wolfram. Predictive reward signal of dopamine neurons. *J. Neurophysiol.* 80: 1–27, 1998. The effects of lesions, receptor blocking, electrical self-stimulation, and drugs of abuse suggest that midbrain dopamine systems are involved in processing reward information and learning approach behavior. Most dopamine neurons show phasic activations after primary liquid and food rewards and conditioned, reward-predicting visual and auditory stimuli. They show biphasic, activation-depression responses after stimuli that resemble reward-predicting stimuli or are novel or particularly salient. However, only few phasic activations follow aversive stimuli. Thus dopamine neurons label environmental stimuli with appetitive value, predict and detect rewards and signal alerting and motivating events. By failing to discriminate between different rewards, dopamine neurons appear to emit an alerting message about the surprising presence or absence of rewards. All responses to rewards and reward-predicting stimuli depend on event predictability. Dopamine neurons are activated by rewarding events that are better than predicted, remain uninfluenced by events that are as good as predicted, and are depressed by events that are worse than predicted. By signaling rewards according to a prediction error, dopamine responses have the formal characteristics of a teaching signal postulated by reinforcement learning theories. Dopamine responses transfer during learning from primary rewards to reward-predicting stimuli. This may contribute to neuronal mechanisms underlying the retrograde action of rewards, one of the main puzzles in reinforcement learning. The impulse response releases a short pulse of dopamine onto many dendrites, thus broadcasting a rather global reinforcement signal to postsynaptic neurons. This signal may improve approach behavior by providing advance reward information before the behavior occurs, and may contribute to learning by modifying synaptic transmission. The dopamine reward signal is supplemented by activity in neurons in striatum, frontal cortex, and amygdala, which process specific reward information but do not emit a global reward prediction error signal. A cooperation between the different reward signals may assure the use of specific rewards for selectively reinforcing behaviors. Among the other projection systems, noradrenaline neurons predominantly serve attentional mechanisms and nucleus basalis neurons code rewards heterogeneously. Cerebellar climbing fibers signal errors in motor performance or errors in the prediction of aversive events to cerebellar Purkinje cells. Most deficits following dopamine-depleting lesions are not easily explained by a defective reward signal but may reflect the absence of a general enabling function of tonic levels of extracellular dopamine. Thus dopamine systems may have two functions, the phasic transmission of reward information and the tonic enabling of postsynaptic neurons.

INTRODUCTION

When multicellular organisms arose through the evolution of self-reproducing molecules, they developed endogenous, autoregulatory mechanisms assuring that their needs for welfare and survival were met. Subjects engage in various forms of approach behavior to obtain resources for maintaining homeostatic balance and to reproduce. One class of resources is called rewards, which elicit and reinforce approach behavior. The functions of rewards were developed further during the evolution of higher mammals to support more sophisticated forms of individual and social behavior. Thus biological and cognitive needs define the nature of rewards, and the availability of rewards determines some of the basic parameters of the subject's life conditions.

Rewards come in various physical forms, are highly variable in time and depend on the particular environment of the subject. Despite their importance, rewards do not influence the brain through dedicated peripheral receptors tuned to a limited range of physical modalities as is the case for primary sensory systems. Rather, reward information is extracted by the brain from a large variety of polysensory, inhomogeneous, and inconstant stimuli by using particular neuronal mechanisms. The highly variable nature of rewards requires high degrees of adaptation in neuronal systems processing them.

One of the principal neuronal systems involved in processing reward information appears to be the dopamine system. Behavioral studies show that dopamine projections to the striatum and frontal cortex play a central role in mediating the effects of rewards on approach behavior and learning. These results are derived from selective lesions of different components of dopamine systems, systemic and intracerebral administration of direct and indirect dopamine receptor agonist and antagonist drugs, electrical self-stimulation, and self-administration of major drugs of abuse, such as cocaine, amphetamine, opiates, alcohol, and nicotine (Beninger and Hahn 1983; Di Chiara 1995; Fibiger and Phillips 1986; Robbins and Everitt 1992; Robinson and Berridge 1993; Wise 1996; Wise and Hoffman 1992; Wise et al. 1978).

The present article summarizes recent research concerning the signaling of environmental motivating stimuli by dopamine neurons and evaluates the potential functions of these signals for modifying behavioral reactions by reference to anatomic organization, learning theories, artificial neuronal models, other neuronal systems, and deficits after lesions. All known response characteristics of dopamine neurons will be described, but predominantly the responses to reward-related stimuli will be conceptualized because they are the best understood presently. Because of the large amount of data available in the literature, the principal system discussed will be the nigrostriatal dopamine projection, but projections from midbrain dopamine neurons to ventral striatum and frontal cortex also will be considered as far as the present knowledge allows.

REWARDS AND PREDICTIONS

Functions of rewards

Certain objects and events in the environment are of particular motivational significance by their effects on welfare, survival, and reproduction. According to the behavioral reactions elicited, the motivational value of environmental objects can be appetitive (rewarding) or aversive (punishing). (Note that "appetitive" is used synonymous for "rewarding" but not for "preparatory.") Appetitive objects have three separable basic functions. In their first function, rewards elicit approach and consummatory behavior. This is due to the objects being labeled with appetitive value through innate mechanisms or, in most cases, learning. In their second function, rewards increase the frequency and intensity of behavior leading to such objects (learning), and they maintain learned behavior by preventing extinction. Rewards serve as positive reinforcers of behavior in classical and instrumental conditioning procedures. In general incentive learning, environmental stimuli acquire appetitive value following classically conditioned stimulus-reward associations and induce approach behavior (Bindra 1968). In instrumental conditioning, rewards "reinforce" behaviors by strengthening associations between stimuli and behavioral responses (Law of Effect: Thorndike 1911). This is the essence of "coming back for more" and is related to the common notion of rewards being obtained for having done something well. In an instrumental form of incentive learning, rewards are "incentives" and serve as goals of behavior following associations between behavioral responses and outcomes (Dickinson and Balleine 1994). In their third function, rewards induce subjective feelings of pleasure (hedonia) and positive emotional states. Aversive stimuli function in opposite directions. They induce withdrawal responses and act as negative reinforcers by increasing and maintaining avoidance behavior on repeated presentation, thereby reducing the impact of damaging events. Furthermore they induce internal emotional states of anger, fear, and panic.

Functions of predictions

Predictions provide advance information about future stimuli, events, or system states. They provide the basic advantage of gaining time for behavioral reactions. Some forms of predictions attribute motivational values to environmental stimuli by association with particular outcomes, thus identifying objects of vital importance and discriminating them from less valuable objects. Other forms code physical parameters of predicted objects, such as spatial position, velocity, and weight. Predictions allow an organism to evaluate future events before they actually occur, permit the selection and preparation of behavioral reactions, and increase the likelihood of approaching or avoiding objects labeled with motivational values. For example, repeated movements of objects in the same sequence allow one to predict forthcoming positions and already prepare the next movement while pursuing the present object. This reduces reaction time between individual targets, speeds up overall performance, and results in an earlier outcome. Predictive eye movements ameliorate behavioral performance through advance focusing (Flowers and Downing 1978).

At a more advanced level, the advance information provided by predictions allows one to make decisions between alternatives to attain particular system states, approach infrequently occurring goal objects, or avoid irreparable adverse effects. Industrial applications use Internal Model Control

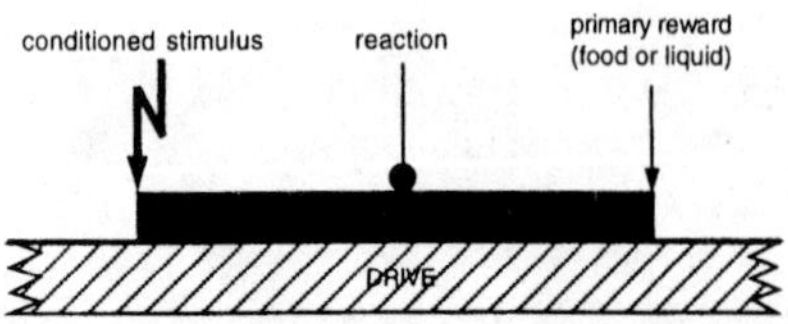

FIG. 1. Processing of appetitive stimuli during learning. An arbitrary stimulus becomes associated with a primary food or liquid reward through repeated, contingent pairing. This conditioned, reward-predicting stimulus induces an internal motivational state by evoking an expectation of the reward, often on the basis of a corresponding hunger or thirst drive, and elicits the behavioral reaction. This scheme replicates basic notions of incentive motivation theory developed by Bindra (1968) and Bolles (1972). It applies to classical conditioning, where reward is automatically delivered after the conditioned stimulus, and to instrumental (operant) conditioning, where reward delivery requires a reaction by the subject to the conditioned stimulus. This scheme applies also to aversive conditioning which is not further elaborated for reasons of brevity.

to predict and react to system states before they actually occur (Garcia et al. 1989). For example, the "fly-by-wire" technique in modern aviation computes predictable forthcoming states of airplanes. Decisions for flying maneuvers take this information into account and help to avoid excessive strain on the mechanical components of the plane, thus reducing weight and increasing the range of operation.

The use of predictive information depends on the nature of the represented future events or system states. Simple representations directly concern the position of upcoming targets and the ensuing behavioral reaction, thus reducing reaction time in a rather automatic fashion. Higher forms of predictions are based on representations permitting logical inference, which can be accessed and treated with varying degrees of intentionality and choice. They often are processed consciously in humans. Before the predicted events or system states occur and behavioral reactions are carried out, such predictions allow one to mentally evaluate various strategies by integrating knowledge from different sources, designing various ways of reaction and comparing the gains and losses from each possible reaction.

Behavioral conditioning

Associative appetitive learning involves the repeated and contingent pairing between an arbitrary stimulus and a primary reward (Fig. 1). This results in increasingly frequent approach behavior induced by the now "conditioned" stimulus, which partly resembles the approach behavior elicited by the primary reward and also is influenced by the nature of the conditioned stimulus. It appears that the conditioned stimulus serves as a predictor of reward and, often on the basis of an appropriate drive, sets an internal motivational state leading to the behavioral reaction. The similarity of approach reactions suggests that some of the general, preparatory components of the behavioral response are transferred from the primary reward to the earliest conditioned, reward-predicting stimulus. Thus the conditioned stimulus acts partly as a motivational substitute for the primary stimulus, probably through Pavlovian learning (Dickinson 1980).

Many so called "unconditioned" food and liquid rewards are probably learned through experience, as every visitor to foreign countries can confirm. The primary reward then might consist of the taste experienced when the object activates the gustatory receptors, but that again may be learned. The ultimate rewarding effect of nutrient objects probably consists in their specific influences on basic biological variables, such as electrolyte, glucose, or amino acid concentrations in plasma and brain. These variables are defined by the vegetative needs of the organism and arise through evolution. Animals avoid nutrients that fail to influence important vegetative variables, for example foods lacking such essential amino acids as histidine (Rogers and Harper 1970), threonine (Hrupka et al. 1997; Wang et al. 1996), or methionine (Delaney and Gelperin 1986). A few primary rewards may be determined by innate instincts and support initial approach behavior and ingestion in early life, whereas the majority of rewards would be learned during the subsequent life experience of the subject. The physical appearance of rewards then could be used for predicting the much slower vegetative effects. This would dramatically accelerate the detection of rewards and constitute a major advantage for survival. Learning of rewards also allows subjects to use a much larger variety of nutrients as effective rewards and thus increase their chance for survival in zones of scarce resources.

ADAPTIVE RESPONSES TO APPETITIVE STIMULI

Cell bodies of dopamine neurons are located mostly in midbrain groups A8 (dorsal to lateral substantia nigra), A9 (pars compacta of substantia nigra), and A10 (ventral tegmental area medial to substantia nigra). These neurons release the neurotransmitter dopamine with nerve impulses from axonal varicosities in the striatum (caudate nucleus, putamen, and ventral striatum including nucleus accumbens) and frontal cortex, to name the most important sites. We record the impulse activity from cell bodies of single dopamine neurons during periods of 20–60 min with moveable microelectrodes from extracellular positions while monkeys learn or perform behavioral tasks. The characteristic polyphasic, relatively long impulses discharged at low frequencies make dopamine neurons easily distinguishable from other midbrain neurons. The employed behavioral paradigms include reaction time tasks, direct and delayed GO-NO GO tasks, spatial delayed response and alternation tasks, air puff and saline active avoidance tasks, operant and classically conditioned visual discrimination tasks, self-initiated movements, and unpredicted delivery of reward in the absence of any formal task. About 100–250 dopamine neurons are studied in each behavioral situation, and fractions of task-modulated neurons refer to these samples.

Initial recording studies searched for correlates of parkinsonian motor and cognitive deficits in dopamine neurons but failed to find clear covariations with arm and eye movements (DeLong et al. 1983; Schultz and Romo 1990; Schultz et al. 1983) or with mnemonic or spatial components of delayed response tasks (Schultz et al. 1993). By contrast, it was found that dopamine neurons were activated in a very distinctive manner by the rewarding characteristics of a wide range of somatosensory, visual, and auditory stimuli.

Activation by primary appetitive stimuli

About 75% of dopamine neurons show phasic activations when animals touch a small morsel of hidden food during exploratory movements in the absence of other phasic stimuli, without being activated by the movement itself (Romo and Schultz 1990). The remaining dopamine neurons do not respond to any of the tested environmental stimuli. Dopamine neurons also are activated by a drop of liquid delivered at the mouth outside of any behavioral task or while learning such different paradigms as visual or auditory reaction time tasks, spatial delayed response or alternation, and visual discrimination, often in the same animal (Fig. 2 *top*) (Hollerman and Schultz 1996; Ljungberg et al. 1991, 1992; Mirenowicz and Schultz 1994; Schultz et al. 1993). The reward responses occur independently of a learning context. Thus dopamine neurons do not appear to discriminate between different food objects and liquid rewards. However, their responses distinguish rewards from nonreward objects (Romo and Schultz 1990). Only 14% of dopamine neurons show the phasic activations when primary aversive stimuli are presented, such as an air puff to the hand or hypertonic saline to the mouth, and most of the activated neurons respond also to rewards (Mirenowicz and Schultz 1996). Although being nonnoxious, these stimuli are aversive in that they disrupt behavior and induce active avoidance reactions. However, dopamine neurons are not entirely insensitive to aversive stimuli, as shown by slow depressions or occasional slow activations after pain pinch stimuli in anesthetized monkeys (Schultz and Romo 1987) and by increased striatal dopamine release after electric shock and tail pinch in awake rats (Abercrombie et al. 1989; Doherty and Gratton 1992; Louilot et al. 1986; Young et al. 1993). This suggests that the phasic responses of dopamine neurons preferentially report environmental stimuli with primary appetitive value, whereas aversive events may be signaled with a considerably slower time course.

Unpredictability of reward

An important feature of dopamine responses is their dependency on event unpredictability. The activations following rewards do not occur when food and liquid rewards are preceded by phasic stimuli that have been conditioned to predict such rewards (Fig. 2, *middle*) (Ljungberg et al. 1992; Mirenowicz and Schultz 1994; Romo and Schultz 1990). One crucial difference between learning and fully acquired behavior is the degree of reward unpredictability. Dopamine neurons are activated by rewards during the learning phase but stop responding after full acquisition of visual and auditory reaction time tasks (Ljungberg et al. 1992; Mirenowicz and Schultz 1994), spatial delayed response tasks (Schultz et al. 1993), and simultaneous visual discriminations (Hollerman and Schultz 1996). The loss of response is not due to a developing general insensitivity to rewards, as activations following rewards delivered outside of tasks do not decrement during several months of experimentation (Mirenowicz and Schultz 1994). The importance of unpredictability includes the time of reward, as demonstrated by transient activations following rewards that are suddenly delivered earlier or later than predicted (Hollerman and Schultz 1996). Taken

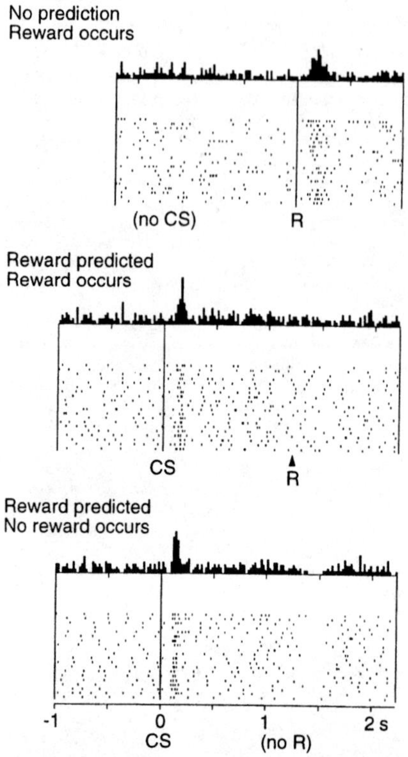

FIG. 2. Dopamine neurons report rewards according to an error in reward prediction. *Top*: drop of liquid occurs although no reward is predicted at this time. Occurrence of reward thus constitutes a positive error in the prediction of reward. Dopamine neuron is activated by the unpredicted occurrence of the liquid. *Middle*: conditioned stimulus predicts a reward, and the reward occurs according to the prediction, hence no error in the prediction of reward. Dopamine neuron fails to be activated by the predicted reward (*right*). It also shows an activation after the reward-predicting stimulus, which occurs irrespective of an error in the prediction of the later reward (*left*). *Bottom*: conditioned stimulus predicts a reward, but the reward fails to occur because of lack of reaction by the animal. Activity of the dopamine neuron is depressed exactly at the time when the reward would have occurred. Note the depression occurring >1 s after the conditioned stimulus without any intervening stimuli, revealing an internal process of reward expectation. Neuronal activity in the 3 graphs follows the equation: dopamine response (Reward) = reward occurred − reward predicted. CS, conditioned stimulus; R, primary reward. Reprinted from Schultz et al. (1997) with permission by American Association for the Advancement of Science.

together, the occurrence of reward, including its time, must be unpredicted to activate dopamine neurons.

Depression by omission of predicted reward

Dopamine neurons are depressed exactly at the time of the usual occurrence of reward when a fully predicted reward fails to occur, even in the absence of an immediately preceding stimulus (Fig. 2, *bottom*). This is observed when animals fail to obtain reward because of erroneous behavior, when liquid flow is stopped by the experimenter despite correct behavior, or when a valve opens audibly without delivering liquid (Hollerman and Schultz 1996; Ljungberg et al. 1991; Schultz et al. 1993). When reward delivery is delayed for 0.5 or 1.0 s, a depression of neuronal activity occurs at the regular time of the reward, and an activation follows the reward at the new time (Hollerman and Schultz 1996). Both responses occur only during a few repetitions until the new time of reward delivery becomes predicted again. By contrast, delivering reward earlier than habitual results in an activation at the new time of reward but fails to induce a depression at the habitual time. This suggests that unusually early reward delivery cancels the reward prediction for the habitual time. Thus dopamine neurons monitor both the occurrence and the time of reward. In the absence of stimuli immediately preceding the omitted reward, the depressions do not constitute a simple neuronal response but reflect an expectation process based on an internal clock tracking the precise time of predicted reward.

Activation by conditioned, reward-predicting stimuli

About 55–70% of dopamine neurons are activated by conditioned visual and auditory stimuli in the various classically or instrumentally conditioned tasks described earlier (Fig. 2, *middle* and *bottom*) (Hollerman and Schultz 1996; Ljungberg et al. 1991, 1992; Mirenowicz and Schultz 1994; Schultz 1986; Schultz and Romo 1990; P. Waelti, J. Mirenowicz, and W. Schultz, unpublished data). The first dopamine responses to conditioned light were reported by Miller et al. (1981) in rats treated with haloperidol, which increased the incidence and spontaneous activity of dopamine neurons but resulted in more sustained responses than in undrugged animals. Although responses occur close to behavioral reactions (Nishino et al. 1987), they are unrelated to arm and eye movements themselves, as they occur also ipsilateral to the moving arm and in trials without arm or eye movements (Schultz and Romo 1990). Conditioned stimuli are somewhat less effective than primary rewards in terms of response magnitude and fractions of neurons activated. Dopamine neurons respond only to the onset of conditioned stimuli and not to their offset, even if stimulus offset predicts the reward (Schultz and Romo 1990). Dopamine neurons do not distinguish between visual and auditory modalities of conditioned appetitive stimuli. However, they discriminate between appetitive and neutral or aversive stimuli as long as they are physically sufficiently dissimilar (Ljungberg et al. 1992; P. Waelti, J. Mirenowicz, and W. Schultz, unpublished data). Only 11% of dopamine neurons, most of them with appetitive responses, show the typical phasic activations also in response to conditioned aversive visual or auditory stimuli in active avoidance tasks in which animals release a key to avoid an air puff or a drop of hypertonic saline (Mirenowicz and Schultz 1996), although such avoidance may be viewed as "rewarding." These few activations are not sufficiently strong to induce an average population response. Thus the phasic responses of dopamine neurons preferentially report environmental stimuli with appetitive motivational value but without discriminating between different sensory modalities.

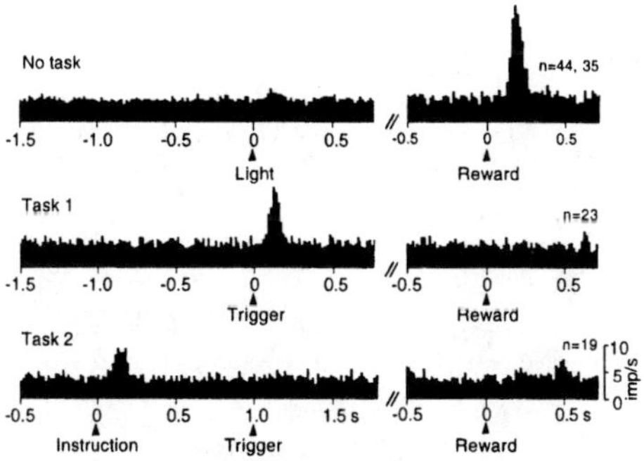

FIG. 3. Dopamine response transfer to earliest predictive stimulus. Responses to unpredicted primary reward transfer to progressively earlier reward-predicting stimuli. All displays show population histograms obtained by averaging normalized perievent time histograms of all dopamine neurons recorded in the behavioral situations indicated, independent of the presence or absence of a response. *Top*: outside of any behavioral task, there is no population response in 44 neurons tested with a small light (data from Ljungberg et al. 1992), but an average response occurs in 35 neurons to a drop of liquid delivered at a spout in front of the animal's mouth (Mirenowicz and Schultz 1994). *Middle*: response to a reward-predicting trigger stimulus in a 2-choice spatial reaching task, but absence of response to reward delivered during established task performance in the same 23 neurons (Schultz et al. 1993). *Bottom*: response to an instruction cue preceding the reward-predicting trigger stimulus by a fixed interval of 1 s in an instructed spatial reaching task (19 neurons) (Schultz et al. 1993). Time base is split because of varying intervals between conditioned stimuli and reward. Reprinted from Schultz et al. (1995b) with permission by MIT Press.

Transfer of activation

During the course of learning, dopamine neurons become gradually activated by conditioned, reward-predicting stimuli and progressively lose their responses to primary food or liquid rewards that become predicted (Hollerman and Schultz 1996; Ljungberg et al. 1992; Mirenowicz and Schultz 1994) (Figs. 2 and 3). During a transient learning period, both rewards and conditioned stimuli elicit dopamine activations. This transfer from primary reward to the conditioned stimulus occurs instantaneously in single dopamine neurons tested in two well-learned tasks employing, respectively, unpredicted and predicted rewards (Romo and Schultz 1990).

Unpredictability of conditioned stimuli

The activations after conditioned, reward-predicting stimuli do not occur when these stimuli themselves are preceded at a fixed interval by phasic conditioned stimuli in fully established behavioral situations. Thus with serial conditioned stimuli, dopamine neurons are activated by the earliest reward-predicting stimulus, whereas all stimuli and rewards following at predictable moments afterwards are ineffective (Fig. 3) (Schultz et al. 1993). Only randomly spaced sequential stimuli elicit individual responses. Also, extensive overtraining with highly stereotyped task performance attenuates the responses to conditioned stimuli, probably because stimuli become predicted by events in the preceding trial (Ljungberg et al. 1992). This suggests that stimulus unpredictability is a common requirement for all stimuli activating dopamine neurons.

Depression by omission of predicted conditioned stimuli

Preliminary data from a previous experiment (Schultz et al. 1993) suggest that dopamine neurons also are depressed when a conditioned, reward-predicting stimulus is predicted itself at a fixed time by a preceding stimulus but fails to occur because of an error of the animal. As with primary rewards, the depressions occur at the time of the usual occurrence of the conditioned stimulus, without being directly elicited by a preceding stimulus. Thus the omission-induced depression may be generalized to all appetitive events.

Activation-depression with response generalization

Dopamine neurons also respond to stimuli that do not predict rewards but closely resemble reward-predicting stimuli occurring in the same context. These responses consist mostly of an activation followed by an immediate depression but may occasionally consist of pure activation or pure depression. The activations are smaller and less frequent than those following reward-predicting stimuli, and the depressions are observed in 30–60% of neurons. Dopamine neurons respond to visual stimuli that are not followed by reward but closely resemble reward-predicting stimuli, despite correct behavioral discrimination (Schultz and Romo 1990). Opening of an empty box fails to activate dopamine neurons but becomes effective in every trial as soon as the box occasionally contains food (Ljungberg et al. 1992; Schultz 1986; Schultz and Romo 1990) or when a neighboring, identical box always containing food opens in random alternation (Schultz and Romo 1990). The empty box elicits weaker activations than the baited box. Animals perform indiscriminate ocular orienting reactions to each box but only approach the baited box with their hand. During learning, dopamine neurons continue to respond to previously conditioned stimuli that lose their reward prediction when reward contingencies change (Schultz et al. 1993) or respond to new stimuli resembling previously conditioned stimuli (Hollerman and Schultz 1996). Responses occur even to aversive stimuli presented in random alternation with physically similar, conditioned appetitive stimuli of the same sensory modality, the aversive response being weaker than the appetitive one (Mirenowicz and Schultz 1996). Responses generalize even to behaviorally extinguished appetitive stimuli. Apparently, neuronal responses generalize to nonappetitive stimuli because of their physical resemblance with appetitive stimuli.

Novelty responses

Novel stimuli elicit activations in dopamine neurons that often are followed by depressions and persist as long as behavioral orienting reactions occur (e.g., ocular saccades). Activations subside together with orienting reactions after several stimulus repetitions, depending on the physical impact of stimuli. Whereas small light-emitting diodes hardly elicit novelty responses, light flashes and the rapid visual and auditory opening of a small box elicit activations that decay gradually to baseline during <100 trials (Ljungberg

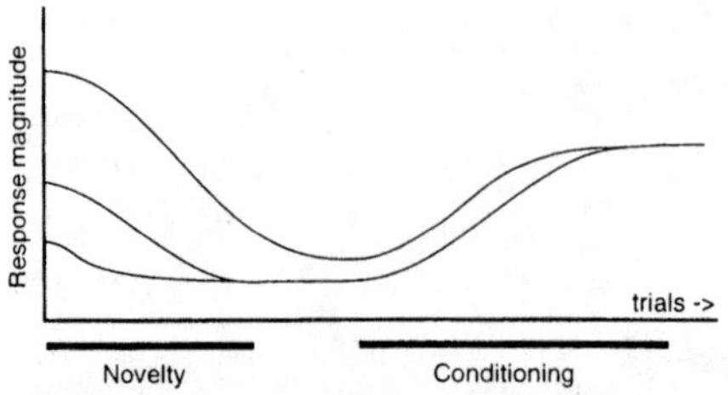

FIG. 4. Time courses of activations of dopamine neurons to novel, alerting, and conditioned stimuli. Activations after novel stimuli decrease with repeated exposure over consecutive trials. Their magnitude depends on the physical salience of stimuli as stronger stimuli induce higher activations that occasionally exceed those after conditioned stimuli. Particularly salient stimuli continue to activate dopamine neurons with limited magnitude even after losing their novelty without being paired with primary rewards. Consistent activations appear again when stimuli become associated with primary rewards. This scheme was contributed by Jose Contreras-Vidal.

et al. 1992). Loud clicks or large pictures immediately in front of an animal elicit strong novelty responses that decay but still induce measurable activations with >1,000 trials (Hollerman and Schultz 1996; Horvitz et al. 1997; Steinfels et al. 1983). Figure 4 shows schematically the different response magnitudes with novel stimuli of different physical salience. Responses decay gradually with repeated exposure but may persist at reduced magnitudes with very salient stimuli. Response magnitudes increase again when the same stimuli are appetitively conditioned. By contrast, responses to novel, even large, stimuli subside rapidly when the stimuli are used for conditioning active avoidance behavior (Mirenowicz and Schultz 1996). Very few neurons (<5%) respond for more than a few trials to conspicuous yet physically weak stimuli, such as crumbling of paper or gross hand movements of the experimenter.

Homogeneous character of responses

The experiments performed so far have revealed that the majority of neurons in midbrain dopamine cell groups A8, A9, and A10 show very similar activations and depressions in a given behavioral situation, whereas the remaining dopamine neurons do not respond at all. There is a tendency for higher fractions of neurons responding in more medial regions of the midbrain, such as the ventral tegmental area and medial substantia nigra, as compared with more lateral regions, which occasionally reach statistical significance (Schultz 1986; Schultz et al. 1993). Response latencies (50–110 ms) and durations (<200 ms) are similar among primary rewards, conditioned stimuli, and novel stimuli. Thus the dopamine response constitutes a relatively homogeneous, scalar population signal. It is graded in magnitude by the responsiveness of individual neurons and by the fraction of responding neurons within the population.

Summary 1: adaptive responses during learning episodes

The characteristics of dopamine responses to reward-related stimuli are best illustrated in learning episodes during that rewards are particularly important for acquiring behavioral responses. The dopamine reward signal undergoes systematic changes during the progress of learning and occurs to the earliest phasic reward-related stimulus, this being either a primary reward or a reward-predicting stimulus (Ljungberg et al. 1992; Mirenowicz and Schultz 1994). During learning, novel, intrinsically neutral stimuli transiently induce responses that weaken soon and disappear (Fig. 4). Primary rewards occur unpredictably during initial pairing with such stimuli and elicit neuronal activations. With repeated pairing, rewards become predicted by conditioned stimuli. Activations after the reward decrease gradually and are transferred to the conditioned, reward-predicting stimulus. If, however, a predicted reward fails to occur because of an error of the animal, dopamine neurons are depressed at the time the reward would have occurred. During repeated learning of tasks (Schultz et al. 1993) or task components (Hollerman and Schultz 1996), the earliest conditioned stimuli activate dopamine neurons during all learning phases because of generalization to previously learned, similar stimuli, whereas subsequent conditioned stimuli and primary rewards activate dopamine neurons only transiently while they are uncertain and new contingencies are being established.

Summary 2: effective stimuli for dopamine neurons

Dopamine responses are elicited by three categories of stimuli. The first category comprises primary rewards and stimuli that have become valid reward predictors through repeated and contingent pairing with rewards. These stimuli form a common class of explicit reward-predicting stimuli, as primary rewards serve as predictors of vegetative rewarding effects. Effective stimuli apparently have an alerting component, as only stimuli with a clear onset are effective. Dopamine neurons show pure activations following explicit reward-predicting stimuli and are depressed when a predicted but omitted reward fails to occur (Fig. 5, *top*).

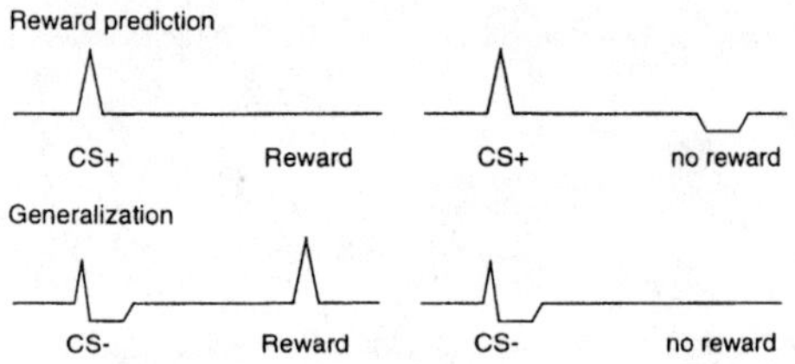

FIG. 5. Schematic display of responses of dopamine neurons to 2 types of conditioned stimuli. *Top*: presentation of an explicit reward-predicting stimulus leads to activation after the stimulus, no response to the predicted reward, and depression when a predicted reward fails to occur. *Bottom*: presentation of a stimulus closely resembling a conditioned, reward-predicting stimulus leads to activation followed by depression, activation after the reward, and no response when no reward occurs. Activation after the stimulus probably reflects response generalization because of physical similarity. This stimulus does not explicitly predict a reward but is related to the reward via its similarity to the stimulus predicting the reward. In comparison with explicit reward-predicting stimuli, activations are lower and often are followed by depressions, thus discriminating between rewarded (CS+) and unrewarded (CS−) conditioned stimuli. This scheme summarizes results from previous and current experiments (Hollerman and Schultz 1996; Ljungberg et al. 1992; Mirenowicz and Schultz 1996; Schultz and Romo 1990; Schultz et al. 1993; P. Waelti and W. Schultz, unpublished results).

The second category comprises stimuli that elicit generalizing responses. These stimuli do not explicitly predict rewards but are effective because of their physical similarity to stimuli that have become explicit reward predictors through conditioning. These stimuli induce activations that are lower in magnitude and engage fewer neurons, as compared with explicit reward-predicting stimuli (Fig. 5, *bottom*). They are frequently followed by immediate depressions. Whereas the initial activation may constitute a generalized appetitive response that signals a possible reward, the subsequent depression may reflect the prediction of no reward in a general reward-predicting context and cancel the erroneous reward assumption. The lack of explicit reward prediction is suggested further by the presence of activation after primary reward and the absence of depression with no reward. Together with the responses to reward-predicting stimuli, it appears as if dopamine activations report an appetitive "tag" affixed to stimuli that are related to rewards.

The third category comprises novel or particularly salient stimuli that are not necessarily related to specific rewards. By eliciting behavioral orienting reactions, these stimuli are alerting and command attention. However, they also have motivating functions and can be rewarding (Fujita 1987). Novel stimuli are potentially appetitive. Novel or particularly salient stimuli induce activations that are frequently followed by depressions, similar to responses to generalizing stimuli.

Thus the phasic responses of dopamine neurons report events with positive and potentially positive motivating effects, such as primary rewards, reward-predicting stimuli, reward-resembling events, and alerting stimuli. However, they do not detect to a large extent events with negative motivating effects, such as aversive stimuli.

Summary 3: the dopamine reward prediction error signal

The dopamine responses to explicit reward-related events can be best conceptualized and understood in terms of formal theories of learning. Dopamine neurons report rewards relative to their prediction rather than signaling primary rewards unconditionally (Fig. 2). The dopamine response is positive (activation) when primary rewards occur without being predicted. The response is nil when rewards occur as predicted. The response is negative (depression) when predicted rewards are omitted. Thus dopamine neurons report primary rewards according to the difference between the occurrence and the prediction of reward, which can be termed an error in the prediction of reward (Schultz et al. 1995b, 1997) and is tentatively formalized as

$$\text{DopamineResponse (Reward)} = \text{RewardOccurred} - \text{RewardPredicted} \quad (1)$$

This suggestion can be extended to conditioned appetitive events that also are reported by dopamine neurons relative to prediction. Thus dopamine neurons may report an error in the prediction of all appetitive events, and *Eq. 1* can be stated in the more general form

$$\text{DopamineResponse (ApEvent)} = \text{ApEventOccurred} - \text{ApEventPredicted} \quad (2)$$

This generalization is compatible with the idea that most rewards actually are conditioned stimuli. With several consecutive, well-established reward-predicting events, only the first event is unpredictable and elicits the dopamine activation.

CONNECTIVITY OF DOPAMINE NEURONS

Origin of the dopamine response

Which anatomic inputs could be responsible for the selectivity and polysensory nature of dopamine responses? Which input activity could lead to the coding of prediction errors, induce the adaptive response transfer to the earliest unpredicted appetitive event and estimate the time of reward?

DORSAL AND VENTRAL STRIATUM. The GABAergic neurons in the striosomes (patches) of the striatum project in a broadly topographic and partly overlapping, interdigitating manner to dopamine neurons in nearly the entire pars compacta of substantia nigra, whereas neurons of the much larger striatal matrix contact predominantly the nondopamine neurons of pars reticulata of substantia nigra, besides their projection to globus pallidus (Gerfen 1984; Hedreen and DeLong 1991; Holstein et al. 1986; Jimenez-Castellanos and Graybiel 1989; Selemon and Goldman-Rakic 1990; Smith and Bolam 1991). Neurons in the ventral striatum project in a nontopographic manner to both pars compacta and pars reticulata of medial substantia nigra and to the ventral tegmental area (Berendse et al. 1992; Haber et al. 1990; Lynd-Balta and Haber 1994; Somogyi et al. 1981). The GABAergic striatonigral projection may exert two distinctively different influences on dopamine neurons, a direct inhibition and an indirect activation (Grace and Bunney 1985; Smith and Grace 1992; Tepper et al. 1995). The latter is mediated by striatal inhibition of pars reticulata neurons and subsequent GABAergic inhibition from local axon collaterals of pars reticulata output neurons onto dopamine neurons. This constitutes a double inhibitory link and results in net activation of dopamine neurons by the striatum. Thus striosomes and ventral striatum may monosynaptically inhibit and the matrix may indirectly activate dopamine neurons.

Dorsal and ventral striatal neurons show a number of activations that might contribute to dopamine reward responses, namely responses to primary rewards (Apicella et al. 1991a; Williams et al. 1993), responses to reward-predicting stimuli (Hollerman et al. 1994; Romo et al. 1992) and sustained activations during the expectation of reward-predicting stimuli and primary rewards (Apicella et al. 1992; Schultz et al. 1992). However, the positions of these neurons relative to striosomes and matrix are unknown, and striatal activations reflecting the time of expected reward have not yet been reported.

The polysensory reward responses might be the result of feature extraction in cortical association areas. Response latencies of 30–75 ms in primary and associative visual cortex (Maunsell and Gibson 1992; Miller et al. 1993) could combine with rapid conduction to striatum and double inhibition of substantia nigra to induce the short dopamine response latencies of <100 ms. Whereas reward-related activity has not been reported for posterior association cortex, neurons in dorsolateral and orbital prefrontal cortex respond to primary rewards and reward-predicting stimuli and show sustained activations during reward expectation (Rolls et al. 1996; Thorpe et al. 1983; Tremblay and Schultz 1995; Watanabe 1996). Some reward responses in frontal cortex depend on reward unpredictability (Matsumoto et al. 1995; L. Tremblay and W. Schultz, unpublished results) or reflect behavioral errors or omitted rewards (Niki and Watanabe 1979; Watanabe 1989). The cortical influence on dopamine neurons would even be faster through a direct projection, originating from prefrontal cortex in rats (Gariano and Groves 1988; Sesack and Pickel 1992; Tong et al. 1996) but being weak in monkeys (Künzle 1978).

NUCLEUS PEDUNCULOPONTINUS. Short latencies of reward responses may be derived from adaptive, feature-processing mechanisms in the brain stem. Nucleus pedunculopontinus is an evolutionary precursor of substantia nigra. In nonmammalian vertebrates, it contains dopamine neurons and projects to the paleostriatum (Lohman and Van Woerden-Verkley 1978). In mammals, this nucleus sends strong excitatory, cholinergic, and glutamatergic influences to a high fraction of dopamine neurons with latencies of ~7 ms (Bolam et al. 1991; Clarke et al. 1987; Futami et al. 1995; Scarnati et al. 1986). Activation of pedunculopontine-dopamine projections induces circling behavior (Niijima and Yoshida 1988), suggesting a functional influence on dopamine neurons.

AMYGDALA. A massive, probably excitatory input to dopamine neurons arises from different nuclei of the amygdala (Gonzalez and Chesselet 1990; Price and Amaral 1981). Amygdala neurons respond to primary rewards and reward-predicting visual and auditory stimuli. The neuronal responses known so far are independent of stimulus unpredictability and do not discriminate well between appetitive and aversive events (Nakamura et al. 1992; Nishijo et al. 1988). Most responses show latencies of 140–310 ms, which are longer than in dopamine neurons, although a few responses occur at latencies of 60–100 ms.

DORSAL RAPHÉ. The monosynaptic projection from dorsal raphé (Corvaja et al. 1993; Nedergaard et al. 1988) has a depressant influence on dopamine neurons (Fibiger et al. 1977; Trent and Tepper 1991). Raphé neurons show short-latency activations after high-intensity environmental stimuli (Heym et al. 1982), allowing them to contribute to dopamine responses after novel or particularly salient stimuli.

SYNTHESIS. A few, well-known input structures are the most likely candidates for mediating the dopamine responses, although additional inputs also may exist. Activations of dopamine neurons by primary rewards and reward-predicting stimuli could be mediated by double inhibitory, net activating input from the striatal matrix (for a simplified diagram, see Fig. 6). Activations also could arise from pedunculopontine nucleus or possibly from reward expectation-related activity in neurons of the subthalamic nucleus projecting to dopamine neurons (Hammond et al. 1983; Matsumura et al. 1992; Smith et al. 1990). The absence of activation with fully predicted rewards could be the result of monosynaptic inhibition from striosomes, cancelling out simultaneously activating matrix input. Depressions at the time of omitted reward could be mediated by inhibitory inputs from neurons

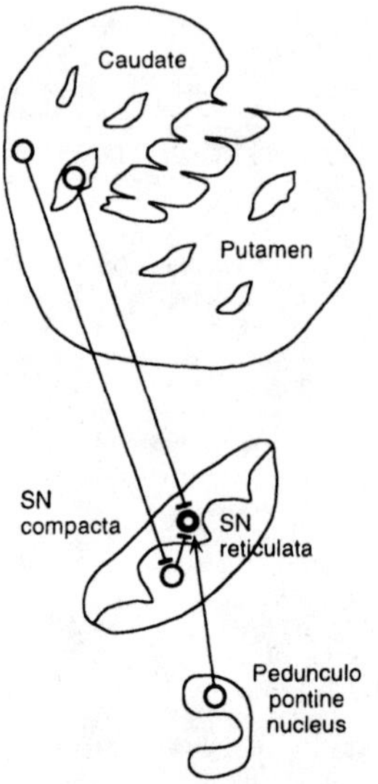

FIG. 6. Simplified diagram of inputs to midbrain dopamine neurons potentially mediating dopamine responses. Only inputs from caudate to substantia nigra (SN) pars compacta and reticulata are shown for reasons of simplicity. Activations may arise by a double inhibitory, net activating influence from GABAergic matrix neurons in caudate and putamen via GABAergic neurons of SN pars reticulata to dopamine neurons of SN pars compacta. Activations also may be mediated by excitatory cholinergic or amino acid-containing projections from nucleus pedunculopontinus. Depressions could be due to monosynaptic GABAergic projections from striosomes (patches) in caudate and putamen to dopamine neurons. Similar projections exist from ventral striatum to dopamine neurons in medial SN pars compacta and group A10 in the ventral tegmental area and from dorsal striatum to group A8 dopamine neurons dorsolateral to SN (Lynd-Balta and Haber 1994). Heavy circle represents dopamine neurons. These projections represent the most likely inputs underlying the dopamine responses, without ruling out inputs from globus pallidus and subthalamic nucleus.

in striatal striosomes (Houk et al. 1995) or globus pallidus (Haber et al. 1993; Hattori et al. 1975; Y. Smith and Bolam 1990, 1991). Convergence between different inputs before or at the level of dopamine neurons could result in the rather complex coding of reward prediction errors and the adaptive response transfer from primary rewards to reward-predicting stimuli.

Phasic dopamine influences on target structures

GLOBAL NATURE OF DOPAMINE SIGNAL. *Divergent projections.* There are ~8,000 dopamine neurons in each substantia nigra of rats (Oorschot 1996) and 80,000–116,000 in macaque monkeys (German et al. 1988; Percheron et al. 1989). Each striatum contains ~2.8 million neurons in rats and 31 million in macaques, resulting in a nigrostriatal divergence factor of 300–400. Each dopamine axon ramifies abundantly in a limited terminal area in striatum and has ~500,000 striatal varicosities from which dopamine is released (Andén

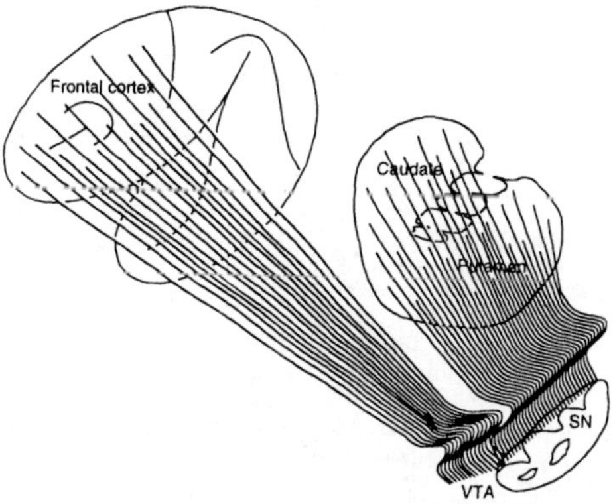

FIG. 7. Global dopamine signal advancing to striatum and cortex. Relatively homogeneous population response of the majority of dopamine neurons to appetitive and alerting stimuli and its progression from substantia nigra to postsynaptic structures can be viewed schematically as a wave of synchronous, parallel activity advancing at a velocity of 1–2 m/s (Schultz and Romo 1987) along the diverging projections from the midbrain to striatum (caudate and putamen) and cortex. Responses are qualitatively indistinguishable between neurons of substantia nigra (SN) pars compacta and ventral tegmental area (VTA). Dopamine innervation of all neurons in striatum and many neurons in frontal cortex would allow the dopamine reinforcement signal to exert a rather global effect. Wave has been compressed to emphasize the parallel nature.

et al. 1966). This results in dopamine input to nearly every striatal neuron (Groves et al. 1995) and a moderately topographic nigrostriatal projection (Lynd-Balta and Haber 1994). The cortical dopamine innervation in monkeys is highest in areas 4 and 6, is still sizeable in frontal, parietal, and temporal lobes, and is lowest in the occipital lobe (Berger et al. 1988; Williams and Goldman-Rakic 1993). Cortical dopamine synapses are predominantly found in layers I and V–VI, contacting a large proportion of cortical neurons there. Together with the rather homogeneous response nature, these data suggest that the dopamine response advances as a simultaneous, parallel wave of activity from the midbrain to striatum and frontal cortex (Fig. 7).

Dopamine release. Impulses of dopamine neurons at intervals of 20–100 ms lead to a much higher dopamine concentration in striatum than the same number of impulses at intervals of 200 ms (Garris and Wightman 1994; Gonon 1988). This nonlinearity is mainly due to the rapid saturation of the dopamine reuptake transporter, which clears the released dopamine from the extrasynaptic region (Chergui et al. 1994). The same effect is observed in nucleus accumbens (Wightman and Zimmerman 1990) and occurs even with longer impulse intervals because of sparser reuptake sites (Garris et al. 1994b; Marshall et al. 1990; Stamford et al. 1988). Dopamine release after an impulse burst of <300 ms is too short for activating the autoreceptor-mediated reduction of release (Chergui et al. 1994) or the even slower enzymatic degradation (Michael et al. 1985). Thus a bursting dopamine response is particularly efficient for releasing dopamine.

Estimates based on in vivo voltammetry suggest that a single impulse releases ~1,000 dopamine molecules at synapses in striatum and nucleus accumbens. This leads to immediate synaptic dopamine concentrations of 0.5–3.0 μM (Garris et al. 1994a; Kawagoe et al. 1992). At 40 μs after release onset, >90% of dopamine has left the synapse, some of the rest being later eliminated by synaptic reuptake (half onset time of 30–37 ms). At 3–9 ms after release onset, dopamine concentrations reach a peak of ~250 nM when all neighboring varicosities simultaneously release dopamine. Concentrations are homogeneous within a sphere of 4 μm diam (Gonon 1997), which is the average distance between varicosities (Doucet et al. 1986; Groves et al. 1995). Maximal diffusion is restricted to 12 μm by the reuptake transporter and is reached in 75 ms after release onset (half transporter onset time of 30–37 ms). Concentrations would be slightly lower and less homogeneous in regions with fewer varicosities or when <100% of dopamine neurons are activated, but they are two to three times higher with impulse bursts. Thus the reward-induced, mildly synchronous, bursting activations in ~75% of dopamine neurons may lead to rather homogeneous concentration peaks in the order of 150–400 nM. Total increases of extracellular dopamine last 200 ms after a single impulse and 500–600 ms after multiple impulses of 20–100 ms intervals applied during 100–200 ms (Chergui et al. 1994; Dugast et al. 1994). The extrasynaptic reuptake transporter (Nirenberg et al. 1996) subsequently brings dopamine concentrations back to their baseline of 5–10 nM (Herrera-Marschitz et al. 1996). Thus in contrast to classic, strictly synaptic neurotransmission, synaptically released dopamine diffuses rapidly into the immediate juxtasynaptic area and reaches short peaks of regionally homogenous extracellular concentrations.

Receptors. Of the two principal types of dopamine receptors, the adenylate cyclase-activating, D1 type receptors constitute ~80% of dopamine receptors in striatum. Of these 80% are in the low-affinity state of 2–4 μM and 20% in the high-affinity state of 9–74 nM (Richfield et al. 1989). The remaining 20% of striatal dopamine receptors belong to the adenylase cyclase-inhibiting D2 type of which 10–0% are in the low-affinity state and 80–90% in the high-affinity state, with similar affinities as D1 receptors. Thus D1 receptors overall have an ~100 times lower affinity than D2 receptors. Striatal D1 receptors are located predominantly on neurons projecting to internal pallidum and substantia nigra pars reticulata, whereas striatal D2 receptors are located mostly on neurons projecting to external pallidum (Bergson et al. 1995; Gerfen et al. 1990; Hersch et al. 1995; Levey et al. 1993). However, the differences in receptor sensitivity may not play a role beyond signal transduction, thus reducing the differences in dopamine sensitivity between the two types of striatal output neurons.

Dopamine is released to 30–40% from synaptic and to 60–70% from extrasynaptic varicosities (Descarries et al. 1996). Synaptically released dopamine acts on postsynaptic dopamine receptors at four anatomically distinct sites in the striatum, namely inside dopamine synapses, immediately adjacent to dopamine synapses, inside corticostriatal glutamate synapses, and at extrasynaptic sites remote from release sites (Fig. 8) (Levey et al. 1993; Sesack et al. 1994; Yung et al. 1995). D1 receptors are localized mainly outside of dopamine synapses (Caillé et al. 1996). The high transient con-

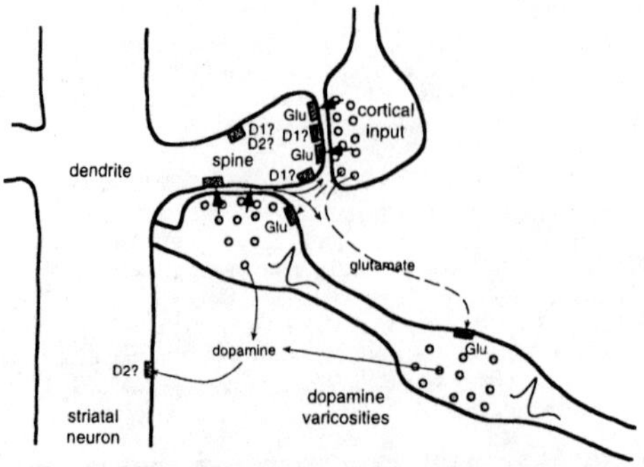

FIG. 8. Influences of dopamine release on typical medium spiny neurons in the dorsal and ventral striatum. Dopamine released by impulses from synaptic varicosities activates a few synaptic receptors (probably of D2 type in the low-affinity state) and diffuses rapidly out of the synapse to reach low affinity D1 type receptors (D1?) that are located nearby, within corticostriatal synapses, or at a limited distance. Phasically increased dopamine activates nearby high-affinity D2 type receptors to saturation (D2?). D2 receptors remain partly activated by the ambient dopamine concentrations after the phasically increased release. Extrasynaptically released dopamine may get diluted by diffusion and activate high-affinity D2 receptors. It should be noted that, in variance with this schematic diagram, most D1 and D2 receptors are located on different neurons. Glutamate released from corticostriatal terminals reaches postsynaptic receptors located on the same dendritic spines as dopamine varicosities. Glutamate also reaches presynaptic dopamine varicosities where it controls dopamine release. Dopamine influences on spiny neurons in frontal cortex are comparable in many respects.

centrations of dopamine after phasic impulse bursts would activate D1 receptors in the immediate vicinity of the active release sites and activate and even saturate D2 receptors everywhere. D2 receptors would remain partly activated when the ambient dopamine concentration returns to baseline after phasic increases.

Summary. The observed, moderately bursting, short-duration, nearly synchronous, response of the majority of dopamine neurons leads to optimal, simultaneous dopamine release from the majority of closely spaced striatal varicosities. The neuronal response induces a short puff of dopamine that is released from extrasynaptic sites or diffuses rapidly from synapses into the juxtasynaptic area. Dopamine quickly reaches regionally homogenous concentrations likely to influence the dendrites of probably all striatal and many cortical neurons. In this way, the reward message in 60–80% of dopamine neurons is broadcast as a divergent, rather global reinforcement signal to the striatum, nucleus accumbens, and frontal cortex, assuring a phasic influence on a maximum number of synapses involved in the processing of stimuli and actions leading to reward (Fig. 7). Dopamine released by neuronal activations after rewards and reward-predicting stimuli would affect juxtasynaptic D1 receptors on striatal neurons projecting to internal pallidum and substantia nigra pars reticulata and all D2 receptors on neurons projecting to external pallidum. The reduction of dopamine release induced by depressions with omitted rewards and reward-predicting stimuli would reduce the tonic stimulation of D2 receptors by ambient dopamine. Thus positive reward prediction errors would influence all types of striatal output neurons, whereas the negative prediction error might predominantly influence neurons projecting to external pallidum.

Potential cocaine mechanisms. Blockade of the dopamine reuptake transporter by drugs like cocaine or amphetamine enhances and prolongs phasic increases in dopamine concentrations (Church et al. 1987a; Giros et al. 1996; Suaud-Chagny et al. 1995). The enhancement would be particularly pronounced when rapid, burst-induced increases in dopamine concentration reach a peak before feedback regulation becomes effective. This mechanism would lead to a massively enhanced dopamine signal after primary rewards and reward-predicting stimuli. It also would increase the somewhat weaker dopamine signal after stimuli resembling rewards, novel stimuli, and particularly salient stimuli that might be frequent in everyday life. The enhancement by cocaine would let these nonrewarding stimuli appear as strong or even stronger than natural rewards without cocaine. Postsynaptic neurons could misinterpret such a signal as a particularly prominent reward-related event and undergo long-term changes in synaptic transmission.

DOPAMINE MEMBRANE ACTIONS. Dopamine actions on striatal neurons depend on the type of receptor activated, are related to the depolarized versus hyperpolarized states of membrane potentials and often involve glutamate receptors. Activation of D1 dopamine receptors enhances the excitation evoked by activation of *N*-methyl-D-aspartate (NMDA) receptors after cortical inputs via L-type Ca^{2+} channels when the membrane potential is in the depolarized state (Cepeda et al. 1993, 1998; Hernandez-Lopez et al. 1997; Kawaguchi et al. 1989). By contrast, D1 activation appears to reduce evoked excitations when the membrane potential is in the hyperpolarized state (Hernandez-Lopez et al. 1997). In vivo dopamine iontophoresis and axonal stimulation induce D1-mediated excitations lasting 100–500 ms beyond dopamine release (Gonon 1997; Williams and Millar 1991). Activation of D2 dopamine receptors reduces Na^+ and N-type Ca^{2+} currents and attenuates excitations evoked by activation of NMDA or α-amino-3-hydroxy-5-methyl-4-isoxazolepropionic acid (AMPA) receptors at any membrane state (Cepeda et al. 1995; Yan et al. 1997). At the systems level, dopamine exerts a focusing effect whereby only the strongest inputs pass through striatum to external and internal pallidum, whereas weaker activity is lost (Brown and Arbuthnott 1983; Filion et al. 1988; Toan and Schultz 1985; Yim and Mogenson 1982). Thus the dopamine released by the dopamine response may lead to an immediate overall reduction in striatal activity, although a facilitatory effect on cortically evoked excitations may be mediated via D1 receptors. The following discussion will show that the effects of dopamine neurotransmission may not be limited to changes in membrane polarization.

DOPAMINE-DEPENDENT PLASTICITY. Tetanic electrical stimulation of cortical or limbic inputs to striatum and nucleus accumbens induces posttetanic depressions lasting several tens of minutes in slices (Calabresi et al. 1992a; Lovinger et al. 1993; Pennartz et al. 1993; Walsh 1993; Wickens et al. 1996). This manipulation also enhances the excitability of corticostriatal terminals (Garcia-Munoz et al. 1992).

Posttetanic potentiation of similar durations is observed in striatum and nucleus accumbens when postsynaptic depolarization is facilitated by removal of magnesium or application of γ-aminobutyric acid (GABA) antagonists (Boeijinga et al. 1993; Calabresi et al. 1992b; Pennartz et al. 1993). D1 or D2 dopamine receptor antagonists or D2 receptor knockout abolish posttetanic corticostriatal depression (Calabresi et al. 1992a; Calabresi et al. 1997; Garcia-Munoz et al. 1992) but do not affect potentiation in nucleus accumbens (Pennartz et al. 1993). Application of dopamine restores striatal posttetanic depression in slices from dopamine-lesioned rats (Calabresi et al. 1992a) but fails to modify posttetanic potentiation (Pennartz et al. 1993). Short pulses of dopamine (5–20 ms) induce long-term potentiation in striatal slices when applied simultaneously with tetanic corticostriatal stimulation and postsynaptic depolarization, complying with a three-factor reinforcement learning rule (Wickens et al. 1996).

Further evidence for dopamine-related synaptic plasticity is found in other brain structures or with different methods. In the hippocampus, posttetanic potentiation is increased by bath application of D1 agonists (Otmakhova and Lisman 1996) and impaired by D1 and D2 receptor blockade (Frey et al. 1990). Burst contingent but not burst noncontingent local applications of dopamine and dopamine agonists increase neuronal bursting in hippocampal slices (Stein et al. 1994). In fish retina, activation of D2 dopamine receptors induces movements of photoreceptors in or out of the pigment epithelium (Rogawski 1987). Posttrial injections of amphetamine and dopamine agonists into rat caudate nucleus improve performance in memory tasks (Packard and White 1991). Dopamine denervations in the striatum reduce the number of dendritic spines (Arbuthnott and Ingham 1993; Anglade et al. 1996; Ingham et al. 1993), suggesting that the dopamine innervation has persistent effects on corticostriatal synapses.

PROCESSING IN STRIATAL NEURONS. An estimated 10,000 cortical terminals and 1,000 dopamine varicosities contact the dendritic spines of each striatal neuron (Doucet et al. 1986; Groves et al. 1995; Wilson 1995). The dense dopamine innervation becomes visible as baskets outlining individual perikarya in pigeon paleostriatum (Wynne and Güntürkün 1995). Dopamine varicosities form synapses on the same dendritic spines of striatal neurons that are contacted by cortical glutamate afferents (Fig. 8) (Bouyer et al. 1984; Freund et al. 1984; Pickel et al. 1981; Smith et al. 1994), and some dopamine receptors are located inside corticostriatal synapses (Levey et al. 1993; Yung et al. 1995). The high number of cortical inputs to striatal neurons, the convergence between dopamine and glutamate inputs at the spines of striatal neurons, and the largely homogeneous dopamine signal reaching probably all striatal neurons are ideal substrates for dopamine-dependent synaptic changes at the spines of striatal neurons. This also may hold for the cortex where dendritic spines are contacted by synaptic inputs from both dopamine and cortical neurons (Goldman-Rakic et al. 1989), although dopamine probably does not influence every cortical neuron.

The basal ganglia are connected by open and closed loops with the cortex and with subcortical limbic structures. The striatum receives to varying degrees inputs from all cortical areas. Basal ganglia outputs are directed predominantly toward frontal cortical areas but also reach the temporal lobe (Middleton and Strick 1996). Many inputs from functionally heterogeneous cortical areas to the striatum are organized in segregated, parallel channels, as are the outputs from internal pallidum directed to different motor cortical areas (Alexander et al. 1986; Hoover and Strick 1993). However, afferents from functionally related but anatomically different cortical areas may converge on striatal neurons. For example, projections from somatotopically related areas of primary somatosensory and motor cortex project to common striatal regions (Flaherty and Graybiel 1993, 1994). Corticostriatal projections diverge into separate striatal "matrisomes" and reconverge in the pallidum, thus increasing the synaptic "surface" for modulatory interactions and associations (Graybiel et al. 1994). This anatomic arrangement would allow the dopamine signal to determine the efficacy of highly structured, task-specific cortical inputs to striatal neurons and exert a widespread influence on forebrain centers involved in the control of behavioral action.

USING THE DOPAMINE REWARD PREDICTION ERROR SIGNAL

Dopamine neurons appear to report appetitive events according to a prediction error (*Eqs. 1* and *2*). Current learning theories and neuronal models demonstrate the crucial importance of prediction errors for learning.

Learning theories

RESCORLA-WAGNER MODEL. Behavioral learning theories formalize the acquisition of associations between arbitrary stimuli and primary motivating events in classical conditioning paradigms. Stimuli gain associative strength over consecutive trials by being repeatedly paired with a primary motivating event

$$\Delta V = \alpha\beta(\lambda - V) \quad (3)$$

where V is current associative strength of the stimulus, λ is maximum associative strength possibly sustained by the primary motivating event, α and β are constants reflecting the salience of conditioned and unconditioned stimuli, respectively (Dickinson 1980; Mackintosh 1975; Pearce and Hall 1980; Rescorla and Wagner 1972). The (λ-V) term indicates the degree to which the primary motivating event occurs unpredictably and represents an error in the prediction of reinforcement. It determines the rate of learning, as associative strength increases when the error term is positive and the conditioned stimulus does not fully predict the reinforcement. When $V = \lambda$, the conditioned stimulus fully predicts the reinforcer, and V will not further increase. Thus learning occurs only when the primary motivating event is not fully predicted by a conditioned stimulus. This interpretation is suggested by the blocking phenomenon, according to which a stimulus fails to gain associative strength when presented together with another stimulus that by itself fully predicts the reinforcer (Kamin 1969). The (λ-V) error term becomes negative when a predicted reinforcer fails to occur, leading to a loss of associative strength of the conditioned stimulus (extinction). Note that these models use the term "reinforcement'' in the broad sense of increasing the frequency and intensity of specific behavior and do not refer to any particular type of learning.

DELTA RULE. The Rescorla-Wagner model relates to the general principle of learning driven by errors between the desired and the actual output, such as the least mean square error procedure (Kalman 1960; Widrow and Sterns 1985). This principle has been applied to neuronal network models in the Delta rule, according to which synaptic weights (ω) are adjusted by

$$\Delta\omega = \eta(t - a)x \quad (4)$$

where t is desired (target) output of the network, a is actual output, and η and x are learning rate and input activation, respectively (Rumelhart et al. 1986; Widrow and Hoff 1960). The desired output (t) is analogous to the outcome (λ), the actual output (a) is analogous to the prediction modified during learning (V), and the delta error term ($\delta = t - a$) is equivalent to the reinforcement error term (λ-V) of the Rescorla-Wagner rule *(Eq. 3)* (Sutton and Barto 1981).

The general dependence on outcome unpredictability relates intuitively to the very essence of learning. If learning involves the acquisition or change of predictions of outcome, no change in predictions and hence no learning will occur when the outcome is perfectly well predicted. This restricts learning to stimuli and behavioral reactions that lead to surprising or altered outcomes, and redundant stimuli preceding outcomes already predicted by other events are not learned. Besides their role in bringing about learning, reinforcers have a second, distinctively different function. When learning is completed, fully predicted reinforcers are crucial for maintaining learned behavior and preventing extinction.

Many forms of learning may involve the reduction of prediction errors. In a general sense, these systems process an external event, generate predictions of this event, compute the error between the event and its prediction, and modify both performance and prediction according to the prediction error. This may not be limited to learning systems dealing with biological reinforcers but concern a much larger variety of neural operations, such as visual recognition in cerebral cortex (Rao and Ballard 1997).

Reinforcement algorithms

UNCONDITIONAL REINFORCEMENT. Neuronal network models can be trained with straightforward reinforcement signals that emit a prediction-independent signal when a behavioral reaction is correctly executed but no signal with an erroneous reaction. Learning in these largely instrumental learning models consists in changing the synaptic weights (ω) of model neurons according to

$$\Delta\omega = \varepsilon rxy \quad (5)$$

where ε is learning rate, r is reinforcement, and x and y are activations of pre- and postsynaptic neurons, respectively, assuring that only synapses participating in the reinforced behavior are modified. A popular example is the associative reward-penalty model (Barto and Anandan 1985). These models acquire skeletal or oculomotor responses, learn sequences, and perform the Wisconsin Card Sorting Test (Arbib and Dominey 1995; Dehaene and Changeux 1991; Dominey et al. 1995; Fagg and Arbib 1992). Processing units in these models acquire similar properties as neurons in parietal association cortex (Mazzoni et al. 1991).

However, the persistence of the teaching signal after learning requires additional algorithms for preventing run away synaptic strengths (Montague and Sejnowski 1994) and for avoiding acquisition of redundant stimuli presented together with reinforcer-predicting stimuli. Previously learned behavior perseveres when contingencies change, as omitted reinforcement fails to induce a negative signal. Learning speed may be increased by adding external information from a teacher (Ballard 1997) and by incorporating information about the past performance (McCallum 1995).

TEMPORAL DIFFERENCE LEARNING. In a particularly efficient class of reinforcement algorithms (Sutton 1988; Sutton and Barto 1981), synaptic weights are modified according to the error in reinforcement prediction computed over consecutive time steps (t) in each trial

$$\hat{r}(t) = r(t) + P(t) - P(t-1) \quad (6)$$

where r is reinforcement and P is reinforcement prediction. $P(t)$ is usually multiplied by a discount factor γ with $0 \leq \gamma < 1$ to account for the decreasing influence of increasingly remote rewards. For reasons of simplicity, γ is set to 1 here. In the case of a single stimulus predicting a single reinforcer, the prediction $P(t-1)$ exists before the time t of reinforcement but terminates at the time of reinforcement $[P(t) = 0]$. This leads to an effective reinforcement signal at the time (t) of reinforcement

$$\hat{r}(t) = r(t) - P(t-1) \quad (6a)$$

The $\hat{r}(t)$ term indicates the difference between actual and predicted reinforcement. During learning, reinforcement is incompletely predicted, the error term is positive when reinforcement occurs, and synaptic weights are increased. After learning, reinforcement is fully predicted by a preceding stimulus $[P(t-1) = r(t)]$, the error term is nil on correct behavior, and synaptic weights remain unchanged. When reinforcement is omitted due to inadequate performance or changed contingencies, the error is negative and synaptic weights are reduced. The $\hat{r}(t)$ term is analogous to the (λ-V) error term of the Rescorla-Wagner model (*Eq. 4*). However, it concerns individual time steps (t) within each trial rather than predictions evolving over consecutive trials. These temporal models of reinforcement capitalize on the fact that the acquired predictions include the exact time of reinforcement (Dickinson et al. 1976; Gallistel 1990; Smith 1968).

The temporal difference (TD) algorithms also employ acquired predictions for changing synaptic weights. In the case of an unpredicted, single conditioned stimulus predicting a single reinforcer, the prediction $P(t)$ begins at time (t), there is no preceding prediction $[P(t-1) = 0]$, and reinforcement has not yet occurred $[r(t) = 0]$. According to *Eq. 6*, the model emits a purely predictive effective reinforcement signal at the time (t) of the prediction

$$\hat{r} = P(t) \quad (6b)$$

In the case of multiple, consecutive predictive stimuli, again with reinforcement absent at the time of predictions, the effective reinforcement signal at the time (t) of the prediction reflects the difference between the current prediction $P(t)$ and the preceding prediction $P(t-1)$

$$\hat{r} = P(t) - P(t-1) \qquad (6c)$$

This constitutes an error term of higher order reinforcement. Similar to fully predicted reinforcers, all predictive stimuli that are fully predicted themselves are cancelled out $[P(t-1) = P(t)]$, resulting in $\hat{r} = 0$ at the times (t) of these stimuli. Only the earliest predictive stimulus contributes to the effective reinforcement signal, as this stimulus $P(t)$ is not predicted by another stimulus $[P(t-1) = 0]$. This results in the same $\hat{r} = P(t)$ at the time (t) of the first prediction as in the case of a single prediction (*Eq. 6b*).

Taken together, the effective reinforcement signal (*Eq. 6*) is composed of the primary reinforcement, which decreases with emerging predictions (*Eq. 6a*) and is replaced gradually by the acquired predictions (*Eqs. 6b* and *6c*). With consecutive predictive stimuli, the effective reinforcement signal moves backward in time from the primary reinforcer to the earliest reinforcer-predicting stimulus. The retrograde transfer results in a more specific assignment of credit to the involved synapses, as predictions occur closer in time to the stimuli and behavioral reactions to be conditioned, as compared with reinforcement at trial end (Sutton and Barto 1981).

Implementations of reinforcement learning algorithms employ the prediction error in two ways, for changing synaptic weights for behavioral output and for acquiring the predictions themselves to continuously compute the prediction error (Fig. 9*A*) (McLaren 1989; Sutton and Barto 1981). These two functions are separated in recent implementations, in which the prediction error is computed in the adaptive critic component and changes the synaptic weights in the actor component mediating behavioral output (Fig. 9*B*) (Barto 1995). A positive error increases the reinforcement prediction of the critic, whereas a negative error from omitted reinforcement reduces the prediction. This renders the effective reinforcement signal highly adaptive.

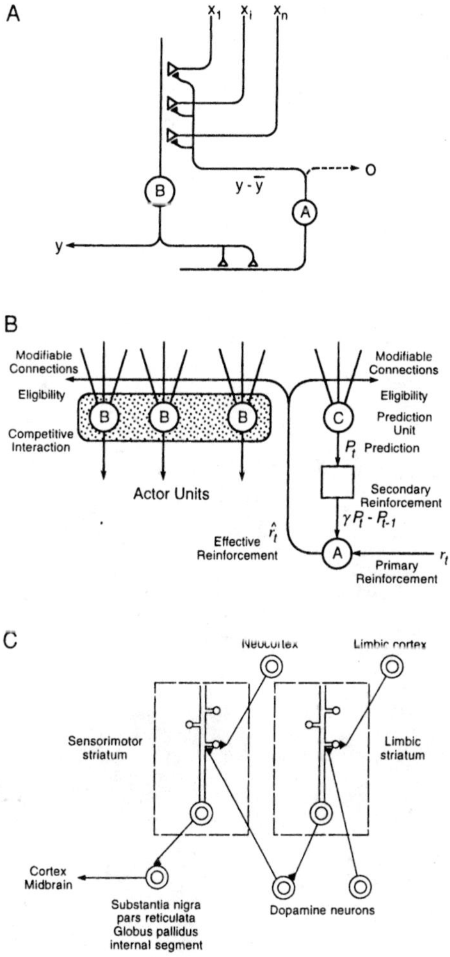

FIG. 9. Basic architectures of neural network models implementing temporal difference algorithms in comparison with basal ganglia connectivity. *A*: in the original implementation the effective teaching signal $y - \bar{y}$ is computed in model neuron *A* and sent to presynaptic terminals of inputs x to neuron *B*, thus influencing $x \rightarrow B$ processing and changing synaptic weights at the $x \rightarrow B$ synapse. Neuron *B* influences behavioral output via axon y and at the same time contributes to the adaptive properties of neuron *A*, namely its response to reinforcer-predicting stimuli. More recent implementations of this simple architecture use neuron *A* rather than neuron *B* for emitting an output *O* of the model (Montague et al. 1996; Schultz et al. 1997). Reprinted from Sutton and Barto (1981) with permission by American Psychological Association. *B*: recent implementation separates the teaching component *A*, called the critic (*right*), from an output component comprised of several processing units *B*, termed the actor (*left*). The effective reinforcement signal $\hat{r}(t)$ is computed by subtracting the temporal difference in weighted reinforcer prediction $\gamma P(t) - P(t-1)$ from primary reinforcement $r(t)$ received from the environment (γ is the discount factor reducing the value of more distant reinforcers). Reinforcer prediction is computed in a separate prediction unit *C*, which is a part of the critic and forms a closed loop with the teaching element *A*, whereas primary reinforcement enters the critic through a separate input r_t. Effective reinforcement signal influences synaptic weights at incoming axons in the actor, which mediates the output and in the adaptive prediction unit of the critic. Reprinted from Barto (1995) with permission by MIT Press. *C*: basic connectivity of the basal ganglia reveals striking similarites with the actor-critic architecture. Dopamine projection emits the reinforcement signal to the striatum and is comparable with the unit *A* in parts *A* and *B*, the limbic striatum (or striosome-patch) takes the position of the prediction unit *C* in the critic, and the sensorimotor striatum (or matrix) resembles the actor units *B*. In the original model (*A*), the single major deviation from established basal ganglia anatomy consists in the influence of neuron *A* being directed at presynaptic terminals, whereas dopamine synapses are located on postsynaptic dendrites of striatal neurons (Freund et al. 1984). Reprinted from Smith and Bolam (1990) with permission by Elsevier Press.

Neurobiological implementations of temporal difference learning

COMPARISON OF DOPAMINE RESPONSE WITH REINFORCEMENT MODELS. The dopamine response coding an error in the prediction of reward (*Eq. 1*) closely resembles the effective error term of animal learning rules (λ-V; *Eq. 4*) and the effective reinforcement signal of TD algorithms at the time (t) of reinforcement [$r(t) - P(t-1)$; *Eq. 6a*], as noted before (Montague et al. 1996). Similarly, the dopamine appetitive event prediction error (*Eq. 2*) resembles the higher order TD reinforcement error [$P(t) - P(t-1)$; *Eq. 6c*]. The nature of the widespread, divergent projections of dopamine neurons to probably all neurons in the striatum and many neurons in frontal cortex is compatible with the notion of a TD global reinforcement signal, which is emitted by the critic for influencing all model neurons in the actor (compare Fig. 7 with Fig. 9*B*). The critic-actor architecture is particularly attractive for neurobiology because of its separate teaching and performance modules. In particular, it resembles closely the connectivity of the basal ganglia, including the reciprocity of striatonigral projections (Fig. 9*C*), as first noted by Houk et al. (1995). The critic simulates dopamine neurons, the reward prediction enters from striosomal striatonigral projections, and the actor resembles striatal matrix neurons with dopamine-dependent plasticity. Interestingly, both dopamine response and theoretical error terms are sign-dependent. They differ from error terms with absolute values that do not discriminate between acquisition and extinction and should have predominantly attentional effects.

APPLICATIONS FOR NEUROBIOLOGICAL PROBLEMS. Although originally developed on the basis of the Rescorla-Wagner model of classical conditioning, models using TD algorithms learn a wide variety of behavioral tasks through basically instrumental forms of conditioning. These tasks reach from balancing a pole on a cart wheel (Barto et al. 1983) to playing world class backgammon (Tesauro 1994). Robots using TD algorithms learn to move about two dimensional space and avoid obstacles, reach and grasp (Fagg 1993) or insert a peg into a hole (Gullapalli et al. 1994). Using the TD reinforcement signal to directly influence and select behavior (Fig. 9*A*), TD models replicate foraging behavior of honeybees (Montague et al. 1995) and simulate human decision making (Montague et al. 1996). TD models with an explicit critic-actor architecture constitute very powerful models that efficiently learn eye movements (Friston et al. 1994; Montague et al. 1993), sequential movements (Fig. 10), and orienting reactions (Contreras-Vidal and Schultz 1996). A recent model added activating-depressing novelty signals for improving the teaching signal, used stimulus and action traces in the critic and actor, and employed winner-take-all rules for improving the teaching signal and for selecting actor neurons with the largest activation. This reproduced in great detail both the responses of dopamine neurons and the learning behavior of animals in delayed response tasks (Suri and Schultz 1996). It is particularly interesting to see that teaching signals using prediction errors result in faster and more complete learning as compared with unconditional reinforcement signals (Fig. 10) (Friston et al. 1994).

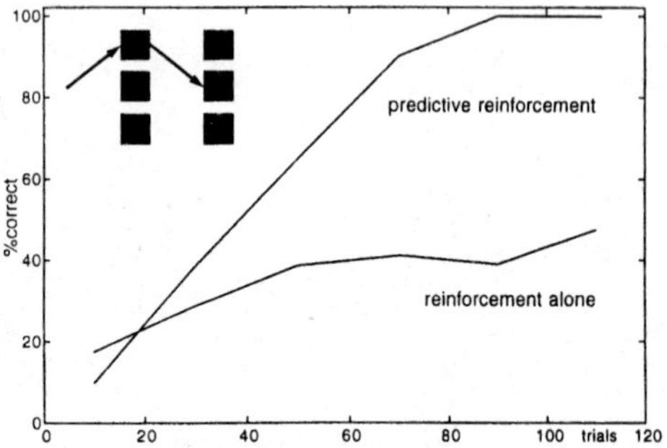

FIG. 10. Advantage of predictive reinforcement signals for learning. A temporal difference model with critic-actor architecture and eligibility trace in the actor was trained in a sequential 2 step-3 choice task (*inset upper left*). Learning advanced faster and reached higher performance when a predictive reinforcement signal was used as teaching signal (adaptive critic, *top*) as compared with using an unconditional reinforcement signal at trial end (*bottom*). This effect becomes progressively more pronounced with longer sequences. Comparable performance with the unconditional reinforcement signal would require a much longer eligibility trace. Data were obtained from 10 simulations (R. Suri and W. Schultz, unpublished observations). A similar improvement in learning with predictive reinforcement was found in a model of oculomotor behavior (Friston et al. 1994).

Possible learning mechanisms using the dopamine signal

The preceding section has shown that the formal prediction error signal emitted by the dopamine response can constitute a particularly suitable teaching signal for model learning. The following sections describe how the biological dopamine response could be potentially used for learning by basal ganglia structures and suggest testable hypotheses.

POSTSYNAPTIC PLASTICITY MEDIATED BY REWARD PREDICTION SIGNAL. Learning would proceed in two steps. The first step involves the acquisition of a dopamine reward-predicting response. In subsequent trials, the predictive dopamine signal would specifically strengthen the synaptic weights (ω) of Hebbian-type corticostriatal synapses that are active at the time of the reward-predicting stimulus, whereas the inactive corticostriatal synapses are left unchanged. This results in the three factor learning rule

$$\Delta\omega = \varepsilon\, \hat{r}\, i\, o \tag{8}$$

where $\hat{r}$ is dopamine reinforcement signal, i is input activity, o is output activity, and ε is learning rate.

In a simplified model, four cortical inputs (i1–i4) contact the dendritic spines of three medium size spiny striatal neurons (o1–o3; Fig. 11). Cortical inputs converge on striatal neurons, each input contacting a different spine. The same spines are unselectively contacted by a common dopamine input R. Activation of dopamine input R indicates that an unpredicted reward-predicting stimulus occurred in the environment, without providing further details (goodness signal). Let us assume that cortical input i2 is activated simultaneously with dopamine neurons and codes one of several specific parameters of the same reward-predicting stimulus, such as its sensory modality, body side, color, texture and position, or a specific parameter of a movement triggered by the stimulus. A set of parameters of this event would be coded by a set of cortical inputs i2. Cortical inputs i1, i3, and i4 unrelated to current stimuli and movements are inactive. The dopamine response leads to unselective dopamine release at all varicosities but would selective strengthen only the active corticostriatal synapses i2–o1 and i2–o2, pro-

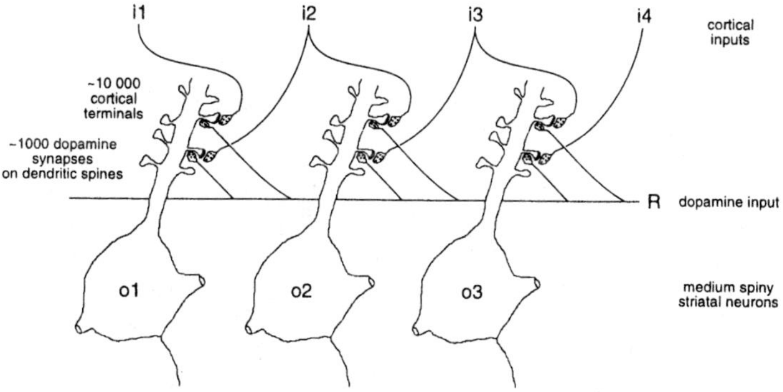

FIG. 11. Differential influences of a global dopamine reinforcement signal on selective corticostriatal activity. Dendritic spines of 3 medium-sized spiny striatal neurons o1, o2, and o3 are contacted by 4 cortical inputs i1, i2, i3, and i4 and by axonal varicosities from a single dopamine neuron R (or from a population of homogenously activated dopamine neurons). Each striatal neuron receives ~10,000 cortical and 1,000 dopamine inputs. At single dendritic spines, different cortical inputs converge with the dopamine input. In 1 version of the model, the dopamine signal enhances simultaneously active corticostriatal transmission relative to nonactive transmission. For example, dopamine input R is active at the same time as cortical input i2, whereas i1, i3, i4 are inactive. This leads to a modification of i2 → o1 and i2 → o2 transmission but leaves i1 → o1, i3 → o2, i3 → o3, and i4 → o3 transmissions unaltered. In a version of the model employing plasticity, synaptic weights of corticostriatal synapses are long-term modified by the dopamine signal according to the same rule. This may occur when dopamine responses to a conditioned stimulus act on corticostriatal synapses that also are activated by this stimulus. In another version employing plasticity, dopamine responses to a primary reward may act backwards in time on corticostriatal synapses that were previously active. These synapses would be made eligible for modification by a hypothetical postsynaptic neuronal trace left from that activity. In comparing the basal ganglia structure with the recent TD model of Fig. 9*B*, dopamine input R replicates the critic with neuron *A*, the striatum with neurons o1–o3 replicates the actor with neuron *B*, cortical inputs i1–i4 replicate the actor input, and the divergent projection of dopamine neurons R on multiple spines of multiple striatal neurons o1–o3 replicates the global influence of the critic on the actor. A similar comparison was made by Houk et al. (1995). This drawing is based on anatomic data by Freund et al. (1984), Smith and Bolam (1990), Flaherty and Graybiel (1993), and Smith et al. (1994).

vided the cortical inputs are strong enough to activate striatal neurons o1 and o2.

This learning mechanism employs the acquired dopamine response at the time of the reward-predicting stimulus as a teaching signal for inducing long-lasting synaptic changes (Fig. 12*A*). Learning of the predictive stimulus or triggered movement is based on the demonstrated acquisition of dopamine response to the reward-predicting stimulus, together with dopamine-dependent plasticity in the striatum. Plasticity changes alternatively might occur in cortical or subcortical structures downstream from striatum after dopamine-mediated short-term enhancement of synaptic transmission in the striatum. The retroactive effects of reward on stimuli and movements preceding the reward are mediated by the response transfer to the earliest reward-predicting stimulus. The dopamine response to predicted or omitted primary reward is not used for plasticity changes in the striatum as it does not occur simultaneously with the events to be conditioned, although it could be involved in computing the dopamine response to the reward-predicting stimulus in analogy to the architecture and mechanism of TD models.

POSTSYNAPTIC PLASTICITY TOGETHER WITH SYNAPTIC ELIGIBILITY TRACE. Learning may occur in a single step if the dopamine reward signal has a retroactive action on striatal synapses. This requires hypothetical traces of synaptic activity that last until reinforcement occurs and makes those synapses eligible for modification by a teaching signal that were active before reinforcement (Hull 1943; Klopf 1982; Sutton and Barto 19811). Synaptic weights (ω) are changed according to

$$\Delta\omega = \varepsilon\, \hat{r}\, h\,(i,\, o) \tag{9}$$

where $\hat{r}$ is dopamine reinforcement signal, $h\,(i, o)$ is eligibility trace of conjoint input and output activity, and ε is learning rate. Potential physiological substrates of eligibility traces consist in prolonged changes in calcium concentration (Wickens and Kötter 1995), formation of calmodulin-dependent protein kinase II (Houk et al. 1995), or sustained neuronal activity found frequently in striatum (Schultz et al. 1995a) and cortex.

Dopamine-dependent plasticity involving eligibility traces constitutes an elegant mechanism for learning sequences backward in time (Sutton and Barto 1981). To start, the dopamine response to the unpredicted primary reward mediates behavioral learning of the immediately preceding event by modifying corticostriatal synaptic efficacy (Fig. 11). At the same time, the dopamine response transfers to the reward-predicting event. A depression at the time of omitted reward prevents learning of erroneous reactions. In the next step, the dopamine response to the unpredicted reward-predicting event mediates learning of the immediately preceding predictive event, and the dopamine response likewise transfers back to that event. As this occurs repeatedly, the dopamine response moves backward in time until no further

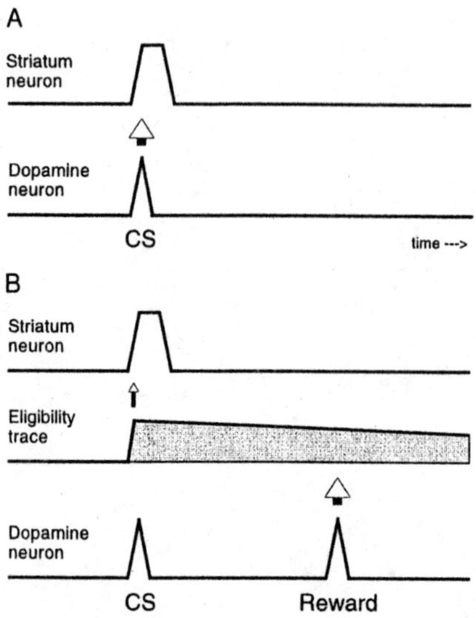

FIG. 12. Influences of dopamine reinforcement signal on possible learning mechanisms in the striatum. *A*: predictive dopamine reward response to a conditioned stimulus (CS) has a direct enhancing or plasticity effect on striatal neurotransmission related to that stimulus. *B*: dopamine response to primary reward has a retrograde plasticity effect on striatal neurotransmission related to the preceding conditioned stimulus. This mechanism is mediated by an eligibility trace outlasting striatal activity. Solid arrows indicate direct effects of dopamine signal on striatal neurotransmission *(A)* or the eligibility trace *(B)*, small arrow in *B* indicates indirect effect on striatal neurotransmission via the eligibility trace.

events precede, allowing at each step the preceding event to acquire reward prediction. This mechanism would be ideally suited for forming behavioral sequences leading to a final reward.

This learning mechanism fully employs the dopamine error in the prediction of appetitive events as retroactive teaching signal inducing long-lasting synaptic changes (Fig. 12*B*). It uses dopamine-dependent plasticity together with striatal elibility traces whose biological suitability for learning remains to be investigated. This results in direct learning by outcome, essentially compatible with the influence of the teaching signal on the actor of TD models. The demonstrated retrograde movement of the dopamine response is used for learning earlier and earlier stimuli.

AN ALTERNATIVE MECHANISM: FACILITATORY INFLUENCE OF PREDICTIVE DOPAMINE SIGNAL. Both mechanisms described above employ the dopamine response as a teaching signal for modifying neurotransmission in the striatum. As the contribution of dopamine-dependent striatal plasticity to learning is not completely understood, another mechanism could be based on the demonstrated plasticity of the dopamine response without requiring striatal plasticity. In a first step, dopamine neurons acquire responses to reward-predicting stimuli. In a subsequent step, the predictive responses could be used to increase the impact of cortical inputs that occur simultaneously at the same dendritic spines of striatal neurons. Postsynaptic activity would change according to

$$\Delta \text{ activity} = \delta \, \hat{r} \, i \qquad (10)$$

where $\hat{r}$ is dopamine reinforcement signal, i is input activity, and δ is an amplification constant. Rather than constituting a teaching signal, the predictive dopamine response provides an enhancing or motivating signal for striatal neurotransmission at the time of the reward-predicting stimulus. With competing stimuli, neuronal inputs occurring simultaneously with the reward-predicting dopamine signal would be processed preferentially. Behavioral reactions would profit from the advance information and become more frequent, faster, and more precise. The facilitatory influence of advance information is demonstrated in behavioral experiments by pairing a conditioned stimulus with lever pressing (Lovibond 1983).

A possible mechanism may employ the focusing effect of dopamine. In the simplified model of Fig. 11, dopamine globally reduces all cortical influences. This lets only the strongest input pass to striatal neurons, whereas the other, weaker inputs become ineffective. This requires a nonlinear, contrast-enhancing mechanism, such as the threshold for generating action potentials. A comparable enhancement of strongest inputs could occur in neurons that would be predominantly excited by dopamine.

This mechanism employs the acquired, reward-predicting dopamine response as a biasing or selection signal for influencing postsynaptic processing (Fig. 12*A*). Improved performance is based entirely on the demonstrated plasticity of dopamine responses and does not require dopamine-dependent plasticity in striatal neurons. The responses to unpredicted or omitted reward occur too late for influencing striatal processing but may help to compute the predictive dopamine response in analogy to TD models.

Electrical stimulation of dopamine neurons as unconditioned stimulus

Electrical stimulation of circumscribed brain regions reliably serves as reinforcement for acquiring and sustaining approach behavior (Olds and Milner 1954). Some very effective self-stimulation sites coincide with dopamine cell bodies and axon bundles in the midbrain (Corbett and Wise 1980), nucleus accumbens (Phillips et al. 1975), striatum (Phillips et al. 1976), and prefrontal cortex (Mora and Myers 1977; Phillips et al. 1979), but also are found in structures unrelated to dopamine systems (White and Milner 1992). Electrical self-stimulation involves the activation of dopamine neurons (Fibiger and Phillips 1986; Wise and Rompré 1989) and is reduced by 6-hydroxydopamine–induced lesions of dopamine axons (Fibiger et al. 1987; Phillips and Fibiger 1978), inhibition of dopamine synthesis (Edmonds and Gallistel 1977), depolarization inactivation of dopamine neurons (Rompré and Wise 1989), and dopamine receptor antagonists administered systemically (Furiezos and Wise 1976) or into nucleus accumbens (Mogenson et al. 1979). Self-stimulation is facilitated with cocaine- or amphetamine-induced increases in extracellular dopamine (Colle and Wise 1980; Stein 1964; Wauquier 1976). Self-stimulation directly increases dopamine utilization in nucleus accumbens, striatum and frontal cortex (Fibiger et al. 1987; Mora and Myers 1977).

It is intriguing to imagine that electrically evoked dopamine impulses and release may serve as unconditioned stimulus in associative learning, similar to stimulation of octopamine neurons in honeybees learning the proboscis reflex (Hammer 1993). However, dopamine-related self-stimulation differs in at least three important aspects from the natural activation of dopamine neurons. Rather than only activating dopamine neurons, natural rewards usually activate several neuronal systems in parallel and allow the distributed coding of different reward components (see further text). Second, electrical stimulation is applied as unconditional reinforcement without reflecting an error in reward prediction. Third, electrical stimulation is only delivered like a reward after a behavioral reaction, rather than at the time of a reward-predicting stimulus. It would be interesting to apply electrical self-stimulation in exactly the same manner as dopamine neurons emit their signal.

Learning deficits with impaired dopamine neurotransmission

Many studies investigated the behavior of animals with impaired dopamine neurotransmission after local or systemic application of dopamine receptor antagonists or destruction of dopamine axons in ventral midbrain, nucleus accumbens, or striatum. Besides observing locomotor and cognitive deficits reminiscent of Parkinsonism, these studies revealed impairments in the processing of reward information. The earliest studies argued for deficits in the subjective, hedonic perception of rewards (Wise 1982; Wise et al. 1978). Further experimentation revealed impaired use of primary rewards and conditioned appetitive stimuli for approach and consummatory behavior (Beninger et al. 1987; Ettenberg 1989; Miller et al. 1990; Salamone 1987; Ungerstedt 1971; Wise and Colle 1984; Wise and Rompre 1989). Many studies described impairments in motivational and attentional processes underlying appetitive learning (Beninger 1983, 1989; Beninger and Hahn 1983; Fibiger and Phillips 1986; LeMoal and Simon 1991; Robbins and Everitt 1992, 1996; White and Milner 1992; Wise 1982). Most learning deficits are associated with impaired dopamine neurotransmission in nucleus accumbens, whereas dorsal striatum impairments lead to sensorimotor deficits (Amalric and Koob 1987; Robbins and Everitt 1992; White 1989). However, the learning of instrumental tasks in general and of discriminative stimulus properties in particular appear to be frequently spared, and it is not entirely resolved whether some of the apparent learning deficits may be confounded by motor performance deficits (Salamone 1992).

Degeneration of dopamine neurons in Parkinson's disease also leads to a number of declarative and procedural learning deficits, including associative learning (Linden et al. 1990; Sprengelmeyer et al. 1995). Deficits are present in trial-and-error learning with immediate reinforcement (Vriezen and Moscovitch 1990) and when associating explicit stimuli with different outcomes (Knowlton et al. 1996), even in early stages of Parkinson's disease without cortical atrophy (Canavan et al. 1989). Parkinsonian patients also show impaired time perception (Pastor et al. 1992). All of these deficits occur in the presence of L-Dopa treatment, which restores tonic striatal dopamine levels without reinstating phasic dopamine signals.

These studies suggest that dopamine neurotransmission plays an important role in the processing of rewards for approach behavior and in forms of learning involving associations between stimuli and rewards, whereas an involvement in more instrumental forms of learning could be questioned. It is unclear whether these deficits reflect a more general behavioral inactivation due to tonically reduced dopamine receptor stimulation rather than the absence of a phasic dopamine reward signal. To resolve this question, as well as more specifically elucidate the role of dopamine in different learning forms, it would be helpful to study learning in those situations in which the phasic dopamine response to appetitive stimuli actually occurs.

Forms of learning possibly mediated by the dopamine signal

The characteristics of dopamine responses and the potential influence of dopamine on striatal neurons may help to delineate some of the learning forms in which dopamine neurons could be involved. The preferential responses to appetitive as opposed to aversive events would favor an involvement in the learning of approach behavior and mediating positive reinforcement effects, rather than withdrawal and punishment. The responses to primary rewards outside of tasks and learning contexts would allow dopamine neurons to play a role in a relatively wide spectrum of learning involving primary rewards, both in classical and instrumental conditioning. The responses to reward-predicting stimuli reflect stimulus-reward associations and would be compatible with an involvement in reward expectation underlying general incentive learning (Bindra 1968). By contrast, dopamine responses do not explicitly code rewards as goal objects, as they only report errors in reward prediction. They also appear to be insensitive to motivational states, thus disfavoring a specific role in state-dependent incentive learning of goal-directed acts (Dickinson and Balleine 1994). The lack of clear relationships to arm and eye movements would disfavor a role in directly mediating the behavioral responses that follow incentive stimuli. However, comparisons between discharges of individual neurons and learning of whole organisms are intrinsically difficult. At the synaptic level, phasically released dopamine reaches many dendrites on probably every striatal neuron and thus could exert a plasticity effect on the large variety of behavioral components involving the striatum, which may include the learning of movements.

The specific conditions in which phasic dopamine signals could play a role in learning are determined by the kinds of stimuli that effectively induce a dopamine response. In the animal laboratory, dopamine responses require the phasic occurrence of appetitive, novel, or particularly salient stimuli, including primary nutrient rewards and reward-predicting stimuli, whereas aversive stimuli do not play a major role. Dopamine responses may occur in all behavioral situations controlled by phasic and explicit outcomes, although higher order conditioned stimuli and secondary reinforcers were not yet tested. Phasic dopamine responses would probably not play a role in forms of learning not mediated by phasically occurring outcomes, and the predictive response would not be able to contribute to learning in situations in which phasic predictive stimuli do not occur, such as relatively slow changes of context. This leads to the interesting question of whether the sparing of some forms of learning by dopamine lesions or neuroleptics might simply reflect the absence of phasic dopamine responses in the first place because the effective stimuli eliciting them were not used.

The involvement of dopamine signals in learning may be illustrated by a theoretical example. Imagine dopamine responses during acquisition of a serial reaction time task when a correct reaction suddenly leads to a nutrient reward. The reward response subsequently is transferred to progressively earlier reward-predicting stimuli. Reaction times improve further with prolonged practice as the spatial positions of targets become increasingly predictable. Although dopamine neurons continue to respond to the reward-predicting stimuli, the further behavioral improvement might be mainly due to the acquisition of predictive processing of spatial positions by other neuronal systems. Thus dopamine responses would occur during the initial, incentive part of learning in which subjects come to approach objects and obtain explicit primary, and possibly conditioned, rewards. They would be less involved in situations in which the progress of learning goes beyond the induction of approach behavior. This would not restrict the dopamine role to initial learning steps, as many situations require to initially learn from examples and only later involve learning by explicit outcomes.

COOPERATION BETWEEN REWARD SIGNALS

Prediction error

The prediction error signal of dopamine neurons would be an excellent indicator of the appetitive value of environmental events relative to prediction but fails to discriminate among foods, liquids, and reward-predicting stimuli and among visual, auditory, and somatosensory modalities. This signal may constitute a reward alert message by which postsynaptic neurons are informed about the surprising appearance or omission of a rewarding or potentially rewarding event without indicating further its identity. It has all the formal characteristics of a powerful reinforcement signal for learning. However, information about the specific nature of rewards is crucial for determining which of the objects should be approached and in which manner. For example, a hungry animal should primarily approach food but not liquid. To discriminate relevant from irrelevant rewards, the dopamine signal needs to be supplemented by additional information. Recent in vivo dialysis experiments showed higher food-induced dopamine release in hungry than in satiated rats (Wilson et al. 1995). This drive dependence of dopamine release may not involve impulse responses, as we have failed to find clear drive dependence with dopamine responses when comparing between early and late periods of individual experimental sessions during which animals became fluid-satiated (J. L. Contreras-Vidal and W. Schultz, unpublished data).

Reward specifics

Information concerning liquid and food rewards also is processed in brain structures other than dopamine neurons, such as dorsal and ventral striatum, subthalamic nucleus, amygdala, dorsolateral prefrontal cortex, orbitofrontal cortex, and anterior cingulate cortex. However, these structures do not appear to emit a global reward prediction error signal similar to dopamine neurons. In primates, these structures process rewards as *1*) transient responses after the delivery of reward (Apicella et al. 1991a,b, 1997; Bowman et al. 1996; Hikosaka et al. 1989; Niki and Watanabe 1979; Nishijo et al. 1988; Tremblay and Schultz 1995; Watanabe 1989), *2*) transient responses to reward-predicting cues (Aosaki et al. 1994; Apicella et al. 1991b; 1996; Hollerman et al. 1994; Nishijo et al. 1988; Thorpe et al. 1983; Tremblay and Schultz 1995; Williams et al. 1993), *3*) sustained activations during the expectation of immediately upcoming rewards (Apicella et al. 1992; Hikosaka et al. 1989; Matsumura et al. 1992; Schultz et al. 1992; Tremblay and Schultz 1995), and *4*) modulations of behavior-related activations by predicted reward (Hollerman et al. 1994; Watanabe 1990, 1996). Many of these neurons differentiate well between different food rewards and between different liquid rewards. Thus they process the specific nature of the rewarding event and may serve the perception of rewards. Some of the reward responses depend on reward unpredictability and are reduced or absent when the reward is predicted by a conditioned stimulus (Apicella et al. 1997; Matsumoto et al. 1995; L. Tremblay and W. Schultz, unpublished data). They may process predictions for specific rewards, although it is unclear whether they signal prediction errors as their responses to omitted rewards are unknown.

Maintaining established performance

Three neuronal mechanisms appear to be important for maintaining established behavioral performance, namely the detection of omitted rewards, the detection of reward-predicting stimuli, and the detection of predicted rewards. Dopamine neurons are depressed when predicted rewards are omitted. This signal could reduce the synaptic efficacy related to erroneous behavioral responses and prevent their repetition. The dopamine response to reward-predicting stimuli is maintained during established behavior and thus continues to serve as advance information. Although fully predicted rewards are not detected by dopamine neurons, they are processed by the nondopaminergic cortical and subcortical systems mentioned above. This would be important for avoiding extinction of learned behavior.

Taken together, it appears that the processing of specific rewards for learning and maintaining approach behavior would profit strongly from a cooperation between dopamine neurons signaling the unpredicted occurrence or omission of reward and neurons in the other structures simultaneously, indicating the specific nature of the reward.

COMPARISONS WITH OTHER PROJECTION SYSTEMS

Noradrenaline neurons

Nearly the entire population of noradrenaline neurons in locus coeruleus in rats, cats, and monkeys shows rather homogeneous, biphasic activating-depressant responses to visual, auditory, and somatosensory stimuli eliciting orienting reactions (Aston-Jones and Bloom 1981; Foote et al. 1980; Rasmussen et al. 1986). Particularly effective are infrequent events to which animals pay attention, such as visual stimuli in an oddball discrimination task (Aston-Jones et al. 1994). Noradrenaline neurons discriminate very well between arousing or motivating and neutral events. They rapidly acquire responses to new target stimuli during reversal and lose responses to previous targets before behavioral reversal is completed (Aston-Jones et al. 1997). Responses occur to free liquid outside of any task and transfer to reward-predicting target stimuli within a task as well as to primary and conditioned aversive stimuli (Aston-Jones et al. 1994; Foote et al. 1980; Rasmussen and Jacobs 1986; Sara and Segal 1991). Responses are often transient and appear to reflect changes in stimulus occurrence or meaning. Activations may occur only for a few trials with repeated presentations of food objects (Vankov et al. 1995) or with conditioned auditory stimuli associated with liquid reward, aversive air puff, or electric foot shock (Rasmussen and Jacobs 1986; Sara and Segal 1991). During conditioning, responses occur to the first few presentations of novel stimuli and reappear transiently whenever reinforcement contingencies change during acquisition, reversal, and extinction (Sara and Segal 1991).

Taken together, the responses of noradrenaline neurons resemble the responses of dopamine neurons in several respects, being activated by primary rewards, reward-predicting stimuli, and novel stimuli and transferring the response from primary to conditioned appetitive events. However, noradrenaline neurons differ from dopamine neurons by responding to a much larger variety of arousing stimuli, by responding well to primary and conditioned aversive stimuli, by discriminating well against neutral stimuli, by rapidly following behavioral reversals, and by showing decrementing responses with repeated stimulus presentation which may require 100 trials for solid appetitive responses (Aston-Jones et al. 1994). Noradrenaline responses are strongly related to the arousing or attention-grabbing properties of stimuli eliciting orienting reactions while being much less focused on appetitive stimulus properties like most dopamine neurons. They are probably driven more by attention-grabbing than motivating components of appetitive events.

Serotonin neurons

Activity in the different raphe nuclei facilitates motor output by setting muscle tone and stereotyped motor activity (Jacobs and Fornal 1993). Dorsal raphe neurons in cats show phasic, nonhabituating responses to visual and auditory stimuli of no particular behavioral meaning (Heym et al. 1982; LeMoal and Olds 1979). These responses resemble responses of dopamine neurons to novel and particularly salient stimuli. Further comparisons would require more detailed experimentation.

Nucleus basalis Meynert

Primate basal forebrain neurons are activated phasically by a large variety of behavioral events including conditioned, reward-predicting stimuli and primary rewards. Many activations depend on memory and associations with reinforcement in discrimination and delayed response tasks. Activations reflect the familiarity of stimuli (Wilson and Rolls 1990a), become more important with stimuli and movements occurring closer to the time of reward (Richardson and DeLong 1990), differentiate well between visual stimuli on the basis of appetitive and aversive associations (Wilson and Rolls 1990b), and change within a few trials during reversal (Wilson and Rolls 1990c). Neurons also are activated by aversive stimuli, predicted visual and auditory stimuli, and movements. They respond frequently to fully predicted rewards in well established behavioral tasks (Mitchell et al. 1987; Richardson and DeLong 1986, 1990), although responses to unpredicted rewards are more abundant in some studies (Richardson and DeLong 1990) but not in others (Wilson and Rolls 1990a–c). In comparison with dopamine neurons, they are activated by a much larger spectrum of stimuli and events, including aversive events, and do not show the rather homogeneous population response to unpredicted rewards and its transfer to reward-predicting stimuli.

Cerebellar climbing fibers

Probably the first error-driven teaching signal in the brain was postulated to involve the projection of climbing fibers from the inferior olive to Purkinje neurons in the cerebellar cortex (Marr 1969), and many cerebellar learning studies are based with this concept (Houk et al. 1996; Ito 1989; Kawato and Gomi 1992; Llinas and Welsh 1993). Climbing fiber inputs to Purkinje neurons transiently change their activity when loads for movements or gains between movements and visual feedback are changed and monkeys adapt to the new situation (Gilbert and Thach 1977; Ojakangas and Ebner 1992). Most of these changes consist of increased activity rather than the activation versus depression responses seen with errors in opposing directions in dopamine neurons. If climbing fiber activation were to serve as teaching signal, conjoint climbing fiber-parallel fiber activation should lead to changes in parallel fiber input to Purkinje neurons. This occurs indeed as long-term depression of parallel fiber input, mainly in in vitro preparations (Ito 1989). However, comparable parallel fiber changes are more difficult to find in behavioral learning situations (Ojakangas and Ebner 1992), leaving the consequences of potential climbing fiber teaching signals open at the moment.

A second argument for a role of climbing fibers in learning involves aversive classical conditioning. A fraction of climbing fibers is activated by aversive air puffs to the cornea. These responses are lost after Pavlovian eyelid conditioning using an auditory stimulus (Sears and Steinmetz 1991), suggesting a relationship to the unpredictability of primary aversive events. After conditioning, neurons in the cerebellar interpositus nucleus respond to the conditioned stimulus (Berthier and Moore 1990; McCormick and Thompson 1984). Lesions of this nucleus or injections of the GABA antagonist bicuculline into the inferior olive prevents the loss of inferior olive air puff responses after conditioning, suggesting that monosynaptic or polysynaptic inhibition from interpositus to inferior olive suppresses responses after conditioning (Thompson and Gluck 1991). This might allow inferior olive neurons to be depressed in the absence of predicted aversive stimuli and thus report a negative error in the prediction of aversive events similar to dopamine neurons.

Thus climbing fibers may report errors in motor performance and errors in the prediction of aversive events, although this may not always involve bidirectional changes as with dopamine neurons. Climbing fibers do not appear to acquire responses to conditioned aversive stimuli, but such responses are found in nucleus interpositus. The computation of aversive prediction errors may involve descending inhibitory inputs to inferior olive neurons, in analogy to striatal projections to dopamine neurons. Thus cerebellar circuits process error signals, albeit differently than dopamine neurons and TD models, and they might implement error learning rules like the Rescorla-Wagner rule (Thompson and Gluck 1991) or the formally equivalent Widrow-Hoff rule (Kawato and Gomi 1992).

DOPAMINE REWARD SIGNAL VERSUS PARKINSONIAN DEFICITS

Impaired dopamine neurotransmission with Parkinson's disease, experimental lesions or neuroleptic treatment is associated with many behavioral deficits in movement (akinesia, tremor, rigidity), cognition (attention, bradyphrenia, planning, learning), and motivation (reduced emotional responses, depression). The range of deficits appears too wide to be simply explained by a malfunctioning dopamine reward signal. Most deficits are considerably ameliorated by systemic dopamine precursor or receptor agonist therapy, although this cannot in a simple manner restitute the phasic information transmission by neuronal impulses. However, many appetitive deficits are not restored by this therapy, such as pharmacologically induced discrimination deficits (Ahlenius 1974) and parkinsonian learning deficits (Canavan et al. 1989; Knowlton et al. 1996; Linden et al. 1990; Sprengelmeyer et al. 1995; Vriezen and Moscovitch 1990).

From these considerations, it appears that dopamine neurotransmission plays two separate functions in the brain, the phasic processing of appetitive and alerting information and the tonic enabling of a wide range of behaviors without temporal coding. Deficits in a similar double dopamine function may underlie the pathophysiology of schizophrenia (Grace 1991). It is interesting to note that phasic changes of dopamine activity may occur at different time scales. Whereas the reward responses follow a time course in the order of tens and hundreds of milliseconds, dopamine release studies with voltammetry and microdialysis concern time scales of minutes and reveal a much wider spectrum of dopamine functions, including the processing of rewards, feeding, drinking, punishments, stress, and social behavior (Abercrombie et al. 1989; Church et al. 1987b; Doherty and Gratton 1992; Louilot et al. 1986; Young et al. 1992, 1993). It appears that dopamine neurotransmission follows at least three time scales with progressively wider roles in behavior, from the fast, rather restricted function of signaling rewards and alerting stimuli via a slower function of processing a considerable range of positively and negatively motivating events to the tonic function of enabling a large variety of motor, cognitive, and motivational processes.

The tonic dopamine function is based on low, sustained, extracellular dopamine concentrations in the striatum (5–10 nM) and other dopamine-innervated areas that are sufficient to stimulate extrasynaptic, mostly D2 type dopamine receptors in their high affinity state (9–74 nM; Fig. 8) (Richfield et al. 1989). This concentration is regulated locally within a narrow range by synaptic overflow and extrasynaptic dopamine release induced by tonic spontaneous impulse activity, reuptake transport, metabolism, autoreceptor-mediated release and synthesis control, and presynaptic glutamate influence on dopamine release (Chesselet 1984). The importance of ambient dopamine concentrations is demonstrated experimentally by the deleterious effects of unphysiologic levels of receptor stimulation. Reduced dopamine receptor stimulation after lesions of dopamine afferents or local administration of dopamine antagonists in prefrontal cortex lead to impaired performance of spatial delayed response tasks in rats and monkeys (Brozoski et al. 1979; Sawaguchi and Goldman-Rakic 1991; Simon et al. 1980). Interestingly, increases of prefrontal dopamine turnover induce similar impairments (Elliott et al. 1997; Murphy et al. 1996). Apparently, the tonic stimulation of dopamine receptors should be neither too low nor too high to assure an optimal function of a given brain region. Changing the influence of well-regulated, ambient dopamine would compromise the correct functioning of striatal and cortical neurons. Different brain regions may require specific levels of dopamine for mediating specific behavioral functions. It may be speculated that ambient dopamine concentrations are also necessary for maintaining striatal synaptic plasticity induced by a dopamine reward signal. A role of tonic dopamine on synaptic plasticity is suggested by the deleterious effects of dopamine receptor blockade or D2 receptor knockout on posttetanic depression (Calabresi et al. 1992a, 1997).

Numerous other neurotransmitters exist also in low ambient concentrations in the extracellular liquid, such as glutamate in striatum (0.9 μM) and cortex (0.6 μM) (Herrera-Marschitz et al. 1996). This may be sufficient to stimulate highly sensitive NMDA receptors (Sands and Barish 1989) but not other glutamate receptor types (Kiskin et al. 1986). Ambient glutamate facilitates action potential activity via NMDA receptor stimulation in hippocampus (Sah et al. 1989) and activates NMDA receptors in cerebral cortex (Blanton and Kriegstein 1992). Tonic glutamate levels are regulated by uptake in cerebellum and increase during phylogenesis, influencing neuronal migration via NMDA receptor stimulation (Rossi and Slater 1993). Other neurotransmitters exist as well in low ambient concentrations, such as aspartate and GABA in striatum and frontal cortex (0.1 μM and 20 nM, respectively) (Herrera-Marschitz et al. 1996), and adenosine in hippocampus where it is involved in presynaptic inhibition (Manzoni et al. 1994). Although incomplete, this list suggests that neurons in many brain structures are permanently bathed in a soup of neurotransmitters that has powerful, specific, physiological effects on neuronal excitability.

Given the general importance of tonic extracellular concentrations of neurotransmitters, it appears that the wide range of parkinsonian symptoms would not be due to deficient transmission of reward information by dopamine neurons but reflect a malfunction of striatal and cortical neurons due to impaired enabling by reduced ambient dopamine.

Dopamine neurons would not be actively involved in the wide range of processes deficient in parkinsonism but simply provide the background concentration of dopamine necessary to maintain proper functioning of striatal and cortical neurons involved in these processes.

I thank Drs. Dana Ballard, Anthony Dickinson, Francois Gonon, David D. Potter, Traverse Slater, Roland E. Suri, Richard S. Sutton, and R. Mark Wightman for enlightening discussions and comments, and also two anonymous referees for extensive comments.

The experimental work was supported by the Swiss National Science Foundation (currently 31.43331.95), the Human Capital and Mobility and the Biomed 2 programs of the European Community via the Swiss Office of Education and Science (CHRX-CT94-0463 via 93.0121 and BMH4-CT95-0608 via 95.0313-1), the James S. McDonnell Foundation, the Roche Research Foundation, the United Parkinson Foundation (Chicago), and the British Council.

Received 20 October 1997; accepted in final form 2 April 1998.

REFERENCES

Abercrombie, E. D., Keefe, K. A., DiFrischia, D. S., and Zigmond, M. J. Differential effect of stress on in vivo dopamine release in striatum, nucleus accumbens, and medial frontal cortex. *J. Neurochem.* 52: 1655–1658, 1989.

Ahlenius, S. Effects of low and high doses of L-dopa on the tetrabenazine or α-methyltyrosine-induced suppression of behaviour in a successive discrimination task. *Psychopharmacologia* 39: 199–212, 1974.

Alexander, G. E., DeLong, M. R., and Strick, P. L. Parallel organization of functionally segregated circuits linking basal ganglia and cortex. *Annu. Rev. Neurosci.* 9: 357–381, 1986.

Amalric, M. and Koob, G. F. Depletion of dopamine in the caudate nucleus but not in nucleus accumbens impairs reaction-time performance. *J. Neurosci.* 7: 2129–2134, 1987.

Andén, N. E., Fuxe, K., Hamberger, B., and Hökfelt, T. A quantitative study on the nigro-neostriatal dopamine neurons. *Acta Physiol. Scand.* 67: 306–312, 1966.

Anglade, P., Mouatt-Prigent, A., Agid, Y., and Hirsch, E. C. Synaptic plasticity in the caudate nucleus of patients with Parkinson's disease. *Neurodegeneration* 5: 121–128, 1996.

Aosaki, T., Tsubokawa, H., Ishida, A., Watanabe, K., Graybiel, A. M., and Kimura, M. Responses of tonically active neurons in the primate's striatum undergo systematic changes during behavioral sensorimotor conditioning. *J. Neurosci.* 14: 3969–3984, 1994.

Apicella, P., Legallet, E., and Trouche, E. Responses of tonically discharging neurons in monkey striatum to visual stimuli presented under passive conditions and during task performance. *Neurosci. Lett.* 203: 147–150, 1996.

Apicella, P., Legallet, E., and Trouche, E. Responses of tonically discharging neurons in the monkey striatum to primary rewards delivered during different behavioral states. *Exp. Brain Res.* 116: 456–466, 1997.

Apicella, P., Ljungberg, T., Scarnati, E., and Schultz, W. Responses to reward in monkey dorsal and ventral striatum. *Exp. Brain Res.* 85: 491–500, 1991a.

Apicella, P., Scarnati, E., Ljungberg, T. and Schultz, W. Neuronal activity in monkey striatum related to the expectation of predictable environmental events. *J. Neurophysiol.* 68: 945–960, 1992.

Apicella, P., Scarnati, E., and Schultz, W. Tonically discharging neurons of monkey striatum respond to preparatory and rewarding stimuli. *Exp. Brain Res.* 84: 672–675, 1991b.

Arbib, M. A. and Dominey, P. F. Modeling the roles of the basal ganglia in timing and sequencing saccadic eye movements. In: *Models of Information Processing in the Basal Ganglia*, edited by J. C. Houk, J. L. Davis, and D. G. Beiser. Cambridge, MA: MIT Press, 1995, p. 149–162.

Arbuthnott, G. W. and Ingham, C. A. The thorny problem of what dopamine does in psychiatric disease. *Prog. Brain Res.* 99: 341–350, 1993.

Aston-Jones, G. and Bloom, F. E. Norepinephrine-containing locus coeruleus neurons in behaving rats exhibit pronounced responses to nonnoxious environmental stimuli. *J. Neurosci.* 1: 887–900, 1981.

Aston-Jones, G., Rajkowski, J., and Kubiak, P. Conditioned responses of monkey locus coeruleus neurons anticipate acquisition of discriminative behavior in a vigilance task. *Neuroscience* 80: 697–716, 1997.

Aston-Jones, G., Rajkowski, J., Kubiak, P., and Alexinsky, T. Locus coeruleus neurons in monkey are selectively activated by attended cues in a vigilance task. *J. Neurosci.* 14: 4467–4480, 1994.

Ballard, D. H. *An Introduction to Neural Computing*. Cambridge, MA: MIT Press, 1997.

Barto, A. G. Adaptive critics and the basal ganglia. In: *Models of Information Processing in the Basal Ganglia*, edited by J. C. Houk, J. L. Davis, and D. G. Beiser. Cambridge, MA: MIT Press, 1995, p. 215–232.

Barto, A. G. and Anandan, P. Pattern-recognizing stochastic learning automata. *IEEE Trasnact. Syst. Man Cybern.* 15: 360–375, 1985.

Barto, A. G., Sutton, R. S., and Anderson, C. W. Neuronlike adaptive elements that can solve difficult learning problems. *IEEE Trans Syst. Man Cybernet.* 13: 834–846, 1983.

Beninger, R. J. The role of dopamine in locomotor activity and learning. *Brain Res. Rev.* 6: 173–196, 1983.

Beninger, R. J. Dissociating the effects of altered dopaminergic function on performance and learning. *Brain Res. Bull.* 23: 365–371, 1989.

Beninger, R. J., Cheng, M., Hahn, B. L., Hoffman, D. C., and Mazurski, E. J. Effects of extinction, pimozide, SCH 23390 and metoclopramide on food-rewarded operant responding of rats. *Psychopharmacology* 92: 343–349, 1987.

Beninger, R. J. and Hahn, B. L. Pimozide blocks establishment but not expression of amphetamine-produced environment-specific conditioning. *Science* 220: 1304–1306, 1983.

Berendse, H. W., Groenewegen, H. J., and Lohman, A. H. M. Compartmental distribution of ventral striatal neurons projecting to the mesencephalon in the rat. *J. Neurosci.* 12: 2079–2103, 1992.

Berger, B., Trottier, S., Verney, C., Gaspar, P., and Alvarez, C. Regional and laminar distribution of the dopamine and serotonin innervation in the macaque cerebral cortex: a radioautographic study. *J. Comp. Neurol.* 273: 99–119, 1988.

Bergson, C., Mrzljak, L., Smiley, J. F., Pappy, M., Levenson, R., and Goldman-Rakic, P. S. Regional, cellular and subcellular variations in the distribution of D_1 and D_5 dopamine receptors in primate brain. *J. Neurosci.* 15: 7821–7836, 1995.

Berthier, N. E. and Moore, J. W. Activity of deep cerebellar nuclear cells during classical conditioning of nictitating membrane extension in rabbits. *Exp. Brain Res.* 83: 44–54, 1990.

Bindra, D. Neuropsychological interpretation of the effects of drive and incentive-motivation on general activity and instrumental behavior. *Psychol. Rev.* 75: 1–22, 1968.

Blanton, M. G. and Kriegstein, A. R. Properties of amino-acid neurotransmitter receptors of embryonic cortical neurons when activated by exogenous and endogenous agonists. *J. Neurophysiol.* 67: 1185–1200, 1992.

Boeijinga, P. H., Mulder, A. B., Pennartz, C.M.A., Manshanden, I., and Lopes da Silva, F. H. Responses of the nucleus accumbens following fornix/fimbria stimulation in the rat. Identification and long-term potentiation of mono- and polysynaptic pathways. *Neuroscience* 53: 1049–1058, 1993.

Bolam, J. P., Francis, C. M., and Henderson, Z. Cholinergic input to dopamine neurons in the substantia nigra: a double immunocytochemical study. *Neuroscience* 41: 483–494, 1991.

Bolles, R. C. Reinforcement, expectancy and learning. *Psychol. Rev.* 79: 394–409, 1972.

Bowman, E. M., Aigner, T. G., and Richmond, B. J. Neural signals in the monkey ventral striatum related to motivation for juice and cocaine rewards. *J. Neurophysiol.* 75: 1061–1073, 1996.

Bouyer, J. J., Park, D. H., Joh, T. H., and Pickel, V. M. Chemical and structural analysis of the relation between cortical inputs and tyrosine hydroxylase-containing terminals in rat neostriatum. *Brain Res.* 302: 267–275, 1984.

Brown, J. R. and Arbuthnott, G. W. The electrophysiology of dopamine (D_2) receptors: a study of the actions of dopamine on corticostriatal transmission. *Neuroscience* 10: 349–355, 1983.

Brozoski, T. J., Brown, R. M., Rosvold, H. E., and Goldman, P. S. Cognitive deficit caused by regional depletion of dopamine in prefrontal cortex of rhesus monkey. *Science* 205: 929–932, 1979.

Caillé, I., Dumartin, B., and Bloch, B. Ultrastructural localization of D1 dopamine receptor immunoreactivity in rat striatonigral neurons and its relation with dopaminergic innervation. *Brain Res.* 730: 17–31, 1996.

Calabresi, P., Maj, R., Pisani, A., Mercuri, N. B., and Bernardi, G. Long-term synaptic depression in the striatum: physiological and pharmacological characterization. *J. Neurosci.* 12: 4224–4233, 1992a.

CALABRESI, P., PISANI, A., MERCURI, N. B., AND BERNARDI, G. Long-term potentiation in the striatum is unmasked by removing the voltage-dependent magnesium block of NMDA receptor channels. *Eur. J. Neurosci.* 4: 929–935, 1992b.

CALABRESI, P., SAIARDI, A., PISANI, A., BAIK, J. H., CENTONZE, D., MERCURI, N. B., BERNARDI, G., AND BORELLI, E. Abnormal synaptic plasticity in the striatum of mice lacking dopamine D2 receptors. *J. Neurosci.* 17: 4536–4544, 1997.

CANAVAN, A.G.M., PASSINGHAM, R. E., MARSDEN, C. D., QUINN, N., WYKE, M., AND POLKEY, C. E. The performance on learning tasks of patients in the early stages of Parkinson's disease. *Neuropsychologia* 27: 141–156, 1989.

CEPEDA, C., BUCHWALD, N. A., AND LEVINE, M. S. Neuromodulatory actions of dopamine in the neostriatum are dependent upon the excitatory aminao acid receptor subtypes activated. *Proc. Natl. Acad. Sci. USA* 90: 9576–9580, 1993.

CEPEDA, C., CHANDLER, S. H., SHUMATE, L. W., AND LEVINE, M. S. Persistent Na^+ conductance in medium-sized neostriatal neurons: characterization using infrared videomicroscopy and whole cell patch-clamp recordings. *J. Neurophysiol.* 74: 1343–1348, 1995.

CEPEDA, C., COLWELL, C. S., ITRI, J. N., CHANDLER, S. H., AND LEVINE, M. S. Dopaminergic modulation of NMDA-induced whole cell currents in neostriatal neurons in slices: contribution of calcium conductances. *J. Neurophysiol.* 79: 82–94, 1998.

CHERGUI, K., SUAUD-CHAGNY, M. F., AND GONON, F. Nonlinear relationship between impulse flow, dopamine release and dopamine elimination in the rat brain in vivo. *Neurocience* 62: 641–645, 1994.

CHESSELET, M. F. Presynaptic regulation of neurotransmitter release in the brain: facts and hypothesis. *Neuroscience* 12: 347–375, 1984.

CHURCH, W. H., JUSTICE, J. B., JR., AND BYRD, L. D. Extracellular dopamine in rat striatum following uptake inhibition by cocaine, nomifensine and benztropine. *Eur. J. Pharmacol.* 139: 345–348, 1987.

CHURCH, W. H., JUSTICE, J. B., JR., AND NEILL, D. B. Detecting behaviorally relevant changes in extracellular dopamine with microdialysis. *Brain Res.* 412: 397–399, 1987.

CLARKE, P.B.S., HOMMER, D. W., PERT, A., AND SKIRBOLL, L. R. Innervation of substantia nigra neurons by cholinergic afferents from pedunculopontine nucleus in the rat: neuroanatomical and electrophysiological evidence. *Neuroscience* 23: 1011–1019, 1987.

COLLE, W. M. AND WISE, R. A. Effects of nucleus accumbens amphetamine on lateral hypothalamus brain stimulation reward. *Brain Res.* 459: 356–360, 1980.

CONTRERAS-VIDAL, J. L. AND SCHULTZ, W. A neural network model of reward-related learning, motivation and orienting behavior. *Soc. Neurosci. Abstr.* 22: 2029, 1996.

CORBETT, D. AND WISE, R. A. Intracranial self-stimulation in relation to the ascending dopaminergic systems of the midbrain: a moveable microelectrode study. *Brain Res.* 185: 1–15, 1980.

CORVAJA, N., DOUCET, G., AND BOLAM, J. P. Ultrastructure and synaptic targets of the raphe-nigral projection in the rat. *Neuroscience* 55: 417–427, 1993.

DEHAENE, S. AND CHANGEUX, J.-P. The Wisconsin Card Sorting Test: theoretical analysis and modeling in a neuronal network. *Cerebr. Cortex* 1: 62–79, 1991.

DELANEY, K. AND GELPERIN, A. Post-ingestive food-aversion learning to amino acid deficient diets by the terrestrial slug Limax maximus. *J. Comp. Physiol. [A]* 159: 281–295, 1986.

DELONG, M. R., CRUTCHER, M. D., AND GEORGOPOULOS, A. P. Relations between movement and single cell discharge in the substantia nigra of the behaving monkey. *J. Neurosci.* 3: 1599–1606, 1983.

DESCARRIES, L., WATKINS, K. C., GARCIA, S., BOSLER, O., AND DOUCET, G. Dual character, asynaptic and synaptic, of the dopamine innervation in adult rat neostriatum: a quantitative autoradiogrphic and immunocytochemical analysis. *J. Comp. Neurol.* 375: 167–186, 1996.

DI CHIARA, G. The role of dopamine in drug abuse viewed from the perspective of its role in motivation. *Drug Alcohol Depend.* 38: 95–137, 1995.

DICKINSON, A. *Contemporary Animal Learning Theory.* Cambridge, UK: Cambridge Univ. Press, 1980.

DICKINSON, A. AND BALLEINE, B. Motivational control of goal-directed action. *Anim. Learn. Behav.* 22: 1–18, 1994.

DICKINSON, A., HALL, G., AND MACKINTOSH, N. J. Surprise and the attenuation of blocking. *J. Exp. Psychol. Anim. Behav. Proc.* 2: 313–322, 1976.

DOHERTY, M. D. AND GRATTON, A. High-speed chronoamperometric measurements of mesolimbic and nigrostriatal dopamine release associated with repeated daily stress. *Brain Res.* 586: 295–302, 1992.

DOMINEY, P., ARBIB, M., AND JOSEPH, J.-P. A model of corticostriatal plasticity for learning oculomotor associations and sequences. *J. Cognit. Neurosci.* 7: 311–336, 1995.

DOUCET, G., DESCARRIES, L., AND GARCIA, S. Quantification of the dopamine innervation in adult rat neostriatum. *Neuroscience* 19: 427–445, 1986.

DUGAST, C., SUAUD-CHAGNY, M. F., AND GONON, F. Continuous in vivo monitoring of evoked dopamine release in the rat nucleus accumbens by amperometry. *Neuroscience* 62: 647–654, 1994.

EDMONDS, D. E. AND GALLISTEL, C. R. Reward versus performance in self-stimulation: electrode-specific effects of α-methyl-p-tyrosine on reward in the rat. *J. Comp. Physiol. Psychol.* 91: 962–974, 1977.

ELLIOTT, R., SAHAKIAN, B. J., MATTHEWS, K., BANNERJEA, A., RIMMER, J., AND ROBBINS, T. W. Effects of methylphenidate on spatial working memory and planning in healthy young adults. *Psychopharmacology* 131: 196–206, 1997.

ETTENBERG, A. Dopamine, neuroleptics and reinforced behavior. *Neurosci. Biobehav. Rev.* 13: 105–111, 1989.

FAGG, A. H. Reinforcement learning for robotic reaching and grasping. In: *New Perspectives in the Control of the Reach to Grasp Movement*, edited by K.M.B. Bennet and U. Castiello. Amsterdam: North-Holland, 1993, p. 281–308.

FAGG, A. H. AND ARBIB, M. A. A model of primate visual-motor conditional learning. *Adapt. Behav.* 1: 3–37, 1992.

FIBIGER, H. C., LEPIANE, F. G., JAKUBOVIC, A., AND PHILLIPS, A. G. The role of dopamine in intracranial self-stimulation of the ventral tegmental area. *J. Neurosci.* 7: 3888–3896, 1987.

FIBIGER, H. C. AND MILLER, J. J. An anatomical and electrophysiological investigation of the serotonergic projection from the dorsal raphé nucleus to the substantia nigra in the rat. *Neuroscience* 2: 975–987, 1977.

FIBIGER, H. C. AND PHILLIPS, A. G. Reward, motivation, cognition: psychobiology of mesotelencephalic dopamine systems. In: *Handbook of Physiology. The Nervous System. Intrinsic Regulatory Systems of the Brain.* Bethesda, MA: Am. Physiol. Soc., 1986, sect. 1, vol. IV, p. 647–675.

FILION, M., TREMBLAY, L., AND BÉDARD, P. J. Abnormal influences of passive limb movement on the activity of globus pallidus neurons in parkinsonian monkey. *Brain Res.* 444: 165–176, 1988.

FLAHERTY, A. W. AND GRAYBIEL, A. Two input systems for body representations in the primate striatal matrix: experimental evidence in the squirrel monkey. *J. Neurosci.* 13: 1120–1137, 1993.

FLAHERTY, A. W. AND GRAYBIEL, A. Input-output organization of the sensorimotor striatum in the squirrel monkey. *J. Neurosci.* 14: 599–610, 1994.

FLOWERS, K. AND DOWNING, A. C. Predictive control of eye movements in Parkinson disease. *Ann. Neurol.* 4: 63–66, 1978.

FOOTE, S. L., ASTON-JONES, G., AND BLOOM, F. E. Impulse activity of locus coeruleus neurons in awake rats and monkeys is a function of sensory stimulation and arousal. *Proc. Natl. Acad. Sci. USA* 77: 3033–3037, 1980.

FREUND, T. F., POWELL, J. F., AND SMITH, A. D. Tyrosine hydroxylase-immunoreactive boutons in synaptic contact with identified striatonigral neurons, with particular reference to dendritic spines. *Neuroscience* 13: 1189–1215, 1984.

FREY, U., SCHROEDER, H., AND MATTHIES, H. Dopaminergic antagonists prevent long-term maintenance of posttetanic LTP in the CA1 region of hippocampal slices. *Brain Res.* 522: 69–75, 1990.

FRISTON, K. J., TONONI, G., REEKE, G. N., JR., SPORNS, O., AND EDELMAN, G. M. Value-dependent selection in the brain: simulation in a synthetic neural model. *Neuroscience* 59: 229–243, 1994.

FUJITA, K. Species recognition by five macaque monkeys. *Primates* 28: 353–366, 1987.

FURIEZOS, G. AND WISE, R. A. Pimozide-induced extinction of intracranial self-stimulation: response patterns rule out motor or performance deficits. *Brain Res.* 103: 377–380, 1976.

FUTAMI, T., TAKAKUSAKI, K., AND KITAI, S. T. Glutamatergic and cholinergic inputs from the pedunculopontine tegmental nucleus to dopamine neurons in the substantia nigra pars compacta. *Neurosci. Res.* 21: 331–342, 1995.

GALLISTEL, C. R. *The Organization of Learning.* Cambridge, MA: MIT Press, 1990.

GARCIA, C. E., PRETT, D. M., AND MORARI, M. Model predictive control: theory and practice—a survey. *Automatica* 25: 335–348, 1989.

GARCIA-MUNOZ, M., YOUNG, S. J., AND GROVES, P. Presynaptic long-term

changes in excitability of the corticostriatal pathway. *Neuroreport* 3: 357–360, 1992.
GARIANO, R. F. AND GROVES, P. M. Burst firing in midbrain dopamine neurons by stimulation of the medial prefrontal and anterior cingulate cortices. *Brain Res.* 462: 194–198, 1988.
GARRIS, P. A., CIOLKOWSKI, E. L., PASTORE, P., AND WIGHTMAN, R. M. Efflux of dopamine from the synaptic cleft in the nucleus accumbens of the rat brain. *J. Neurosci.* 14: 6084–6093, 1994a.
GARRIS, P. A., CIOLKOWSKI, E. L., AND WIGHTMAN, R. M. Heterogeneity of evoked dopamine overflow within the striatal and striatoamygdaloid regions. *Neuroscience* 59: 417–427, 1994b.
GARRIS, P. A. AND WIGHTMAN, R. M. Different kinetics govern dopaminergic transmission in the amygdala, prefrontal cortex, and striatum: an in vivo voltammetric study. *J. Neurosci.* 14: 442–450, 1994.
GERFEN, C. R. The neostriatal mosaic: compartmentalization of corticostriatal input and striatonigral output systems. *Nature* 311: 461–464, 1984.
GERFEN, C. R., ENGBER, T. M., MAHAN, L. C., SUSEL, Z., CHASE, T. N., MONSMA, F. J., JR., AND SIBLEY, D. R. D1 and D2 dopamine receptor-regulated gene expression of striatonigral and striatopallidal neurons. *Science* 250: 1429–1432, 1990.
GERMAN, D. C., DUBACH, M., ASKARI, S., SPECIALE, S. G., AND BOWDEN, D. M. 1-methyl-4-phenyl-1,2,3,6-tetrahydropyridine (MPTP)-induced parkinsonian syndrome in macaca fascicularis: which midbrain dopaminergic neurons are lost? *Neuroscience* 24: 161–174, 1988.
GILBERT, P.F.C. AND THACH, W. T. Purkinje cell activity during motor learning. *Brain Res.* 128: 309–328, 1977.
GIROS, B., JABER, M., JONES, S. R., WIGHTMAN, R. M., AND CARON, M. G. Hyperlocomotion and indifference to cocaine and amphetamine in mice lacking the dopamine transporter. *Nature* 379: 606–612, 1996.
GOLDMAN-RAKIC, P. S., LERANTH, C., WILLIAMS, M. S., MONS, N., AND GEFFARD, M. Dopamine synaptic complex with pyramidal neurons in primate cerebral cortex. *Proc. Natl. Acad. Sci. USA* 86: 9015–9019, 1989.
GONON, F. Nonlinear relationship between impulse flow and dopamine released by rat midbrain dopaminergic neurons as studied by in vivo electrochemistry. *Neuroscience* 24: 19–28, 1988.
GONON, F. Prolonged and extrasynaptic excitatory action of dopamine mediated by D1 receptors in the rat striatum in vivo. *J. Neurosci.* 17: 5972–5978, 1997.
GONZALES, C. AND CHESSELET, M.-F. Amygdalonigral pathway: An anterograde study in the rat with *Phaseolus vulgaris* Leucoagglutinin (PHA-L). *J. Comp. Neurol.* 297: 182–200, 1990.
GRACE, A. A. Phasic versus tonic dopamine release and the modulation of dopamine system responsivity: a hypothesis for the etiology of schizophrenia. *Neuroscience* 41: 1–24, 1991.
GRACE, A. A. AND BUNNEY, B. S. Opposing effects of striatonigral feedback pathways on midbrain dopamine cell activity. *Brain Res.* 333: 271–284, 1985.
GRAYBIEL, A. M., AOSAKI, T., FLAHERTY, A. W., AND KIMURA, M. The basal ganglia and adaptive motor control. *Science* 265: 1826–1831, 1994.
GROVES, P. M., GARCIA-MUNOZ, M., LINDER, J. C., MANLEY, M. S., MARTONE, M. E., AND YOUNG, S. J. Elements of the intrinsic organization and information processing in the neostriatum. In: *Models of Information Processing in the Basal Ganglia,* edited by J. C. Houk, J. L. Davis, and D. G. Beiser. Cambridge, MA: MIT Press, 1995, p. 51–96.
GULLAPALLI, V., BARTO, A. G., AND GRUPEN, R. A. Learning admittance mapping for force-guided assembly. In: *Proceedings of the 1994 International Conference on Robotics and Automation.* Los Alamitos, CA: Computer Society Press, 1994, p. 2633–2638.
HABER, S. N., LYND, E., KLEIN, C., AND GROENEWEGEN, H. J. Topographic organization of the ventral striatal efferent projections in the rhesus monkey: an autoradiographic tracing study. *J. Comp. Neurol.* 293: 282–298, 1990.
HABER, S., LYND-BALTA, E., AND MITCHELL, S. J. The organization of the descending ventral pallidal projections in the monkey. *J. Comp. Neurol.* 329: 111–128, 1993.
HAMMER, M. An identified neuron mediates the unconditioned stimulus in associative olfactory learning in honeybees. *Nature* 366: 59–63, 1993.
HAMMOND, C., SHIBAZAKI, T., AND ROUZAIRE-DUBOIS, B. Branched output neurons of the rat subthalamic nucleus: electrophysiological study of the synaptic effects on identified cells in the two main target nuclei, the entopeduncular nucleus and the substantia nigra. *Neuroscience* 9: 511–520, 1983.
HATTORI, T., FIBIGER, H. C., AND MCGEER, P. L. Demonstration of a pallido-nigral projection innervating dopaminergic neurons. *J. Comp. Neurol.* 162: 487–504, 1975.
HEDREEN, J. C. AND DELONG, M. R. Organization of striatopallidal, striatonigral and nigrostriatal projections in the macaque. *J. Comp. Neurol.* 304: 569–595, 1991.
HERNANDEZ-LOPEZ, S., BARGAS, J., SURMEIER, D. J., REYES, A., AND GALARRAGA, E. D1 receptor activation enhances evoked discharge in neostriatal medium spiny neurons by modulating an L-type Ca^{2+} conductance. *J. Neurosci.* 17: 3334–3342, 1997.
HERRERA-MARSCHITZ, M., YOU, Z. B., GOINY, M., MEANA, J. J., SILVEIRA, R., GODUKHIN, O. V., CHEN, Y., ESPINOZA, S., PETTERSSON, E., LOIDL, C. F., LUBEC, G., ANDERSSON, K., NYLANDER, I., TERENIUS, L., AND UNGERSTEDT, U. On the origin of extracellular glutamate levels monitored in the basal ganglia of the rat by in vivo microdialysis. *J. Neurochem.* 66: 1726–1735, 1996.
HERSCH, S. M., CILIAX, B. J., GUTEKUNST, C.-A., REES, H. D., HEILMAN, C. J., YUNG, K. K. L., BOLAM, J. P., INCE, E., YI, H. AND LEVEY, A. I. Electron microscopic analysis of D1 and D2 dopamine receptor proteins in the dorsal striatum and their synaptic relationships with motor corticostriatal afferents. *J. Neurosci.* 15: 5222–5237, 1995.
HEYM, J. TRULSON, M. E., AND JACOBS, B. L. Raphe unit activity in freely moving cats: effects of phasic auditory and visual stimuli. *Brain Res.* 232: 29–39, 1982.
HIKOSAKA, O., SAKAMOTO, M., AND USUI, S. Functional properties of monkey caudate neurons. III. Activities related to expectation of target and reward. *J. Neurophysiol.* 61: 814–832, 1989.
HOLLERMAN, J. R. AND SCHULTZ, W. Activity of dopamine neurons during learning in a familiar task context. *Soc. Neurosci. Abstr.* 22: 1388, 1996.
HOLLERMAN, J. R., TREMBLAY, L., AND SCHULTZ, W. Reward dependency of several types of neuronal activity in primate striatum. *Soc. Neurosci. Abstr.* 20: 780, 1994.
HOLSTEIN, G. R., PASIK, P., AND HAMORI, J. Synapses between GABA-immunoreactive axonal and dendritic elements in monkey substantia nigra. *Neurosci. Lett.* 66: 316–322, 1986.
HOOVER, J. E. AND STRICK, P. L. Multiple output channels in the basal ganglia. *Science* 259: 819–821, 1993.
HORVITZ, J. C., STEWART, T., AND JACOBS, B. L. Burst activity of ventral tegmental dopamine neurons is elicited by sensory stimuli in the awake cat. *Brain Res.* 759: 251–258, 1997.
HOUK, J. C., ADAMS, J. L., AND BARTO, A. G. A model of how the basal ganglia generate and use neural signals that predict reinforcement. In: *Models of Information Processing in the Basal Ganglia,* edited by J. C. Houk, J. L. Davis, and D. G. Beiser. Cambridge, MA: MIT Press, 1995, p. 249–270.
HOUK, J. C., BUCKINGHAM, J. T., AND BARTO, A. G. Models of the cerebellum and motor learning. *Behav. Brain Sci.* 19: 368–383, 1996.
HRUPKA, B. J., LIN, Y. M., GIETZEN, D. W., AND ROGERS, Q. R. Small changes in essential amino acid concentrations alter diet selection in amino acid-deficient rats. *J. Nutr.* 127: 777–784, 1997.
HULL, C. L. *Principles of Behavior.* New York: Appleton-Century-Crofts, 1943.
INGHAM, C. A., HOOD, S. H., WEENINK, A., VAN MALDEGEM, B., AND ARBUTHNOTT, G. W. Morphological changes in the rat neostriatum after unilateral 6-hydroxydopamine injections into the nigrostriatal pathway. *Exp. Brain Res.* 93: 17–27, 1993.
ITO, M. Long-term depression. *Annu. Rev. Neurosci.* 12: 85–102, 1989.
JACOBS, B. L. AND FORNAL, C. A. 5-HT and motor control: a hypothesis. *Trends Neurosci.* 16: 346–352, 1993.
JIMENEZ-CASTELLANOS, J. AND GRAYBIEL, A. M. Evidence that histochemically distinct zones of the primate substantia nigra pars compacta are related to patterned distributions of nigrostriatal projection neurons and striatonigral fibers. *Exp. Brain Res.* 74: 227–238, 1989.
KALMAN, R. E. A new approach to linear filtering and prediction problems. *J. Basic Eng. Trans. ASME* 82: 35–45, 1960.
KAMIN, L. J. Selective association and conditioning. In: *Fundamental Issues in Instrumental Learning,* edited by N. J. Mackintosh and W. K. Honig. Halifax, Canada: Dalhousie University Press, 1969, p. 42–64.
KAWAGOE, K. T., GARRIS, P. A., WIEDEMANN, D. J., AND WIGHTMAN, R. M. Regulation of transient dopamine concentration gradients in the microenvironment surrounding nerve terminals in the rat striatum. *Neuroscience* 51: 55–64, 1992.
KAWAGUCHI, Y., WILSON, C. J., AND EMSON, P. C. Intracellular recording of identified neostriatal patch and matrix spiny cells in a slice preparation preserving cortical inputs. *J. Neurophysiol.* 62: 1052–1068, 1989.

KAWATO, M. AND GOMI, H. The cerebellum and VOR/OKR learning models. *Trends Neurosci.* 15: 445–453, 1992.

KISKIN, N. I., KRISHTAL, O. A., AND TSYNDRENKO, A. Y. Excitatory amino acid receptors in hippocampal neurons: kainate fails to desensitize them. *Neurosci. Lett.* 63: 225–230, 1986.

KLOPF, A. H. *The Hedonistic Neuron: A Theory of Memory, Learning and Intelligence*. Washington, DC: Hemisphere, 1982.

KNOWLTON, B. J., MANGELS, J. A., AND SQUIRE, L. R. A neostriatal habit learning system in humans. *Science* 273: 1399–1402, 1996.

KÜNZLE, H. An autoradiographic analysis of the efferent connections from premotor and adjacent prefrontal regions (areas 6 and 9) in *Macaca fascicularis. Brain Behav. Evol.* 15: 185–234, 1978.

LEMOAL, M. AND OLDS, M. E. Peripheral auditory input to the midbrain limbic area and related structures. *Brain Res.* 167: 1–17, 1979.

LEMOAL, M. AND SIMON, H. Mesocorticolimbic dopaminergic network: functional and regulatory roles. *Physiol. Rev.* 71: 155–234, 1991.

LEVEY, A. I., HERSCH, S. M., RYE, D. B., SUNAHARA, R. K., NIZNIK, H. B., KITT, C. A., PRICE, D. L., MAGGIO, R., BRANN, M. R., AND CILIAX, B. J. Localisation of D1 and D2 dopamine receptors in brain with subtype-specific antibodies. *Proc. Natl. Acad. Sci. USA* 90: 8861–8865, 1993.

LINDEN, A., BRACKE-TOLKMITT, R., LUTZENBERGER, W., CANAVAN, A. G. M., SCHOLZ, E., DIENER, H. C., AND BIRBAUMER, N. Slow cortical potentials in parkinsonian patients during the course of an associative learning task. *J. Psychophysiol.* 4: 145–162, 1990.

LJUNGBERG, T., APICELLA, P., AND SCHULTZ, W. Responses of monkey midbrain dopamine neurons during delayed alternation performance. *Brain Res.* 586: 337–341, 1991.

LJUNGBERG, T., APICELLA, P., AND SCHULTZ, W. Responses of monkey dopamine neurons during learning of behavioral reactions. *J. Neurophysiol.* 67: 145–163, 1992.

LLINAS, R. AND WELSH, J. P. On the cerebellum and motor learning. *Curr. Opin. Neurobiol.* 3: 958–965, 1993.

LOHMAN, A.H.M. AND VAN WOERDEN-VERKLEY, I. Ascending connections to the forebrain in the tegu lizard. *J. Comp. Neurol.* 182: 555–594, 1978.

LOUILOT, A., LEMOAL, M. AND SIMON, H. Differential reactivity of dopaminergic neurons in the nucleus accumbens in response to different behavioral situations. An in vivo voltammetric study in free moving rats. *Brain Res.* 397: 395–400, 1986.

LOVIBOND, P. F. Facilitation of instrumental behavior by a Pavlovian appetitive conditioned stimulus. *J. Exp. Psychol. Anim. Behav. Proc.* 9: 225–247, 1983.

LOVINGER, D. M., TYLER, E. C., AND MERRITT, A. Short- and long-term synaptic depression in rat neostriatum. *J. Neurophysiol.* 70: 1937–1949, 1993.

LYND-BALTA, E. AND HABER, S. N. Primate striatonigral projections: a comparison of the sensorimotor-related striatum and the ventral striatum. *J. Comp. Neurol.* 345: 562–578, 1994.

MACKINTOSH, N. J. A theory of attention: variations in the associability of stimulus with reinforcement. *Psychol. Rev.* 82: 276–298, 1975.

MANZONI, O. J., MANABE, T., AND NICOLL, R. A. Release of adenosine by activation of NMDA receptors in the hippocampus. *Science* 265: 2098–2101, 1994.

MARR, D. A theory of cerebellar cortex. *J. Physiol. (Lond.)* 202: 437–470, 1969.

MARSHALL, J. F., O'DELL, S. J., NAVARRETE, R. AND ROSENSTEIN, A. J. Dopamine high-affinity transport site topography in rat brain: major differences between dorsal and ventral striatum. *Neuroscience* 37: 11–21, 1990.

MATSUMOTO, K., NAKAMURA, K., MIKAMI, A., AND KUBOTA, K. Response to unpredictable water delivery into the mouth of visually responsive neurons in the orbitofontal cortex of monkeys. *Abstr. Satellite Symp. IBR Meeting in Honor of Prof. Kubota, Inuyama, Japan*, P-14, 1995.

MATSUMURA, M., KOJIMA, J., GARDINER, T. W., AND HIKOSAKA, O. Visual and oculomotor functions of monkey subthalamic nucleus. *J. Neurophysiol.* 67: 1615–1632, 1992.

MAUNSELL, J.H.R. AND GIBSON, J. R. Visual response latencies in striate cortex of the macaque monkey. *J. Neurophysiol.* 68: 1332–1344, 1992.

MAZZONI, P., ANDERSEN, R. A., AND JORDAN, M. I. A more biologically plausible learning rule than backpropagation applied to a network model of cortical area 7. *Cereb. Cortex* 1: 293–307, 1991.

MCCALLUM, A. K. *Reinforcement learning with selective perception and hidden states* (PhD thesis). Rochester, NY: Univ. Rochester, 1995.

MCCORMICK, D. A. AND THOMPSON, R. F. Neuronal responses of the rabbit cerebellum during acquisition and peformance of a classically conditioned nictitating membrane-eyelid response. *J. Neurosci.* 4: 2811–2822, 1984.

MCLAREN, I. The computational unit as an assembly of neurones: an implementation of an error correcting learning algorithm. In: *The Computing Neuron*, edited by R. Durbin, C. Miall, and G. Mitchison. Amsterdam: Addison-Wesley, 1989 p. 160–178.

MICHAEL, A. C., JUSTICE, J. B., JR., AND NEILL, D. B. In vivo voltammetric determination of the kinetics of dopamine metabolism in the rat. *Neurosci. Lett.* 56: 365–369, 1985.

MIDDLETON, F. A. AND STRICK, P. L. The temporal lobe is a target of output from the basal ganglia. *Proc. Natl. Acad. Sci. USA* 93: 8683–8687, 1996.

MILLER, E. K., LI, L., AND DESIMONE, R. Activity of neurons in anterior inferior temporal cortex during a short-term memory task. *J. Neurosci.* 13: 1460–1478, 1993.

MILLER, J. D., SANGHERA, M. K., AND GERMAN, D. C. Mesencephalic dopaminergic unit activity in the behaviorally conditioned rat. *Life Sci.* 29: 1255–1263, 1981.

MILLER, R., WICKENS, J. R., AND BENINGER, R. J. Dopamine D-1 and D-2 receptors in relation to reward and performance: a case for the D-1 receptor as a primary site of therapeutic action of neuroleptic drugs. *Prog. Neurobiol.* 34: 143–183, 1990.

MIRENOWICZ, J. AND SCHULTZ, W. Importance of unpredictability for reward responses in primate dopamine neurons. *J. Neurophysiol.* 72: 1024–1027, 1994.

MIRENOWICZ, J. AND SCHULTZ, W. Preferential activation of midbrain dopamine neurons by appetitive rather than aversive stimuli. *Nature* 379: 449–451, 1996.

MITCHELL, S. J., RICHARDSON, R. T., BAKER, F. H., AND DELONG, M. R. The primate globus pallidus: neuronal activity related to direction of movement. *Exp. Brain Res.* 68: 491–505, 1987.

MOGENSON, G. J., TAKIGAWA, M., ROBERTSON, A., AND WU, M. Self-stimulation of the nucleus accumbens and ventral tegmental area of Tsai attenuated by microinjections of spiroperidol into the nucleus accumbens. *Brain Res.* 171: 247–259, 1979.

MONTAGUE, P. R., DAYAN, P., NOWLAN, S. J., POUGET, A., AND SEJNOWSKI, T. J. Using aperiodic reinforcement for directed self-organization during development. In: *Neural Information Processing Systems 5*, edited by S. J. Hanson, J. D. Cowan, and C. L. Giles. San Mateo, CA: Morgan Kaufmann, 1993, p. 969–976.

MONTAGUE, P. R., DAYAN, P., PERSON, C., AND SEJNOWSKI, T. J. Bee foraging in uncertain environments using predictive hebbian learning. *Nature* 377: 725–728, 1995.

MONTAGUE, P. R., DAYAN, P., AND SEJNOWSKI, T. J. A framework for mesencephalic dopamine systems based on predictive Hebbian learning. *J. Neurosci.* 16: 1936–1947, 1996.

MONTAGUE, P. R. AND SEJNOWSKI, T. J. The predictive brain: temporal coincidence and temporal order in synaptic learning mechanisms. *Learn. Memory* 1: 1–33, 1994.

MORA, F. AND MYERS, R. D. Brain self-stimulation: direct evidence for the involvement of dopamine in the prefrontal cortex. *Science* 197: 1387–1389, 1977.

MURPHY, B. L., ARNSTEN, A. F., GOLDMAN-RAKIC, P. S., AND ROTH, R. H. Increased dopamine turnover in the prefrontal cortex impairs spatial working memory performance in rats and monkeys. *Proc. Natl. Acad. Sci. USA* 93: 1325–1329, 1996.

NAKAMURA, K., MIKAMI, A., AND KUBOTA, K. Activity of single neurons in the monkey amygdala during performance of a visual discrimination task. *J. Neurophysiol.* 67: 1447–1463, 1992.

NEDERGAARD, S., BOLAM, J. P., AND GREENFIELD, S. A. Facilitation of dendritic calcium conductance by 5-hydroxytryptamine in the substantia nigra. *Nature* 333: 174–177, 1988.

NIIJIMA, K. AND YOSHIDA, M. Activation of mesencephalic dopamine neurons by chemical stimulation of the nucleus tegmenti pedunculopontinus pars compacta. *Brain Res.* 451: 163–171, 1988.

NIKI, H. AND WATANABE, M. Prefrontal and cingulate unit activity during timing behavior in the monkey. *Brain Res.* 171: 213–224, 1979.

NIRENBERG, M. J., VAUGHAN, R. A., UHL, G. R., KUHAR, M. J., AND PICKEL, V. M. The dopamine transporter is localized to dendritic and axonal plasma membranes of nigrostriatal dopaminergic neurons. *J. Neurosci.* 16: 436–447, 1996.

NISHIJO, H., ONO, T., AND NISHINO, H. Topographic distribution of modality-specific amygdalar neurons in alert monkey. *J. Neurosci.* 8: 3556–3569, 1988.

NISHINO, H., ONO, T., MURAMOTO, K. I., FUKUDA, M., AND SASAKI, K.

Neuronal activity in the ventral tegmental area (VTA) during motivated bar press feeding behavior in the monkey. *Brain Res.* 413: 302–313, 1987.

OJAKANGAS, C. L. AND EBNER, T. J. Purkinje cell complex and simple spike changes during a voluntary arm movement learning task in the monkey. *J. Neurophysiol.* 68: 2222–2236, 1992.

OLDS, J. AND MILNER, P. Positive reinforcement produced by electrical stimulation of septal area and other regions of rat brain. *J. Comp. Physiol. Psychol.* 47: 419–427, 1954.

OORSCHOT, D. E. Total number of neurons in the neostriatal, pallidal, subthalamic, and substantia nigral nuclei of the rat basal ganglia: a stereological study using the Cavalieri and optical disector methods. *J. Comp. Neurol.* 366: 580–599, 1996.

OTMAKHOVA, N. A. AND LISMAN, J. E. D1/D5 dopamine recetor activation increases the magnitude of early long-term potentiation at CA1 hippocampal synapses. *J. Neurosci.* 16: 7478–7486, 1996.

PACKARD, M. G. AND WHITE, N. M. Dissociation of hippocampus and caudate nucleus memory systems by posttraining intracerebral injection of dopamine agonists. *Behav. Neurosci.* 105: 295–306, 1991.

PASTOR, M. A., ARTIEDA, J., JAHANSHAHI, M., AND OBESO, J. A. Time estimation and reproduction is abnormal in Parkinson's disease. *Brain* 115: 211–225, 1992.

PEARCE, J. M. AND HALL, G. A model for Pavlovian conditioning: variations in the effectiveness of conditioned but not of unconditioned stimuli. *Psychol. Rev.* 87: 532–552, 1980.

PENNARTZ, C.M.A., AMEERUN, R. F., GROENEWEGEN, H. J., AND LOPES DA SILVA, F. H. Synaptic plasticity in an in vitro slice preparation of the rat nucleus accumbens. *Eur. J. Neurosci.* 5: 107–117, 1993.

PERCHERON, G., FRANCOIS, C., YELNIK, J., AND FENELON, G. The primate nigro-striato-pallido-nigral system. Not a mere loop. In: *Neural Mechanisms in Disorders of Movement*, edited by A. R. Crossman and M. A. Sambrook. London: John Libbey, 1989, p. 103–109.

PHILLIPS, A. G., BROOKE, S. M., AND FIBIGER, H. C. Effects of amphetamine isomers and neuroleptics on self-stimulation from the nucleus accumbens and dorsal noradrenergic bundle. *Brain Res.* 85: 13–22, 1975.

PHILLIPS, A. G., CARTER, D. A., AND FIBIGER, H. C. Dopaminergic substrates of intracranial self-stimulation in the caudate nucleus. *Brain Res.* 104: 221–232, 1976.

PHILLIPS, A. G. AND FIBIGER, H. C. The role of dopamine in mediating self-stimulation in the ventral tegmentum, nucleus accumbens, and medial prefrontal cortex. *Can. J. Psychol.* 32: 58–66, 1978.

PHILLIPS, A. G., MORA, F., AND ROLLS, E. T. Intracranial self-stimulation in orbitofrontal cortex and caudate nucleus of rhesus monkey: effects of apomorphine, pimozide, and spiroperidol. *Psychopharmacology* 62: 79–82, 1979.

PICKEL, V. M., BECKLEY, S. C., JOH, T. H., AND REIS, D. J. Ultrastructural immunocytochemical localization of tyrosine hydroxylase in the neostriatum. *Brain Res.* 225: 373–385, 1981.

PRICE, J. L. AND AMARAL, D. G. An autoradiographic study of the projections of the central nucleus of the monkey amygdala. *J. Neurosci.* 1: 1242–1259, 1981.

RAO, R.P.N. AND BALLARD, D. H. Dynamic model of visual recognition predicts neural response properties in the visual cortex. *Neural Computat.* 9: 721–763, 1997.

RASMUSSEN, K. AND JACOBS, B. L. Single unit activity of locus coeruleus neurons in the freely moving cat. II. Conditioning and pharmacological studies. *Brain Res.* 371: 335–344, 1986.

RASMUSSEN, K., MORILAK, D. A., AND JACOBS, B. L. Single unit activity of locus coeruleus neurons in the freely moving cat. I. During naturalistic behaviors and in response to simple and complex stimuli. *Brain Res.* 371: 324–334, 1986.

RESCORLA, R. A. AND WAGNER, A. R. A theory of Pavlovian conditioning: variations in the effectiveness of reinforcement and nonreinforcement. In: *Classical Conditioning II: Current Research and Theory*, edited by A. H. Black and W. F. Prokasy. New York: Appleton Century Crofts, 1972, p. 64–99.

RICHARDSON, R. T. AND DELONG, M. R. Nucleus basalis of Meynert neuronal activity during a delayed response task in monkey. *Brain Res.* 399: 364–368, 1986.

RICHARDSON, R. T. AND DELONG, M. R. Context-dependent responses of primate nucleus basalis neurons in a go/no-go task. *J. Neurosci.* 10: 2528–2540, 1990.

RICHFIELD, E. K., PENNNEY, J. B., AND YOUNG, A. B. Anatomical and affinity state comparisons between dopamine D1 and D2 receptors in the rat central nervous system. *Neuroscience* 30: 767–777, 1989.

ROBBINS, T. W. AND EVERITT, B. J. Functions of dopamine in the dorsal and ventral striatum. *Semin. Neurosci.* 4: 119–128, 1992.

ROBBINS, T. W. AND EVERITT, B. J. Neurobehavioural mechanisms of reward and motivation. *Curr. Opin. Neurobiol.* 6: 228–236, 1996.

ROBINSON, T. E. AND BERRIDGE, K. C. The neural basis for drug craving: an incentive-sensitization theory of addiction. *Brain Res. Rev.* 18: 247–291, 1993.

ROGAWSKI, M. A. New directions in neurotransmitter action: dopamine provides some important clues. *Trends Neurosci.* 10: 200–205, 1987.

ROGERS, Q. R. AND HARPER, A. E. Selection of a solution containing histidine by rats fed a histidine-imbalanced diet. *J. Comp. Physiol. Psychol.* 72: 66–71, 1970.

ROLLS, E. T., CRITCHLEY, H. D., MASON, R., AND WAKEMAN, E. A. Orbitofrontal cortex neurons: role in olfactory and visual association learning. *J. Neurophysiol.* 75: 1970–1981, 1996.

ROMO, R., SCARNATI, E., AND SCHULTZ, W. Role of primate basal ganglia and frontal cortex in the internal generation of movements: comparisons in striatal neurons activated during stimulus-induced movement initiation and execution. *Exp. Brain Res.* 91: 385–395, 1992.

ROMO, R. AND SCHULTZ, W. Dopamine neurons of the monkey midbrain: contingencies of responses to active touch during self-initiated arm movements. *J. Neurophysiol.* 63: 592–606, 1990.

ROMPRÉ, P.-P. AND WISE, R. A. Behavioral evidence for midbrain dopamine depolarization inactivation. *Brain Res.* 477: 152–156, 1989.

ROSSI, D. J. AND SLATER, N. T. The developmental onset of NMDA receptor channel activity during neuronal migration. *Neuropharmacology* 32: 1239–1248, 1993.

RUMELHART, D. E., HINTON, G. E., AND WILLIAMS, R. J. Learning internal representations by error propagation. In: *Parallel Distributed Processing I*, edited by D. E. Rumelhart and J. L. McClelland. Cambridge, MA: MIT Press, 1986, p. 318–362.

SAH, P., HESTRIN, S., AND NICOLL, R. A. Tonic activation of NMDA receptors by ambient glutamate enhances excitability of neurons. *Science* 246: 815–818, 1989.

SALAMONE, J. D. The actions of neuroleptic drugs on appetitive instrumental behaviors. In: *Handbook of Psychopharmacology*, edited by L. L. Iversen, S. D. Iversen, and S. H. Snyder. New York: Plenum, 1987, vol. 19, p. 576–608.

SALAMONE, J. D. Complex motor and sensorimotor functions of striatal and accumbens dopamine: involvement in instrumental behavior processes. *Psychopharmacology* 107: 160–174, 1992.

SANDS, S. B. AND BARISH, M. E. A quantitative description of excitatory amino acid neurotransmitter responses on cultured ambryonic Yenopus spinal neurons. *Brain Res.* 502: 375–386, 1989.

SARA, S. J. AND SEGAL, M. Plasticity of sensory responses of locus coeruleus neurons in the behaving rat: implications for cognition. *Prog. Brain Res.* 88: 571–585, 1991.

SAWAGUCHI, T. AND GOLDMAN-RAKIC, P. S. D1 Dopamine receptors in prefrontal cortex: involvement in working memory. *Science* 251: 947–950, 1991.

SCARNATI, E., PROIA, A., CAMPANA, E., AND PACITTI, C. A microiontophoretic study on the nature of the putative synaptic neurotransmitter involved in the pedunculopontine-substantia nigra pars compacta excitatory pathway of the rat. *Exp. Brain Res.* 62: 470–478, 1986.

SCHULTZ, W. Responses of midbrain dopamine neurons to behavioral trigger stimuli in the monkey. *J. Neurophysiol.* 56: 1439–1462, 1986.

SCHULTZ, W., APICELLA, P., AND LJUNGBERG, T. Responses of monkey dopamine neurons to reward and conditioned stimuli during successive steps of learning a delayed response task. *J. Neurosci.* 13: 900–913, 1993.

SCHULTZ, W., APICELLA, P., ROMO, R., AND SCARNATI, E. Context-dependent activity in primate striatum reflecting past and future behavioral events. In: *Models of Information Processing in the Basal Ganglia*, edited by J. C. Houk, J. L. Davis, and D. G. Beiser. Cambridge, MA: MIT Press, 1995a, p. 11–28.

SCHULTZ, W., APICELLA, P., SCARNATI, E., AND LJUNGBERG, T. Neuronal activity in monkey ventral striatum related to the expectation of reward. *J. Neurosci.* 12: 4595–4610, 1992.

SCHULTZ, W., DAYAN, P., AND MONTAGUE, R. R. A neural substrate of prediction and reward. *Science* 275: 1593–1599, 1997.

SCHULTZ, W. AND ROMO, R. Responses of nigrostriatal dopamine neurons to high intensity somatosensory stimulation in the anesthetized monkey. *J. Neurophysiol.* 57: 201–217, 1987.

SCHULTZ, W. AND ROMO, R. Dopamine neurons of the monkey midbrain: contingencies of responses to stimuli eliciting immediate behavioral reactions. *J. Neurophysiol.* 63: 607–624, 1990.

SCHULTZ, W., ROMO, R., LJUNGBERG, T., MIRENOWICZ, J., HOLLERMAN, J. R., AND DICKINSON, A. Reward-related signals carried by dopamine neurons. In: *Models of Information Processing in the Basal Ganglia,* edited by J. C. Houk, J. L. Davis, and D. G. Beiser. Cambrdige, MA: MIT Press, 1995b, p. 233–248.

SCHULTZ, W., RUFFIEUX, A., AND AEBISCHER, P. The activity of pars compacta neurons of the monkey substantia nigra in relation to motor activation. *Exp. Brain Res.* 51: 377–387, 1983.

SEARS, L. L. AND STEINMETZ, J. E. Dorsal accessory inferior olive activity diminishes during acquisition of the rabbit classically conditioned eyelid response. *Brain Res.* 545: 114–122, 1991.

SELEMON, L. D. AND GOLDMAN-RAKIC, P. S. Topographic intermingling of striatonigral and striatopallidal neurons in the rhesus monkey. *J. Comp. Neurol.* 297: 359–376, 1990.

SESACK, S. R., AOKI, C., AND PICKEL, V. M. Ultrastructural localization of D2 receptor-like immunoreactivity in midbrain dopamine neurons and their striatal targets. *J. Neurosci.* 14: 88–106, 1994.

SESACK, S. R. AND PICKEL, V. M. Prefrontal cortical efferents in the rat synapse on unlabelled neuron targets of catecholamine terminals in the nucleus accumbens septi and on dopamine neurons in the ventral tegmental area. *J. Comp. Neurol.* 320: 145–160, 1992.

SIMON, H., SCATTON, B., AND LEMOAL, M. Dopaminergic A10 neurons are involved in cognitive functions. *Nature* 286: 150–151, 1980.

SMITH, A. D. AND BOLAM, J. P. The neural network of the basal ganglia as revealed by the study of synaptic connections of identified neurones. *Trends Neurosci.* 13: 259–265, 1990.

SMITH, I. D. AND GRACE, A. A. Role of the subthalamic nucleus in the regulation of nigral dopamine neuron activity. *Synapse* 12: 287–303, 1992.

SMITH, M. C. CS-US interval and US intensity in classical conditioning of the rabbit's nictitating membrane response. *J. Comp. Physiol. Psychol.* 66: 679–687, 1968.

SMITH, Y., BENNETT, B. D., BOLAM, J. P., PARENT, A., AND SADIKOT, A. F. Synaptic relationships between dopaminergic afferents and cortical or thalamic input in the sensorimotor territory of the striatum in monkey. *J. Comp. Neurol.* 344: 1–19, 1994.

SMITH, Y. AND BOLAM, J. P. The output neurones and the dopaminergic neurones of the substantia nigra receive a GABA-containing input from the globus pallidus in the rat. *J. Comp. Neurol.* 296: 47–64, 1990.

SMITH, Y. AND BOLAM, J. P. Convergence of synaptic inputs from the striatum and the globus pallidus onto identified nigrocollicular cells in the rat: a double anterograde labelling study. *Neuroscience* 44: 45–73, 1991.

SMITH, Y., HAZRATI, L.-N., AND PARENT, A. Efferent projections of the subthalmaic nucleus in the squirrel monkey as studied by the PHA-L anterograde tracing method. *J. Comp. Neurol.* 294: 306–323, 1990.

SOMOGYI, P., BOLAM, J. P., TOTTERDELL, S., AND SMITH, A. D. Monosynaptic input from the nucleus accumbens—ventral striatum region to retrogradely labelled nigrostriatal neurones. *Brain Res.* 217: 245–263, 1981.

SPRENGELMEYER, R., CANAVAN, A.G.M., LANGE, H. W., AND HÖMBERG, V. Associative learning in degenerative neostriatal disorders: contrasts in explicit and implicit remembering between Parkinson's and Huntington's disease patients. *Mov. Disord.* 10: 85–91, 1995.

SURMEIER, D. J., EBERWINE, J., WILSON, C. J., STEFANI, A., AND KITAI, S. T. Dopamine receptor subtypes colocalize in rat striatonigral neurons. *Proc. Natl. Acad. Sci. USA* 89: 10178–10182, 1992.

STAMFORD, J. A., KRUK, Z. L., PALIJ, P., AND MILLAR, J. Diffusion and uptake of dopamine in rat caudate and nucleus accumbens compared using fast cyclic voltammetry. *Brain Res.* 448: 381–385, 1988.

STEIN, L. Self-stimulation of the brain and the central stimulant action of amphetamine. *Federation Proc.* 23: 836–841, 1964.

STEIN, L., XUE, B. G., AND BELLUZZI, J. D. In vitro reinforcement of hippocampal bursting: a search for Skinner's atoms of behavior. *J. Exp. Anal. Behav.* 61: 155–168, 1994.

STEINFELS, G. F., HEYM, J., STRECKER, R. E., AND JACOBS, B. L. Behavioral correlates of dopaminergic unit activity in freely moving cats. *Brain Res.* 258: 217–228, 1983.

SUAUD-CHAGNY, M. F., DUGAST, C., CHERGUI, K., MSGHINA, M., AND GONON, F. Uptake of dopamine released by impulse flow in the rat mesolimbic and striatal system in vivo. *J. Neurochem.* 65: 2603–2611, 1995.

SURI, R. E. AND SCHULTZ, W. A neural learning model based on the activity of primate dopamine neurons. *Soc. Neurosci. Abstr.* 22: 1389, 1996.

SUTTON, R. S. Learning to predict by the method of temporal difference. *Machine Learn.* 3: 9–44, 1988.

SUTTON, R. S. AND BARTO, A. G. Toward a modern theory of adaptive networks: expectation and prediction. *Psychol. Rev.* 88: 135–170, 1981.

TEPPER, J. M, MARTIN, L. P., AND ANDERSON, D. R. $GABA_A$ receptor-mediated inhibition of rat substantia nigra dopaminergic neurons by pars reticulata projection neurons. *J. Neurosci.* 15: 3092–3103, 1995.

TESAURO, G. TD-Gammon, a self-teaching backgammon program, achieves master-level play. *Neural Comp.* 6: 215–219, 1994.

THOMPSON, R. F. AND GLUCK, M. A. Brain substrates of basic associative learning and memory. In: *Perspectives on Cognitive Neuroscience,* edited by R. G. Lister and H. J. Weingartner. New York: Oxford Univ. Press, 1991, p. 25–45.

THORNDIKE, E. L. *Animal Intelligence: Experimental Studies.* New York: MacMillan, 1911.

THORPE, S. J., ROLLS, E. T., AND MADDISON, S. The orbitofrontal cortex: neuronal activity in the behaving monkey. *Exp. Brain Res.* 49: 93–115, 1983.

TOAN, D. L. AND SCHULTZ, W. Responses of rat pallidum cells to cortex stimulation and effects of altered dopaminergic activity. *Neuroscience* 15: 683–694, 1985.

TONG, Z.-Y., OVERTON, P. G., AND CLARK, D. Stimulation of the prefrontal cortex in the rat induces patterns of activity in midbrain dopaminergic neurons which resemble natural burst events. *Synapse* 22: 195–208, 1996.

TREMBLAY, L. AND SCHULTZ, W. Processing of reward-related information in primate orbitofrontal neurons. *Soc. Neurosci. Abstr.* 21: 952, 1995.

TRENT, F. AND TEPPER, J. M. Dorsal raphé stimulation modifies striatal-evoked antidromic invasion of nigral dopamine neurons in vivo. *Exp. Brain Res.* 84: 620–630, 1991.

UNGERSTEDT, U. Adipsia and aphagia after 6-hydroxydopamine induced degeneration of the nigro-striatal dopamine system. *Acta Physiol. Scand. Suppl.* 367: 95–117, 1971.

VANKOV, A., HERVÉ-MINVIELLE, A., AND SARA, S. J. Response to novelty and its rapid habituation in locus coeruleus neurons of the freely exploring rat. *Eur. J. Neurosci.* 7: 1180–1187, 1995.

VRIEZEN, E. R. AND MOSCOVITCH, M. Memory for temporal order and conditional associative-learning in patients with Parkinson's disease. *Neuropsychologia* 28: 1283–1293, 1990.

WALSH, J. P. Depression of excitatory synaptic input in rat striatal neurons. *Brain Res.* 608: 123–128, 1993.

WANG, Y., CUMMINGS, S. L., AND GIETZEN, D. W. Temporal-spatial pattern of c-fos expression in the rat brain in response to indispensable amino acid deficiency. I. The initial recognition phase. *Mol. Brain Res.* 40: 27–34, 1996.

WATANABE, M. The appropriateness of behavioral responses coded in post-trial activity of primate prefrontal units. *Neurosci. Lett.* 101: 113–117, 1989.

WATANABE, M. Prefrontal unit activity during associative learning in the monkey. *Exp. Brain Res.* 80: 296–309, 1990.

WATANABE, M. Reward expectancy in primate prefrontal neurons. *Nature* 382: 629–632, 1996.

WAUQUIER, A. The influence of psychoactive drugs on brain self-stimulation in rats: a review. In: *Brain Stimulation Reward,* edited by A. Wauquier and E. T. Rolls. New York: Elsevier, 1976, p. 123–170.

WHITE, N. M. Reward or reinforcement: what's the difference? *Neurosci. Biobehav. Rev.* 13: 181–186, 1989.

WHITE, N. W. AND MILNER, P. M. The psychobiology of reinforcers. *Annu. Rev. Psychol.* 43: 443–471, 1992.

WIGHTMAN, R. M. AND ZIMMERMAN, J. B. Control of dopamine extracellular concentration in rat striatum by impulse flow and uptake. *Brain Res. Rev.* 15: 135–144, 1990.

WICKENS, J. R., BEGG, A. J., AND ARBUTHNOTT, G. W. Dopamine reverses the depression of rat corticostriatal synapses which normally follows high-frequency stimulation of cortex in vitro. *Neuroscience* 70: 1–5, 1996.

WICKENS, J. AND KÖTTER, R. Cellular models of reinforcement. In: *Models of Information Processing in the Basal Ganglia,* edited by J. C. Houk, J. L. Davis, and D. G. Beiser. Cambridge, MA: MIT Press, 1995, p. 187–214.

Widrow, G. and Hoff, M. E. Adaptive switching circuits. *IRE Western Electronic Show Conven., Conven. Rec.* part 4: 96–104, 1960.

Widrow, G. and Sterns, S. D. *Adaptive Signal Processing.* Englewood Cliffs, NJ: Prentice-Hall, 1985.

Williams, S. M. and Goldman-Rakic, P. S. Characterization of the dopaminergic innervation of the primate frontal cortex using a dopamine-specific antibody. *Cereb. Cortex* 3: 199–222, 1993.

Williams, G. V. and Millar, J. Concentration-dependent actions of stimulated dopamine release on neuronal activity in rat striatum. *Neuroscience* 39: 1–16, 1990.

Williams, G. V., Rolls, E. T., Leonard, C. M., and Stern, C. Neuronal responses in the ventral striatum of the behaving monkey. *Behav. Brain Res.* 55: 243–252, 1993.

Wilson, C., Nomikos, G. G., Collu, M., and Fibiger, H. C. Dopaminergic correlates of motivated behavior: importance of drive. *J. Neurosci.* 15: 5169–5178, 1995.

Wilson, C. J. The contribution of cortical neurons to the firing pattern of striatal spiny neurons. In: *Models of Information Processing in the Basal Ganglia,* edited by J. C. Houk, J. L. Davis, and D. G. Beiser. Cambridge, MA: MIT Press, 1995, p. 29–50.

Wilson, F.A.W. and Rolls, E. T. Neuronal responses related to the novelty and familiarity of visual stimuli in the substantia innominata, diagonal band of Broca and periventricular region of the primate forebrain. *Exp. Brain Res.* 80: 104–120, 1990a.

Wilson, F.A.W. and Rolls, E. T. Neuronal responses related to reinforcement in the primate basal forebrain. *Brain Res.* 509: 213–231, 1990b.

Wilson, F.A.W. and Rolls, E. T. Learning and memory is reflected in the responses of reinforcement-related neurons in the primate basal forebrain. *J. Neurosci.* 10: 1254–1267, 1990c.

Wise, R. A. Neuroleptics and operant behavior: the anhedonia hypothesis. *Behav. Brain Sci.* 5: 39–87, 1982.

Wise, R. A. Neurobiology of addiction. *Curr. Opin. Neurobiol.* 6: 243–251, 1996.

Wise, R. A. and Colle, L. Pimozide attenuates free feeding: "best scores" analysis reveals a motivational deficit. *Psychopharmacologia* 84: 446–451, 1984.

Wise, R. A. and Hoffman, D. C. Localization of drug reward mechanisms by intracranial injections. *Synapse* 10: 247–263, 1992.

Wise, R. A. and Rompre, P.-P. Brain dopamine and reward. *Annu. Rev. Psychol.* 40: 191–225, 1989.

Wise, R. A., Spindler, J., de Wit, H., and Gerber, G. J. Neuroleptic-induced "anhedonia" in rats: pimozide blocks reward quality of food. *Science* 201: 262–264, 1978.

Wynne, B. and Güntürkün, O. Dopaminergic innervation of the telencephalon of the pigeon (*Columba liva*): a study with antibodies against tyrosine hydroxylase and dopamine. *J. Comp. Neurol.* 357: 446–464, 1995.

Yan, Z., Song, W. J., and Surmeier, D. J. D2 dopamine receptors reduce N-type Ca^{2+} currents in rat neostriatal cholinergic interneurons through a membrane-delimited, protein-kinase-C-insensitive pathway. *J. Neurophysiol.* 77: 1003–1015, 1997.

Yim, C. Y. and Mogenson, G. J. Response of nucleus accumbens neurons to amygdala stimulation and its modification by dopamine. *Brain Res.* 239: 401–415, 1982.

Young, A.M.J., Joseph, M. H., and Gray, J. A. Increased dopamine release in vivo in nucleus accumbens and caudate nucleus of the rat during drinking: a microdialysis study. *Neuroscience* 48: 871–876, 1992.

Young, A.M.J., Joseph, M. H., and Gray, J. A. Latent inhibition of conditioned dopamine release in rat nucleus accumbens. *Neuroscience* 54: 5–9, 1993.

Yung, K.K.L., Bolam, J. P., Smith, A. D., Hersch, S. M., Ciliax, B. J., and Levey, A. I. Immunocytochemical localization of D1 and D2 dopamine receptors in the basal ganglia of the rat: light and electron microscopy. *Neuroscience* 65: 709–730, 1995.

Prediction of Reinforcing Responses to Psychostimulants in Humans by Brain Dopamine D_2 Receptor Levels

Nora D. Volkow, M.D., Gene-Jack Wang, M.D., Joanna S. Fowler, Ph.D., Jean Logan, Ph.D., Samuel J. Gatley, Ph.D., Andrew Gifford, Ph.D., Robert Hitzemann, Ph.D., Yu-Shin Ding, Ph.D., and Naomi Pappas, M.S.

Objective: This study assessed whether brain dopamine D_2 receptor levels, which show significant intersubject variability, predict reinforcing responses to psychostimulants in humans. **Method:** [^{11}C]Raclopride and positron emission tomography were used to measure D_2 receptor levels in 23 healthy men (mean age=34 years, SD=7) who had no drug abuse histories in order to assess if there were differences between the subjects who liked and those who disliked the effects of intravenous methylphenidate (0.5 mg/kg). **Results:** Subjects who liked the effects of methylphenidate had significantly lower D_2 receptor levels (mean=2.72 B_{max}/K_d, SD=0.3) than subjects who disliked its effects (mean=3.16, SD=0.3). Moreover, the higher the D_2 levels found, the more intense were methylphenidate's unpleasant effects. **Conclusions:** These results provide preliminary evidence that D_2 receptor levels predict response to psychostimulants in humans and that low D_2 receptors may contribute to psychostimulant abuse by favoring pleasant response.

(Am J Psychiatry 1999; 156:1440–1443)

One of the most challenging problems in the neurobiology of drug addiction is understanding why some individuals abuse drugs, whereas others do not. It has been hypothesized that low levels of dopamine D_2 receptors predispose subjects to use drugs as a means of compensating for the decrease in activation of reward circuits activated by these receptors (1). However, the data supporting D_2 receptor level involvement in predisposition to drug addiction are controversial (2), and the involvement of D_2 receptor levels in the reinforcing responses to drugs in humans has not been demonstrated.

In the present study, we used [^{11}C]raclopride and positron emission tomography (PET) to determine if there were differences in striatal D_2 receptor levels between subjects who reported the effects of methylphenidate (a psychostimulant drug that, like cocaine, blocks the dopamine transporters [3]) as pleasant and those who reported them as unpleasant and to assess whether D_2 receptor levels predict behavioral responses to methylphenidate, which differ markedly among subjects (4, 5). Although raclopride binds to both D_2 and D_3 receptors, the striatal concentration of D_3 receptors is very low (≈1% of D_2 receptors) (6), so that the PET measurements mainly reflect binding to D_2 receptors.

METHOD

Twenty-three male subjects (mean age=34 years, mean SD=7) without psychiatric, neurological, or medical disease or drug abuse

Received Nov. 16, 1998; revision received Feb. 12, 1999; accepted Feb. 23, 1999. From the Medical and Chemistry Departments, Brookhaven National Laboratory, Upton, N.Y.; and the Department of Psychiatry, State University of New York at Stony Brook. Address reprint requests to Dr. Volkow, Medical Department, Bldg. 490, Upton, NY 11973; volkow@bnl.gov (e-mail).

Supported in part by U.S. Department of Energy contract ACO2-76CH00016 and National Institute on Drug Abuse grant DA-06891.

The authors thank David Alexoff, Robert Carciello, Paula Cervany, Richard Ferrieri, Payton King, Alex Levy, Robert MacGregor, Noelwah Netusil, Carol Redvanly, David Schlyer, Colleen Shea, Donald Warner, and Cristopher Wong for their help.

FIGURE 1. Distribution Volume Images of [^{11}C]Raclopride at the Levels of the Striatum (left) and Cerebellum (right) in a Healthy Male Subject Who Reported the Effects of Methylphenidate as Pleasant and in a Healthy Male Subject Who Reported Them as Unpleasant[a]

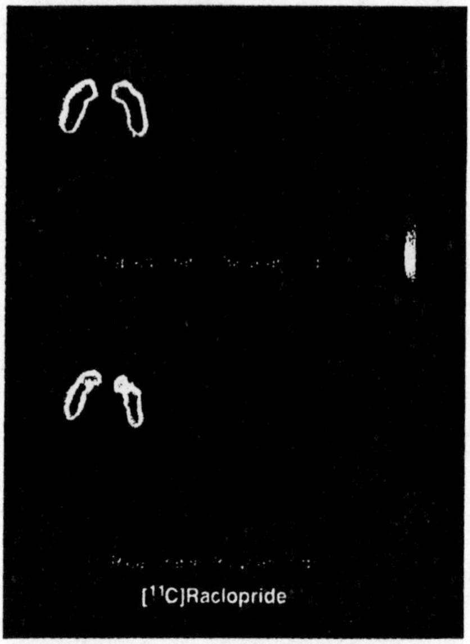

[a] The images have been normalized to the cerebellar activity of each subject because this reflects nonspecific binding. Notice the lower activity in the striatum of the subject who reported the effects of methylphenidate as pleasant than in the striatum of the subject who reported them as unpleasant. 100% = 25 ml/mg; 10% = 0.4 ml/mg.

or dependence (except nicotine) were studied. Subjects were scanned by using a CTI 931 tomograph (Siemens, Nashville) after intravenous injection of 4–10 mCi of [^{11}C]raclopride (specific activity=0.5–1.5 Ci/μM) (7). On a different day, subjects were given an intravenous dose of methylphenidate (0.5 mg/kg) after being told they would receive either placebo or methylphenidate. Behavioral effects were measured by using analogue self-rating scales for pleasant (happiness, mood, sexual desire, and desire for methylphenidate) and unpleasant (annoyance, distrust, anxiety, loss of control, and restlessness) drug effects, scored from 0 to 10 minutes before and 27 minutes after methylphenidate treatment (8). At the end of the study, subjects were asked if the effects of methylphenidate were pleasant or unpleasant. Written informed consent was obtained from all subjects after procedures had been fully explained.

Regions in the striatum and cerebellum were outlined on the individual's summed [^{11}C]raclopride image (between 15 and 54 minutes after injection of the radiotracer) and were then projected into the dynamic images to generate time activity curves (7). These time activity curves, along with the time activity curves for the amount of unchanged tracer in plasma, were used to obtain distribution volumes (equilibrium measurement of the ratio of tissue concentration to plasma concentration) and to compute the B_{max}/K_d (ratio of the distribution volume in the striatum to that in the cerebellum minus 1) (9). This method has been shown to yield reliable and accurate es-

FIGURE 2. D_2 Receptor Levels (B_{max}/K_d) in 23 Healthy Male Subjects Who Reported the Effects of Methylphenidate as Pleasant, Unpleasant, or Neutral[a]

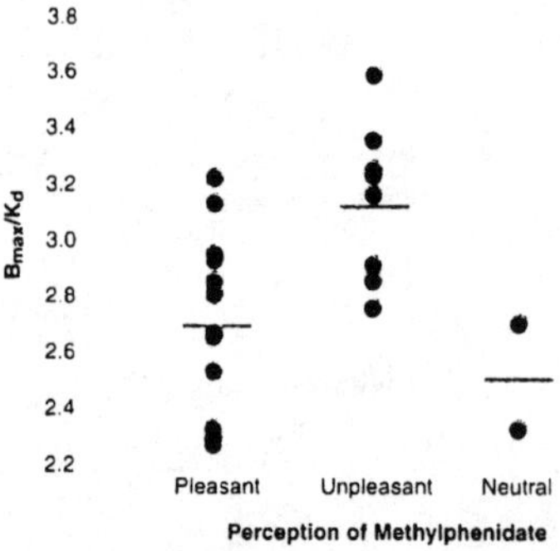

[a] B_{max}/K_d values were lower in subjects who reported the effects of methylphenidate as pleasant than in those who reported them as unpleasant. The horizontal lines represent the means for the B_{max}/K_d estimates for the different groups.

timates of B_{max}/K_d (10). Differences in B_{max}/K_d between the subjects who liked and those who disliked the effects of methylphenidate were compared by using Student's t tests (two-tailed); Pearson product-moment correlations were used to compute correlations between D_2 receptor levels and methylphenidate-induced behavioral changes (ratings after methylphenidate treatment minus baseline ratings). Significance was set at $p<0.01$.

RESULTS

Twelve subjects described the effects of methylphenidate as pleasant, nine described them as unpleasant, and two responded neutrally. There were no differences in demographic characteristics, smoking status, or plasma methylphenidate concentrations between individuals who liked and those who disliked the effects of methylphenidate.

Subjects who liked the effects of methylphenidate had significantly lower levels of D_2 receptors (mean=2.72 B_{max}/K_d, SD=0.32) than did subjects who disliked the effects (mean=3.16, SD=0.26) (t=3.3, df=19, $p<0.004$) (figure 1 and figure 2). The levels of D_2 receptors were correlated negatively with methylphenidate-induced increases in the self-rating scales for happiness (r=–0.58, df=22, $p<0.005$) and increases in the self-rating scales for mood (r=–0.52, df=12, p=0.01) and positively correlated with the methylphenidate-induced increases in the self-rating scales for annoyance (r=0.53, df=22, p=0.01) and distrust (r=0.66, df=12, $p<0.001$). Although the results were not significant ($p>0.05<0.20$), the correlations with D_2 receptor levels for the other pleasant drug effects were positive, and those for the other unpleasant effects were negative (figure 3).

FIGURE 3. Regression Slopes and Correlations Between the Behavioral Effects of Methylphenidate[a] and the Measures of Dopamine D_2 Receptor Levels (B_{max}/K_d) in 23 Healthy Male Subjects

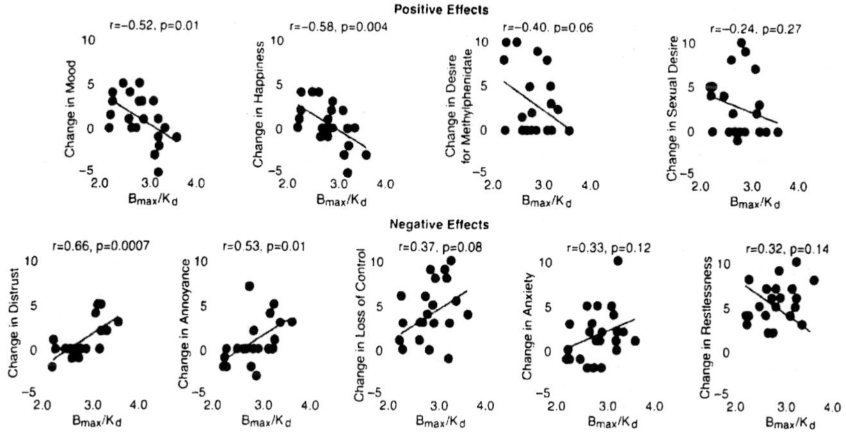

[a] Ratings after methylphenidate treatment minus baseline ratings.

DISCUSSION

The differences in response to methylphenidate between subjects with high and low D_2 receptor levels can be explained by the hypothesis that there is an optimal range in which D_2 receptor stimulation can be perceived as reinforcing; too little may not be sufficient, but too much may be aversive (11). Thus, it is possible that in subjects with high D_2 receptor levels, a small dose of methylphenidate may be perceived as pleasant. If D_2 receptor levels modulate sensitivity to physiological reinforcers (12), then one could postulate that low D_2 receptor levels would predispose a subject to use drugs as a means of compensating for decreased activation of reward circuits (1). Alternatively, low D_2 receptor levels could predispose individuals to psychostimulant abuse by favoring initial pleasant drug responses, which have been shown to predict future drug use (13), and/or high D_2 receptor levels may protect against drug abuse by favoring unpleasant drug responses.

Subjects who reported the effects of methylphenidate as pleasant, as most cocaine abusers do (13), had D_2 receptor levels similar to those previously reported in cocaine abusers (B_{max}/K_d=2.6, SD=0.3) (14). Thus, these results bring to light the possibility that low D_2 receptor levels in cocaine abusers may have antedated their cocaine use and may have contributed to their cocaine abuse. However, even if this possibility were to be corroborated, the fact that the subjects who liked methylphenidate had D_2 receptor levels similar to those found in cocaine addicts but were not drug abusers suggests that additional variables are involved in the vulnerability to drug abuse.

These results are highly suggestive of an involvement of D_2 receptor levels in the perception of the reinforcing effects of psychostimulants. These results agree with those from studies in laboratory animals indicating that D_2 receptor levels mediate reinforcing responses to drugs of abuse. This is evidenced by the decrease in the reinforcing effects of alcohol and morphine in mice who lack D_2 receptors (D_2 receptor knockout) (15, 16) and by the decrease in the reinforcing effects of cocaine in animals given drugs that block D_2 receptors (17, 18). While the studies on the effects of D_2 receptor antagonists in the reinforcing effects of psychostimulants in humans have not been as conclusive as those in laboratory animals, they have shown a decrease in the subjective ratings of pleasant sensations and of the craving induced by cocaine (19, 20). The lower efficacy of D_2 receptor antagonists reported in human studies may reflect the fact that the doses used were lower than those used in laboratory animals.

Although analogue scales for self-reports of drug effects have been shown to be reliable and consistent across studies and to predict administration of drugs in human subjects (21), this study would have benefited had these measures been corroborated by other behavioral instruments—e.g., the Profile of Mood States.

This is the first evidence in humans showing an association between D_2 receptor levels in brain and the reinforcing responses to psychostimulants. Further studies are required to determine the involvement of D_2 receptors in the predisposition to drug abuse.

REFERENCES

1. Blum K, Cull JC, Braverman ER, Comings DE: Reward deficiency syndrome. Am Sci 1996; 84:132–145
2. Goldman D, Urbanek M, Guenther D, Robin R, Long JC: A functionally deficient DRD2 variant [Ser311Cys] is not linked to alcoholism and substance abuse. Alcohol 1998; 16:47–52
3. Ritz MC, Lamb RJ, Goldberg SR, Kuhar MJ: Cocaine receptors on dopamine transporters are related to self-administration of cocaine. Science 1987; 237:1219–1223
4. Joyce PR, Donald RA, Nicholls MG, Lievesey JH, Abbott RM: Endocrine and behavioral responses to methylphenidate in normal subjects. Biol Psychiatry 1986; 21:1015–1023
5. Chait LD: Reinforcing and subjective effects of methylphenidate in humans. Behav Pharmacol 1994; 5:281–288
6. Sokoloff P, Schwartz JC: Novel dopamine receptors half a decade later. Trends Pharmacol Sci 1995; 16:270–275
7. Volkow ND, Fowler JS, Wang GJ, Dewey SL, Schlyer D, MacGregor R, Logan J, Alexoff D, Shea C, Hitzemann R, Angrist B, Wolf AP: Reproducibility of repeated measures of ^{11}C raclopride binding in the human brain. J Nucl Med 1993; 34:609–613
8. Wang G-J, Volkow ND, Hitzemann RJ, Wong C, Angrist B, Burr G, Pascani K, Pappas N, Lu A, Cooper T, Lieberman JA: Behavioral and cardiovascular effects of intravenous methylphenidate in normal subjects and cocaine abusers. Eur Addict Res 1997; 3:49–54
9. Logan J, Fowler JS, Volkow ND, Wolf AP, Dewey SL, Schlyer DJ, MacGregor RR, Hitzemann R, Bendriem B, Gatley SJ, Christman DR: Graphical analysis of reversible radioligand binding from time-activity measurements applied to [N-^{11}C-methyl]cocaine PET studies in human subjects. J Cereb Blood Flow Metab 1990; 10:740–747
10. Endres CJ, Carson RE: Assessment of dynamic neurotransmitter changes with bolus or infusion delivery of neuroreceptor ligands. J Cereb Blood Flow Metab 1998; 18:1196–1210
11. Glick SD, Raucci J, Wang S, Keller RW Jr, Carlson JN: Neurochemical predisposition to self-administer cocaine in rats: individual differences in dopamine and its metabolites. Brain Res 1994; 653:148–154
12. Chausmer AL, Ettenberg A: A role for D2, but not D1, dopamine receptors in the response-reinstating effects of food reinforcement. Pharmacol Biochem Behav 1997; 57:681–685
13. Davidson ES, Finch JF, Schenk S: Variability in subjective responses to cocaine: initial experiences of college students. Addict Behav 1993; 18:445–453
14. Volkow ND, Wang GJ, Fowler JS, Logan J, Gatley SJ, Hitzemann R, Chen AD, Dewey SL, Pappas N: Decreased striatal dopaminergic responsivity in detoxified cocaine abusers. Nature 1997; 386:830–833
15. Phillips TJ, Brown KJ, Burkhart-Kasch S, Wenger CD, Kelly MA, Rubinstein M, Grandy DK, Low MJ: Alcohol preference and sensitivity are markedly reduced in mice lacking D2 receptors. Nat Neurosci 1998; 1:610–615
16. Maldonado R, Saiardi A, Valverde O, Samad TA, Roques BP, Borrelli E: Absence of opiate rewarding effects in mice lacking dopamine D2 receptors. Nature 1997; 388:586–589
17. De Wit H, Wise RA: Blockade of cocaine reinforcement in rats with the dopamine receptor blocker pimozide, but not with the noradrenergic blockers phentolamine or phenoxybenzamine. Can J Psychol 1977; 31:195–203
18. Spealman RD: Antagonism of behavioral effects of cocaine by selective dopamine receptor blockers. Psychopharmacology (Berl) 1990; 101:142–145
19. Berger SP, Hall S, Mickalian JD, Reid MS, Crawford CA, Delucchi K, Carr K, Hall S: Haloperidol antagonism of cue-elicited cocaine craving. Lancet 1996; 347:504–508
20. Sherer MA, Kumor KM, Jaffe JH: Effects of intravenous cocaine are partially attenuated by haloperidol. Psychiatry Res 1989; 27:117–125
21. Fischman MW, Foltin RW: Utility of subjective-effects measurements in assessing abuse liability of drugs in humans. Br J Addict 1991; 86:1563–1570

Addiction (1996) 91(7), 921–949

SCIENTIFIC HORIZONS

Addictive drugs as reinforcers: multiple partial actions on memory systems

NORMAN M. WHITE

Department of Psychology, McGill University, Montreal, Quebec, Canada

Abstract

This review applies some new experimental findings and theoretical ideas about how reinforcers act on the neural mechanisms of learning and memory to the problem of how addictive drugs affect behaviour. A basic assumption of this analysis is that all changes in behaviour, including those involved in drug addiction and the initiation of drug self-administration, require the storage of new information in the nervous system. Animal studies suggest that such information is processed in several (this review deals with three) more or less independent learning and memory systems in the mammalian brain. Reinforcers can interact with these systems in three ways: they activate neural substrates of observable approach or escape responses, they produce unobservable internal states that can be perceived as rewarding or aversive, and they modulate or enhance the information stored in each of the memory systems. It is suggested that each addictive drug maintains its own self-administration by mimicking some subset of these actions. Evidence supporting the notion of multiple memory systems and data on the actions of several drugs (amphetamine, cocaine, nicotine, alcohol and morphine) on these systems are briefly reviewed. The utility of the concept of "reward" for understanding the effects of drugs on behaviour is discussed. Evidence demonstrating actions of drugs on multiple neural substrates of reinforcement suggests that no single factor is likely to explain either addictive behaviour in general or self-administration in particular. Some of the findings on the development and maintenance of self-administration by animals of the five exemplar drugs are discussed in the context of these ideas.

Introduction

This review explores the application of some recent experimental work on learning and memory in animals to understanding the biological bases of drug addiction. The concept of "reinforcement", the notion that certain events promote changes in behaviour, plays a central role in applying these experimental findings to drug addiction. The findings suggest that reinforcement is not a unitary process. Rather, it comprises several independent functions, some or all of which can be active simultaneously. This means that an addictive substance may cause changes in behaviour by initiating several different kinds of reinforcement processes. Each of these processes influences behaviour in specific ways.

The notion that drugs act as reinforcers is not new (e.g. Wise & Stein, 1970; Crow, 1973; Di Chiara, Acquas & Carboni, 1992; Wise *et al.*,

Correspondence to: Norman White, Department of Psychology, McGill University, 1205 Dr Penfield Avenue, Montreal, Quebec H3A 1B1, Canada. Tel: 01-514-398-6082; fax: 01-514-398-4896; e-mail: nwhite@psych.mcgill.ca

0965–2140/96/070921–29 $8.00 © Society for the Study of Addiction to Alcohol and Other Drugs

Carfax Publishing Company

1992), nor is the idea that drugs have different kinds of effects on behaviour. The present approach to these issues may be distinguished from earlier ones in several ways. A basic assumption is that all changes in behaviour involve the storage of new information in the nervous system; a process commonly called "learning and memory". Therefore, understanding learning and memory processes is essential to the analysis of changes in behaviour produced by addictive drugs. The present scheme is based on a theory of multiple parallel learning and memory systems. Each system is identified with a specific set of brain structures. Each acquires a different type of information and influences behaviour in a different way.

Reinforcers have different functions in each system. Although an understanding of the functions of naturally occurring reinforcers within each of these systems provides an important basis for analysing the effects of addictive drugs on behaviour, drugs are not treated as straightforward substitutes for natural reinforcers. Instead, addictive drugs are seen to mimic certain specific effects of reinforcers. Because each drug has a unique set of pharmacological actions, each has the potential to produce a different subset of the effects of naturally occurring reinforcers. This view focuses attention on specification of the neural substrates on which each drug acts and on the behavioural consequences of these actions.

Perhaps the best known application of the concept of reinforcement to the problem of explaining the effects of drugs on behaviour is based on a purely behavioural definition of reinforcers (Skinner, 1938) as events that follow a response and increase the probability that it will be repeated in similar situations. While unobjectionable as a description, this definition is incompatible with the present goal of specifying how each reinforcing action of each drug alters behaviour. In line with this objective, this review describes three specific behavioural actions of reinforcers, describes how certain drugs can have each of these same effects on behaviour and presents evidence contributing to identification of the neural substrates of these behaviour-altering effects of drugs and reinforcers.

Two of the actions of reinforcers involve two classes of responses they elicit, a property sometimes described by the term "incentive" (Bindra, 1969, 1978; Trowill, Panksepp & Gandelman, 1969; Milner, 1977; Toates, 1986). One class consists of skeletal responses that take the form of observable approach or escape behaviours, the other consists of unobservable patterns of autonomic and central responses that can be perceived as rewarding or aversive affective states (Young, 1959; Cabanac, Minaire & Adair, 1968; Cabanac & Ferber, 1987; Wise, 1982). These response-eliciting actions of reinforcers produce behaviour change by a process called "classical conditioning". While an organism is exposed to the incentive properties of a reinforcer (or an addictive drug) neutral cues that are present may acquire the property of eliciting responses that are similar to those produced by the reinforcer or drug. These cues then become *conditioned incentives* or secondary reinforcers. This process requires the storage of a neural representation of the relationship between the conditioned incentive cues and the conditioned responses they elicit. Therefore, describing the reinforcement process alone cannot provide a complete explanation of the behaviour change (White & Milner, 1992) produced by reinforcers or addictive drugs. Such an explanation can come only from an understanding of how reinforcement effects interact with learning and memory processes.

The third action of reinforcers is their function as *memory modulators*, or improvers (Thorndike, 1911; Landauer, 1969; Gold & McGaugh, 1975; McGaugh & Gold, 1989). Both reinforcers and drugs act on the neural substrates of memory to enhance or strengthen memories that have recently been acquired. In this way, both reinforcers and drugs increase the degree of control that experiences, including drug-related experiences, exert on future behaviour.

At the most general level, reinforcers function within learning and memory systems. They constitute part of experience, they elicit responses and they act to promote the storage of new information. This review attempts to apply what is known about how naturally occurring reinforcers interact with learning and memory systems to understanding the effects of addictive drugs on behaviour. After considering how drugs act on the nervous system and how this action can be studied in the context of reinforcement and memory, the hypothesis of multiple memory systems and their neural substrates will be reviewed. Evidence that drugs have effects on each of these systems will be presented, leading to an examination of how this analysis provides a basis for understanding the addictive process. Obviously, given the present state of knowledge, this understanding will remain incomplete.

Self-administration and drug action

Addictive drugs are self-administered by humans. Although social and economic influences may lead to an individual's first contact with an addictive drug, the present account has nothing to say about these factors. Once such a drug has entered an individual's body it has the potential to affect behaviour by its pharmacological actions on neural substrates of reinforcement and their interaction with learning and memory systems.

The fact that laboratory animals self-administer many addictive drugs by bar-pressing in operant chambers suggests that at least some of these processes of behaviour change can be studied in this animal model. Among the drugs that are generally agreed to be addictive to humans, laboratory rats self-administer amphetamine (Pickens & Harris, 1968; Pickens & Thompson, 1971; Yokel & Wise, 1975), cocaine (Pickens & Thompson, 1968; Roberts, Corcoran & Fibiger, 1977; Roberts & Koob, 1982), nicotine (Corrigall *et al.*, 1992), alcohol (Amit *et al.*, 1977; Weiss *et al.*, 1992; Samson *et al.*, 1993; Boyle *et al.*, 1994) and morphine (Weeks & Collins, 1968; Smith & Davis, 1973; Bozarth & Wise, 1981). Findings about the effects of these drugs, primarily on the behaviour of laboratory rats, are used in the following discussions as illustrations of how addictive drugs act on neural systems to initiate behavioural processes that promote their self-administration. The findings described suggest that these drugs can act variously on the neural substrates that mediate the two incentive functions of reinforcers (skeletal and internal affective responses), as well as mimicking the memory modulating effects of reinforcers. Although any one of these actions could result in self-administration, the findings suggest that most drugs simultaneously activate more than one of these processes.

Except in the laboratory drugs are invariably self-administered by systemic routes, leading to their spread throughout the body and, more particularly, to all parts of the nervous system. These include the neural systems that mediate the effects of reinforcers on behaviour. These neural systems contain and relate to each other via synaptic mechanisms. The fact that these synapses involve chemical neurotransmission of different types at different stages of the reinforcement and memory processes provides the basis for the effects of drugs on the systems. Drugs act at synapses that correspond in some way to their pharmacological properties. The probability that any drug acts at exactly the same series of synapses activated by any naturally occurring reinforcer is low. A drug is more likely to activate a pattern of synapses that only partially corresponds to that activated by any natural reinforcer. Furthermore, a systemically-administered drug may act at more than one site, initiating more than one behavioural process. Accordingly, drugs should be expected to reproduce some part or parts of the natural reinforcement process, fail to produce other parts, and possibly counteract still others. Because of these partial effects on reinforcement processes addictive drugs have the potential to produce unnatural, unexpected and even bizarre combinations of behavioural effects.

Direct intracerebral administration of addictive drugs has been used in attempts to localize their sites of action in the nervous system (e.g. Wise & Hoffman, 1992). According to the present scheme, by acting at a particular synapse a drug that alters behaviour initiates a reinforcement process that then interacts with a learning and memory system. There is no reason to presume that the pharmacological properties of the synapses mediating the latter processes are the same as those of the synapses that were initially activated by the drug. Therefore, information obtained with intracerebral administration of addictive drugs can pertain only to the first stage of the process by which they alter behaviour; that is, to the initial action of the drug on the nervous system.

Information about subsequent stages of the processes of behavioural change initiated by drugs can be obtained with other kinds of manipulations, including primarily various lesion techniques. Disruption of the behaviour-altering action of an addictive drug by damage to a particular brain structure suggests the involvement of that structure either in the initial action of the drug or in the subsequent learning and memory process that mediates the change in behaviour. Similarities in the patterns of lesion effects on drug-related behaviours and on learning and memory processes involving naturally occurring reinforcers lead to inferences about the memory processes that mediate the behavioural changes produced by addictive drugs.

In the following sections these processes are examined in two stages: first the three functions of reinforcers will be discussed in more detail; secondly the effects of these reinforcement functions on learning and memory systems will be described.

Behavioural effects of reinforcers

Incentive actions

The neural systems that control normal behaviour receive and process different types of information: an important distinction among these is that between external and internal sources. Environmental stimuli, or cues, constitute information from external sources. Most external cues have no immediate effect on behaviour, although organisms can learn about their presence in any situation (see *Declarative learning*). In this sense, they have purely informational properties. As already discussed, other external cues have the capacity to elicit behaviour with little or no previous experience. Examples of the latter include food, water, sexual partners and painful events. Because of this capacity we distinguish such cues and call them "reinforcers". If a reinforcer elicits approach responses we label it a positive incentive or a "reward'; if it elicits escape responses we label it "aversive" or "punishing".

Note that these labels are based on observable skeletal responses (approach and escape) and usually carry with them assumptions about the internal affective states elicited by reinforcers. These internal states are made up of a variety of reinforcer-elicited autonomic and central neural responses and are not usually directly observable. They are thought to be the basis of the perceived affective properties of reinforcers (Izard, 1972; Malmo, 1975; Candland *et al.*, 1977). Although it is an assumption, it seems a very reasonable one that naturally occurring reinforcers simultaneously elicit corresponding skeletal responses and internal states (White, Messier & Carr, 1987). Thus, it seems likely that approach responses are elicited together with unobservable internal states that are perceived as rewarding (Glickman & Schiff, 1967), and escape responses are elicited together with unobservable internal states that are perceived as aversive.

In summary, it can be inferred that reinforcers activate the neural substrates of two kinds of responses: observable approach or escape behaviour and an array of less observable or unobservable internal states, some of which are perceived as positive or negative affect. The activation of these substrates also initiates a learning process by which neutral cues come to activate the same substrates, leading to the same or similar responses. This type of learning is discussed under the heading of *Conditioned incentive learning*. This is one of three types of learning in the present scheme.

Drugs and incentive actions

Given the ways in which addictive drugs act on neural substrates it seems unlikely that the fixed relationship between observed responses and internal states elicited by natural reinforcers is always maintained when the substrates are activated by these drugs. Thus, an addictive drug may act at synapses in the neural substrate that mediates approach responses normally activated by reinforcers with positive incentive properties (note that in the absence of an external cue, no identifiable approach response would actually occur in this situation (White, Messier & Carr, 1987). At the same time, the same drug might also act at other synapses mediating internal states that are perceived as either rewarding or aversive, and the nature of these internal states may change with repeated exposure to the drug. Evidence suggesting the simultaneous presence of observable approach responses and incompatible aversive internal affective states will be described.

As is the case for naturally occurring reinforcers, the direct action of drugs on synapses that are parts of neural substrates mediating skeletal and affective responses leads to conditioned incentive learning. As a result of this process neutral cues in the environment come to elicit similar patterns of neural activity and the skeletal and affective responses produced by these patterns of activity.

Drugs can also produce other kinds of unlearned internal affective states. One class of such effects occurs as part of the constellation of withdrawal symptoms produced when a drug is withheld from a dependent individual. These states are generally thought to be perceived as aversive. Changes in the neural response to drugs as a result of use (e.g. "incentive sensitization; Robinson & Berridge, 1993); or "anhedonia"; (Wise, 1982) or disuse (e.g. "craving"; Kozlowski & Wilkinson, 1987), have also been hypothesized to produce affective states that influence drug self-administration.

In the present scheme, internal affective states, however they are produced, come to influence behaviour as an individual learns about their relationship to external cues and events. In the case of affective states involving addictive drugs, knowledge of this relationship leads to behaviours that maximize rewarding states and/or minimize aversive states (often referred to as "self-medication"). The process of learning about these internal states and their relationships to external cues is discussed under the heading of *Declarative learning*. Declarative learning is the second of the three kinds of learning in the present scheme.

Memory-modulating action

For some time after the neural representation of a memory is formed it is subject to alteration by the occurrence of certain events. This phenomenon was originally discovered by observing the disrupting effects of trauma on memory for immediately preceding experiences, and it was later shown that electroconvulsive shock and other events have similar effects (McGaugh, 1966; McGaugh & Herz, 1972). These findings led to the theory of memory consolidation, the idea that when memories are first formed the neural change that represents them is labile and subject to influence by external events. With the passage of time the neural representation becomes more permanent and resistant to the influence of the same events.

Although some kinds of events disrupt memory, others such as eating (Huston, Mondadori & Waser, 1974), drinking a sucrose solution (Messier & White, 1984) and foot-shock (White & Legree, 1984) have been shown to improve or enhance memories when they occur during the immediate post-training period. One interpretation of these effects is that they are due to acceleration or promotion of the consolidation process. Enhancement leads to an increase in the probability that the memory will influence future behaviour; therefore, memory enhancement is one of the defining properties of reinforcing events (Gold & McGaugh, 1975; Huston, Mueller & Mondadori, 1977; Huston & Oitzl, 1989; White & Milner, 1992). This effect of reinforcers is similar to that originally described by Thorndike (1898), who called the enhancing action of reinforcers "stamping in" of memories.

A number of addictive drugs have memory-enhancing properties as demonstrated in the laboratory using post-training administration techniques that limit their effects to memory consolidation. These include amphetamine (Doty & Doty, 1966; Martinez *et al.*, 1980; Packard, Williams & McGaugh, 1992), cocaine (Janak, Keppel & Martinez, 1992; Weinberger *et al.*, 1992), nicotine (Garg & Holland, 1968; Evangelista, Gattoni & Izquierdo, 1970; Faiman, De Erausquin & Baratti, 1991) and alcohol (Alkana & Parker, 1979; Parker *et al.*, 1980; Lamberty *et al.*, 1990). Post-training administration of morphine can also enhance memory in some circumstances (White, Major & Siegel, 1978; Staubli & Huston, 1980), but it has also been reported that morphine impairs memory (Messing *et al.*, 1981; Introini-Collison, McGaugh & Baratti, 1985) and that the opiate antagonists naloxone (Messing *et al.*, 1979; Gallagher, King & Young, 1983; Messing, Rijk & Rigter, 1983; Tomaz, Aguiar & Nogueira, 1990) and naltrexone (Messing, Rijk & Rigter, 1983; Introini-Collison *et al.*, 1985; Castellano *et al.*, 1989; Canli, Cook & Miczek, 1990) enhance memory. In all of these experiments the drugs were administered systemically and enhancement was demonstrated in a variety of different learning situations. Therefore it is not possible to determine where in the nervous system the drugs acted to enhance the memories.

There is some evidence that drugs can produce these modulatory effects by acting directly on neural substrates of memory. There is other evidence that some drugs can act on a central memory modulating mechanism that may affect the memories stored in several different systems. These effects will be discussed for each type of memory to be considered here.

Summary

A summary of the three actions of reinforcers described here is presented in Fig. 1. The figure illustrates the present account of how these actions affect each of three learning and memory

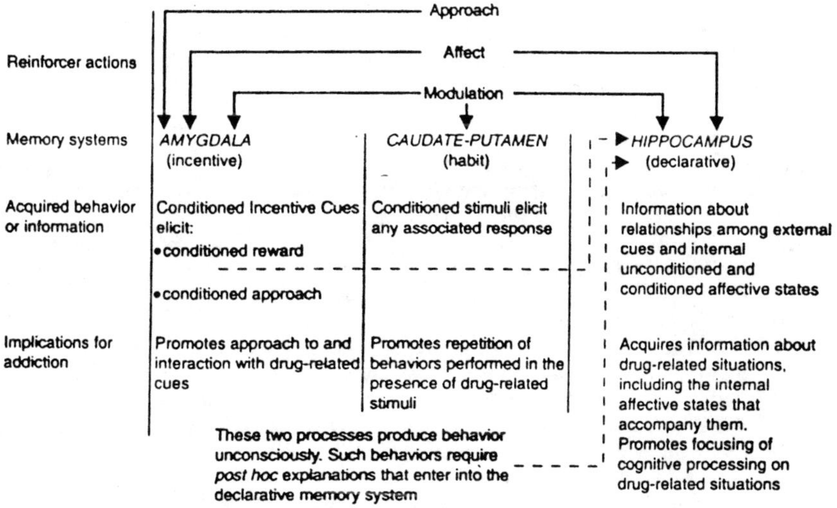

Figure 1. *Schematic representation of proposed processes underlying drug addiction. The three actions of reinforcers are listed in the horizontal band at the top, labelled "Reinforcer actions" (in the column on the left). Each addictive drug is capable of mimicking some or all of these functions of natural reinforcers. These reinforcing actions influence behaviour by acting on learning and memory systems. The systems are shown in the band labelled "Memory systems". Each system is named for a brain structure that is central to it. Each system acquires a different type of behaviour or information: a one-word description of the kind of learning mediated in each system is below the name of its central structure. Evidence for the existence of these systems and the kinds of behaviour they produce is discussed in the text. These behaviours are described in the band labelled "Acquired behavior or information". The role of each of these behaviours in the addictive process is described in the band labelled "Implications for addiction". Most addictive drugs initiate more than one of these processes.*

systems (named for their central neural structures, to be discussed in the next section), and summarizes the implications for addictive behaviour of each of these effects.

By their pharmacological action on synapses in the neural systems mediating the influence of naturally occurring reinforcers on behaviour, addictive drugs can produce some subset of the behavioural effects of reinforcers, sometimes in unnatural combinations. The nature of the behaviour change produced by any drug will depend on some interaction between the behaviour required to obtain the drug and the specific reinforcement substrates on which the particular drug acts. In the case of a standard laboratory behaviour such as drug self-administration by rats bar-pressing in an operant chamber, this means that each self-administered drug may promote the behaviour by a different combination of actions on reinforcement and memory substrates. Furthermore, in other behavioural tests that may engage different learning and memory systems the same drug may influence behaviour by its action on different reinforcement or memory substrates. In humans the constellation of the neural substrates on which a particular drug acts and of the behaviours required to obtain the drug will result in learning some combination of drug-taking and other behaviours labelled with the term "addiction".

The following sections present a description of the evidence for multiple effects of naturally occurring reinforcers and of how drugs mimic these effects.

Multiple memory systems: substrates for actions of reinforcers and drugs

The idea that the mammalian brain contains several more or less independent neural systems, each of which is simultaneously engaged in processing a different type of information about an individual's external experience, internal states, behaviour and thoughts can be described as a form of "parallel processing". Although the complete neural systems are not precisely defined, a structure central to each system has been identified. These are the amygdala, the caudate nucleus–putamen complex (dorsal neostriatum) and the hippocampus. Each of the neural systems is named for one of these structures but the structures perform the functions attributed to them together with other brain areas with which they enjoy close anatomical relationships. Memory-related functions are attributed to the central structure of each system on the basis of evidence that manipulations (electrical stimulation or microinjections of neuro-active substances) limited to them, can either impair or enhance memory consolidation (Kesner & Wilburn, 1974; White & Milner, 1992).

The present version of the multiple memory systems hypothesis is based on a series of recent experiments (Packard, Hirsh & White, 1989; Packard & White, 1990, 1991; McDonald & White, 1993, 1994; White & McDonald, 1993) involving the learning of different behavioural tasks by rats. Each behavioural task was designed to provide a different kind of information about the location of food on a maze. The hypothesis was tested that the specific kind of information provided in each task was acquired and stored by a different memory system. This was done by determining the effects of a series of artificially produced lesions to the central structures of each memory system on the animals' ability to acquire and remember the information available in each task. The results led to inferences about the kind of information learned by each of the neural systems.

The results of these experiments, taken together with the work of others, suggest that a neural system in which the amygdala has a central function mediates *conditioned incentive learning* of both skeletal responses and internal affective states (Jones & Mishkin, 1972; Squire & Zola-Morgan, 1991; Davis, 1992). A different neural system, in which the hippocampus is the main structure, mediates *declarative learning:* the acquisition of information about the relationship among external cues and events, including their relationship to internal affective states (Hirsh, 1980; Hirsh & Krajden, 1982; Olton, 1982; Mishkin & Petri, 1984). A third neural system, that includes the matrix compartment of caudate–putamen (White, 1989), mediates stimulus–response (S–R) associations that are expressed in behaviour as *habit learning* (Divac, 1968; Mishkin, Malamut & Bachevalier, 1984; Prado-Alcala, 1985). Although this almost certainly does not exhaust the list of the kinds of learning that go on in the mammalian nervous system a consideration of the interactions of drugs with these neural systems accounts for most of the major behavioural changes involved in drug addiction.

These conclusions are used in the following sections as the basis for describing the mnemonic functions of each of the neural systems. The action of reinforcers within each of these systems is also described and evidence for each of these actions of addictive drugs is reviewed. This evidence shows that the integrity of the memory systems is critical for mediating the effects of the drugs on behaviour, and is therefore consistent with the idea that the behavioural changes produced by addictive drugs can be understood in terms of their actions on these systems.

Conditioned incentive learning

As already described, neutral stimuli that are present when a reinforcer acts on a neural substrate of approach behaviour or elicits an internal state that is perceived as rewarding can acquire the ability to elicit similar responses in the absence of the reinforcer. The type of learning in which reinforcers play this role was originally described by Pavlov (1927) whose famous experiments with conditioned salivation involved one of the autonomic components of the set of responses elicited by food in hungry dogs. The combination of these incentive reinforcement and learning processes can result in both behavioural (White, Messier & Carr, 1987) and internal (Stewart & Eikelboom, 1987; Stewart, 1992) responses in the presence of conditioned incentive cues, but in the absence of the reinforcer that originally elicited them.

The most common laboratory demonstration of positive conditioned incentive effects is the conditioned cue preference (CCP) task (often called "conditioned place preference"), in which animals are exposed to a reinforcer in the presence of neutral cues; on future occasions the animals approach the formerly neutral cues, which now qualify as conditioned incentive cues.

This behaviour is impaired by lesions of the amygdala (Everitt *et al.*, 1991; McDonald &

White, 1993), nucleus accumbens (Everitt *et al.*, 1991) and tegmental pedunculopontine nucleus (Bechara & van der Kooy, 1992). These structures may all be parts of a neural system that acquires classically conditioned observable approach and unobservable internal responses. Approach behaviour in the CCP task is not impaired by lesions of the hippocampus or caudate–putamen systems (White & McDonald, 1993).

A similar experimental paradigm has been used to condition taste cues to aversive internal states (Garcia & Kimeldorf, 1957; Nachman & Ashe, 1973; Garcia, Hankins & Rusiniak, 1976). In these experiments animals are given the opportunity to eat or drink a substance with a novel (usually preferred) taste and are then made ill, often with radiation or lithium chloride injections. In tests given one or more days later, the animals decrease their consumption of the substance. This type of learning is called conditioned taste aversion (CTA).

The CTA can be differentiated from the CCP in two ways. First, in contrast to the CCP, CTAs are not readily elicited by conditioned external cues (Garcia & Koelling, 1966; Reicher & Holman, 1977; Sherman *et al.*, 1980b; Stefurak, Martin & van der Kooy, 1990). Neutral or even rewarding taste cues are most easily conditioned in the CTA paradigm, suggesting that these conditioned incentive cues elicit aversive internal states. Secondly, CTAs are blocked by lesions of the basolateral nucleus of the amygdala (Nachman & Ashe, 1974; Elkins, 1980; Dunn & Everitt, 1988; Yamamoto & Fujimoto, 1991), while the CCP is eliminated by lesions of the lateral nucleus of the amygdala (McDonald & White, 1993). This difference suggests that positive and negative incentive learning are mediated by different neural substrates.

A number of addictive drugs produce CCPs; that is, cues that are present when the drug is active acquire the capacity to elicit conditioned approach responses or rewarding internal states, or both. At the same time, there is evidence that the same drugs also produce aversive internal states in CTA paradigms. In the present scheme simultaneously existing CCPs and CTAs are seen as the results of partial pharmacological actions on reinforcement substrates. Thus, a drug may act simultaneously on a neural substrate of approach (activation of which will in future be elicited by conditioned external, or distal cues) and on a neural substrate of aversion (activation of which will in future be elicited by conditioned taste, or proximal cues). Since different types of conditioned cues activate the two types of conditioned responses (approach/reward and aversion) they generally do not interfere with each other. Although it is not clear that effects of this kind are produced by any naturally occurring reinforcer, they have been reported for most addictive drugs, as will now be described.

Amphetamine. Systemic administration of amphetamine produces both a CCP (Phillips, Spyraki & Fibiger, 1982; Spyraki, Fibiger & Phillips, 1982b) and a CTA (LeBlanc & Cappell, 1974; Stolerman & D'Mello, 1978), and both of these conditioned responses can be acquired simultaneously (Reicher & Holman, 1977; Sherman *et al.*, 1980b). Microinjection of amphetamine into nucleus accumbens produces a CCP but no effect in a conditioned taste test; in contrast, microinjection into area postrema produces a CTA but no effect in a conditioned cue test (Carr & White, 1986). These direct actions of the drug at different brain sites suggest that the effects on behaviour in the CCP and CTA paradigms are mediated by different neural systems.

Dopaminergic transmission in nucleus accumbens is critical for both acquisition and expression of the amphetamine CCP (Spyraki, Fibiger & Phillips, 1982b; Hiroi & White, 1990, 1991a). Lesions of the lateral nucleus of the amygdala (Hiroi & White, 1991b) and of the tegmental pedunculopontine nucleus (Bechara & van der Kooy, 1989) block the amphetamine CCP. These findings suggest that conditioned incentive responses to distal cues are produced by a neural process that is initiated by the action of amphetamine in nucleus accumbens and involves the relationship of this structure to the lateral nucleus of amygdala and pedunculopontine nucleus (White & Hiroi, 1993). By this process the drug may produce a conditioned approach response and rewarding internal conditioned incentive responses. The drug also appears to act on a neural system that may involve area postrema to produce an aversive state that can be elicited by conditioned taste cues, but not by distal environmental cues.

Cocaine. Cocaine produces a CPP when injected intraperitoneally (Brown & Fibiger,

1993), subcutaneously (Isaac *et al.*, 1989), intravenously (Mucha *et al.*, 1982), or into the ventricles of the brain (Morency & Beninger, 1986). However, micro-injections of cocaine into nucleus accumbens do not produce a CCP (Hemby *et al.*, 1992), and the precise location of the central action of this drug in producing the CCP is unknown.

The CCP produced by intraperitoneal cocaine is blocked by lesions of the amygdala that include the lateral nucleus (Brown & Fibiger, 1993) and the CCP produced by subcutaneous injections is blocked by lesions of the prefrontal cortex (Isaac *et al.*, 1989), suggesting that the behaviour involves classically conditioned responses mediated by a neural system that includes these two brain areas.

The intraperitoneal CCP is not blocked by systemically administered dopamine agonists, or by dopamine-specific lesions of nucleus accumbens (Spyraki, Fibiger & Phillips, 1982a). In contrast, the CCPs produced by intravenous and intraventricular cocaine are blocked by systemically administered dopamine antagonists (Spyraki, Nomikos & Varonos, 1987) suggesting that the CCPs produced by these injection routes are mediated by different mechanisms. There is currently no evidence on the possible involvement of the amygdala in the intravenous or intraventricular CCPs.

Systemically administered cocaine also produces a CTA, and this behaviour is acquired simultaneously with the CCP (Smith & Holman, 1987; Ferrari, O'Connor & Riley, 1991). Lesions of the pre-frontal cortex have no effect on the CTA (Isaac *et al.*, 1989).

These findings suggest that cocaine may act to produce a CCP in two ways. Intraperitoneally administered cocaine may activate a rewarding internal state that can be conditioned to external cues by a neural system that includes amygdala and prefrontal cortex, but that may not include nucleus accumbens or involve dopamine. At the same time, the effect of dopamine antagonists on the CCP observed with intravenous or central administration of cocaine suggests that the drug can also act on a dopaminergic system. The lack of information about the involvement of specific neural systems in the cocaine CCP produced by these injection routes leaves the possibility open that in these cases the drug may also act on an amygdala-based learning system to produce a conditioned approach response. Cocaine also acts on an unknown substrate of aversion; these responses can be elicited by conditioned taste cues, but not by external cues.

Nicotine. Although there are several contradictory reports, there is no clear published evidence that systemically administered nicotine produces a CCP (Clarke & Fibiger, 1987; Stolerman & Shoaib, 1991) in a properly controlled paradigm. However, microinjections of nicotine into the ventricles or into the tegmental pedunculopontine nucleus produce a CCP (Iwamoto, 1990). Systemic injections of nicotine produce a CTA (Jensen *et al.*, 1990; Ossenkopp & Giugno, 1990), and this effect is blocked by intraventricular injection of a nicotinic antagonist (Reavill *et al.*, 1986).

These findings suggest that the direct pharmacological activation of nicotinic acetylcholine receptors, some of which may be located in the pedunculopontine nucleus, may produce conditioned incentive behaviours with external cues as the conditioned stimuli. However, the failure to observe a CCP following systemic injections of nicotine suggests that the drug probably does not act on this substrate when delivered by this route. Alternatively, systemic administration may permit an action of nicotine on a different substrate that promotes some behavioural tendency opposing the centrally mediated conditioned approach/reward response. The drug may produce a peripherally mediated aversive internal response (or an escape response) that can be associated with conditioned external cues. An aversive conditioned internal state can also be elicited by conditioned taste cues.

Alcohol. Alcohol produces a CCP in mice (Cunningham *et al.*, 1992; Cunningham & Prather, 1992) which is not blocked by dopamine antagonists (Cunningham *et al.*, 1992). In rats it produces conditioned cue aversions (Cunningham, 1979), even when the drug is self-administered (Stewart & Grupp, 1989). Alcohol also produces a CTA in rats (Cunningham, 1979). The evidence that this drug activates escape and/or aversive substrates that can be elicited by both conditioned external and conditioned taste cues suggests that alcohol does not act on the neural substrate of conditioned approach/reward in rats. Alcohol does appear to activate an internal aversive state that can be elicited by conditioned taste cues and, possibly, also by conditioned external cues.

Morphine. Morphine produces a CCP when injected systemically (Beach, 1957; Mucha *et al.*, 1982) and when microinjected into nucleus accumbens (van der Kooy *et al.*, 1982), ventral tegmental area (Wise & Hoffman, 1992) or hippocampus (Corrigall & Linseman, 1988). Systemic morphine also produces a CTA (LeBlanc & Cappell, 1974; Sherman *et al.*, 1980a), probably by an action on peripheral (Bechara & van der Kooy, 1985, 1987) and central (Suzuki *et al.*, 1993; Ableitner & Herz, 1989) kappa receptors. The CCP and the CTA are acquired simultaneously (White, Sklar & Amit, 1977).

The CCP produced by systemically administered morphine in certain situations is blocked by lesions of the amygdala (McDonald, Hansen & White, unpublished data) and by lesions of the hippocampal system (Olmstead & Franklin, 1994). It is also blocked by lesions of the pedunculopontine nucleus (Bechara & van der Kooy, 1989; Olmstead & Franklin, 1993). Thus morphine may act initially in nucleus accumbens, ventral tegmental area and hippocampus to initiate a process that involves the pedunculopontine nucleus, as well as amygdala- and hippocampus-based learning to produce the CCP. The involvement of the amygdala in the morphine CCP suggests that the drug may produce conditioned approach responses. The involvement of the hippocampus suggests that it may also produce conditioned internal responses that are perceived as rewarding. As will be described under *Declarative learning* (and as illustrated in Fig. 1), the hippocampal system may be involved in the CCP based on conditioned reward (as opposed to conditioned approach) as the substrate mediating learning about the place in the apparatus that produces the strongest conditioned rewarding effect—presumably the place closest to the conditioned incentive cues—thereby maximizing the conditioned reward experienced.

The morphine-produced internal aversive state may be partly mediated by agranular insular cortex (Mackey, Keller & van der Kooy, 1986). This internal response can be activated by conditioned taste cues, but not by external cues.

Memory-modulating effects in the amygdala. There is evidence for two kinds of memory-modulation processes involving the amygdala. First, post-training administration of amphetamine facilitates acquisition of the CCP (White & Carr, 1985). This finding is indirect evidence that the presence of an addictive drug can act to modulate the memory of the conditioned responses mediated in the amygdala-based memory system. However, at present there is little direct evidence (e.g. Izquierdo *et al.*, 1992) for task specific modulatory effects of memories thought to depend on the amygdala system. Further research on this possibility will be required.

It has also been suggested that the amygdala mediates the modulatory action of certain drugs on memories that may be processed in other neural systems (McGaugh *et al.*, 1990; Izquierdo *et al.*, 1992). Of the drugs under discussion here, there is evidence that amphetamine (Packard, Cahill & McGaugh, 1993) has this kind of effect. Memory-modulating effects of opiate antagonists on aversively motivated tasks are also mediated in the amygdala (Castellano, Libri & Ammassari-Teule, 1988; Introini-Collison, Nagahara & McGaugh, 1989).

Contribution to self-administration. The amygdala-based incentive conditioning processes described here can contribute to self-administration in two ways. First, activation of the neural substrate of approach behaviour by a drug in the presence of an array of neutral cues can cause those cues to acquire the capacity to elicit an approach response, even if the response was never actually performed. As a result of this process an individual would have a tendency to approach and interact with these conditioned cues. It should be noted that this behaviour is not the result of any conscious planning in either animals or humans. On the contrary, in humans it is a type of behaviour that would require the attribution of a cause or reason *after* it had been performed (see Fig. 1).

The second way in which amygdala-based processes can contribute to self-administration is by incentive conditioning of internal affective states. Cues that are present while a drug is pharmacologically active can elicit conditioned internal responses that are perceived as being rewarding or aversive (McAuliffe & Gordon, 1974; Kliner & Pickens, 1982; Lamb *et al.*, 1991). In turn, these conditioned affective states can affect behaviour as the individual learns about behaviours that can alter them (see Fig. 1). As already described for morphine, in the case of the CCP this may involve learning about the location in the apparatus that maximizes conditioned reward. This secondary process involves hippocampal-based declarative learning, described in the next section.

The operation of these behavioural processes would produce behaviours that are typical of addiction in humans: a increase in the probability of approach to and association with drug-related cues, together with a *post hoc* attribution of a rational basis for the behaviour.

Declarative learning

As already described, most external cues have no direct effects on behaviour in the absence of experience (although some may initially elicit orientating responses). However, this does not mean that nothing is learned about these cues. There is ample evidence that both animals (e.g. Kimble, 1981; Hirsh & Krajden, 1982) and humans (Squire & Zola-Morgan, 1991) learn about the relationships among cues even when those cues are of no consequence. This type of learning was originally described by Tolman (1948; 1949), who labelled it "stimulus–stimulus" (S–S) to describe the fact that it involves learning about relationships among cues and events. In contrast to conditioned incentive and habit learning (see next section), declarative learning does not include information about responses or any particular behaviour. Rather, information about cues in the environment is used to generate appropriate behaviours when required. The term "declarative memory" was proposed (Cohen & Squire, 1980) to suggest this property.

Findings from experiments with humans (Penfield & Milner, 1958; Milner, Corkin & Teuber, 1968), with non-human primates (Mishkin & Petri, 1984; Mishkin, Malamut & Bachevalier, 1984; Murray, 1990; Gaffan, 1987; Squire, Knowlton & Musen, 1993) and with rats (Hirsh, 1974; Olton & Samuelson, 1976; Olton, Walker & Gage, 1978) are consistent with the suggestion that declarative learning is mediated by a neural system that includes the hippocampus and may describe complex cognitive learning in humans. Learning in the hippocampal system occurs very rapidly with relatively little experience (e.g. Sharp, McNaughton & Barnes, 1985; Breese, Hampson & Deadwyler, 1989). This property is important for understanding the development of addictive behaviours to be discussed in a subsequent section.

This view of the neural basis of declarative learning implies that the system of which the hippocampus forms a part can quickly acquire information of a general kind about all situations that are experienced. To the extent that information stored in this system includes knowledge of relationships among external events relevant to the situation in which a drug is obtained (e.g. the social situation), declarative learning can contribute to the addictive process on this general level.

Declarative learning involving internal affective states. A more specific role for hippocampus-based declarative learning in drug addiction may be its interaction with the array of unobservable central and autonomic responses thought to constitute the affective states produced by the use and disuse of drugs. In addition to learning about the relationships among external cues there is evidence that this system can acquire information about the relationship between external cues and internal states (Hirsh, Leber & Gillman, 1978; Hirsh, Holt & Mosseri, 1978; Hirsh, Davis & Holt, 1979; Davidson & Jarrard, 1993). In the present scheme, this function of the hippocampal system is what allows individuals to learn about the connection between environmental cues and the affective states produced by drugs. The behaviours generated as a consequence of learning about how a particular environment can be manipulated to control an affective state result in the form of drug-taking often called "self-medication".

Internal affective states, whether they are produced by drug use, by disuse, or by conditioned cues, cannot directly produce any behaviour on their own. An individual experiencing such a state for the first time must learn through experience what behaviours operate on its environment to change the affective state in a desired way. In the most straightforward situation of this kind an individual experiencing positive affect produced by a drug could learn about this property of the drug and how to obtain and use it to produce the rewarding state. Learning about the relationship between the internal state and the external situation in which the drug can be obtained is seen here as an instance of hippocampal-based declarative learning. The process is illustrated in Fig. 1.

A similar type of declarative learning could also occur with respect to conditioned rewarding cues. As already described for the morphine CCP, individuals could learn to maximize their contact with conditioned incentive cues as a way of increasing the amount of conditioned reward they experience.

Several theories of drug addiction are based upon the presumed desire of drug-dependent individuals experiencing withdrawal symptoms to alleviate these aversive affective states (e.g. (Littleton, 1991; Koob, 1992a, 1992b; Markou & Koob, 1992). Indeed, the motivating effect of aversive withdrawal symptoms is probably the oldest and most obvious explanation for addictive behaviour. According to the present scheme, such behaviours are the result of hippocampus-based declarative learning about how to alleviate the aversive affective state that accompanies withdrawal.

In another group of related theories of drug addiction, some combination of conditioned and unconditioned changes in the affective state produced by the repeated self-administration of a drug or by ceasing to use a drug after a period of continuous self-administration contributes to the initiation or maintenance (or both) of addictive behaviours. This kind of process is suggested by concepts such as "incentive sensitization" (Robinson & Berridge, 1993), "craving" (e.g. Kozlowski & Wilkinson, 1987; Wise, 1988) and "anhedonia" (Wise *et al.*, 1978; Wise, 1982). According to the present hypothesis, these affective states can influence behaviour only as the individual experiencing them learns about how to manipulate them by interacting with its environment. This involves hippocampus-based declarative learning.

Many authors (e.g. Stewart, de Witt & Eikelboom, 1984; Wise, 1988; Lamb *et al.*, 1991; West, 1991; Di Chiara *et al.*, 1992; Robinson & Berridge, 1993) have questioned the idea that internal affective states produced by either naturally occurring reinforcers or addictive drugs are a major part of the process by which these events change behaviour, suggesting that the "motivational" (West, 1991) actions of reinforcers—in the present analysis, conditioned incentive learning and habit learning—are the major agents of behaviour change in drug-related situations. While these forms of learning are important in the present scheme, an additional process involving hippocampus-based declarative learning about directly produced and conditioned internal affective states is equally important.

Modulation of hippocampal learning. Although there is no reason to believe that enhancement of hippocampus based memories by either reinforcers or drugs is necessary for this system to acquire new information, such an action could increase the influence of drug-related declarative learning on behaviour when it included information about the relationship between external stimuli and drug-produced, internal affective states.

Amphetamine is the only drug under consideration here for which there is direct evidence of hippocampal memory enhancing effects (Packard & White, 1991). Post-training intrahippocampal injections of amphetamine or the dopamine receptor-specific agonists SKF-38393 or LY-171555 enhanced memory in the win-shift radial maze task, suggesting the involvement of dopaminergic function.

There is also evidence for the involvement of cholinergic (Singh, Ott & Matthies, 1974; Grecksch, Ott & Matthies, 1978; Jaffard *et al.*, 1980; Jaffard & Destrade, 1982; Ridley, Aitken and Baker, 1989; Izquierdo *et al.*, 1992; Ohno, Yamamoto & Watanabe, 1993) and noradrenergic (Harley, Milway & Lacaille, 1989; Johnston, Hopkins & Gray, 1989; Izquierdo *et al.*, 1992) mechanisms in the mediation of memory processes by the hippocampus. Certain addictive drugs interact with these dopaminergic, cholinergic and noradrenergic mechanisms in hippocampus. Cocaine increases hippocampal acetylcholine release (Imperato, Obinu & Gessa, 1993). Nicotine increases both acetylcholine (Toide & Arima, 1989) and noradrenaline (Brazell, Mitchell & Gray, 1991) release as well as catecholamine synthesis (Mitchell *et al.*, 1989) in hippocampus. Alcohol has been reported to decrease hippocampal choline uptake (Hunt, Majchrowicz & Dalton, 1979). Morphine withdrawal increases hippocampal noradrenaline release (Silverstone, Done & Sharp, 1993).

Several of these drugs also have effects on neural activity in the hippocampus that may be related to its memory functions. Cocaine increases non-specific hippocampal neural activity

(Rector, Poe & Harper, 1993) and can also increase the bursting rate of CA1 pyramidal neurons when pressure-injected onto single cells in an operant conditioning paradigm (Stein & Belluzzi, 1989). Nicotine increases the size of the population spike recorded in the CA1 field of hippocampal slices (Freund, Jungschaffer & Collins, 1990), and alcohol alters the excitability of hippocampal neurons (Urrutia & Gruol, 1992). Morphine affects the firing rates of hippocampal neurones (Dafny *et al.*, 1979) and increases the size of the field potentials produced in CA1 by stimulation of striatum radiatum and in dentate gyrus by stimulation of perforant path (Linseman & Corrigall, 1982).

The effects of these drugs on various hippocampal functions suggest the possibility that they may act on the memory storage process in this system. Direct evidence for this possibility will have to await the appropriate experiments.

Contribution to self-administration. In the present scheme, hippocampally mediated declarative learning contributes to the self-administration of addictive drugs by acquiring information about the relationships among features of external situations and the internal affective states produced by the drugs. These affective states can be produced directly by the drugs themselves, by withdrawing a drug from a dependent individual, or by the presence of conditioned cues. Thus, the scheme assigns the hippocampal system the role of *learning about* the relationship of affective states to external cues.

Two points of comparison between this learning process and amygdala-based incentive learning and caudate–putamen-based habit learning should be noted. First, information acquired by the hippocampal system is fully accessible to consciousness. Therefore, in humans, the reasons for behaviours initiated on the basis of declarative learning are fully apparent to the individual concerned. In contrast, the amygdala- and caudate-based learning processes are not accessible to consciousness. Behaviours produced by these systems therefore require the attribution of *post hoc* explanations by the individual concerned (see Fig. 1).

Secondly, compared with the amygdala- and caudate–putamen—mediated motivational effects of drugs, which act directly to produce specific drug-related responses, information acquired by the hippocampal system has the potential to generate much more complex, cognitively controlled behaviour in drug-related situations. Once this type of information has been acquired by the hippocampal system, the modulating action of some addictive drugs might improve memory for this information thereby increasing the tendency for the system to recall contextually relevant information. This would increase the incidence of drug-related cognitions and behaviour and reduce the importance of thoughts and behaviour related to other contexts. This is typical of addiction.

Habit learning

Habits (Mishkin & Petri, 1984; Zola-Morgan & Squire, 1993) are well-learned sequences of behaviour that are elicited automatically by the appropriate stimuli. The study of this form of learning (sometimes called "S–R learning") is the basis of a large field of experimentation based on "associative" learning theories (e.g. Estes, 1991). In this form of learning, S–R associations (i.e. the "bonds" between the neural representations of a stimulus and a response) are strengthened slightly each time the response occurs in the presence of the stimulus and is followed by reinforcement. Because of this incremental accretion of "habit strength" (Hull, 1943) acquisition of S–R habits occurs relatively slowly.

Data from a number of sources (Divac, 1968; Petri & Mishkin, 1993), including observations in humans (Butters *et al.*, 1986) and experiments on primates (Mishkin, Malamut & Bachevalier, 1984; Wang, Aigner & Mishkin, 1990) and rats (Packard, Hirsh & White, 1989; Packard & White, 1990; McDonald & White, 1993) suggest that this type of learning is mediated by a neural system that includes the caudate–putamen complex. The idea that sensorimotor, or stimulus–response, associations are mediated by the caudate–putamen has been put forward a number of times on the basis of anatomical, pharmacological and behavioural evidence (Groves, 1983; Mishkin, Malamut & Bachevalier, 1984; Alexander, DeLong & Strick, 1986; Phillips & Carr, 1987; Gerfen, 1992). For these associations to influence future behaviour some process must act to give them a degree of permanency. This occurs as a result of the memory-modulating action of reinforcers in the caudate–putamen.

Of the drugs under consideration here, direct

evidence for caudate–putamen—specific memory-enhancing effects is available only for amphetamine (Carr & White, 1984; Viaud & White, 1989a; Packard & White, 1991). Findings in these and other studies (Packard & White, 1989; White, 1988, 1989; White & Viaud, 1991) suggest that this effect of amphetamine is a result of its dopamine agonist properties. Other evidence (Haycock *et al.*, 1973; Prado-Alcala & Cobos-Zapiain, 1977; Prado-Alcala & Cobos-Zapiain, 1979; Prado-Alcala, 1985; Robbins & Everitt, 1987; Viaud & White, 1989b; Viaud, unpublished PhD thesis, 1991) suggests that cholinergic mechanisms in the caudate-putamen are also involved in the memory-related functions of this neural system. Several other addictive drugs are known to affect these two neurochemical substrates in caudate–putamen. Cocaine increases levels of extracelluar dopamine in caudate–putamen when administered systemically (Hurd *et al.*, 1990; Kuczenski, Segal & Aizenstein, 1991) or centrally (Manley *et al.*, 1992), and increases acetylcholine levels in this structure (Imperato, Obinu & Gessa, 1993). Cocaine also induces a high level of expression of the immediate early gene c-*fos* (a proposed measure of neural activation) throughout the striatum (Graybiel, Moratalla & Robertson, 1990). Nicotine also acts to increase dopamine levels in caudate–putamen when administered systemically (Damsma *et al.*, 1988; Toide & Arima, 1989) or when injected into substantia nigra (Blaha & Winn, 1993). Alcohol has been reported to increase levels of acetylcholine (Parker *et al.*, 1978; Jope & Jenden, 1981) and high affinity choline uptake (Hunt, Majchrowicz & Dalton, 1979; Jope & Jenden, 1981) in caudate–putamen. Morphine has been reported to have no effect on dopamine release in caudate–putamen (Moleman & Bruinvels, 1979; Wood & Rao, 1991), but there is evidence that this drug increases dopamine turnover (Smith *et al.*, 1980) and dopamine-sensitive adenylate cyclase (Iwatsubo & Clouet, 1975) levels in caudate–putamen, suggesting that morphine does affect dopamine activity levels and/or sensitivity to dopamine in this system.

The effects of these drugs on dopamine and/or acetylcholine systems in the caudate-putamen suggest the possibility that some of them may act in this structure to strengthen S–R associations. Direct evidence for this possibility awaits the relevant behavioural experiments.

Contribution to self-administration. The act of drug self-administration by animals or humans involves behaviours that occur in the presence of stimuli, leading to the formation of S–R associations. To the extent that the drugs discussed here act on the caudate–putamen to enhance this type of memory, these S–R associations would be incrementally strengthened each time the self-administration behaviour occurs, increasing the probability that the behaviour would be repeated in the presence of the stimuli. In this way, one of the effects of addictive drugs is to reinforce directly the behaviour that leads to their own self-administration, creating habits with powerful control over behaviour. Behaviours produced in this way in humans would occur without prior planning by the individual concerned and would therefore require the fabrication of a reason for their occurrence (Fig. 1).

Self-administration

A central feature of the argument made here is that there are multiple causes for the addictive properties of drugs. The argument is based on an analysis of how drugs act on the neural substrates of behaviour change. The analysis suggests that several more or less independent neural systems may acquire different types of information about an individual's ongoing experiences, and that reinforcers have a different function in each system. An addictive drug may mimic some or all of the effects of reinforcers on these systems. An explanation for the development of addictive behaviour (including self-administration of any drug) may then be found in the multiple parallel actions of that drug on the neural systems that mediate learned changes in behaviour.

The concept of "reward" (and its instantiation in the mesolimbic dopamine system) is often used to describe the property of reinforcers that alters behaviour and, more specifically, the capacity of drugs to promote their own self-administration. From the perspective of the present analysis it can be argued that the use of this concept may actually impede understanding of how drugs affect behaviour. The evidence presented suggests that such understanding will require a considerably more precise specification of the diverse effects of each drug on each of several neural systems—as well as a description of the behavioural processes produced by each of these effects—than can be accommodated by the single unidimensional concept of reward. On the basis of the fact that they are self-administered, all five of the drugs discussed here have been said to have rewarding properties. However, the evidence presented casts doubt on this assertion and shows that many behaviours including self-administration may be acquired and maintained in more than one way by more than one neural system, and that these processes do not necessarily involve positive affect, or reward. Therefore, an understanding of how drugs promote self-administration requires a precise analysis of how each drug acts to change each kind of behaviour.

In the following selective review, evidence concerning the intravenous self-administration of the exemplar drugs coincides on some points with what is known about the neural mediation of the reinforcement and learning processes for each of the drugs. Some of these points are mentioned here; however in many instances there is clearly a lack of evidence connecting the reinforcing effects and the self-administration of these drugs. In these cases the possible involvement of such mechanisms, as indicated by evidence reviewed in previous sections, is also suggested.

Amphetamine. Amphetamine is intravenously self-administered by monkeys (Wilson & Schuster, 1972; Balster & Schuster, 1973), and experiments with rats demonstrated the critical involvement of dopamine systems (Yokel & Wise, 1975, 1978) in this behaviour. Rats self-administer amphetamine directly into nucleus accumbens (Hoebel *et al.*, 1983) and dopamine-specific lesions of nucleus accumbens eliminate intravenous amphetamine self-administration (Lyness, Friedle & Moore, 1979). These manipulations are similar to those described in the discussion of the amphetamine CCP; the fact that they have the same effects on that behaviour and on self-administration is consistent with the suggestion that conditioned incentive effects of amphetamine mediate its self-administration (White & Hiroi, 1993), although the lack of evidence for the involvement of the lateral nucleus of the amygdala in the latter behaviour is a significant lacuna in this hypothesis.

Dopamine-specific lesions of the basolateral amygdala decrease the threshold dose for amphetamine self-administration (Deminiere *et al.*, 1988), suggesting the possibility that this part of the amygdala may mediate conditioned aversive effects of the drug as it does certain other conditioned aversive effects (Maeda, Morimoto & Yanagimoto, 1993; Fanselow & Kim, 1994).

Data reviewed earlier suggest that, in addition to its effects on the nucleus accumbens–amygdala system, the behaviour-altering actions of amphetamine may also be promoted by its memory-improving action in both hippocampus (on information about environmental cues that can be used to manipulate the direct and conditioned affective states produced by the drug) and caudate–putamen (on S–R sequences that include self-administration responses). Further research with self-administration and other paradigms will be required to test these hypotheses.

This evidence suggests that amphetamine self-administration is initially reinforced by a direct action of the drug on the neural substrates of conditioned incentive learning (probably the conditioned approach response). Continued self-administration promoted by the initial experience with the drug would lead to learning about how to obtain the drug to control the affective states its use or lack of use may produce and, after more experience, would also lead to a strongly reinforced self-administration habit.

Cocaine. In the laboratory cocaine is self-administered intravenously (Wilson & Schuster, 1972; Balster & Schuster, 1973; Roberts, Loh & Vickers, 1989). The drug is also self-administered directly into the medial prefrontal cortex and dopamine specific lesions of this brain area block the behaviour (Goeders & Smith, 1983). In medial prefrontal cortex, cocaine has been shown to act on the terminals of dopaminergic neurones to release dopamine, which acts on post-synaptic D_2 receptors (Goeders & Smith, 1986). Although cocaine is not self-administered directly into nucleus accumbens (Goeders & Smith, 1983), dopamine specific lesions of this brain area attenuate or block intravenous cocaine self-administration (Roberts, Corcoran & Fibiger, 1977; Roberts *et al.*, 1980; Pettit *et al.*, 1984; Caine & Koob, 1994), as does injection of a dopamine antagonist into nucleus accumbens (McGregor & Roberts, 1993). Injections of a dopamine antagonist into the basolateral amygdala (which very likely also affected the lateral nucleus) also appeared to decrease the tendency of self-administered cocaine to maintain bar pressing (McGregor & Roberts, 1993). Consistent with these findings, systemically administered dopamine antagonists also impair cocaine self-administration (Woolverton & Virus, 1989; Corrigall & Coen, 1991a), possibly because of their actions on dopaminergic mechanisms in medial pre-frontal cortex, nucleus accumbens and amygdala.

The facts that both the cocaine CCP and self-administration are impaired by lesions of the medial prefrontal cortex, that nucleus accumbens dopamine function is essential to both behaviours, and that the amygdala participates in both behaviours all implicate conditioned incentive learning in cocaine self-administration. Some of these incentive functions are similar to those that contribute to amphetamine self administration; however, there is no evidence that medial prefrontal cortex is involved in the incentive functions of the latter drug. Further research will be required to understand how the action of cocaine on prefrontal cortex interacts with the amygdala–nucleus accumbens incentive learning system.

There is also a report that cocaine is self-administered directly into the hippocampus (Stein & Belluzzi, 1989) suggesting the possibility that the drug could have direct effects on this structure. These could be of a directly rewarding nature or they could be modulatory, acting to improve the retention of information associated with self-administration. This may include learning about the affective consequences of the use and disuse of cocaine, as well as information about any conditioned affective responses produced by the drug. As already discussed, it is also possible that cocaine can have a modulatory effect on the caudate–putamen, increasing the influence of self-administration habits on behaviour.

Amphetamine and cocaine both appear to act on more than one of the neural systems described here to promote self-administration. This is consistent with their high addiction liability. It also means that once established addiction to these drugs would be very difficult to eliminate. Treatments aimed at any one of the behavioural processes that reinforce the taking of these drugs are unlikely to be effective.

Nicotine. Although tobacco products in various forms are clearly addictive (Lemaire & Meisch, 1985) there has been some controversy over whether or not a reinforcing effect resulting from a pharmacological action of nicotine is the major reason for this addiction (Goldberg & Henningfield, 1988; Corrigall, 1991). When animals are required to perform a simple operant response to receive a single intravenous injection of nicotine (e.g. Cox, Goldstein & Nelson, 1984), their response rates are low. However, higher rates have been reported when animals were pretrained to perform an operant response for food (Corrigall & Coen, 1989) or another drug (e.g. cocaine, Henningfield & Goldberg, 1983) and then switched to performing the same response for nicotine. Responding is further improved if the nicotine is available on a second order schedule (Doughtery *et al.*, 1981; Henningfield & Goldberg, 1988) so that environmental cues, in some cases explicit cues (Sliffer, 1983), become an important part of the self-administration situation.

Given the lack of evidence for reinforcing effects of nicotine in behavioural paradigms that measure incentive reward (e.g. the CCP), the findings on self-administration of this drug are perhaps not surprising. Possibly a clue to the nature of nicotine's reinforcing effect is the fact that self-administration of the drug is facilitated by pretraining of the response and by associating that response with a specific cue or with the cues that are produced by a second-order reinforcement schedule. The facilitatory effect of explicit specification of the stimuli and responses that must be associated to obtain nicotine suggests that the primary reinforcing action of nicotine may be its memory modulating action on stimulus–response sequences in the caudate–putamen. The behavioural topology of nicotine self-administration: slow acquisition of responding and slow cessation of responding when the drug is withdrawn (e.g. Corrigall & Coen, 1989), is consistent with the presence of a habit that is incrementally strengthened by responding in the presence of reinforcement and weakened by responding in the absence of reinforcement.

Nicotine self-administration is attenuated by systemic administration of a dopamine antagonist (Corrigall & Coen, 1991b) and by dopamine-specific lesions of nucleus accumbens (Corrigall *et al.*, 1992). In both these cases, self-administration declined in a manner that suggested extinction of an S–R habit. Evidence that the effects of acetylcholine manipulations on memory in the caudate nucleus (Robbins & Everitt, 1987; Viaud, unpublished PhD thesis, 1991) may depend on dopamine function are consistent with the possibility that the dopamine system is required to mediate the suggested memory-improving action of nicotine.

This hypothesis about the reinforcing action of nicotine implies that the initial development of tobacco addiction may depend solely on the modulation by nicotine of a caudate–putamen-based self-administration habit, made up of a series of reinforced S–R associations. This would account for the relatively slow development of the behaviour in both animals and humans. As with other drugs, as the tobacco self-administration habit is reinforced by repetitive behaviour and increasingly large doses of the drug are taken, direct and conditioned affective states associated with the use and disuse of nicotine and the other components of tobacco smoke may eventually develop. Behaviours that lead to manipulation of these states would be the result of hippocampus-based declarative learning. The combination of these learning processes initiated by nicotine would form the basis of addiction to tobacco.

The fundamental characteristic of nicotine (or tobacco) self-administration in the addicted organism, implied by its S–R nature, is that specific stimuli will most effectively elicit self-administration and that this behaviour will be independent of the reinforcer that originally strengthened the S–R association for a considerable length of time after the reinforcer is removed from the situation. Therefore, the most successful treatment may be the cessation of smoking followed by some form of support for coping with this strong, persistent behavioural tendency.

Alcohol. There are reported failures to observe intravenous self-administration of alcohol by laboratory animals (DeNoble, Mele & Porter, 1985), although relatively weak self-administration of the drug by this route has been reported within a narrow dose range (Lyness & Smith, 1992). On the grounds that alcohol is self-administered orally by humans, the bulk of research with this drug has been devoted to developing ways to get animals—primarily rats—to drink it, and with assessing the validity of the behaviours so produced as animal "models" of alcoholism in humans. Much like humans, rats do not immediately consume large quantities of alcohol when given the opportunity to do so. An early study showing that rats bar-press more for simultaneous access to drinking water and an intragastric infusion of alcohol than for simultaneous access to drinking alcohol and intragastric water (Amit & Stern, 1969) suggests strongly that this is because of its aversive taste.

Rats can be induced to drink fairly large quantities of alcohol using a variety of different techniques. The simplest of these involves presenting the animals with alcohol to drink (in addition to normal access to food and water) either continuously, on alternate days (sometimes in gradually increasing concentrations), or for brief periods daily (Sinclair, 1974; Brown & Amit, 1977; Boyle *et al.*, 1994). Regardless of how the alcohol is presented, rats tend to consume pharmacologically active amounts of the drug during short bursts of drinking that occur throughout the day (Gill, France & Amit, 1986), and almost all rats increase their consumption after 8 to 12 days of exposure, albeit to different degrees. In one study in which increasing concentrations were presented on alternate days, all rats eventually took at least 50% of their total daily liquid intake as alcohol at concentrations that ranged between 14% and 33% (Brown & Amit, 1977).

Other methods used to increase rats' consumption of alcohol include schedule-induced polydipsia (Meisch & Thompson, 1971), training them to bar-press for water and then substituting alcohol for the water (Meisch & Beardsley, 1975), and the so-called "fading" technique (Samson *et al.*, 1987; Samson, Pfeffer & Tolliver, 1988; Grant & Johanson, 1988). In this latter procedure animals are trained to perform some response for a potent reward such as a sucrose solution; alcohol is then gradually substituted for the training reinforcer and maintains robust responding that responds to dose manipulations. However, none of these methods increases rats' consumption of alcohol more than the straightforward presentation of the drug itself.

Neither intravenous (Lyness & Smith, 1992) nor oral (Rassnick, Stinus & Koob, 1993) self-administration of alcohol is affected by dopamine-specific lesions of nucleus accumbens. Earlier work (Amit *et al.*, 1977; Brown *et al.*, 1977) had shown that antagonism of the noradrenergic, but not of the dopamine system reduces oral alcohol consumption in rats. These observations are consistent with the failure of alcohol to produce a CCP in rats and with the conclusion that the drug does not interact with the amygdala-based incentive learning system.

The oral self-administration of alcohol is reduced to various degrees by drugs that antagonize the GABA or serotonin receptor systems (McBride *et al.*, 1988; Lyness & Smith, 1992; Rassnick *et al.*, 1992). Self-administration is also reduced by the partial inverse benzodiazepine receptor agonist, Ro 15-4513 (Samson *et al.*, 1987, 1989). Interestingly, this drug failed to affect an alcohol CCP in alcohol preferring mice (Risinger *et al.*, 1992), a finding that is consistent with the conclusion that the incentive reward system is not involved in the mediation of alcohol's reinforcing action.

Possibly related to the importance of these receptor systems, there is evidence that alcohol self-administration may be promoted by its apparent ability to relieve aversive states related to anxiety (Schuckit & Monteiro, 1988; George, 1993; Mollenauer *et al.*, 1993). Learning about the effect of alcohol consumption on such aversive affective states might also promote self-administration, and this type of reinforcing effect may depend on hippocampus-based declarative learning.

The recent demonstration that Tryon maze-bright rats exposed to increasing concentrations of alcohol on alternate days are among the largest rodent consumers of alcohol ever reported (Amit & Smith, 1992) is consistent with this hypothesis. This strain was bred for its ability to perform well on mazes (Innis, 1992) and it is well-known that the spatial learning ability rats use to solve mazes is a function of the hippocampus (O'Keefe & Nadel, 1978). If the maze-bright rats do in fact have superior hippocampal function, this facility may also account for their exceptional ability to associate the affective state produced by alcohol with the features of the environment that can be manipulated to obtain the drug.

These considerations suggest that in humans the initiation of alcohol self-administration could be largely due to declarative learning based on its anxiety reduction or other perceptible properties, and that these effects may also be important for maintaining the behaviour. The data from animal studies suggest that with repeated use the drug may reinforce a self-administration habit and aversive responses due to withdrawal may also develop that would be subject to hippocampus-based declarative learning. Based on these proposed mechanisms, alcohol self-administration may be treatable by a combination of behaviour therapy for the habit-based behaviour, and counselling to identify and remove sources of anxiety.

Morphine. Morphine is self-administered systemically by laboratory animals (e.g. Weeks, 1962; Weeks & Collins, 1968; Woods & Schuster, 1971; Smith *et al.*, 1980, 1985); in all of these cases the animals were made "dependent" on morphine to some degree with a course of non-contingent injections before the start of self-administration training. In non-dependent animals morphine is self-administered intraventricularly (Amit, Brown & Sklar, 1976) and directly into ventral tegmental area (Bozarth & Wise, 1981; Bozarth & Wise, 1988; Welzl, Kuhn & Huston, 1989; Devine & Wise, 1994), lateral hypothalamus (Olds, 1979; Cazala, Darracq & Saint-Marc, 1987; Balleine, 1992), and nucleus accumbens (Olds, 1982). The functional relevance of the findings for the two latter areas has been questioned because of the high doses required to observe the effect (Wise, 1989). The observation that the intracerebral self-administration of morphine is blocked by naloxone (Bozarth & Wise, 1981, 1988; Olds, 1979; Cazala, Darracq & Saint-Marc, 1987) is consistent with the hypothesis that an action of morphine on opiate receptors in one or more of these brain areas mediates these effects.

Lesions of nucleus accumbens that destroy cell bodies (Smith *et al.*, 1985; Dworkin *et al.*, 1988b) produce small increases in the dose of morphine required to maintain self-administration, but lesions of the same brain area that destroy only the terminals of dopamine-containing neurones have no effect on morphine self-administration (Dworkin *et al.*, 1988a). This suggests that although some nucleus accumbens mechanism may contribute to morphine self-administration, this contribution is modest and may not involve dopamine. The latter suggestion is supported by evidence that dopamine is not involved in the conditioned incentive effects of morphine in non-dependent animals (Bechara & van der Kooy, 1992). In these respects the role of the nucleus accumbens in morphine self-administration differs from its role in both amphetamine and cocaine self-administration, even though this brain area may be involved in the mediation of some form of conditioned incentive behaviours with all three drugs.

As suggested in the section on conditioned incentive behaviours, the morphine CCP may involve hippocampus-based learning about conditioned reward, while the amphetamine and cocaine CCPs may depend primarily on conditioned approach behaviours, which do not involve the hippocampal learning system. Further investigation will be required to test the hypothesis that hippocampus-based learning about amygdala-based conditioned reward contributes to morphine self-administration.

Other properties of morphine that involve affective states include its analgesic action, its alleviation of morphine withdrawal symptoms (most laboratory demonstrations of intravenous morphine self-administration start by making the animals "dependent" on the drug) and its property of relieving social isolation stress (Panksepp *et al.*, 1978). Learning about any or all of these actions of morphine—a function that may involve the memory system that includes the hippocampus—could lead to its self-administration.

Lesions of the caudate–putamen in rats that have acquired morphine self-administration produce an immediate 10-fold decrease in the dose of the drug required to maintain self-administration, and a decrease in the threshold dose for initiating the behaviour in naive animals (Glick, Cox & Crane, 1975); see also (Linseman, 1976). This finding suggests that the caudate–putamen memory system does not participate in morphine self-administration. Moreover, the size and rapidity of the apparent increase in sensitivity to morphine is not entirely consistent with a biochemical change following neural damage. As an alternative, it is possible that destruction of the caudate memory system eliminates a substrate of behaviours that compete with morphine-reinforced self-administration (e.g. McDonald & White, 1994), resulting in an immediate facilitation of the behaviour.

The available data on morphine suggest that initiation of its self-administration may be based on declarative learning about its anxiety reducing and its rewarding and conditioned rewarding properties, and that these processes may also be the ones that maintain the behaviour, even if the affective processes themselves change with repeated use of the drug. It is important to note that although morphine is an opiate drug these suggestions do not necessarily apply to other drugs in this class.

Conclusion

These preliminary attempts to specify the neural substrates of action and the behavioural processes initiated by the reinforcing effects of five addictive drugs suggest that each affects a unique combination of substrates and has a different set of actions. According to the present analysis a detailed experimental examination of the interaction of each drug with the neural substrates of each of the three learning and memory systems will be required to understand the addictive process in each case. The analysis leads to many predictions about these interactions that are experimentally testable. The improved understanding of the process by which each drug promotes behaviour change that should result from these experiments will, in turn, lead to the development of treatment strategies that focus specifically on the behavioural processes controlled by each drug. In addition to pharmacological treatments the useful strategies are likely to include various methods promoting extinction of drug-related behaviours (e.g. O'Brien & Childress, 1991; O'Brien *et al.*, 1992) as well as more cognitive or psychodynamic approaches (e.g. Drummond, 1991; Falkowski, 1991) as well as new treatments that may be suggested by the present approach to understanding drug addiction.

Acknowledgements

I am grateful to Frances Abbott, Zalman Amit, Paul Clarke, Keith Franklin, Noboru Hiroi and Robert McDonald for their comments on earlier versions of this manuscript and for useful discussions on its content. Preparation of the manuscript was supported by grants from Fonds FCAR, Province of Quebec, and from the Natural Sciences and Engineering Research Council, and the Medical Research Council of Canada.

References

ABLEITNER, A. & HERZ, A. (1989) Limbic brain structures are important sites of kappa-opioid receptor-mediated actions in the rat: a [14C]-2-deoxyglucose study, *Brain Research*, 478, 326–336.

Alexander, G. E., DeLong, M. R. & Strick, P. L. (1986) Parallel organization of functionally segregated circuits linking basal ganglia and cortex, *Annual Review of Neuroscience*, 9, 357–381.

Alkana, R. L. & Parker, E. S. (1979) Memory facilitation by post-training injection of ethanol, *Psychopharmacology*, 66, 117–119.

Amit, Z. & Stern, M. H. (1969) Alcohol ingestion without oropharyngeal sensations, *Psychonomic Science*, 15, 162–163.

Amit, Z. & Smith, B. R. (1992) Differential ethanol intake in Tryon maze-bright and Tryon maze-dull rats: implications for the validity of the animal model of selectively bred rats for high ethanol consumption, *Psychopharmacology*, 108, 136–140.

Amit, Z., Brown, Z. & Sklar, L. S. (1976) Intraventricular self-administration of morphine in naive laboratory rats, *Psychopharmacology*, 48, 291–294.

Amit, Z., Brown, Z. W., Levitan, D. E. & Vgren, S.-O. (1977) Noradrenergic mediation of the positive reinforcing properties of ethanol: I. Suppression of ethanol consumption in laboratory rats following dopamine-beta-hydroxylase inhibition, *Archives Internationales de Pharmacodynamie et de Therapie*, 230, 65–75.

Balleine, B. (1992) Instrumental performance following a shift in primary motivation depends on incentive learning, *Journal of Experimental Psychology: Animal Behavior Processes*, 18, 236–250.

Balster, R. L. & Schuster, C. R. (1973) A comparison of d-amphetamine, l-amphetamine, and methamphetamine self-administration in rhesus monkeys, *Pharmacology, Biochemistry and Behavior*, 1, 67–71.

Beach, H. D. (1957) Morphine addiction in rats, *Canadian Journal of Psychology*, 11, 104–112.

Bechara, A. & van der Kooy, D. (1985) Opposite motivational effects of endogenous opiods in brain and periphery, *Nature*, 314, 533–534.

Bechara, A. & van der Kooy, D. (1987) Kappa receptors mediate the peripheral aversive effects of opiates, *Pharmacology, Biochemistry and Behavior*, 28, 227–233.

Bechara, A. & van der Kooy, D. (1989) The tegmental pedunculopontine nucleus: a brain-stem output of the limbic system critical for the conditioned place preferences produced by morphine and amphetamine, *Journal of Neuroscience*, 9, 3400–3409.

Bechara, A. & van der Kooy, D. (1992) A single brain stem substrate mediates the motivational effects of both opiates and food in nondeprived rats but not in deprived rats, *Behavioral Neuroscience*, 106, 351–363.

Bindra, D. (1969) The interrelated mechanisms of reinforcement and motivation, and the nature of their influence on response, *Nebraska Symposium on Motivation*, 17, 1–37.

Bindra, D. (1978) How adaptive behavior is produced: a perceptual–motivational alternative to response-reinforcement, *Behavioral and Brain Sciences*, 1, 41–91.

Blaha, C. D. & Winn, P. (1993) Modulation of dopamine efflux in the striatum following cholinergic stimulation of the substantia nigra in intact and pedunculopontine tegmental nucleus-lesioned rats, *Journal of Neuroscience*, 13, 1035–1044.

Boyle, A. E., Smith, B. R., Spivak, K. & Amit, Z. (1994) Voluntary ethanol consumption in rats: The importance of the exposure paradigm in determining final intake outcome, *Behavioural Pharmacology*, 5, 502–512.

Bozarth, M. A. & Wise, R. A. (1981) Intracranial self-administration of morphine into the ventral tegmental area in rats, *Life Sciences*, 28, 551–555.

Bozarth, M. A. & Wise, R. A. (1988) Anatomically distinct opiate receptor fields mediate reward and physical dependence, *Science*, 224, 516–517.

Brazell, M. P., Mitchell, S. N. & Gray, J. A. (1991) Effect of acute administration of nicotine on *in vivo* release of noradrenaline in the hippocampus of freely-moving rats: a dose-response and antagonist study, *Neuropharmacology*, 30, 823–833.

Breese, C. R., Hampson, R. E. & Deadwyler, S. A. (1989) Hippocampal place cells: stereotypy and plasticity, *Journal of Neuroscience*, 9, 1097–1111.

Brown, E. E. & Fibiger, H. C. (1993) Differential effects of excitotoxic lesions of the amygdala on cocaine-induced conditioned locomotion and conditioned place preference, *Psychopharmacology*, 113, 123–130.

Brown, Z. W. & Amit, Z. (1977) The effects of selective catecholamine depletions by 6-hydroxy-dopamine on ethanol preference in rats, *Neuroscience Letters*, 5, 333–336.

Brown, Z. W., Amit, Z., Levitan, D. E., Vgren, S.-O. & Sutherland, E. A. (1977) Noradrenergic mediation of the positive reinforcing properties of ethanol: II. Extinction of ethanol drinking behavior in laboratory rats by inhibition of dopamine-beta-hydroxylase. Implications for treatment procedures in human alcoholics, *Archives Internationales de Pharmacodynamie et de Therapie*, 230, 76–82.

Butters, N., Martone, M., White, B., Granholm, E. & Wolfe, J. (1986) Clinical validators: comparisons of demented and amnesic patients, in: Poon, L. (Ed.) *Handbook of Clinical Assessment of Memory*, 337–352 (Washington, American Psychological Association).

Cabanac, M. & Ferber, C. (1987) Pleasure and preference in a two-dimensional sensory space, *Appetite*, 8, 15–28.

Cabanac, M., Minaire, Y. & Adair, E. R. (1968) Influence of internal factors on the pleasantness of a gustative sweet sensation, *Communications in Behavioral Biology*, 1, 77–82.

Caine, S. B. & Koob, G. F. (1994) Effects of mesolimbic dopamine depletion on responding maintained by cocaine and food, *Journal of the Experimental Analysis of Behavior*, 61, 213–221.

Candland, D. K., Fell, J. P., Keen, E., Leshner, A. I., Tarpy, R. M. & Plutchik, R. (1977) *Emotion* (Monterey, CA, Brooks-Cole).

Canli, T., Cook, R. G. & Miczek, K. A. (1990) Opiate antagonists enhance the working memory of rats in the radial maze, *Pharmacology, Biochemistry and Behavior*, 36, 521–525.

Carr, G. D. & White, N. M. (1984) The relationship between stereotypy and memory improvement produced by amphetamine, *Psychopharmacology*, 82, 203–209.

CARR, G. D. & WHITE, N. M. (1986) Anatomical dissociation of amphetamine's rewarding and aversive effects: an intracranial microinjection study, *Psychopharmacology*, 89, 340–346.

CASTELLANO, C., LIBRI, V. & AMMASSARI-TEULE, M. (1988) The amygdala mediates the impairing effect of the selective k-opioid receptor agonist U-50, 488 on memory in CD1 mice, *Behavioural Brain Research*, 30, 251–258.

CASTELLANO, C., INTROINI-COLLISON, I. B., PAVONE, F. & MCGAUGH, J. L. (1989) Effects of naloxone and naltrexone on memory consolidation in CD1 mice: involvement of GABAergic mechanisms, *Pharmacology, Biochemistry and Behavior*, 32, 563–567.

CAZALA, P., DARRACQ, C. & SAINT-MARC, M. (1987) Self-administration of morphine into the lateral hypothalamus in the mouse, *Brain Research*, 416, 283–288.

CLARKE, P. B. S. & FIBIGER, H. C. (1987) Apparent absence of nicotine-induced conditioned place preference in rats, *Psychopharmacology*, 92, 84–88.

COHEN, N. J. & SQUIRE, L. R. (1980) Preserved learning and retention of pattern-analyzing skill in amnesia: dissociation of knowing how and knowing what, *Science*, 210, 207–209.

CORRIGALL, W. A. (1991) Understanding brain mechanisms in nicotine reinforcement, *British Journal of Addictions*, 86, 507–510.

CORRIGALL, W. A. & COEN, K. M. (1989) Nicotine maintains robust self-administration in rats on a limited-access schedule, *Psychopharmacology*, 99, 473–478.

CORRIGALL, W. A. & COEN, K. M. (1991a) Cocaine self-administration is increased by both D1 and D2 dopamine antagonists, *Pharmacology, Biochemistry and Behavior*, 39, 799–802.

CORRIGALL, W. A. & COEN, K. M. (1991b) Selective dopamine antagonists reduce nicotine self-administration, *Psychopharmacology*, 104, 171–176.

CORRIGALL, W. A. & LINSEMAN, M. A. (1988) Conditioned place preference produced by intra-hippocampal morphine, *Pharmacology, Biochemistry and Behavior*, 30, 787–789.

CORRIGALL, W. A., FRANKLIN, K. B. J., COEN, K. M. & CLARKE, P. B. S. (1992) The mesolimbic dopaminergic system is implicated in the reinforcing effects of nicotine, *Psychopharmacology*, 107, 285–289.

COX, B. M., GOLDSTEIN, A. & NELSON, W. T. (1984) Nicotine self-administration in rats, *British Journal of Pharmacology*, 83, 49–55.

CROW, T. J. (1973) Catecholamine-containing neurones and electrical self-stimulation: 2. A theoretical interpretation and some psychiatric implications, *Psychological Medicine*, 3, 66–73.

CUNNINGHAM, C. L. (1979) Flavor and location aversions produced by ethanol, *Behavioral and Neural Biology*, 27, 362–367.

CUNNINGHAM, C. L. & PRATHER, L. K. (1992) Conditioning trial duration affects ethanol-induced conditioned place preference in mice, *Animal Learning and Behavior*, 20, 187–194.

CUNNINGHAM, C. L., MALOTT, D. H., DICKINSON, S. D. & RISINGER, F. O. (1992) Haloperidol does not alter expression of ethanol-induced conditioned place preference, *Behavioural Brain Research*, 50, 1–5.

DAFNY, N., BROWN, M., BURKS, T. F. & RIGOR, B. M. (1979) Patterns of unit responses to incremental doses of morphine in central gray, reticular formation, medial thalamus, caudate nucleus, hypothalamus, septum and hippocampus in unanesthetized rats, *Neuropharmacology*, 18, 489–495.

DAMSMA, G., WESTERINK, B. H. C., DE VRIES, J. B. & HORN, A. S. (1988) The effect of systemically applied cholinergic drugs on the striatal release of dopamine and its metabolites, as determined by automated brain dialysis in conscious rats, *Neuroscience Letters*, 89, 349–354.

DAVIDSON, T. L. & JARRARD, L. E. (1993) A role for hippocampus in the utilization of hunger signals, *Behavioral and Neural Biology*, 59, 167–171.

DAVIS, M. (1992) The role of the amygdala in fear and anxiety, *Annual Review of Neuroscience*, 15, 353–375.

DEMINIERE, J. M., TAGHZOUTI, K., TASSIN, J. P., LE MOAL, M. & SIMON, H. (1988) Increased sensitivity to amphetamine and facilitation of amphetamine self-administration after 6-hydroxydopamine lesions of the amygdala, *Psychopharmacology*, 94, 232–236.

DENOBLE, V. J., MELE, P. C. & PORTER, J. H. (1985) Intravenous self-administration of pentobarbital and ethanol in rats, *Pharmacology, Biochemistry and Behavior*, 23, 759–763.

DEVINE, D. P. & WISE, R. A. (1994) Self-administration of morphine, DAMGO, and DPDPE into the ventral tegmental area of rats, *Journal of Neuroscience*, 14, 1978–1984.

DICHIARA, G., ACQUAS, E. & CARBONI, E. (1992) Drug motivation and abuse: a neurobiological perspective, *Annals of the New York Academy of Sciences*, 654, 207–219.

DIVAC, I. (1968) Functions of the caudate nucleus, *Acta Biologiae Experimentalis (Warsaw)*, 28, 107–120.

DOTY, B. & DOTY, L. (1966) Facilitating effects of amphetamine on avoidance conditioning in relation to age and problem difficulty, *Psychopharmacology*, 9, 234–241.

DOUGHTERY, J., MILLER, D., TODD, G. & KOSTENBAUDER, H. B. (1981) Reinforcing and other behavioral effects of nicotine, *Neuroscience and Biobehavioral Reviews*, 5, 487–495.

DRUMMOND, D. C. (1991) Individual therapy with drug-takers: getting started, in: GLASS, I. B. (Ed.) *Addiction Behaviour*, pp. 240–243 (London, Tavistock/Routledge).

DUNN, L. T. & EVERITT, B. J. (1988) Double dissociations of the effects of amygdala and insular cortex lesions on conditioned taste aversion, passive avoidance and neophobia in the rat using the excitotoxin ibotenic acid, *Behavioral Neuroscience*, 102, 3–23.

DWORKIN, S. I., GUERIN, G. F., CO, C., GOEDERS, N. E. & SMITH, J. E. (1988a) Lack of an effect of 6-hydroxydopamine lesions of the nucleus accumbens on intravenous morphine self-administration, *Pharmacology, Biochemistry and Behavior*, 30, 1051–1057.

DWORKIN, S. I., GUERIN, G. F., GOEDERS, N. E. & SMITH, J. E. (1988b) Kainic acid lesions of the nucleus accumbens selectively attenuate morphine self-administration, *Pharmacology, Biochemistry and Behavior*, 29, 175–181.

ELKINS, R. L. (1980) Attenuation of X-ray-induced taste aversions by olfactory-bulb or amygdaloid lesions, *Physiology and Behavior*, 24, 515–521.

ESTES, W. K. (1991) Cognitive architectures from the standpoint of an experimental psychologist, *Annual Review of Psychology*, 42, 1–28.

EVANGELISTA, A. M., GATTONI, R. C. & IZQUIERDO, I. (1970) Effect of amphetamine, nicotine and hexamethonium on performance of a conditioned response during acquisition and retention trials, *Psychopharmacology*, 3, 91–96.

EVERITT, B. J., MORRIS, K. A., O'BRIEN, A. & ROBBINS, T. W. (1991) The basolateral amygdala–ventral striatal system and conditioned place preference: further evidence of limbic–striatal interactions underlying reward-related processes, *Neuroscience*, 42, 1–18.

FAIMAN, C. P., DE ERAUSQUIN, G. A. & BARATTI, C. M. (1991) The enhancement of retention induced by vasopressin in mice may be mediated by an activation of central nicotinic cholinergic mechanisms, *Behavioral and Neural Biology*, 56, 183–199.

FALKOWSKI, W. (1991) Group psychotherapy for alcoholics and drug addicts, in: GLASS, I. B. (Ed.) *Addiction Behaviour*, pp. 244–248 (London, Tavistock/Routledge).

FANSELOW, M. S. & KIM, J. J. (1994) Acquisition of contextual Pavlovian fear conditioning is blocked by application of an NMDA receptor antagonist D, L-2-amino-5-phosphonovaleric acid to the basolateral amygdala, *Behavioral Neuroscience*, 108, 210–212.

FERRARI, C. M., O'CONNOR, D. A. & RILEY, A. L. (1991) Cocaine-induced taste aversions: effect of route of administration, *Pharmacology, Biochemistry and Behavior*, 38, 267–271.

FREUND, R. K., JUNGSCHAFFER, D. A. & COLLINS, A. C. (1990) Nicotine effects in mouse hippocampus are blocked by mecamylamine, but not other nicotinic antagonists, *Brain Research*, 511, 187–191.

GAFFAN, D. (1987) Amnesia, personal memory and the hippocampus: experimental neuropsychological studies in monkeys, in: STAHL, S. M., IVERSEN, S. D. & GOODMAN, E. C. (Eds) *Cognitive Neurochemistry*, pp. 46–56 (Oxford, Oxford University Press).

GALLAGHER, M., KING, R. A. & YOUNG, N. B. (1983) Opiate antagonists improve spatial memory, *Science*, 221, 975–976.

GARCIA, J. & KOELLING, R. A. (1966) Relationship of cue to consequence in avoidance learning, *Psychonomic Science*, 7, 439–450.

GARCIA, J., HANKINS, W. G. & RUSINIAK, K. W. (1976) Flavor aversion studies, *Science*, 192, 265–266.

GARCIA, J. & KIMELDORF, D. J. (1957) Temporal relationship within the conditioning of a saccharine aversion through radiation exposure, *Journal of Comparative and Physiological Psychology*, 50, 180–183.

GARG, M. & HOLLAND, H. C. (1968) Consolidation and maze learning: a further study of post-trial injections of a stimulant drug (nicotine), *International Journal of Neuropharmacology*, 7, 55–59.

GEORGE, F. R. (1993) Genetic models in the study of alcoholism and substance abuse mechanisms, *Progress in Neuropsychopharmacology and Biological Psychiatry*, 17, 345–361.

GERFEN, C. R. (1992) The neostriatal mosaic: Multiple levels of compartmental organization in the basal ganglia, *Annual Review of Neuroscience*, 15, 285–320.

GILL, K., FRANCE, C. & AMIT, Z. (1986) Voluntary ethanol consumption in rats: an examination of blood/brain ethanol levels and behavior, *Alcoholism: Clinical and Experimental Research*, 10, 457–462.

GLICK, S. D., COX, R. D. & CRANE, A. M. (1975) Changes in morphine self-administration and morphine dependence after lesions of the caudate nucleus in rats, *Psychopharmacology*, 41, 219–224.

GLICKMAN, S. E. & SCHIFF, B. B. (1967) A biological theory of reinforcement, *Psychological Review*, 74, 81–109.

GOEDERS, N. E. & SMITH, J. E. (1983) Cortical dopaminergic involvement in cocaine reinforcement, *Science*, 221, 773–775.

GOEDERS, N. E. & SMITH, J. E. (1986) Reinforcing properties of cocaine in the medial prefrontal cortex: primary action on presynaptic dopaminergic terminals, *Pharmacology, Biochemistry and Behavior*, 25, 191–199.

GOLD, P. E. & MCGAUGH, J. L. (1975) A single trace, two process view of memory storage processes, in: DEUTSCH, D. & DEUTSCH, J. A. (Eds) *Short Term Memory* (New York, Academic Press).

GOLDBERG, S. R. & HENNINGFIELD, J. E. (1988) Reinforcing effects of nicotine in humans and experimental animals responding under intermittent schedules of iv drug injection, *Pharmacology, Biochemistry and Behavior*, 30, 227–234.

GRANT, K. A. & JOHANSON, C. E. (1988) Oral ethanol self-administration in free-feeding rhesus monkeys, *Alcoholism: Clinical and Experimental Research*, 12, 780–784.

GRAYBIEL, A. M., MORATALLA, R. & ROBERTSON, H. A. (1990) Amphetamine and cocaine induce drug-specific activation of the c-*fos* gene in striosome-matrix compartments and limbic subdivisions of the striatum, *Proceedings of the National Academy of Sciences, USA*, 87, 6912–6916.

GRECKSCH, G., OTT, T. & MATTHIES, H. (1978) Influence of post-training intrahippocampally applied oxotremorine on the consolidation of a brightness discrimination, *Pharmacology, Biochemistry and Behavior*, 8, 215–218.

GROVES, P. M. (1983) A theory of the functional organization of the neostriatum and the neostriatal control of voluntary movement, *Brain Research Reviews*, 5, 109–132.

HARLEY, C., MILWAY, J. S. & LACAILLE, J. C. (1989) Locus coeruleus potentiation of dentate gyrus responses: evidence for two systems, *Brain Research Bulletin*, 22, 643–650.

HAYCOCK, J. W., DEADWYLER, S. A., SIDEROFF, S. I. & MCGAUGH, J. L. (1973) Retrograde amnesia and cholinergic systems in the caudate–putamen complex and dorsal hippocampus of the rat, *Experimental Neurology*, 41, 201–213.

HEMBY, S. E., JONES, G. H., JUSTICE, JR, J. B. & NEILL, D. B. (1992) Conditioned locomotor activity but not conditioned place preference following intra-accumbens infusions of cocaine, *Psychopharmacology*, 106, 330–336.

HENNINGFIELD, J. E. & GOLDBERG, S. R. (1983) Nicotine as a reinforcer in human subjects and laboraary animals, *Pharmacology, Biochemistry and Behavior*, 19, 989–992.

HENNINGFIELD, J. E. & GOLDBERG, S. R. (1988) Pharmacologic determinants of tobacco self-administration by humans, *Pharmacology, Biochemistry and Behavior*, 30, 221–226.

HIROI, N. & WHITE, N. M. (1990) The reserpine-sensitive dopamine pool mediates (+)-amphetamine-conditioned reward in the place preference paradigm, *Brain Research*, 510, 33–42.

HIROI, N. & WHITE, N. M. (1991a) The amphetamine conditioned place preference: differential involvement of dopamine receptor subtypes and two dopaminergic terminal areas, *Brain Research*, 552, 141–152.

HIROI, N. & WHITE, N. M. (1991b) The lateral nucleus of the amygdala mediates expression of the amphetamine conditioned place preference, *Journal of Neuroscience*, 11, 2107–2116.

HIRSH, R. (1974) The hippocampus and contextual retrieval of information from memory: a theory, *Behavioral Biology*, 12, 421–444.

HIRSH, R. (1980) The hippocampus, conditional operations and cognition, *Physiological Psychology*, 8, 175–182.

HIRSH, R. & KRAJDEN, J. (1982) The hippocampus and the expression of knowledge, in: ISAACSON, R. L. & SPEAR, N. E. (Eds) *The Expression of Knowledge*, pp. 213–241 (New York, Plenum).

HIRSH, R., DAVIS, R. E. & HOLT, L. (1979) Fornix-thalamus fibers, motivational states, and contextual retrieval, *Experimental Neurology*, 65, 373–390.

HIRSH, R., HOLT, L. & MOSSERI, A. (1978) Hippocampal mossy fibers motivation states and contextual retrieval, *Experimental Neurology*, 62, 68–79.

HIRSH, R., LEBER, B. & GILLMAN, R. (1978) Fornix fibers and motivational states as controllers of behavior: a study stimulated by the contextual retrieval theory, *Behavioral Biology*, 22, 463–475.

HOEBEL, B. G., MONACO, A. P., HERNANDEZ, L., AULISI, E. F., STANLEY, B. G. & LENARD, L. G. (1983) Self-injection of amphetamine directly into the brain, *Psychopharmacology*, 81, 158–163.

HULL, C. L. (1943) *Principles of Behavior* (New York, Appleton-Century-Crofts).

HUNT, W. A., MAJCHROWICZ, E. & DALTON, T. K. (1979) Alterations in high-affinity choline uptake in brain after acute and chronic ethanol treatment, *Journal of Pharmacology and Experimental Therapeutics*, 210, 259–263.

HURD, Y. L., WEISS, F., KOOB, G. & UNGERSTEDT, U. (1990) The influence of cocaine self-administration on *in vivo* dopamine and acetylcholine neurotransmission in rat caudate–putamen, *Neuroscience Letters*, 109, 227–233.

HUSTON, J. P. & OITZL, M.-S. (1989) The relationship between reinforcement and memory: parallels in the rewarding and mnemonic effects of the neuropeptide substance P, *Neuroscience and Biobehavioral Reviews*, 13, 171–180.

HUSTON, J. P., MONDADORI, C. & WASER, P. G. (1974) Facilitation of learning by reward of post-trial memory processes, *Experientia*, 30, 1038–1040.

HUSTON, J. P., MUELLER, C. C. & MONDADORI, C. (1977) Memory facilitation by posttrial hypothalamic stimulation and other reinforcers: a central theory of reinforcement, *Biobehavioral Reviews*, 1, 143–150.

IMPERATO, A., OBINU, M. C. & GESSA, G. L. (1993) Effects of cocaine and amphetamine on acetylcholine release in the hippocampus and caudate nucleus, *European Journal of Pharmacology*, 238, 377–381.

INNIS, N. K. (1992) Tolman and Tryon, *American Psychologist*, 47, 190–197.

INTROINI-COLLISON, I. B., NAGAHARA, A. H. & MCGAUGH, J. L. (1989) Memory enhancement with intra-amygdala post-training naloxone is blocked by concurrent administration of propranolol, *Brain Research*, 476, 94–101.

INTROINI-COLLISON, I. B., MCGAUGH, J. L. & BARATTI, C. M. (1985) Pharmacological evidence of a central effect of naltrexone, morphine, and beta-endorphin and a peripheral effect of met- and leu-enkephalin on retention of an inhibitory avoidance response in mice, *Behavioral and Neural Biology*, 44, 434–446.

ISAAC, W. L., NONNEMAN, A. J., NEISWANDER, J., LANDERS, T. & BARDO, M. T. (1989) Prefrontal cortex lesions differentially disrupt cocaine reinforced conditioned place preference but not conditioned taste aversion, *Behavioral Neuroscience*, 103, 345–355.

IWAMOTO, E. T. (1990) Nicotine conditions place preferences after intracerebral admininstration in rats, *Psychopharmacology*, 100, 251–257.

IWATSUBO, K. & CLOUET, D. H. (1975) Dopamine-sensitive adenylate cyclase of the caudate nucleus of rats treated with morphine or haloperidol, *Biochemical Pharmacology*, 24, 1499–1503.

IZARD, C. E. (1972) *Patterns of Emotions* (New York, Academic).

IZQUIERDO, I., DA CUNHA, C., ROSAT, R., JERUSALINSKY, D., FERREIRA, M. B. C. & MEDINA, J. H. (1992) Neurotransmitter receptors involved in post-training memory processing by the amygdala, medial septum, and hippocampus of the rat, *Behavioral and Neural Biology*, 58, 16–26.

JAFFARD. R. & DESTRADE, C. (1982) Learning and memory processes as related to genotypic or experimental variations of hippocampal and cholinergic activity in inbred strains of mice, in: LEIBLICH, I. (Ed.) *Genetics of the Brain*, pp. 299–322 (Amsterdam, Elsevier Biomedical Press).

JAFFARD, R., DESTRADE, C., SOUMIREU-MOURAT, B., DURKIN, T. & EBEL, A. (1980) Changes in hippocampal cholinergic activity following learning in mice, *Neuroscience Letters*, 19, 349–352.

JANAK, P. H., KEPPEL, G. & MARTINEZ JR, J. L. (1992) Cocaine enhances retention of avoidance conditioning in rats, *Psychopharmacology*, 106, 383–387.

JENSEN, R. A., GILBERT, D. G., MELISKA, C. J., LANDRUM, T. A. & SZARY, A. B. (1990) Characterization of a dose–response curve for nicotine-induced conditioned taste aversion in rats: relationship to elevation of plasma endorphin concentration, *Behavioral and Neural Biology*, 53, 428–440.

JOHNSTON, D., HOPKINS, W. F. & GRAY, R. (1989) The role of norepinephrine in long-term potentiation at mossy-fiber synapses in the hippocampus, in: BYRNE, J. H. & BERRY, W. O. (Eds) *Neural Models of*

Plasticity, 307–328 (San Diego, CA, Academic Press).

JONES, B. & MISHKIN, M. (1972) Limbic lesions and the problem of stimulus–reinforcement associations, *Experimental Neurology*, 36, 362–377.

JOPE, R. J. & JENDEN, D. J. (1981) Effects of acute ethanol treatment on cholinergic functions in rats, *Substances Alcohol Actions/Misuses*, 2, 15–23.

KESNER, R. P. & WILBURN, M. W. (1974) A review of electrical stimulation of the brain in the context of learning and retention, *Behavioral Biology*, 10, 259–292.

KIMBLE, D. P. (1981) Latent learning in hippocampally lesioned rats, *Physiology and Behavior*, 26, 1055–1059.

KLINER, D. J. & PICKENS, R. (1982) Indicated preference for drugs of abuse, *International Journal of the Addictions*, 17, 543–547.

KOOB, G. F. (1992a) Drugs of abuse: anatomy, pharmacology and function of reward pathways, *Trends in Pharmacological Sciences*, 13, 177–184.

KOOB, G. F. (1992b) Neural mechanisms of drug reinforcement, *Annals of the New York Academy of Sciences*, 654, 171–191.

KOZLOWSKI, L. T. & WILKINSON, D. A. (1987) Use and misuse of the concept of craving by alcohol, tobacco and drug researchers, *British Journal of Addictions*, 82, 31–36.

KUCZENSKI, R., SEGAL, D. S. & AIZENSTEIN, M. L. (1991) Amphetamine, cocaine, and fencamfamine: relationship between locomotor and stereotypy response profiles and caudate and accumbens dopamine dynamics, *Journal of Neuroscience*, 11, 2703–2712.

LAMB, R. J., PRESTON, K. L., SCHINDLER, C. W. *et al.* (1991) The reinforcing and subjective effects of morphine in post-addicts: a dose–response study, *Journal of Pharmacology and Experimental Therapeutics*, 259, 1165–1173.

LAMBERTY, G. J., BECKWITH, B. E., PETROS, T. V. & ROSS, A. R. (1990) Posttrial treatment with ethanol enhances recall of prose narratives, *Physiology and Behavior*, 48, 653–658.

LANDAUER, T. K. (1969) Reinforcement as consolidation, *Psychological Review*, 76, 82–96.

LEBLANC, A. E. & CAPPELL, H. (1974) Attenuation of punishing effects of morphine and amphetamine by chronic prior treatment, *Journal of Comparative and Physiological Psychology*, 87, 691–698.

LEMAIRE, G. A. & MEISCH, R. A. (1985) Oral drug self-administration in rhesus monkeys: interactions between drug amount and fixed ratio size, *Journal of the Experimental Analysis of Behavior*, 44, 377–389.

LINSEMAN, M. A. (1976) Effects of lesions of the caudate nucleus on morphine dependence in the rat, *Pharmacology, Biochemistry and Behavior*, 5, 465–472.

LINSEMAN, M. A. & CORRIGALL, W. A. (1982) Effects of morphine on CA1 versus dentate hippocampal field potentials following systemic administration in freely-moving rats, *Neuropharmacology*, 21, 361–366.

LITTLETON, J. (1991) Drug dependence as pharmacological adaptation, in: GLASS, I. B. (Ed.) *Addiction Behaviours*, 11–14 (London, Tavistock/Routledge).

LYNESS, W. H. & SMITH, F. L. (1992) Influence of dopaminergic and serotonergic neurons on intravenous ethanol self-administration in the rat, *Pharmacology, Biochemistry and Behavior*, 42, 187–192.

LYNESS, W. H., FRIEDLE, N. M. & MOORE, K. E. (1979) Destruction of dopaminergic nerve terminals in nucleus accumbens: effect on d-amphetamine self-administration, *Pharmacology, Biochemistry and Behavior*, 11, 553–556.

MACKEY, W. B., KELLER, J. & VAN DER KOOY, D. (1986) Visceral cortex lesions block conditioned taste aversions induced by morphine, *Pharmacology, Biochemistry and Behavior*, 24, 71–78.

MAEDA, H., MORIMOTO, H. & YANAGIMOTO, K. (1993) Response characteristics of amygdaloid neurons provoked by emotionally significant environmental stimuli in cats, with special reference to response durations, *Canadian Journal of Physiology and Pharmacology*, 71, 374–378.

MALMO, R. B. (1975) *On Emotions, Needs, and Our Archaic Brain* (New York, Holt, Rinehart & Winston).

MANLEY, L. D., KUCZENSKI, R., SEGAL, D. S., YOUNG, S. J. & GROVES, P. M. (1992) Effects of frequency and pattern of medial forebrain bundle stimulation on caudate dialysate dopamine and serotonin, *Journal of Neurochemistry*, 58, 1491–1498.

MARKOU, A. & KOOB, G. F. (1992) Construct validity of a self-stimulation threshold paradigm: effects of reward and performance manipulations, *Physiology and Behavior*, 51, 111–119.

MARTINEZ, J. L., VASQUEZ, B. J., RIGTER, H., ET AL. (1980) Attenuation of amphetamine-induced enhancement of learning by adrenal demedullation, *Brain Research*, 195, 433–443.

MCAULIFFE, W. E. & GORDON, R. A. (1974) A test of Lindesmith's theory of addiction: the frequency of euphoria among long-term addicts, *American Journal of Sociology*, 79, 795–840.

MCBRIDE, W. J., MURPHY, J. M., LUMENG, L. & LI, T.-K. (1988) Effects of RO 15–4513, fluoxetine and desipramine on the intake of ethanol, water and food by the alcohol-preferring (P) and -nonpreferring (NP) lines of rats, *Pharmacology, Biochemistry and Behavior*, 30, 1045–1050.

MCDONALD, R. J. & WHITE, N. M. (1993) A triple dissociation of memory systems: hippocampus, amygdala and dorsal striatum, *Behavioral Neuroscience*, 107, 3–22.

MCDONALD, R. J. & WHITE, N. M. (1994) Parallel information processing in the water maze: evidence for independent memory systems involving dorsal striatum and hippocampus, *Behavioral and Neural Biology*, 61, 260–270.

MCGAUGH, J. L. (1966) Time dependent processes in memory storage, *Science*, 153, 1351–1358.

MCGAUGH, J. L. & GOLD, P. E. (1989) Hormonal modulation of memory, in: BRUSH, R. B. & LEVINE, S. (Eds) *Psychoendocrinology*, 305–339 (New York, Academic).

MCGAUGH, J. L. & HERZ, M. J. (1972) *Memory Consolidation* (San Francisco, Albion).

MCGAUGH, J. L., INTROINI-COLLISON, I. B., NAGAHARA, A. H., CAHILL, L., BRIONI, J. D. & CASTELLANO, C. (1990) Involvement of the amygdaloid complex in neuromodulatory influences on memory average, *Neuroscience and Biobehavioral Reviews*, 14, 425–431.

McGregor, A. & Roberts, D. C. S. (1993) Dopaminergic antagonism within the nucleus accumbens or the amygdala produces differential effects on intravenous cocaine self-administration under fixed and progressive ratio schedules of reinforcement, *Brain Research*, 624, 245–252.

Meisch, R. A. & Beardsley, P. (1975) Ethanol as a reinforcer for rats: effects of concurrent access to water and alternate positions of water and ethanol, *Psychopharmacology*, 43, 19–23.

Meisch, R. A. & Thompson, T. (1971) Ethanol intake in the absence of concurrent food reinforcement, *Psychopharmacology*, 22, 72–79.

Messier, C. & White, N. M. (1984) Contingent and non-contingent actions of sucrose and saccharin reinforcers: effects on taste preference and memory, *Physiology and Behavior*, 32, 195–203.

Messing, R. B., Jensen, R. A., Martinez, J. L. *et al.* (1979) Naloxone enhancement of memory, *Behavioral and Neural Biology*, 27, 266–275.

Messing, R. B., Rijk, H. & Rigter, H. (1983) Facilitation of hot plate response learning by pre- and post-training naltrexone administration, *Psychopharmacology*, 81, 33–36.

Messing, R. B., Jensen, R. A., Vasquez, B. J., Martinez, J. L., Spiehler, V. R. & McGaugh, J. L. (1981) Opiate modulation of memory, in: Martinez, J. L., Jensen, R. A., Messing, R. B., Rigter, H. & McGaugh, J. L. (Eds) *Endogenous Peptides in Learning and Memory Processes*, pp. 431–443 (New York, Academic Press).

Milner, P. M. (1977) Theories of reinforcement, drive and motivation, in: Iversen, L. L., Iversen, S. D. & Snyder, S. H. (Eds) *Handbook of Psychopharmacology, Vol 7: Principles of Behavioral Pharmacology*, 181–200 (New York, Plenum Press).

Milner, B., Corkin, S. & Teuber, H.-L. (1968) Further analysis of the hippocampal amnesic syndrome: 14-year follow-up study of H.M, *Neuropsychologia*, 6, 215–234.

Mishkin, M. & Petri, H. L. (1984) Memories and habits: some implications for the analysis of learning and retention, in: Squire, L. R. & Butters, N. (Eds) *Neuropsychology of Memory*, pp. 287–296 (New York, Guilford Press).

Mishkin, M., Malamut, B. & Bachevalier, J. (1984) Memories and habits: two neural systems, in: Lynch, G., McGaugh, J. L. & Weinberger, N. M. (Eds) *Neurobiology of Human Memory and Learning*, pp. 65–77 (New York, Guilford Press).

Mitchell, S. N., Brazell, M. P., Joseph, M. H., Alavijeh, M. S. & Gray, J. A. (1989) Regionally specific effects of acute and chronic nicotine on rates of catecholamine and 5-hydroxytriptamine synthesis in rat brain, *European Journal of Pharmacology*, 167, 311–322.

Moleman, P. & Bruinvels, J. (1979) Effect of morphine on dopaminergic neurons in the rat basal forebrain and striatum, *Journal of Neural Transmission*, 46, 225–237.

Mollenauer, S., Bryson, R., Robison, M., Sardo, J. & Coleman, C. (1993) EtOH self-administration in anticipation of noise stress in C57BL/6J mice, *Pharmacology, Biochemistry and Behavior*, 46, 35–38.

Morency, M. A. & Beninger, R. J. (1986) Dopaminergic substrates of cocaine-induced place conditioning, *Brain Research*, 399, 33–41.

Mucha, R. F., van der Kooy, D., O'Shaughnessy, M. & Bucenieks, P. (1982) Drug reinforcement studied by the use of place conditioning in rat, *Brain Research*, 243, 91–105.

Murray, E. A. (1990) Representational memory in nonhuman primates, in: Kesner, R. P. & Olton, D. S. (Eds) *Neurobiology of Comparative Cognition*, 127–155 (Hilldale, NJ, Earlbaum).

Nachman, M. & Ashe, J. H. (1973) Learned taste aversions in rats as a function of dosage, concentration, and route of administration of LiCl, *Physiology and Behavior*, 10, 73–78.

Nachman, M. & Ashe, J. H. (1974) Effects of basolateral amygdala lesions on neophobia, learned taste aversions, and sodium appetite in rats, *Journal of Comparative and Physiological Psychology*, 87, 622–643.

O'Brien, C. P. & Childress, A. R. (1991) Behaviour therapy of drug dependence, in: Glass, I. B. (Ed.) *Addiction Behaviour*, pp. 230–235 (London, Tavistock/Routledge).

O'Brien, C. P., Childress, A. R., McLellan, A. T. & Ehrman, R. (1992) Classical conditioning in drug-dependent humans, *Annals of the New York Academy of Sciences*, 654, 400–415.

O'Keefe, J. & Nadel, L. (1978) *The Hippocampus as a Cognitive Map* (Oxford, Oxford University Press).

Ohno, M., Yamamoto, T. & Watanabe, S. (1993) Blockade of hippocampal nicotinic receptors impairs working memory but not reference memory in rats, *Pharmacology, Biochemistry and Behavior*, 45, 89–93.

Olds, M. E. (1979) Hypothalamic substrate for the positive reinforcing properties of morphine in the rat, *Brain Research*, 168, 351–360.

Olds, M. E. (1982) Reinforcing effects of morphine in the nucleus accumbens, *Brain Research*, 237, 429–440.

Olmstead, M. C. & Franklin, K. B. J. (1993) Effects of pedunculopontine tegmental nucleus lesions on morphine-induced conditioned place preference and analgesia in the formalin test, *Neuroscience*, 57, 411–418.

Olmstead, M. C. & Franklin, K. G. B. (1994) The development of a conditioned place preference (CPP) to morphine: I. Effects of lesions of various CNS sites, *Society for Neuroscience Abstracts*, 20, 1230 (Abstract).

Olton, D. S. (1982) Spatially organized behaviors of animals: behavioral and neurological studies, in: Potegal, M. (Ed.) *Spatial Abilities: Develop Physiological Foundations*, pp. 335–360 (New York, Academic Press).

Olton, D. S. & Samuelson, R. J. (1976) Remembrances of places past: spatial memory in the rat, *Journal of Experimental Psychology: Animal Behavior Processes*, 2, 97–116.

Olton, D. S., Walker, J. A. & Gage, F. H. (1978) Hippocampal connections and spatial discrimination, *Brain Research*, 139, 295–308.

Ossenkopp, K.-P. & Giugno, L. (1990) Nicotine-induced conditioned taste aversions are enhanced in rats with lesions of the area postrema, *Pharmacology, Biochemistry and Behavior*, 36, 625–630.

Packard, M. G. & White, N. M. (1989) Memory facilitation produced by dopamine receptor agonists: role of receptor subtype and mnemonic requirements, *Pharmacology, Biochemistry and Behavior*, 33, 511–518.

Packard, M. G. & White, N. M. (1990) Lesions of the caudate nucleus selectively impair 'reference memory' acquisition in the radial maze, *Behavioral and Neural Biology*, 53, 39–50.

Packard, M. G. & White, N. M. (1991) Dissociation of hippocampal and caudate nucleus memory systems by post-training intracerebral injection of dopamine agonists, *Behavioral Neuroscience*, 105, 295–306.

Packard, M. G., Cahill, L. & McGaugh, J. L. (1993) Effects of post-training d-amphetamine injections into hippocampus, amygdala and caudate nucleus on retention in spatial and cued water maze tasks, *Society for Neuroscience Abstracts*, 19, 1226.

Packard, M. G., Hirsh, R. & White, N. M. (1989) Differential effects of fornix and caudate nucleus lesions on two radial maze tasks: evidence for multiple memory systems, *Journal of Neuroscience*, 9, 1465–1472.

Packard, M. G., Williams, C. L. & McGaugh, J. L. (1992) Enhancement of win-shift radial maze retention by peripheral posttraining administration of *d*-amphetamine and 4-OH amphetamine, *Psychobiology*, 20, 280–285.

Panksepp, J., Herman, B. H., Connor, R., Bishop, P. & Scott, J. P. (1978) The biology of social attachments: opiates alleviate separation distress, *Biological Psychiatry*, 13, 607–618.

Parker, E. S., Birnbaum, I. M., Weingartner, H., Hartley, J. T., Stillman, R. C. & Wyatt, R. J. (1980) Retrograde enhancement of human memory with alcohol, *Psychopharmacology*, 69, 219–222.

Parker, T. H., Roberts, R. K., Henderson, G. I., Hoyumpa, A. M., Schmidt, D. E. & Schenker, S. (1978) The effects of ethanol on cerebral regional acetylcholine concentration and utilization, *Proceedings of the Society for Experimental Biology and Medicine*, 159, 270–275.

Pavlov, I. P. (1927) *Conditioned Reflexes* (Oxford, Oxford University Press).

Penfield, W. & Milner, B. (1958) Memory deficit produced by bilateral lesions in the hippocampal zone, *Archives of Neurology and Psychiatry*, 79, 475–497.

Petri, H. L. & Mishkin, M. (1993) Behaviorism, cognitivism and the neuropsychology of memory, *American Scientist*, 82, 30–37.

Pettit, H. O., Ettenberg, A., Bloom, F. E. & Koob, G. F. (1984) Destruction of dopamine in the nucleus accumbens selectively attenuates cocaine but not heroin self-administration in rats, *Psychopharmacology*, 84, 167–173.

Phillips, A. G. & Carr, G. D. (1987) Cognition and the basal ganglia: a possible substrate for procedural knowledge, *Canadian Journal of Neurological Science*, 14, 381–385.

Phillips, A. G., Spyraki, C. & Fibiger, H. C. (1982) Conditioned place preference with amphetamine and opiates as reward stimuli: attenuation by haloperidol, in: Hoebel, B. G. & Novin, D. (Eds) *The Neural Basis of Feeding and Reward*, pp. 455–464 (Brunswick, ME, Haer Institute).

Pickens, R. & Harris, W. C. (1968) Self-administration of d-amphetamine by rats, *Psychopharmacologia*, 12, 158–163.

Pickens, R. & Thompson, T. (1968) Cocaine reinforced behavior in rats: effects of reinforcement magnitude and fixed ratio size, *Journal of Pharmacology and Experimental Therapeutics*, 161, 122–129.

Pickens, R. & Thompson, T. (1971) Characteristics of stimulant drug reinforcement, in: Thompson, T. & Pickens, R. (Eds) *Stimulus Properties of Drugs*, pp. 177–192 (New York, Appleton-Century-Crofts).

Prado-Alcala, R. A. (1985) Is cholinergic activity of the caudate nucleus involved in memory? *Life Sciences*, 37, 2135–2142.

Prado-Alcala, R. A. & Cobos-Zapiain, G. G. (1977) Learning deficits induced by cholinergic blockade of the caudate nucleus as a function of experience, *Brain Research*, 138, 190–196.

Prado-Alcala, R. A. & Cobos-Zapiain, G. G. (1979) Improvement of learned behavior through cholinergic stimulation of the caudate nucleus, *Neuroscience Letters*, 14, 253–258.

Rassnick, S., Stinus, L. & Koob, G. F. (1993) The effects of 6-hydroxydopamine lesions of the nucleus accumbens and the mesolimbic dopamine system on oral self-administration of ethanol in the rat, *Brain Research*, 623, 16–24.

Rassnick, S., D'Amico, E., Riley, E., Pulvirenti, L., Zieglgansberger, W. & Koob, G. F. (1992) GABA and nucleus accumbens glutamate neurotransmission modulate ethanol self-administration in rats, *Annals of the New York Academy of Sciences*, 654, 502–505.

Reavill, C., Stolerman, I. P., Kumar, R. & Garcha, H. S. (1986) Chlorisondamine blocks acquisition of the conditioned taste aversion produced by (−)-nicotine, *Neuropharmacology*, 25, 1067–1069.

Rector, D. M., Poe, G. R. & Harper, R. M. (1993) Imaging of hippocampal and neocortical neural activity following intravenous cocaine administration in freely behaving cats, *Neuroscience*, 54, 633–641.

Reicher, M. A. & Holman, E. W. (1977) Location preference and flavor aversion reinforced by amphetamine in rats, *Animal Learning and Behavior*, 5, 343–346.

Ridley, R. M., Aitken, D. M. & Baker, H. F. (1989) Learning about rules but not about reward is impaired following lesions of the cholinergic projection to the hippocampus, *Brain Research*, 502, 306–318.

Risinger, F. O., Malott, D. H., Riley, A. L. & Cunningham, C. L. (1992) Effect of Ro 15-4513 on ethanol-induced conditioned place preference, *Pharmacology, Biochemistry and Behavior*, 43, 97–102.

Robbins, T. W. & Everitt, B. J. (1987) Comparative functions of the central noradrenergic, dopaminergic and cholinergic systems, *Neuropharmacology*, 78, 893–901.

Roberts, D. C. S. & Koob, G. F. (1982) Disruption of cocaine self-administration following 6-hydroxydopamine lesions of the ventral tegmental area in rats, *Pharmacology, Biochemistry and Behavior*, 17, 901–904.

Roberts, D. C. S., Corcoran, M. E. & Fibiger, H. C. (1977) On the role of ascending catecholaminergic systems in intravenous self-administration of cocaine, *Pharmacology, Biochemistry and Behavior*, 6, 615–620.

Roberts, D. C. S., Koob, G. F., Klonoff, P. & Fibiger, H. C. (1980) Extinction and recovery of cocaine self-administration following 6-hydroxydopamine lesions of the nucleus accumbens, *Pharmacology, Biochemistry and Behavior*, 12, 781–787.

Roberts, D. C. S., Loh, E. A. & Vickers, G. (1989) Self-administration of cocaine on a progressive ratio schedule in rats: dose-response relationship and effect of haloperidol pretreatment, *Psychopharmacology*, 97, 535–538.

Robinson, T. E. & Berridge, K. C. (1993) The neural basis of drug craving: an incentive-sensitization theory of addiction, *Brain Research Reviews*, 18, 247–291.

Samson, H. H., Haraguchi, M., Tolliver, G. A. & Sadeghi, K. G. (1989) Antagonism of ethanol-reinforced behavior by the benzodiazepine inverse agonists RO 15-4513 and FG 7142: relation to sucrose reinforcement, *Pharmacology, Biochemistry and Behavior*, 33, 601–608.

Samson, H. H., Hodge, C. W., Tolliver, G. A. & Haraguchi, M. (1993) Effect of dopamine agonists and antagonists on ethanol-reinforced behavior: the involvement of the nucleus accumbens, *Brain Research Bulletin*, 30, 133–141.

Samson, H. H., Pfeffer, A. O. & Tolliver, G. A. (1988) Oral ethanol self-administration in rats: models of alcohol-seeking behavior, *Alcoholism: Clinical and Experimental Research*, 12, 591–598.

Samson, H. H., Tolliver, G. A., Pfeffer, A. O., Sadeghi, K. G. & Mills, F. G. (1987) Oral ethanol reinforcement in the rat: effect of the partial inverse benzodiazepine agonist RO 15-4513, *Pharmacology, Biochemistry and Behavior*, 27, 517–519.

Schuckit, M. A. & Monteiro, M. G. (1988) Alcoholism, anxiety and depression, *British Journal of Addictions*, 83, 1373–1380.

Sharp, P. E., McNaughton, B. L. & Barnes, C. A. (1985) Enhancement of hippocampal field potentials in rats exposed to a complex, novel environment, *Brain Research*, 339, 361

Sherman, J. E., Pickman, C., Rice, A., Liebeskind, J. C. & Holman, E. W. (1980a) Rewarding and aversive effects of morphine: temporal and pharmacological properties, *Pharmacology, Biochemistry and Behavior*, 13, 501–515.

Sherman, J. E., Roberts, T., Roskam, S. E. & Holman, E. W. (1980b) Temporal properties of the rewarding and aversive effects of amphetamine in rats, *Pharmacology, Biochemistry and Behavior*, 13, 597–599.

Silverstone, P. H., Done, C. & Sharp, T. (1993) *In vivo* monoamine release during naloxone-precipitated morphine withdrawal, *NeuroReport*, 4, 1043–1045.

Sinclair, J. D. (1974) Rats learning to work for alcohol, *Nature*, 249, 590–592.

Singh, H. K., Ott, T. & Matthies, H. (1974) Effect of intrahippocampal injection of atropine on different phases of a learning experiment, *Psychopharmacology*, 38, 247–258.

Skinner, B. F. (1938) *The Behavior of Organisms* (New York, Appleton-Century-Crofts).

Sliffer, B. L. (1983) Schedule-induction of nicotine self-administration, *Pharmacology, Biochemistry and Behavior*, 19, 1005–1009.

Smith, S. G. & Davis, W. M. (1973) Behavioral control by stimuli associated with acquisition of morphine, *Behavioral Biology*, 9, 777–780.

Smith, C. A. & Holman, E. W. (1987) Rewarding and aversive effects of stimulant drugs in infant rats, *Pharmacology, Biochemistry and Behavior*, 26, 211–215.

Smith, J. E., Co, C., Freeman, M. E., Sands, M. P. & Lane, J. D. (1980) Neurotransmitter turnover in rat striatum is correlated with morphine self-administration, *Nature*, 287, 152–154.

Smith, J. E., Guerin, G. F., Co, C., Barr, T. S. & Lane, J. D. (1985) Effects of 6-OHDA lesions of the central medial nucleus accumbens on rat intravenous morphine self-administration, *Pharmacology, Biochemistry and Behavior*, 23, 843–849.

Spyraki, C., Fibiger, H. C. & Phillips, A. G. (1982a) Cocaine-induced place preference conditioning: lack of effects of neuroleptics and 6-hydroxydopamine lesions, *Brain Research*, 253, 195–203.

Spyraki, C., Fibiger, H. C. & Phillips, A. G. (1982b) Dopaminergic substrates of amphetamine-induced place preference conditioning, *Brain Research*, 253, 185–193.

Spyraki, C., Nomikos, G. G. & Varonos, D. D. (1987) Intravenous cocaine-induced place preference: attenuation by haloperidol, *Behavioural Brain Research*, 26, 57–62.

Squire, L. R., Knowlton, B. & Musen, G. (1993) The structure and organization of memory, *Annual Review of Psychology*, 44, 453–495.

Squire, L. R. & Zola-Morgan, S. (1991) The medial temporal lobe memory system, *Science*, 253, 1380–1386.

Staubli, U. & Huston, J. P. (1980) Avoidance learning enhanced by post-trial morphine injection, *Behavioral and Neural Biology*, 28, 487–490.

Stefurak, T. L., Martin, G. & van der Kooy, D. (1990) The representation in memory of morphine's unconditioned motivational effects depends on the nature of the conditioned stimulus, *Psychobiology*, 18, 435–442.

Stein, L. & Belluzzi, J. D. (1989) Cellular investigations of behavioral reinforcement, *Neuroscience and Biobehavioral Reviews*, 13, 69–80.

Stewart, J. (1992) Neurobiology of conditioning to drugs of abuse, *Annals of the New York Academy of Sciences*, 654, 335–346.

Stewart, J. & Eikelboom, R. (1987) Conditioned drug effects, in: Iversen, L. L., Iversen, S. D. & Snyder, S. H. (Eds) *Handbook of Psychopharmacology*, Vol. 19, 1–57 (New York, Plenum).

Stewart, R. B. & Grupp, L. A. (1989) Conditioned place aversion mediated by self-administered ethanol in the rat: a consideration of blood ethanol levels,

Pharmacology, Biochemistry and Behavior, 32, 431–437.

STEWART, J., DE WITT, H. & EIKELBOOM, R. (1984) Role of unconditioned and conditioned drug effects in the self-administration of opiates and stimulants, *Psychological Review*, 91, 251–268.

STOLERMAN, I. P. & D'MELLO, G. D. (1978) Amphetamine-induced taste aversion demonstrated with operant behaviour, *Pharmacology, Biochemistry and Behavior*, 8, 107–111.

STOLERMAN, I. P. & SHOAIB, M. (1991) The neurobiology of tobacco addiction, *Trends in Pharmacological Sciences*, 12, 467–473.

SUZUKI, T., FUNADA, M., NARITA, M., MISAWA, M. & NAGASE, H. (1993) Morphine-induced place preference in the CXBK mouse: characteristics of mu opioid receptor subtypes, *Brain Research*, 602, 45–52.

THORNDIKE, E. L. (1898) Animal intelligence. An experimental study of the associative processes in animals, *Psychological Monographs*, 2, 1–109.

THORNDIKE, E. L. (1911) *Animal Intelligence* (New York, Macmillan)

TOATES, F. M. (1986) *Motivational Systems* (Cambridge, UK, Cambridge University Press).

TOIDE, K. & ARIMA, T. (1989) Effects of cholinergic drugs on extracellular levels of acetylcholine and choline in rat cortex, hippocampus and striatum studied by brain dialysis, *European Journal of Pharmacology*, 173, 133–141.

TOLMAN, E. C. (1948) Cognitive maps in rats and men, *Psychological Review*, 56, 144–155.

TOLMAN, E. C. (1949) There is more than one kind of learning, *Psychological Review*, 56, 144–155.

TOMAZ, C., AGUIAR, M. S. & NOGUEIRA, P. J. C. (1990) Facilitation of memory by peripheral administration of substance P and naloxone using avoidance and habituation learning tasks, *Neuroscience and Biobehavioral Reviews*, 14, 447–453.

TROWILL, J. A., PANKSEPP, J. & GANDELMAN, R. (1969) An incentive model of rewarding brain stimulation, *Psychological Review*, 76, 264–281.

URRUTIA, A. & GRUOL, D. L. (1992) Acute alcohol alters the excitability of cerebellar Pukinje neurons and hippocampal neurons in culture, *Brain Research*, 569, 26–37.

VAN DER KOOY, D., MUCHA, R. F., O'SHAUGHNESSY, M. & BUCENIEKS, P. (1982) Reinforcing effects of brain microinjections of morphine revealed by conditioned place preference, *Brain Research*, 243, 107–117.

VIAUD, M. D. & WHITE, N. M. (1989a) Dissociation of visual and olfactory conditioning in the neostriatum of rats, *Behavioural Brain Research*, 32, 31–42.

VIAUD, M. D. & WHITE, N. M. (1989b) Differential effects of scopolamine injected into neostriatum on acquisition, consolidation and retrieval of conditioned emotional responses, *Society for Neuroscience Abstracts*, 15, 734 (Abstract).

WANG, J., AIGNER, T. & MISHKIN, M. (1990) Effects of neostriatal lesions on visual habit formation in rhesus monkeys, *Society for Neuroscience Abstracts*, 16, 617

WEEKS, J. R. (1962) Experimental morphine addiction: method for automatic intravenous injections in unrestrained rats, *Science*, 138, 143–144.

WEEKS, J. R. & COLLINS, R. J. (1968) Patterns of intravenous self-injection by morphine addicted rats, in: WICKLER, A. (Ed.) *The Addictive States*, 288–298 (Baltimore, Williams & Wilkins).

WEINBERGER, S. B., RIEDEL, C. A., JANAK, P. H. & MARTINEZ, JR., J. L. (1992) Cocaine enhances one-way avoidance responding in mice, *Pharmacology, Biochemistry and Behavior*, 41, 851–854.

WEISS, F., HURD, Y. L., UNGERSTEDT, U., MARKOU, A., PLOTSKY, P. M. & KOOB, G. F. (1992) Neurochemical correlates of cocaine and ethanol self-administration, *Annals of the New York Academy of Sciences*, 654, 220–241.

WELZL, H., KUHN, G. & HUSTON, J. P. (1989) Self-administration of small amounts of morphine through glass micropipettes into the ventral tegmental area of the rat, *Neuropharmacology*, 28, 1017–1023.

WEST, R. (1991) Psychological theories of addiction, in: GLASS, I. B. (Ed.) *Addiction Behaviour*, pp. 20–24 (London, Tavistock/Routledge).

WHITE, N. M. (1988) Effect of nigrostriatal dopamine depletion on the post-training, memory improving action of amphetamine, *Life Sciences*, 43, 7–12.

WHITE, N. M. (1989) A functional hypothesis concerning the striatal matrix and patches: mediation of S–R memory and reward, *Life Sciences*, 45, 1943–1957.

WHITE, N. M. & CARR, G. D. (1985) The conditioned place preference is affected by two independent reinforcement processes, *Pharmacology, Biochemistry and Behavior*, 23, 37–42.

WHITE, N. M. & HIROI, N. (1993) Amphetamine conditioned cue preference and the neurobiology of drug seeking, *Seminars in the Neurosciences*, 5, 329–336.

WHITE, N. M. & LEGREE, P. (1984) Effect of post-training exposure to an aversive stimulus on retention, *Physiological Psychology*, 12, 233–236.

WHITE, N. M., MAJOR, R. & SIEGEL, J. (1978) Effect of morphine on one-trial appetitive learning, *Life Sciences*, 23, 1967–1972.

WHITE, N. M. & MCDONALD, R. J. (1993) Acquisition of a spatial conditioned place preference is impaired by amygdala lesions and improved by fornix lesions, *Behavioural Brain Research*, 55, 269–281.

WHITE, N. M. & MILNER, P. M. (1992) The psychobiology of reinforcers, *Annual Review of Psychology*, 43, 443–471.

WHITE, N. M. & VIAUD, M. D. (1991) Localized intracaudate dopamine D2 receptor activation during the post-training period improves memory for visual or olfactory conditioned emotional responses in rats, *Behavioral and Neural Biology*, 55, 255–269.

WHITE, N. M., MESSIER, C. & CARR, G. D. (1987) Operationalizing and measuring the organizing influence of drugs on behavior, in: BOZARTH, M. A. (Ed.) *Methods of Measuring the Reinforcing Properties of Abused Drugs*, pp. 591–618 (New York, Springer-Verlag).

WHITE, N. M., SKLAR, L. & AMIT, Z. (1977) The reinforcing action of morphine and its paradoxical side effect, *Psychopharmacology*, 52, 63–66.

WILSON, M. C. & SCHUSTER, C. R. (1972) The effects of chlorpromazine on psychomotor stimulant self-administration in the rhesus monkey, *Psychopharmacology*, 26, 115–126.

WISE, C. D. & STEIN, L. (1970) Amphetamine: facilitation of behavior by augmented release of norepinephrine from the medial forebrain bundle, in: COSTA, E. & GARATTINI, S. (Eds) *Amphetamines and Related Compounds*, pp. 463–485 (New York, Raven Press).

WISE, R. A. (1982) Neuroleptics and operant behavior: the anhedonia hypothesis, *Behavioral and Brain Sciences*, 5, 39–87.

WISE, R. A. (1988) The neurobiology of craving: implications for the understanding and treatment of addiction, *Journal of Abnormal Psychology*, 97, 118–132.

WISE, R. A. (1989) Opiate reward: sites and substrates, *Neuroscience and Biobehavioral Reviews*, 13, 129–133.

WISE, R. A. & HOFFMAN, D. C. (1992) Localization of drug reward mechanisms by intracranial injections, *Synapse*, 10, 247–263.

WISE, R. A., BAUCO, P., CARLEZON JR W. A. & TROJNIAR, W. (1992) Self-stimulation and drug reward mechanisms, *Annals of the New York Academy of Sciences*, 654, 192–198.

WISE, R. A., SPINDLER, J., DE WITT, H. & GERBER, G. J. (1978) Neuroleptic-induced "anhedonia" in rats: pimozide blocks reward quality of food, *Science*, 201, 262–264.

WOOD, P. L. & RAO, T. S. (1991) Morphine stimulation of mesolimbic and mesocortical but not nigrostriatal dopamine release in the rat as reflected by changes in 3-methoxytyramine levels, *Neuropharmacology*, 30, 399–401.

WOODS, J. H. & SCHUSTER, C. R. (1971) Opiates as reinforcing stimuli, in: THOMPSON, T. & PICKENS, R. (Eds) *Stimulus Properties of Drugs*, pp. 163–175 (New York, Appleton-Century-Crofts).

WOOLVERTON, W. L. & VIRUS, R. M. (1989) The effects of a D_1 and a D_2 dopamine antagonist on behavior maintained by cocaine or food, *Pharmacology, Biochemistry and Behavior*, 32, 691–697.

YAMAMOTO, T. & FUJIMOTO, Y. (1991) Brain mechanisms of taste aversion learning in the rat, *Brain Research Bulletin*, 27, 403–406.

YOKEL, R. A. & WISE, R. A. (1975) Increased lever pressing for amphetamine after pimozide in rats: implications for a dopamine theory of reward, *Science*, 187, 547–549.

YOKEL, R. A. & WISE, R. A. (1978) Amphetamine-type reinforcement by dopaminergic agonists in the rat, *Psychopharmacology*, 58, 289–296.

YOUNG, P. T. (1959) The role of affective processes in learning and motivation, *Psychological Review*, 66, 104–125.

ZOLA-MORGAN, S. & SQUIRE, L. R. (1993) Neuroanatomy of memory, *Annual Review of Neuroscience*, 16, 547–563.

Acknowledgments

Warner, L.A., Kessler, R.C., Hughes, M., Anthony, J.C., Nelson, C.B. "Prevalence and Correlates of Drug Use and Dependence in the United States: Results from the National Comorbidity Survey." *Arch Gen Psychiatry* 52, 3 (1995): 219–229. Reprinted with the permission of American Medical Association.

Sigvardsson, S., Bohman, M., and Cloninger, C.R. "Replication of the Stockholm Adoption Study of Alcoholism Confirmatory Cross-Fostering Analysis." *Archives of General Psychology* 53 (1996): 681–687. Reprinted with the permission of American Medical Association.

Merikangas, K.R., Stolar, M., Stevens, D.E., Goulet, J., Preisig, M.A., Fenton, B., Zhang, H., O'Malley, S.S., Rounsaville, B.J. "Familial Transmission of Substance Use Disorders." *Arch Gen Psychiatry* 55, 11 (1998): 973–979. Reprinted with the permission of American Medical Association.

McLellan, A.T., Lewis, D.C., O'Brien, C.P., Kleber, H.D. "Drug Dependence, a Chronic Medical Illness: Implications for Treatment, Insurance, and Outcomes Evaluation." *JAMA* 284, 13 (2000): 1689–1695. Copyright 2000. The American Medical Association.

Vaillant, G.E. "A Long-Term Follow-up of Male Alcohol Abuse." *Arch Gen Psychiatry* 53 (1996): 243–249. Reprinted with the permission of American Medical Association.

Nesse, R.M. "An Evolutionary Perspective on Substance Abuse." *Ethology and Sociobiology* 15 (1994): 339–348. Copyright 1994. Reprinted with permission from Elsevier Science.

O'Brien, C.P., Childress, A.R., Ehrman, R., and Robbins, S.J. "Conditioning Factors in Drug Abuse: Can They Explain Compulsion?" *Journal of Psychopharmacology* 12, 1 (1998): 15–22. Reprinted with the permission of Sage Publications Ltd.

Robinson, T.E., and Berridge, K.C. "The Neural Basis of Drug Craving: An Incentive Sensitization Theory of Addiction." *Brain Res Brain Res Rev* 18, 3 (1993): 247–291. Reprinted with the permission of Elsevier Science BV.

Tiffany, S.T. "A Cognitive Model of Drug Urges and Drug-Use Behavior: Role of Automatic and Nonautomatic Processes." *Psychological Review* 97, 2 (1990): 147–168. Copyright © 1990 by the American Psychological Association. Reprinted with permission.

Volkow, N.D., Wang, G.-J., Fowler, J.S., Logan, J., Gatley, S.J., Hitzemann, R., Chen, A.D., Dewey, S.L., and Pappas, N. "Decreased Striatal Dopaminergic Responsiveness in Detoxified Cocaine-Dependent Subjects." *Nature* 386 (1997): 830–833. Reprinted by permission from Nature Vol. 386 pp. 830–833 Copyright © 1997. Macmillan Magazines Ltd.

Berridge, K.C., and Robinson, T.E. "What Is the Role of Dopamine in Reward: Hedonic Impact, Reward Learning, or Incentive Salience?" *Brain Res Brain Res Rev* 28 (1998): 309–369. Reprinted with the permission of Elsevier Science BV.

Breiter, H.C., Gollub, R.L., Weisskoff, R.M., Kennedy, D.N., Makris, N., Berke, J.D., Goodman, J.M., Kantor, H.L., Gastfriend, D.R., Riorden, J.P., Mathew, R.T., Rosen, B.R., and Hyman, S.E. "Acute Effects of Cocaine on Human Brain Activity and Emotion." *Neuron* 19 (1997): 591–611. Reprinted from *Neuron*, 19, "Acute effects of cocaine on human brain activity and emotion" 591–611, Copyright 1997, with permission from Elsevier Science.

Kendler, K.S., Karkowski, L.M., Neale, M.C., and Prescott, C.A. "Illicit Psychoactive Substance Use, Heavy Use, Abuse, and Dependence in a US Population-Based Sample of Male Twins." *Arch Gen Psychiatry* 57 (2000): 261–269. Reprinted with the permission of American Medical Association.

Schultz, W. "Predictive Reward Signal of Dopamine Neurons." *J Neurophysiol* 80 (1998): 1–27. Reprinted with the permission of American Physiological Society.

Volkow, N.D., Wang, G.J., Fowler, J.S., Logan, J., Gatley, S.J., Gifford, A., Hitzemann, R., Ding, Y.S., and Pappas, N. "Prediction of Reinforcing Responses to Psychostimulants in Humans by Brain Dopamine D2 Receptor Levels." *Am. J. Psychiatry* 156 (1999): 1440–1443. *Am J Psychiatry* 156 (1999): 1440–1443. Copyright 1999, the American Psychiatric Association. Reprinted by permission.

White, N.M. "Addictive Drugs as Reinforcers: Multiple Partial Actions on Memory Systems." *Addiction* 91 (1996): 921–949. Reprinted with the permission of Taylor & Francis Ltd. http://www.tandf.co.uk.